Food Guide Pyramid
A Guide to Daily Food Choices

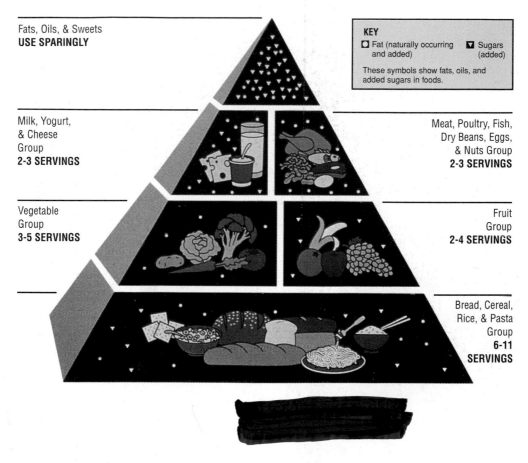

Fats, Oils, & Sweets
USE SPARINGLY

KEY
□ Fat (naturally occurring and added)   ▼ Sugars (added)
These symbols show fats, oils, and added sugars in foods.

Milk, Yogurt, & Cheese Group
2-3 SERVINGS

Meat, Poultry, Fish, Dry Beans, Eggs, & Nuts Group
2-3 SERVINGS

Vegetable Group
3-5 SERVINGS

Fruit Group
2-4 SERVINGS

Bread, Cereal, Rice, & Pasta Group
6-11 SERVINGS

Nutrition Essentials and Diet Therapy

Brenda Purdy

Eighth Edition

Nutrition Essentials and Diet Therapy

Nancy J. Peckenpaugh, MSEd, RD, CDN, CDE
Dietitian in Private Practice, Lifetime Nutrition Services
Dietitian, Office of Dr. Adam Law and Dryden Family Medicine
Tompkins County Head Start and
The Special Children's Center Nutrition Consultant
Ithaca, New York

Charlotte M. Poleman, RD, CDN
Formerly Community Dietitian and Nutrition Consultant for
Broome Developmental Services and Area Nursing Homes
Ithaca, New York

W.B. SAUNDERS COMPANY
A Division of Harcourt Brace & Company
Philadelphia   London   Toronto   Montreal   Sydney   Tokyo

W.B. Saunders Company

A Division of Harcourt Brace & Company

The Curtis Center
Independence Square West
Philadelphia, Pennsylvania 19106–3399

Library of Congress Cataloging-in-Publication Data

Peckenpaugh, Nancy J.
    Nutrition : essentials and diet therapy / Nancy J. Peckenpaugh.
Charlotte M. Poleman. — 8th ed.
        p.   cm.
    Includes bibliographical references and index.
    ISBN 0–7216–7707–X
    1. Diet therapy. 2. Nutrition. I. Poleman, Charlotte M.
II. Title.
    [DNLM: 1. Nutrition nurses' instruction. 2. Diet Therapy nurses'
instruction. QU 145 P367n 1999]
RM216.P67   1999
613.2—dc21
DNLM/DLC   98–48476

NUTRITION ESSENTIALS AND DIET THERAPY   ISBN   0–7216–7707–X

Printed in the United States of America.

Last digit is the print number: 9   8   7   6   5   4   3   2   1

To my Scottish and Welsh ancestors, who showed me the need for good nutrition, and to my grandmother (whose parents were German immigrants), who helped me learn to love lima beans, sauerkraut, and spinach with vinegar.
Nancy J. Peckenpaugh

To my husband, Tom, whose professional work in the economics of food and agriculture in developing countries has been a positive influence for me while co-authoring many editions of this book.
Charlotte M. Poleman

Preface

Every year we learn something significantly new about nutrition. Ongoing research at every level, from the biochemical to the sociocultural, expands our knowledge base in this important discipline. While this new knowledge increases our potential for improving the care we bring to our patients, it also makes the teaching and learning of nutrition more complex and difficult, particularly given the limited class time devoted to nutrition in the education of health care professionals. In writing the Eighth Edition of *Nutrition Essentials and Diet Therapy*, our objective has been to provide a concise, focused, and practical approach to basic health care nutrition.

In providing a better focus, we concentrate on what is most important for the health care provider to know about the nutrition basics and the application of nutrition knowledge. We rigorously reviewed and revised the previous edition to this end:

- To provide a focused examination of the nutrients, we continued to combine the five nutrient chapters into two: Chapter 3, *Carbohydrate, Protein, and Fat: The Energy Macronutrients of Balanced Meals;* and Chapter 5, *Food as the Source of Vitamins, Minerals, Phytochemicals, and Water.* We combined these chapters in order to emphasize that foods provide a compilation of nutrients, thus helping the student to better apply theory to practice. The nutrient chapters are still subdivided, allowing instructors the option of teaching these nutrients separately.
- The section on the life cycle continues to follow the section on disease management. This allows discussion on how disease management influences life cycle concerns, with an emphasis on family impact.
- Repetition was reduced in the book in order to better meet the needs of restricted class time while allowing for coverage of new and updated content.
- Popular features of the book have been retained, including Facts & Fallacies, question format for the major headings, and basic readability.

Features in the New Edition

To make the text more practical and appealing, we incorporated the following features:

- *Colorful illustrations, tables, and design* throughout the book add visual appeal and make the content more interesting for the student. In particular, the color photographs give students a realistic view of nutrition and clinical applications.
- *Critical Thinking Case Studies* at the end of each chapter portray multicultural scenarios of health and nutrition. The critical thinking questions give students the opportunity to apply the concepts from each chapter to clinical situations.
- *Teaching Pearls* incorporate counseling and patient teaching skills for promotion of positive nutrition practices.

Discussions of important topics have been substantially updated and expanded, including those dealing with diabetes mellitus, such as carbohydrate counting and insulin pump therapy, HIV and AIDS, eating disorders, dental health, and nutritional support. We added new emphasis on the research of the genetics of alcoholism, which has an impact on nutritional well-being.

We expanded the discussion of insulin resistance syndrome and its impact on a variety of health conditions, such as cardiovascular disease, central obesity, and Type 2 diabetes. As our food supply changes throughout the world, both in quantity and quality, there is a strong correlation between the development of obesity, diabetes, cardiovascular disease, and cancer. It is now recognized that a worldwide epidemic of diabetes is occurring at the same time that our food habits are changing and physical activity is declining. This increased rate of diabetes due to changing to a more Westernized lifestyle has been shown in the Pima Indians, Alaskan Eskimos, Australian Aborigines, and many other populations.

Instructional Materials

As in previous editions, a separate Instructor's Manual is available. This helpful supplement includes answers to the text questions, suggested reading materials, sources of audiovisual aids, and sample test questions and answers. It also provides a guide for using the Critical Thinking Case Studies in classroom discussion.

Also available with the new edition is a package of 29 colorful transparency overheads. Featuring illustrations from the textbook, this visual package will enhance your lectures.

Our guiding principle throughout the writing of this text has been that nutrition is and increasingly will be one of the core disciplines for health care as we move into the 21st century. Not everyone takes medications, not everyone undergoes surgery or other extraordinary procedures, but everyone needs good nutrition. It is the single most important factor in the care of the well and the ill client. Medical nutrition therapy saves health care dollars while improving the quality of lives. As previously stated, our aim has been to make this body of information more accessible and useful to the people who need it most, the health care providers. We would be very interested in your views concerning how well we have met this objective and how we might better meet it in future editions. Please write to us in care of W.B. Saunders Company with your suggestions.

Nancy J. Peckenpaugh, MSEd, RD, CDN, CDE

Charlotte M. Poleman, RD, CDN

Acknowledgments

We continue to pay tribute to the original author, Alberta Shackelton, who helped pioneer the advanced instruction of nutrition at Rutgers University with the first publication of this nursing textbook in 1929—back when butter was a food group! The enthusiastic support of the staff at the Tompkins Day Treatment Program in their assistance in providing photographs used in the text is fully appreciated. The insight of Dr. Adam Law, endocrinologist, into lipid disorders related to the insulin resistance syndrome and insulin pump therapy for diabetes management was invaluable in the preparation of this edition. The authors further thank the dedicated staff at W.B. Saunders Company, especially Senior Nursing Editor Maura Connor and Editorial Assistant Amelia Cullinan, for their expertise during the revision process.

Nancy J. Peckenpaugh, MSEd, RD, CDN, CDE

Charlotte M. Poleman, RD, CDN

Reviewers

Shirley A. Anderson, MSN
Kirkwood Community College
Cedar Rapids, Iowa

Marjorie L. Bender, PhD, RD
Nutritionist, Lower Savannah Health
    District
Aiken, South Carolina;
Adjunct Instructor, Georgia Military
    College
Fort Gordon Branch
Fort Gordon, Georgia

John E. Buynak, RN, CMA
Berks Technical Institute
Wyomissing, Pennsylvania

Sharon Fulling, MSN
Assistant Dean/Director of Nursing &
    HPER
Mississippi County Community College
Blytheville, Arkansas

Nancy L. Lyons, BSN, RN
Instructor
School of Practical Nursing
Holy Name Hospital
Teaneck, New Jersey

Shirley D. Miller, PhD, RN, MEd
Okefenokee Technical Institute
Waycross, Georgia

Melanie Shuran, PhD, RD, LD
Finch University of Health Sciences/The
    Chicago Medical School
North Chicago, Illinois

Barbara T. Silver, BSN, RN
Berger Pines School of Practical Nursing
Paramus, New Jersey

Contents

Section **Lifespan and Wellness Concerns in Promoting Health and Managing Illness 329**

Appendixes

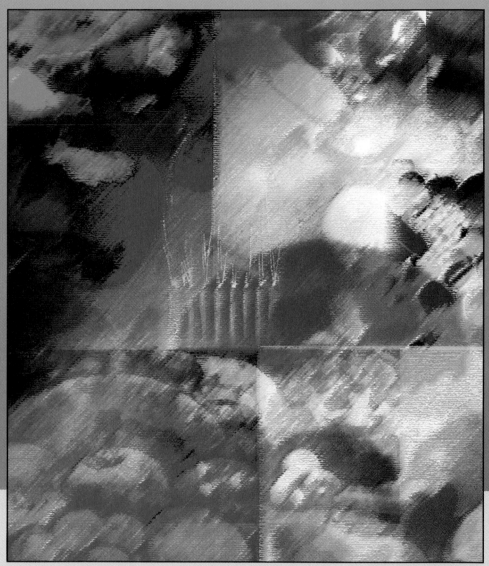

The Art of Nutrition

Section 1

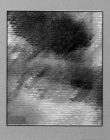

1

The Basics of Nutrition and Health in a Family Meal Environment

Objectives

After completing this chapter, you should be able to:

- Identify biopsychosocial influences on nutritional intake and health.
- Define terms used in the study of nutrition.
- Describe the role of vegetarianism on health.
- Describe the impact of snacking on health.
- Describe how to include fast foods in a healthy diet.
- Describe the impact of alcohol on health.
- Identify your personal strengths and weaknesses in nutrition knowledge and application.

Terms to Identify

Beta-carotene	Grazing	Medical nutrition therapy
Biopsychosocial	Learned food aversion	Nutrient density
Chronic disease	Legumes	Vegan
Cleft palate	Medical geneology	Vegetarian
Empty kilocalories		

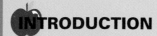

INTRODUCTION

We are a nation of immigrants and, as such, our genetically based health problems can be traced back to our roots of our many heritages whether our families originate from Northern Europe, Southern Europe, Africa, or other parts of the world. Even Native Americans are believed to have originally migrated from Asia. Though we may be Americans we all share different family biopsychosocial factors (differences in genetics and in psychological and social factors—see

Chapter 2 for more information). Even if there is not a direct familial link, "unrelated members of an ethnic group or race with common ancestry share a common gene pool and, hence, may resemble one another (biochemically and physically) more than they resemble people from other groups. High blood pressure, obesity, hyperlipidemia, atherosclerosis, and various cancers appear to aggregate in families for genetic reasons rather than merely because of common environment" (National Reseach Council, 1989). This is referred to as **medical geneology.**

Around the world it has been shown that a change to a more Westernized diet and lifestyle with increased kcalories, fat, sugar, and reduced fiber and activity level results in obesity and increased rates of diabetes. This is described as having a genetic predisposition to obesity and diabetes, which the environment brings out. This tendency has been found among persons whose ancestors came from areas near the equator, including persons of African, Spanish, Pacific Island, and Native American heritage. More recently it has been noted that Alaskan natives, who prior to 1957 had low rates of obesity and diabetes, now face rampant growth of both conditions (Murphy et al., 1995).

One theory of why these populations and others are at increased risk today is due to their exposure to historical cycles of famine. Those who survived probably had a genetically programmed ability to maintain body mass (weight) during times of famine and an easy ability to gain weight during times of plenty. Although the underlying genetics that allowed many of our ancestors to survive during times of famine was beneficial then, those same genetics may lead to chronic health conditions within our current food-oriented society.

As we learn more about medical geneology, our ability to provide precise and accurate information about nutrition will be increased for various population groups whose nutritional needs differ from the population at large. For example, the simple public health message that encourages a low-fat and high-carbohydrate diet can be detrimental for people with the insulin resistance syndrome (diagnosis includes high blood levels of triglycerides; see Chapters 8 and 9).

A return to or maintenance of plant-based diets is being promoted around the world. Traditional ethnic cooking is often based around legumes that have been a mainstay of cooking for centuries. Other traditional food habits—such as eating dandelion greens, having baked beans every Saturday, or taking a spoonful of cod liver oil—are seldom found today in the United States. The change in our food supply and the nutrients we consume continues to impact world health. Hawaii, for example, with one of the highest rates of obesity worldwide since the diet changed to one high in fat and sugar, has been advocating a return to traditional Hawaiian foods.

Owing to the complexities of medical geneolgy, along with diverse family structures that include single parents, grandparents with custody, foster and adoptive parents and remarried families with diverse lifestyles and food habits, effective nutrition intervention is as much an art as it is a science. Food choices are influenced by our family eating habits, which often have strong historical and cultural roots but are also impacted by television advertising and fast-paced lifestyles. Food choices and biological health needs may be in conflict.

WHAT ARE BIOPSYCHOSOCIAL CONCERNS IN HEALTH CARE?

Biopsychosocial concerns address the interplay between environmental (external) and internal forces. For example, the diagnosis of diabetes is primarily a biochemical or internal problem, but for the person hearing this diagnosis it involves psychological issues of acceptance versus denial and social concerns of healthy living in an environment that may be stressful and that may provide little opportunity for low-fat, low-sugar food choices (external problems or social forces). The biochemical problem of either very-high or very-low blood sugars can also affect the ability to think (cognitive functioning) and emotions. The incidence of depression, for example, increases with poor blood sugar control. The nurse or other health care professional who is aware of the interplay between external and internal forces will be a much more effective team member in the health care system.

WHAT ARE THE BASIC TERMS TO UNDERSTAND IN THE STUDY OF NUTRITION?

1. *Nutrition* is the sum of the processes by which the body uses food for energy, maintenance, and growth.
2. *Malnutrition* is a state in which a prolonged lack of one or more nutrients retards physical development or causes the appearance of specific clinical conditions (e.g., anemia, goiter, rickets). Excess nutrient intake creates another form of malnutrition when it leads to conditions such as obesity, heart disease, hypertension, and hypercholesterolemia.
3. *Optimal nutrition* means that a person is receiving and using the essential nutrients to maintain health and well-being at the highest possible level.
4. *Nutritional status* is the condition of the body as it relates to the consumption and use of food. *Good nutritional status* refers to the intake of a balanced diet containing all the essential nutrients necessary to meet the body's requirements for energy, maintenance, and growth. This means the body requirements are being met. *Poor nutritional status* refers to inadequate intake (or use) of nutrients to meet the body's requirements for energy, maintenance, and growth. In nursing terms, intake is less than the body requirements. A person who is malnourished has a poor nutritional status (see the section on nutritional assessment in Chapter 7).
5. A *nutrient* is a chemical substance that is present in food and needed by the body. Proteins, carbohydrates, fats, minerals, trace elements, vitamins, and water are included in the more than 50 known nutrients needed by the body.
6. A *kilocalorie* (or kcalorie) is a unit of measure used to express the fuel value of carbohydrates, fats, and proteins. The large calorie (or kilocalorie [kcal]) used in nutrition represents the amount of heat necessary to raise the temperature of 1 kg of water 1° C. One pound of body fat equals 3500 kilocalories.
7. *Health* is currently recognized as being more than the absence of disease. High-level wellness is present when an individual is actively engaged in moving toward the fulfillment of his or her potential.

8. *Public health* is the field of medicine that is concerned with safeguarding and improving the health of the community as a whole. Public health nurses may work out of public health departments or private health organizations.

9. *Holistic health* is a system of preventive medicine that takes into account the whole individual: it promotes personal responsibility for well-being and acknowledges the total influences—biological, psychological, and social—that affect health, including nutrition, exercise, and emotional well-being.

10. *Medical nutrition therapy* (referred to in the past as diet therapy) is the treatment of disease through nutritional therapy by registered dietitians or RDs. Registered dietitians are uniquely qualified to provide medical nutrition therapy due to extensive training in food composition and preparation, nutrition and biochemistry, anatomy and physiology, as well as life-cycle concerns and disease states.

HOW DO FOOD AND DIETARY PATTERNS DEVELOP?

Sound nutriton begins in infancy through the impact of food culture. Persons of various ethnic heritage and cultural communities consume differing types and amounts of foods. The family affects the growing child's meal environment and exposure to food.

In the ideal scenario, the infant is exposed to a variety of foods and is fed in a manner that promotes positive meal association. The infant then is more likely to become a child who learns to like a variety of foods that are of high quality and dense in nutrients. Because the child has been allowed to eat on the basis of his or her own hunger and satiety cues in a positive meal environment, eating takes place according to growth needs, and thus an appropriate quantity of food intake is maintained (see Chapter 17 for more detailed information on child development and nutritional needs).

Many factors can change this ideal scenario. Children may have food allergies or food intolerances, and these foods become associated with physical discomfort. Learned food aversions fall into this classification. For example, a food that is eaten prior to the onset of an illness that is unrelated to the food (such as a viral illness) becomes mistakenly associated with the illness. If this food is avoided in the future, it is appropriately termed a **learned food aversion.**

Many barriers to adequate nutrient intake are external in nature, and may stem from a variety of causes:

- *Economic* (inadequate money to purchase food)
- *Physical* (lack of food storage facilities or physical impairment such as **cleft palate**—a birth defect in which there is an opening in the roof of the mouth, lips, or both)
- *Cultural* (lack of exposure to a variety of food because of limited parental offerings or overemphasis on meat or high-fat and high-sugar foods)
- *Ecological* (droughts, floods)
- *Emotional* (television advertisements depicting nonnutritious foods as appealing)
- *Religious* (adherence to restrictive food codes)
- *Political* (food boycotts, forced starvation for military purposes)

How Can the Health Care Professional Facilitate Positive Meal Environments?

The health care professional can help promote harmonious family mealtimes, which will allow the innate satiety cues to function more effectively and also promote the association of eating with positive feelings, by making the following recommendations to family members:

- Focus on positive conversations during mealtimes; avoid points of potential conflict and friction.
- Use soft music, candles, or both to facilitate a quiet, relaxed atmosphere.
- Eat as a family as much as possible in contrast to eating on the run.
- Encourage children to eat with the family but do not force them to eat; encourage the *one-taste rule* and emphasize that tastes are learned.
- Serve food that looks appealing by using a combination of colors, textures, and sizes (e.g., orange carrot "coins," white chicken, crisp lettuce wedges, warm biscuits, and cold milk).
- Watch portion sizes; smaller portions are useful for small appetites and for weight control.
- Provide rest and calming activities just prior to and after meals.

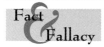

Fallacy: Children who do not "clean their plates" should not have dessert.

Fact: This commonly practiced fallacy may work in the short term to coerce children to eat their meals, but the long-term implications outweigh any benefits. This approach implicitly conveys to children that desserts have more value than other foods, because dessert is being used as a reward. Parents should be reminded that desserts can be nutritious, such as fresh, juicy fruit, a colorful fruit salad, or a piece of pumpkin pie or carrot cake. The "clean the plate" philosophy can also contribute to overeating and excess weight gain. Children (and many adults) need to learn to stop eating when they are comfortably full.

What Are Some Cultural and Societal Influences on Nutritional Intake?

Changing Food Habits in the United States

Because more women are working outside of the home, increasing numbers of men are now shopping for and preparing food (Fig. 1–1). Changing demographics also has an impact on the nutritional status of the United States as a whole, which in turn affects food choices. The increasing number of elderly and minority persons affects the rate of chronic health concerns. Households composed of single persons are growing, with an increased demand for more ready-to-use foods, which are often high in fat and salt.

Americans now eat far more sugar than our ancestors did. A big part of this increased sugar intake is through added sugar, such as high-fructose corn syrup,

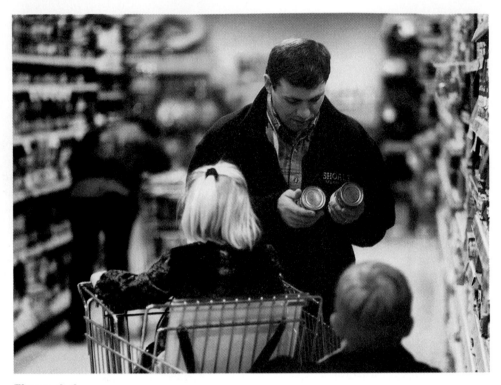

Figure 1–1
Men are becoming more involved in food shopping and meal preparation, which has increased their concern with the nutritional value of foods.

in the food supply. Consumption of these sugars dramatically increased with regular soft drinks up from 23.8 gallons per capita in 1970 to 40.3 gallons today; the consumption of corn syrup and sweeteners also rose, up from 3.2 pounds per capita to an amazing 138 pounds by 1994 (Family Economics and Nutrition Review, 1997).

Unfortunately, our society tends to overvalue many foods with empty kilocalories. Schools often reward academic achievement with candy, divorced parents may give their children extra "treats" in an attempt to lessen their guilt, and television advertisements tell us "Go ahead, you deserve it!" Because of this reward system and because people like the taste of sweets, many Americans overconsume low-nutrient foods that are high in fat and sugar.

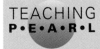

TEACHING
P•E•A•R•L   A useful analogy to use with children is to explain that some foods (those high in fat and sugar—shown in the tip of the Food Guide Pyramid to portray that they should be consumed in a small amount) help us grow outward whereas plant foods (in the lower part of the Food Guide Pyramid) help us grow upward. Using your hands to describe these changes graphically is very effective in aiding children's understanding.

Impact of Regional, Ethnic, Cultural, and Religious Dietary Habits in Studying Nutrition and Meal Planning. In many countries and cultures it is still common to find daily use of legumes (dried beans and peas) and greens. Lentils are one of the oldest foods known, having been eaten for at least 8000 years. From Northern Africa, through the Mediterranean, to Syria, people commonly sit down to half a plate of spinach, not a small dollop as Americans typically eat, if they eat it at all. In England, people to this day love baked beans on toast. Sardines, salmon, herring, mackerel, anchovies, cod (and cod liver oil) were basic foods to many of our ancestors, although they no longer are commonly consumed. Religious holiday food choices have long been practiced, such as 24-hour fasting for the Jewish holiday Yom Kippur, abstaining from meat on Fridays among Catholics (which has developed into the "Friday Fishfry"), or "giving up chocolate" for Lent.

The population of the United States includes many ethnic groups. They come from all parts of the world and have varied eating habits. Immigrants from Yugoslavia at the turn of the century did not know how to eat a banana. Currently, many young Americans have never had a variety of vegetables such as Swiss chard or lentils, or even basic vegetables such as brussel sprouts and broccoli. Persons from the South are more likely than others to eat okra, collard greens, kale, pinto beans, and black-eyed peas. Those who were born before World War II (before the process of hydrogenation was introduced) remember stirring their peanut butter. Some ethnic foods, such as Italian and Mexican, have become popular with broad groups of Americans. Unfortunately, these foods often become "Americanized" with excess amounts of cheese and meat added. Chinese meals in China are low in fat, but Chinese restaurants in the United States increasingly serve food high in fat. One Chinese buffet restaurant in the United States was recently observed to have chocolate cake and green jello.

Foods familiar in other countries may be rare and expensive in the United States and consequently may be omitted from the diet after immigration. If an ethnic group does give up some of its own food habits and adopts those of the new country, the poorest of the new country's nutritional habits are frequently chosen, such as a preference for excessive sweets and fats. This trend was found among second- and third-generation Mexican families living in California, whose diet, as compared with the traditional diet in Mexico, showed a decrease in **beta-carotene** foods such as dark green leafy vegetables and deep orange vegetables and fruits (beta-carotene turns into vitamin A in the body), in conjunction with increased sugar and fat (Romero-Gwynn et al., 1993).

The lure of foods advertised on television, which are often high in fat and sugar, also needs to be considered. It is important to acknowledge this desire to try new foods, but consumers also must focus on maintaining the low-fat, low-sugar, low-salt, and high-fiber foundation of the diet according to the Dietary Guidelines for all Americans. Table 1–1 shows how the five food groups of the Food Guide Pyramid are incorporated into different types of eating patterns. A typical day's diet for any ethnic, regional, or religious group may be evaluated nutritionally by checking it against an acceptable meal plan such as the Food Guide Pyramid.

Table 1-1
Ethnic and Regional Food Patterns According to the Basic Food Groups of the Food Guide Pyramid

Ethnic Group	Bread and Cereal	Eggs, Meat, Fish, Poultry	Dairy Products	Fruits and Vegetables	Seasonings and Fats
Italian	Northern Italy Crusty white bread Cornmeal and rice Southern Italy Pasta	Beef, chicken, eggs, fish, anchovies	Milk in coffee, cheese	Broccoli, zucchini, other squash, eggplant, artichokes, string beans, legumes,* tomatoes, peppers, asparagus, fresh fruit	Olives and olive oil, balsamic vinegar, salt, pepper, garlic, capers, basil
Puerto Rican	Rice, beans, noodles, spaghetti, oatmeal, cornmeal	Dry salted codfish, meat, salt pork, sausage, chicken, beef	Hot milk in coffee	Starchy root vegetables, green bananas, plantains, legumes,* tomatoes, green pepper, onion, pineapple, papaya, citrus fruits	Lard, herbs, oil, vinegar
Near Eastern	Bulgur (wheat)	Lamb, mutton, chicken, fish, eggs	Fermented milk, sour cream, yogurt, cheese	Nuts, grape leaves	Sheep's butter, olive oil
Greek	Plain wheat bread, phyllo dough	Lamb, pork, poultry, eggs, organ meats	Yogurt, cheese, butter	Onions, tomatoes, legumes,* fresh fruit	Olive oil, parsley, lemon, vinegar
Mexican	Lime-treated corn tortillas	Little meat (ground beef or pork), poultry, fish	Cheese, evaporated milk as beverage for infants	Pinto beans,* tomatoes, potatoes, onions, lettuce, black beans	Chili pepper, salt, garlic
Chinese	Rice, wheat, millet, corn, noodles	Little meat and no beef, fish (including raw fish) eggs of hen, duck, and pigeon, tofu and soybeans	Water buffalo milk occasionally, soybean milk, cheese	Soybeans,* soybean sprouts, bamboo sprouts, soy curd cooked in lime water, radish leaves, legumes,* vegetables, fruits	Sesame seeds, ginger, almonds, soy sauce, peanut oil
African American	Hot breads, pastries, cakes, cereals, white rice	Chicken, salt pork, ham, bacon, sausage	Milk and milk products (often lactase-free)	Kale, mustard, turnip greens, cabbage, hominy grits, sweet potatoes, watermelon	Molasses
Jewish	Noodles, crusty white seed rolls, rye bread, pumpernickel bread	Kosher meat (from forequarters and organs from beef, lamb, veal) Fish (except shellfish)	Milk and milk products Milk not eaten at same meal as meat	Vegetables— usually cooked with meat Fruits	

*Legumes are also counted as a meat substitute.

What Are Some Positive Ethnic Eating Habits That Follow the Dietary Guidelines for Americans?

International research suggests that Americans might benefit by eating more like people in other countries, for example, those described here (Broihier, 1993):

Chinese. Studies show that the Chinese have lower blood cholesterol levels and about one-tenth the incidence of heart disease of Americans. They also have a lower cancer rate. Chinese meals focus on rice and vegetables with soybean foods, such as tofu, serving as the primary daily protein source. Only 15 to 25 percent of the Chinese diet comes from fat.

French. The French have a low risk of heart disease, second only to the Japanese. The fat content of the French diet has only equaled ours since the 1980s, and their rate of heart disease may not have had time to catch up with the American rate, thus explaining their paradox of their high-fat diet with their low rates of heart disease. The French, however, eat small amounts of meat and plenty of vegetables. Wine provides phytochemicals that are believed to reduce the risk of heart disease. Further, the French tend not to eat rich desserts on a regular basis, and it is difficult to find a soda pop or a junk food aisle in France. As a rule, the French eat less shortening, oil, eggs, and sugar than Americans do.

Japanese. The Japanese have the lowest rate of heart disease in the world, as well as a generally low cancer risk. The Japanese diet centers around rice and vegetables but also includes lots of noodles, seaweed, fish, and soybean products including tofu.

Mediterranean Region. Both Greeks and southern Italians have low rates of heart disease. The traditional Mediterranean diet is based around "beans and greens." The consumption of lean red meat is usually limited to a few times per month, and fish is eaten about once a week. Sweets are eaten in small amounts on special occasions only. Olives and olive oil are used liberally but they are low in saturated fat and cholesterol-free yet high in monounsaturated fats. The amount of cheese used is much more moderate in these countries than in the United States.

WHAT IS THE IMPACT OF VEGETARIANISM ON HEALTH?

Who Follows Vegetarian Diets?

The number of vegetarians has increased rapidly over the past few decades. It is now estimated that at least 12 million Americans consider themselves **vegetarians,** and a significant number of new vegetarians are teenagers. One study found that 4 percent of teenagers, most of whom were girls, followed a vegetarian diet (Reilly, 1997). Two religious groups that forego consumption of meat and other animal products are Seventh Day Adventists and Muslims. Many persons of the Jewish faith adopt a vegetarian eating plan to help follow a kosher diet. Others follow vegetarian diets for health, political, cultural, or economic reasons, or a combination of these. People who follow a vegetarian diet that is planned around legumes, whole grains, a variety of fruits and vegetables, and low-fat milk products can improve their health through the reduction in cholesterol levels. However, just because a person avoids meat does not mean he or she is following a healthy diet. Humans cannot survive on chocolate alone!

How Do Vegetarian Diets Differ?

There are three main classifications of vegetarian diets:

1. *Lacto-ovo vegetarian.* Plant foods (whole grains, legumes, fruits, and vegetables) are supplemented with dairy products and eggs. This is probably the most common type of vegetarian diet. *Lacto* comes from the word *lactose* (milk sugar) and *ovo* comes from *ovum* (egg). Lacto-ovo vegetarians often also eat fish and chicken.
2. *Lacto-vegetarian.* Dairy products are included, but eggs are not.
3. *Total vegetarian* **(vegan).** Animal food sources (including eggs and dairy products) are completely excluded. For this reason, the diet may be low or inadequate in iodine, vitamin B_{12}, iron, calcium, zinc, riboflavin, and vitamin D. Good meal planning can allow for a healthy vegan diet that includes legumes, nuts, whole grains, and soy products for complementary proteins over the course of the day.

Nutritious Sample Menu for a Vegan Diet

Breakfast

Oatmeal with soy milk	Orange juice
Whole wheat toast with peanut butter	Half a grapefruit
	Herbal tea

Lunch

Minestrone soup	Whole wheat bread
Apple slices	Glass of soy milk
Pecans and raisins	

Supper

Tofu stir-fry with snow peas and carrot wedges	Couscous
Fresh spinach salad with croutons and dressing	Cantaloupe wedges
	Herbal iced tea

Snack

Almonds	Glass of soy milk
Whole-wheat crackers	

How Should One Plan a Vegetarian Diet?

Because meat provides protein, a variety of B vitamins, and minerals, alternative foods high in these nutrients need to be included in the diet for health (Table 1–2). The minimum amount of meat in the Food Guide Pyramid is 4 oz daily or the equivalent amount in meat substitutes. Meat is replaced with an increased intake of **legumes** (dried beans and peas), nuts, meat analogs such as soybean burgers, eggs, and milk products. One-half cup of legumes is equivalent to 1 oz of meat. One egg, ¼ cup nuts, 2 tablespoons of peanut butter, or 1 cup of milk contains a similar amount of protein as 1 oz of meat. The minimum number of servings (2 cups of milk and 4 oz of meat equivalent) will meet protein needs. Soymilk may replace cow's milk as a high source of protein and calcium.

Vegans (those persons who eliminate all animal products from the diet) need to emphasize legumes, nuts, and whole grains to meet the dietary need for complete protein. These foods are also high in B vitamins and minerals. Calcium is a particular nutritional challenge for vegans because they avoid milk products. Soy remains the best alternative, but other food alternatives are available (see the list of vegetarian calcium sources in Table 1–3). If adequate calcium intake is not possible, supplementation may be required. Foods fortified with vitamin B_{12} should be included. Brewer's yeast is a natural source of vitamin B_{12}. A spread used to put on crackers in England, Marmite™, is a yeast product that contains vitamin B_{12}. Marmite™ may be found in larger U.S. grocery stores carrying British foods.

Because of their restrictive food code, it is of the utmost importance that vegetarians primarily consume **nutrient-dense** foods (foods that have high amounts of nutrients in relation to the total kilocalories). The use of whole grains is critical to provide all of the needed essential amino acids for complementary protein. **Empty kilocalorie** foods (foods high in kilocalories but low in nutrients) should be avoided, unless kilocalorie needs are high and all essential nutrients are being consumed in the diet.

Table 1–2
Food Sources for Important Nutrients in the Vegetarian Diet

Nutrient	Sources
Calcium*	Milk and milk products, particularly cheese and yogurt; fortified soy milk; dark green leafy vegetables such as parsley, kale, and mustard, dandelion, and collard greens
Iron	Legumes, dark green leafy and other vegetables, whole-grain or enriched cereals or breads, some nuts, and dried fruits (Many factors may affect absorption of this nutrient)
Riboflavin (Vitamin B_2)	Milk, legumes, whole grains, and certain vegetables
Vitamin B_{12}	Milk and eggs, fortified soybean milk, and fortified soya products, Marmite™
Zinc	Nuts, beans, wheat germ, and cheese
Protein	Eggs, milk, nuts and seeds, legumes, especially soybeans and tofu

*See Table 1–3.

Table 1–3
Sources of Calcium in the Vegetarian Diet

Food Source	Average Calcium (mg)
4 oz tofu	110
½ cup almonds	175
½ cup peanuts	50
1 cup greens (except spinach)	200
1 cup dried apricots	100
1 cup dates	130
1 tbsp blackstrap molasses	135
½ cup oysters	110
3 oz salmon	165
3 oz sardines	370

By combining different foods in vegetarian diets, complete proteins can be formed from the available amino acids over a 24-hour period. Emphasis should be on the inclusion of legumes and whole grains at a minimum and if possible the inclusion of eggs, dairy, and nuts can help ensure adequate protein.

HOW DOES SNACKING AFFECT NUTRITION?

Many people find it more convenient to eat when they can, and snacking has become part of our culture. The term **grazing** is sometimes applied to the frequent all-day eating in which many people engage. The daily coffee break is a popular custom for people in all walks of life.

When one eats generally does not matter for the healthy population. Rather, it is more important to consider *what* is eaten, and *how much*, remembering the principles of moderation, balance, and variety. Three meals daily may be satisfactory for some people, but others find that the best way to receive adequate and appropriate amounts of kilocalories and nutrients is to eat more often. Snacking can be beneficial for children and the older adult alike, especially if appetites are small in relation to physical needs. As a general rule, snacks with low nutrient density should not replace nutrient-dense foods.

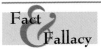
Fact & Fallacy

Fallacy: A late-night snack or meal causes weight gain.

Fact: The time when food is eaten has little impact on weight. What is more important is the total kilocalorie and fat content of meals and snacks. Saving all the day's kilocalories for one late-night meal may be a problem. Rather, the kilocalories should be spread out over the day, with inclusion of at least three meals throughout the day. This can help promote a higher metabolic rate (see Chapters 4 and 20).

How Should Snacks Be Chosen?

There is no single perfect snack, but some snacks are more nutritious than others, and careful selection is necessary to avoid potential problems. Snacks should be planned according to the needs of each member of the family. An individual who nibbles food during food preparation or cleanup may find it easy to put on unwanted pounds and hard to succeed in a weight-reduction program. Conversely, planned snacking can be an effective means for meeting the energy and nutrient needs of a growing or very active child or adolescent and may be an effective weight-management strategy.

Snacks should be chosen from the five food groups. Foods such as sticky sweets, which have been found to increase susceptibility to tooth decay, should be avoided. A piece of fresh fruit or a handful of low-fat, whole-grain crackers can be an appropriate snack. Rinsing the mouth with water is important after any kind of carbohydrate-based snack to help prevent dental decay (see Chapter 19).

HOW DO FAST FOODS AFFECT NUTRITION?

People of various cultures eat at fast-food restaurants (Fig. 1–2). Remembering the goal of balance, variety, and moderation, fast-food meals can safely be included in the diet. Obesity can result with excess fat and sugar intake.

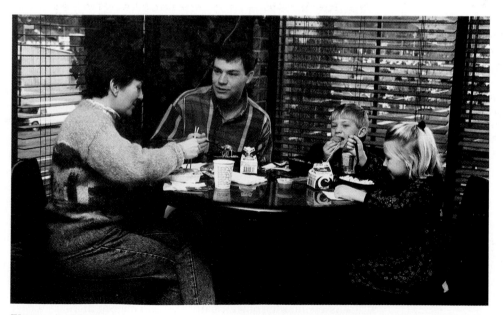

Figure 1–2
Restaurant eating is often a family socialization experience in the United States.

Nutritious Menu Including Fast Food

Breakfast (at home)
Toasted English muffin with
  natural peanut butter
Banana slices dipped in wheat
  germ*

Glass of 1 percent or skim milk

Lunch (cafeteria)
Chili con carne
Mixed salad greens with Italian
  dressing

Piece of cornbread
Glass of 1 percent or skim milk or
  8 oz yogurt

Afternoon Snack
Bunch of grapes (brought from
  home)

Supper (fast-food restaurant)
Small cheeseburger
Small orange juice
Coleslaw

Soft ice cream or frozen yogurt for
  dessert

Snack (at home)
Herb-seasoned low-fat popcorn

Small glass apple cider

*Wheat germ has a nutty flavor and crunchy texture and is found in the cereal section of the grocery store. One tablespoon contains about 10 percent of the recommended dietary allowance for vitamin B_1, folic acid, vitamin E, zinc, and phosphorus. It is also high in magnesium.

What Is the Definition of Fast Foods?

It is unfortunate that fast foods are often referred to as *junk food*. Junk foods usually are thought of as being low in nutrient density, especially for the amount of kcalories such as high-sugar or high-fat foods. Although these types of foods can be found in any restaurant, low-fat meal choices can be found on fast-food menus. The Food Guide Pyramid concept can easily be applied to fast food. To illustrate: a small cheeseburger on a bun with lettuce, tomato, and onion, plus juice, represents the five food groups; a taco is composed of a shell made from grain, along with ground beef, shredded cheese, shredded lettuce, and tomato; pizza has a crust made from grain, plus tomato sauce, cheese, and various vegetable and meat toppings; a typical fried chicken dinner with mashed potato, coleslaw, a roll, and a glass of milk also represents at least four of the five food groups. To help include fast foods in a manner consistent with the Food Guide Pyramid, the following tips may help:

- Focus on smaller portions of meat and cheese dishes.
- Remove the skin from cooked chicken.
- Look for bean-based dishes and salads or other vegetables or fruits.

- Use lemon instead of salad dressing or butter.
- Choose a small or low-sugar beverage.

Fast foods can also meet the nutrient density criteria required by the U.S. Department of Agriculture for Type A school lunches by providing one-third of the recommended dietary allowance (RDA) for selected nutrients and if chosen wisely can fit into the Dietary Guidelines for all Americans. Serving sizes are important; one lettuce leaf does not equal one serving of vegetable. See Appendix 4 for a nutritional analysis of selected fast-food restaurants.

HOW DOES ALCOHOL INTERFERE WITH NUTRITIONAL STATUS?

Excessive alcohol consumption affects health under two general, broad modes. One is the altered food intake resulting from factors such as decreased or increased appetite, replacement of the kilocalories in food for those in alcohol (concern for weight control or loss of appetite for food associated with heavy intake of alcohol), or the use of available food money for alcohol. The other major impact is impaired absorption, reduced storage, altered metabolic needs, and impaired use of nutrients. Thiamine deficiency is often a result of excess alcohol and too little food (see Chapter 4). A moderate amount of alcohol is acceptable and potentially desirable as long as there is little risk of alcohol abuse.

WHAT IS THE ROLE OF THE NURSE OR OTHER HEALTH CARE PROFESSIONAL IN THE FAMILY MEAL ENVIRONMENT?

Family eating behaviors fall in a spectrum from ideal to poor. The ideal diet consists of a balance of high-quality, nutritionally dense foods in appropriate quantities and variety to support normal growth and repair while inhibiting the development of chronic disease. Most families have a combination of ideal and poor food habits. All health care professionals can reinforce the positive food habits by giving ideas about how to incorporate well-liked nutritious foods into one's daily lifestyle.

The nurse plays a vital role in assessing and identifying patient and family needs, while facilitating solutions in a counseling approach. Meal planning can be relatively simple when few or no negative forces are influencing a family. The more likely scenario, however, is a combination of internal and external barriers to good nutrition, which can best be overcome through a total health care team approach. Many community services are available that can complement the skills of the health care team.

A nurse's contacts with patients in any situation provide unlimited teaching opportunities to promote better nutrition. The nurse's own dietary habits, attitudes and state of nutrition are reflected in his or her interest and approach when helping patients understand the importance of a basic normal or modified diet. Success will more likely occur if the nurse starts with good attitudes about the importance of nutrition. By having a good basic knowledge of nutrition and by keeping informed, the nurse can do much to combat the misinformation forced on the public by slanted advertising, food faddists, quacks, and self-termed untrained "health specialists," among others.

What Is Your Nutrition IQ as You Begin the Study of Nutrition?

Some of the following statements are true, and some are false. Read each question and then write your answer in the blank before you consult the list of correct answers on page 19. Relevant chapter numbers are provided for further information.

1. _____ A daily diet for weight reduction should have adequate amounts of protein, carbohydrates, fat, minerals, and vitamins but should furnish less than the daily requirements for kilocalories. (Chapter 20)
2. _____ Margarine and butter contain the same number of calories. (Chapter 3)
3. _____ Food allergies and food intolerances are the same thing. (Chapter 15)
4. _____ A well person who eats the right kinds and amounts of foods every day generally does not need to take vitamin pills to meet the RDA. (Chapter 5)
5. _____ Skipping meals is a good way to lose weight safely. (Chapter 20)
6. _____ Children should not have dessert unless they clean their plates. (Fact & Fallacy, Chapter 1)
7. _____ Calcium supplements are the best way to increase calcium intake if one does not like milk. (Chapter 5)
8. _____ The risk of heart disease can be reduced by following a diet low in saturated fat, cholesterol, and sodium. (Chapter 8)
9. _____ White bread is the same as wheat bread. (Chapter 3)
10. _____ Olives, olive oil, avocados, and most nuts are low in saturated fat and moderate amounts are fine for a low-cholesterol diet. (Chapter 3)
11. _____ People with diverticulosis should eat dried beans and peas because they are high in fiber, dependent on individual tolerance. (Chapter 11)
12. _____ An obese woman should lose weight if she becomes pregnant. (Chapter 16)
13. _____ Children should be forced to eat vegetables for their own good. (Chapter 17)
14. _____ Baby teeth are not important and therefore good dental care and oral hygiene should wait until children are old enough to brush their own teeth. (Chapter 19)
15. _____ It is possible for elderly people to develop muscle mass. (Chapter 21)
16. _____ Not all food additives are harmful. (Chapter 22)
17. _____ If a survivor of breast cancer gains weight, it is always due to consumption of too many kilocalories. (Chapter 12)

18. _____ Natural sweets like honey may be eaten freely by people with diabetes. (Chapter 9)
19. _____ Drinking water at mealtimes may aid digestion if the water is not used to wash down food. (Chapter 4)
20. _____ A teenager needs more milk every day than does a preschooler. (Chapter 17)

Number correct answers _____
Number incorrect answers _____
How good do you think your Nutrition Score is? _____

Correct Answers to the Nutrition IQ

1. T	8. T	15. T
2. T	9. T	16. T
3. F	10. T	17. F
4. T	11. T	18. F
5. F	12. F	19. T
6. F	13. F	20. T
7. F	14. F	

Critical Thinking

Case Study

During a physical exam prior to his upcoming wedding, Patrick learned that he has a high cholesterol and triglyceride level. Now Patrick is wondering if his Irish heritage could have something to do with his cholesterol problem. His dad never mentioned any health problems and seemed healthy except for his huge belly. Patrick wanted to talk with his fiancé about his doctor's visit, because she would be able to help him figure out how he was going to eat now. In thinking about how her mother was preparing his favorite meal tonight of boiled ham and cabbage, Patrick figured it might be his last piece of meat for awhile, because his doctor told him to stop eating meat. Patrick knew his fiancé's family had returned to a more traditional Italian style of eating with lots of "beans and greens" because of her dad's diabetes and high cholesterol.

Applications

1. How might you feel if your doctor told you that you could no longer eat meat, especially if you grew up in a "meat and potato" family? What health professional can provide individualized guidance on how much meat can be included in a low-fat, low-cholesterol diet?
2. Describe how family and culture influence food choices.

Study Questions and Classroom Activities

1. Explain what is meant by the following statement: "Good meal planning is both a science and an art."
2. How would you advise a patient to overcome food dislikes or avoidances?
3. Analyze food advertisements in magazines. To whom are the ads appealing? How?
4. Become familiar with the ethnic, religious, or regional diet assigned you by the instructor and summarize information about it to present to the class. Be prepared to discuss this ethnic diet in terms of the five food groups of the Food Guide Pyramid and Dietary Guidelines for Americans (see Chapter 6). What are the good points? How could the diet be improved? Each student in the class will then use the following chart to record important information about each diet presented in class.

Ethnic Dietary Habits

Regional or ethnic diet (list foods):

Characteristics and main dish:

Good nutritional features:

Desirable nutritional improvements:

5. Students might tell about the food customs and dietary habits of their country or countries of heritage and possibly demonstrate the ethnic dishes popular in their personal family meals. Markets of a city, ethnic food sections of large grocery stores, and ethnic restaurants afford good opportunities for learning about foods used by families with different ethnic backgrounds. The class might prepare a traditional Italian/Mediterranean meal or determine if any traditional Italian foods (such as bean-based dishes) can be found on local menus.

"My Food and Nutrition Experience Diary"

To help make you food-and-nutrition minded as you study nutrition, (1) jot down in the space provided any food and nutrition comments, questions, or experiences you encounter in discussions with individuals out of a classroom setting and later as you give nutritional care to patients (checking menus, setting up or observing and serving trays, feeding patients, and so on) and (2) assemble in a notebook (preferable), folder, or file box any available food and nutrition booklets, clippings, or other printed materials.

Date   **Food and Nutrition Experience**   **Comments**

References

Broihier CA: Environmental Nutrition. April 1993; 16(4):1–4.

Family Economics and Nutrition Review: U.S. per Capita Food Consumption. 1997; 10(1):38–41.

Murphy NJ, Schraer CD, Thiele MC, Boyko EJ, Bulkow LR, Doty BJ: Dietary change and obesity associated with glucose intolerance in Alaska Natives. J Am Diet Assoc. 1995; 95(6):676–682.

National Research Council, Committee on Diet and Health: Diet and Health. Washington, DC, National Academy Press, 1989; pp. 87, 94.

Reilly L: Bites of passage. Vegetarian Times. November 1997; 78–85.

Romero-Gwynn E, Gwynn D, Grivetti L, et al.: Dietary acculturation among Latinos of Mexican descent. Nutrition Today. July/August 1993; 6–12.

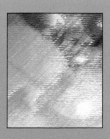

2

The Nutrition Care Process as Used by Health Care Professionals

Objectives

After completing this chapter, you should be able to:

- Describe what total health care means and how best to utilize this approach.
- Describe the steps of the nursing process as it relates to nutrition care.
- Describe the implications of the health belief model for patient compliance.
- Describe good interviewing skills.
- Describe appropriate nutrition interventions for families.
- Describe the role of the patient in facilitating compliance in health care and nutrition.

Terms to Identify

Active listening	Cognitive	Nursing process
Activities of daily living (ADL)	Expanded Food and Nutrition Education Program (EFNEP)	Nutrition care process
Affective		Nutrition Program for the Elderly
Albumin	Health belief model	Psychomotor
American Heart Association	"I" versus "You" statements	Women, Infants, and Children (WIC)
Assessment	Metabolic	Supplemental Food
Change agent	Nonverbal communication	Program
Cholesterol		

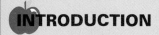

INTRODUCTION

Imagine yourself, as a health care professional, meeting a new patient or consumer. What do you say? Where do you begin? What questions should you ask? How do you help the person to be open about expressing their health and nutrition needs and concerns? Do you present yourself as very professional and aloof, informal and witty, or perhaps a combination? What are you trying to achieve through contact with the patient? These are just some of the questions that face a new nurse or practicing health care professional.

HOW IS NUTRITION AN ASPECT OF TOTAL HEALTH CARE?

The total needs and care of the patient as a person and community member, rather than in terms of diagnosis, continue to be emphasized in health care education. Nutrition is considered an integral part of patient care, along with the physical, social, psychiatric, and economic aspects. The patient (the term *patient* will be used throughout this book to mean client, consumer, and so on) requires adequate nutritional intake to maintain an already good nutritional state or to improve a poor one. For many patients, food is the single most important factor used to restore good health.

Patient-centered educational activities are the accepted approach in choosing learning experiences by the health professional. As a result, the patient has a better understanding of medical nutrition therapy in illness and recovery as well as in everyday living. Nutrition education strategies, as noted in the sections titled "Teaching Pearls" provided throughout this textbook, can later be applied in patient education settings.

Improvement in food selection patterns for bettering one's health frequently means changing habits of long standing. This is a slow, step-by-step, almost never-ending process necessitating a real desire to change, a deep conviction that change is important, and the willingness to substitute desirable food habits for undesirable ones. Health care professionals dealing with nutritional improvement, although primarily concerned with the **metabolic** (biochemical) role of food in health, must also have some understanding of the circumstances under which dietary habits are acquired and the various meanings that food may have for different individuals. This is especially true in dealing with patients who suffer from a disorder or disease that requires drastic, long-term changes in dietary habits.

A registered dietitian is of special importance when there are complex factors or medical conditions that interfere with nutritional status. Other professionals may need to be consulted as well, such as the family physician (for medically related factors), the occupational therapist or speech pathologist (for physical factors such as cleft palate), and the social worker or mental health worker (for negative family dynamics and finances). To make the best use of these professional resources, the nurse should first identify the patient's nutritional needs by describing the factors that are negatively influencing the family's ability to feed itself adequately. This role particularly suits the nurse or other health care professional who has frequent, regular contact with patients.

What Is the Health Care Team?

The health care team comprises all the health care professionals that work with a given patient or patients and their families toward the common goal of patient health. This includes the medical part of the team (physician, nurse, dietitian, physical therapist, and pharmacist), the social professionals (social worker, psychologist, occupational therapist), and other community resource personnel who play a role in facilitating good health. Because each type of health care professional has a unique perspective on needs assessment and health care planning, a team approach is most effective in eliciting positive changes in a person's well-being.

The patient should also be considered part of the health care team. The patient may arguably be the most important member of the health care team. This is especially true in managing chronic illness, when the patient must make day-to-day management decisions regarding lifestyle changes. Lifestyle changes, no matter how small, can have either a positive or a negative impact on health. It is critical that patients feel they have choices in their health care intervention, and they should be considered integral to the health care team in the planning and implementation stage. The patient needs to be encouraged to contribute fully to the assessment phase and be actively involved in the planning stage. This will increase patient cooperation and health outcomes by facilitating compliance through identifying realistic health care changes.

The Physician

Generally the person with the most broad-based knowledge related to patient health care is the medical doctor (MD), otherwise referred to as the physician. The physician knows the patient's medical history and has a general understanding of the relationship between disease states and other health concerns. Often, however, it is in the best interest of the patient for the physician to refer patients to other complementary health services, such as a registered dietitian for medical nutrition therapy. Doctors may not have the office time or the skills that an occupational therapist might provide. The physician needs to be kept abreast of the health services the patient receives. This may be in the form of written documentation in a hospitalized patient's chart, through standardized written correspondence from a community agency or other health care provider, or through telephone contact when there is an urgent need to discuss patient needs between the physician and the health care provider. Final health care decisions often are in the realm of the physician, who should be kept informed of concerns of the health care team and their recommendations for individual patient care.

The Nurse

The nurse generally has the most contact with individual patients and their families. The nurse can provide other members of the health care team with good insight into patient needs because of this in-depth patient contact. Ongoing assessment and monitoring of patient eating habits and health status are important roles of the nurse.

The Social Worker

The social worker is the health care professional who has expertise in the area of community resources including financial, counseling, technical support, and educational services. The social worker often can help patients identify and express barriers—whether perceived or actual—they may be facing in order to meet the goal of achieving health and wellness. Many times the patient is not ready to hear health care advice because of the need to resolve and come to terms with a chronic or acute illness.

The Physical Therapist

Assisting in promoting mobility and physical movement to control pain is part of the role of the physical therapist, or PT. A physical therapist may be involved with helping a person enhance the physical capabilities that have been impaired due to illness or trauma. The PT may promote exercise that is appropriate for the individual to promote weight loss or increase muscle strength.

The Occupational Therapist

The occupational therapist, or OT, emphasizes the remaining strengths of the individual and identifies adaptive devices that would enhance independent functioning, such as large-handled spoons and reaching devices. The OT works to increase the amount or types of **activities of daily living** (**ADL**) a patient is involved with, such as personal hygiene and eating. This is of particular importance after a person has suffered a stroke or other physical injury that impairs or prevents independent living.

The Speech Pathologist

The professional to consult when assessing the seemingly simple act of swallowing is the speech pathologist. Swallowing, a series of interrelated steps, can be seriously impaired due to stroke or other neurological damage (see Chapter 11). Aspiration of food (inhaling food into the lungs) is of serious consequence and can lead to partial or full airway obstruction or pneumonia. A speech pathologist can help determine the degree of risk for aspiration and make appropriate care plans that other health care professionals can use in developing their plans. For example, the physical therapist may be enlisted to help the patient position correctly for good swallowing, the occupational therapist may promote eating utensils designed for special feeding needs, and the dietitian may need to plan certain food consistencies to facilitate effective swallowing.

The Pharmacist

The registered pharmacist is responsible for preparing the nutritional solutions that the physician orders. These solutions are administered through veins or enteral routes (see Chapter 14). The dietitian often makes recommendations in consultation with the physician on the solution used in order to provide appropriate amounts of nutrients for the specific patient's needs. Because of the pharmacist's specialized knowledge about drugs and their actions, she or he is able to serve as a resource person concerning drug and nutrient interactions.

The Registered Dietitian

The registered dietitian, or RD, is the health care professional best qualified to interpret the science of how food is used by the body in health and disease states and to evaluate how changes in the diet can improve a patient's health status. The RD is trained to work with culturally diverse populations in adapting customary foods to meet ongoing health concerns for effective medical nutrition therapy.

The Nutritionist

A nutritionist is an educator, as well as a counselor, who usually works in a public health setting and who typically has at least a bachelor's degree in nutrition. The legal credential certified or licensed nutritionist is used in some states to help indicate qualified nutritionists. All RDs are nutritionists.

THE NUTRITION CARE PLANNING PROCESS

What Are Assessment Strategies?

The **nutrition care process** of assessment, planning, intervention, and evaluation is the same as the **nursing process** with the omission of diagnosis. It is both a science and an art. By following the steps of the nursing process you will be a more effective health care professional. With practice and experience it will become easier, but your own unique style can either help or hinder the process of patient nutrition health care. Being very observant of **nonverbal communication** (facial expressions or other body language) and verbal communication from the patients you work with can guide you to becoming an effective change agent in patient compliance. A positive **change agent** is one who is directly and indirectly involved in promoting improved health of patients and consumers. Nurses and other health care professionals need to become culturally competent. Awareness of each individual patient's sociocultural background is important for planning sensitive and tactful interventions and to best promote patient health (Schiavenato, 1997). Cultural assessments are not limited to a specific ethnic group, because every patient has values, beliefs, and practices that need to be assessed (Narayan, 1997).

Generally, each step of the nursing process or nutrition care process should be followed in order. There is also a degree of integration between each step of the process, and the process is usually repeated several times during the course of patient intervention. This chapter emphasizes the importance of developing patient rapport by using good communication skills in the process of assessment, planning, intervention, and evaluation.

The **assessment** phase involves knowing the patient's initial medical and nutritional status. Knowledge of any previous or current health concerns is important in determining the best course of action. One simple assessment is determining if the patient is overweight or underweight or has had a change in weight that may be indicative of a problem. Lab values—such as those for hemoglobin (to determine iron status), **albumin** (to determine protein status), cholesterol and other blood fats such as triglycerides, blood glucose, and other lab values—can help determine health needs that should be addressed in the later intervention phase. Other specific indicators for the assessment of nutritional status are covered in Chapter 7. These physical findings relate to the *bio* part of biopsychosocial concerns.

For effective intervention, assessment should also include the psychosocial issues that may be contributing to physical health concerns and may need to be addressed before realistic changes can take place in patient health care. For example, social events or poor self-esteem may be causing negative food choices. This part of the assessment phase requires excellent communication skills to promote patient disclosure of potentially sensitive and personal lifestyle issues. Developing rapport and trust is critical to effective nutrition assessment and intervention. The more thorough the assessment phase, the more likely that appropriate and well-focused intervention strategies can be identified and implemented. A "hit-or-miss" intervention plan is not only potentially a waste of time, energy, and money but can even be harmful to the patient.

The health belief model, as discussed in a later section, complements the nursing process by assessing health values and beliefs prior to intervention. Family health history and heritage may give further useful information that can help the patient understand the need for making changes.

What Are Planning Strategies?

The planning stage of the nursing process brings together all the findings of the assessment phase, starting with identifying priority health concerns, long-term health goals, and short-term objectives. Identifying small, achievable, and measurable objectives aimed at long-term goals and specified health outcomes is important for facilitating behavioral change by patients. When the health care professional is clear on goals and rationale for change, appropriate objectives and means of intervention can be determined.

Objectives are the steps needed to achieve long-term health goals. They should include measurable action verbs combined in a statement of intent or expected health outcome. For example, the action verbs *to identify, to state,* and *to demonstrate* can all be used in patient objectives. The expected time frame for achievement of the objectives is sometimes also included. Objectives might read as follows. The patient will

- Identify foods high in salt using food labels.
- Substitute low-salt foods for high-salt foods.
- Determine foods high in sugar versus foods high in fiber.
- Correlate after-meal blood glucose values to meal intake.
- Describe low-fat food alternatives.

These objectives might be evaluated or measured through follow-up counseling sessions, through observation, or from improved lab values. Although objectives are aimed at short-term, measurable activities or outcomes, goals should be more broad based, such as "Patient will achieve a triglyceride level less than 200 mg/dL." It is important to write out the planning process to increase the effectiveness of the intervention, and to communicate the care plan to other members of the health care team.

The short-term objectives may need to be prioritized, starting with the most important change. A patient is more likely to implement easy changes than more complex changes or too many changes at once. As objectives are met in the intervention and evaluation phases, the patient should receive positive reinforcement for these changes and then be encouraged to meet the others as needed.

The evaluation plan is also determined prior to the intervention phase. Evaluation ultimately means changes in lab values or other clinical health outcomes. Because money is limited, the health care field now demands effective patient intervention and documented positive health outcomes.

The intervention phase can begin once the planned health outcomes are written or at least thought out or expressed verbally with the patient. A review with the patient of goals, objectives, and means of evaluation as based on the assessment phase can help promote compliance.

What Are Intervention Strategies?

Intervention approaches often begin with simple, brief reinforcing messages. One question might be "Have you tried the new low-fat snacks of hot pretzels or herb-seasoned popcorn? They are really delicious." A more general question might also be asked, such as "Have you ever tried to lower your fat or sugar intake?" Suggestions can then be built on the patient's earlier attempts or changes in eating habits.

Patient retention of information is enhanced by combining different modes of information given. It is known that people remember best what they have heard, seen, and practiced. Therefore, verbal reinforcement of written educational material is more effective than simply giving patients a brochure. Reviewing food labels and having patients describe the amount of sodium, sugar, or fat in the food product is another exercise that can be very effective in patient compliance. Asking patients what has been successful in the past in their attempts to improve their health is also useful. This allows reinforcement of the positive attempts or changes made in the past.

Through identifying individual or group goals and objectives, messages can be kept to a few key points. Prioritizing messages and offering sequential information needed to elicit patient health and eating changes are important. Simple concepts can later be built upon with more complex concepts. For example, decision-making skills regarding meal planning are advanced concepts and need to be stressed after there is a general understanding of the rationale for change. Messages given should offer positive reinforcement for behavior change. Scare tactics can cause inappropriate behaviors for health improvement, such as denial or tuning out the message. Follow-up reinforcement or referral to other appropriate services can assist patients to continue developing more positive health habits (see Table 2–1).

Table 2–1
Common Family Nutrition Problems and Possible Solutions

Problem	Referrals to or Sources of Solutions
Inadequate economic resources for purchasing food	The Food Stamp Program The **Women, Infants, and Children (WIC) Supplemental Food Program**—a program for lower-income families that includes food coupons and nutrition education Food pantries and soup kitchens The **Expanded Food and Nutrition Education Program (EFNEP)**—a program of the Cooperative Extension Service that can be referred to for budgeting assistance Use food models to determine if excess intake in one food group (such as meat) can be reduced to allow for increase in other foods
Physical constraints to obtaining food	**Nutrition Program for the Elderly** for meal delivery for homebound older adults Local grocery stores with delivery service Public Health Nursing for professional home-based assessment
Inadequate cooking equipment or storage facilities	EFNEP for recipes and meal ideas
Food dislikes	A qualified nutritionist (or registered dietitian) for food alternatives Explain that tastes are learned; suggest the one-taste approach to facilitate acceptance

Inadequate time to prepare food	Suggest use of nutritious but convenient food ideas
	  Vitamin A ideas: carrot sticks, apricots, cantaloupe, watermelon
	  Protein ideas: cheese (low-fat or moderate amounts of natural cheese), peanut butter, eggs, or egg whites

Too much sodium in diet	The local **American Heart Association (AHA),** an organization promoting heart health, for recipe ideas A registered dietitian for individualized meal plans and behavioral change strategies Suggest use of frozen or fresh vegetables, Swiss cheese instead of high-sodium processed cheese, spices and herbs or jelly to enhance the natural flavor of food Explain that our taste for salt is both learned and unlearned Explain that salt substitutes should be used only on the advice of a medical doctor because of potential harm from the potassium content
Too much sugar in diet	Encourage gradual sugar reduction while tastes change: use of ½ or ¾ of usual amount in baking or at the table; suggest use of fresh fruit or fruit canned in light syrup Explain that spices such as cinnamon or nutmeg can enhance the natural flavor without added sugar Encourage the use of ice water, flavored waters, iced tea, or diet soda as a replacement for soft drinks
Too much cholesterol, fat, and saturated fat	The American Heart Association for recipe ideas Suggest a gradual change from 4 percent (whole milk) to 2 percent (reduced-fat) to 1 percent (low-fat) or skim milk (fat-free) while tastes change Suggest use of less butter, margarine, mayonnaise, and oil Explain that although cholesterol is found only in animal foods, saturated fats should be mainly avoided; food products with ingredient labels that say *liquid oil* are better than those that say *hydrogenated* oil (see Chapters 3 and 8 for more details)
Negative effects of commercials on food-buying practices	Explain that advertisements are meant to sell products; they generally are not concerned with healthy dietary habits Explain to children that many foods they see advertised help them to grow outward, not upward (a representation with your hands can be helpful to children)

What Are Evaluation Strategies?

The final step of evaluation should be considered during the planning and intervention phases. The effectiveness of the plan in terms of the patient's progress must then be documented and evaluated by information and skills gained by the patient and by the outcomes of lab blood tests or other measures, as set forth in the specific patient goals and objectives. Examples might be achieving a 10 percent weight loss, a fasting blood sugar level under 110 mg/dL, or a blood cholesterol level of less than 200 mg/dL. The evaluation process can help the health care professional determine if further intervention is needed.

Many forms of evaluation may be performed. Measuring health outcomes is one important form, which might be done with ongoing, informal evaluation through observation, such as at mealtimes or in other social settings, or through informal conversation such as a discussion of food likes and dislikes. More formal evaluation may involve monitoring lab values. Monitoring the growth in children and weight changes in adults is a simple but effective means of measuring nutritional status. Evaluation may also focus on knowledge gained through verbal or written questions. Before-and-after tests can evaluate the outcome of a planned intervention but should be used with caution, as many adults do not like to be quizzed.

The nutrition care plan (see Chapter 7, Fig. 7–4) should always be incorporated into the total patient care plan. This plan should be formulated by the health care team as soon as possible to establish patient-centered goals to be met before discharge. The physician will then review the plan.

In summary, the nutrition care planning process includes (1) making a nutrition assessment, (2) identifying nutritional needs, (3) planning how to meet nutritional needs using goals and objectives, (4) carrying out the plan of care, (5) evaluating nutritional care, and (6) planning nutrition discharge (see Chapter 7).

WHAT IS THE HEALTH BELIEF MODEL?

The **health belief model** was originally described by Rosenstock in 1977 and is based on the theory that a patient makes health decisions in line with personal health values and the perceived benefits. The health belief model suggests that people need to believe that they are susceptible to illness, that they can make changes in their lifestyle, and that changing their lifestyle will make a positive impact on their health. The patient needs to weigh the health benefits against the social or financial costs of changing or maintaining current health and nutrition habits.

The cost of change, aside from the monetary aspect of health care services, relates to the social cost of eating differently from others and the psychological cost of changing food habits. For example, a person may feel that quality of life is more important than quantity of life to the point of refusing to attempt any lifestyle changes. The person's motivation to make lifestyle changes should be determined prior to the intervention phase. Providing a diet sheet of foods to avoid can be wasteful and possibly harmful psychologically if the person does not have confidence in his or her ability to make changes in eating habits. This approach may negatively impact patients' trust in their health care provider if information given is not realistic for them.

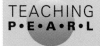

TEACHING
P•E•A•R•L

Quality of life versus quantity of life might be addressed by asking an assessment question such as "How do you feel about eating less cheese and butter to bring down your cholesterol level?" You might add the statement, "Eating less fat will also help you lose weight and thus bring down your triglyceride level. Are you willing to try low-fat cheese and to use less butter?"

INTERVIEWING AND COMMUNICATION SKILLS

How Are Good Communication Skills Important in Health Care?

Both the assessment phase and the intervention phase require using good communication skills with patients. The planning stage also requires good written and verbal communication skills in working with other health care professionals in the coordination of patient care. Nonverbal communication is also involved. Using an authoritative manner is not as effective as using an empathetic approach along with active listening techniques.

To promote patient discussion of personal health concerns, the following strategies are helpful (Fig. 2–1):

- Use a warm, friendly, positive approach.
- Sit in comfortable proximity, neither too close nor too far away.
- Use good eye contact, with eyes intent but not staring.
- Face the patient and lean forward.
- Have arms unfolded and resting in a relaxed manner.
- Carefully listen to what the patient is saying, using affirming responses to encourage the patient to clarify comments made.
- Allow pauses in the conversation; take as long a pause as needed to consider how to best make replies—it shows that you are interested in giving correct and appropriate replies.

Terminology used in the intervention stage can further promote or hinder patient openness. Using overly technical medical jargon can discourage the patient's understanding and willingness to ask questions. As much as possible, the health care professional should use terms and expressions that are understood and used by the patient in everyday settings. Observing the nonverbal communication signals that the patient exhibits can assist the health care professional in determining and fine-tuning messages given based on patient needs. A patient who initially is very talkative but who becomes very quiet or begins to look at the clock is sending a powerful message. The health care professional needs to observe the patient's verbal and nonverbal communication and respond accordingly.

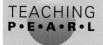 Using simple analogies can diffuse any growing tension and help redirect the message based on the patient's needs. In describing complex medical conditions you might say, "There are little doors into the body's cells that allow insulin and sugar to get in. The insulin is sometimes referred to as the key that allows glucose through the doors of the cell. These doors are called receptor sites if you do much reading on diabetes." (See Chapter 9.)

What Are Some Interviewing Tips?

In the process of nutritional assessment, the following three realms should not be overlooked in patient care: (1) **cognitive** (knowledge), (2) **affective** (attitudes), and (3) **psychomotor** or behavioral (behaviors). Does the family have adequate knowledge about good nutritional practices? Does the family value good nutrition? What constraints does the family have in gaining access to and consuming a balanced diet? What is the patient's family meal environment in general? Can the patient shop and cook? Is the patient's ability to chew, swallow, and digest food appropriate?

A variety of interviewing and assessment methods can be used to identify these three areas, such as diet history (see Chapter 7) and active listening–type

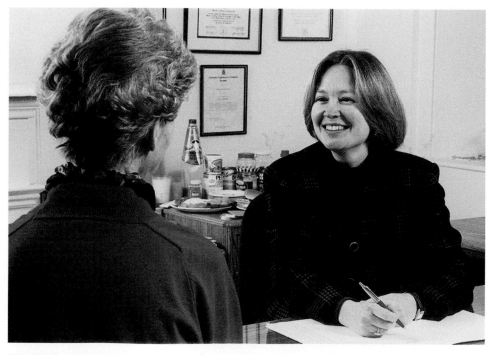

Figure 2–1
Effective nutrition care starts with good patient communication and rapport development.

questions (see the next section). It is important to be aware that patients sometimes combine misconceptions with accurate information. Asking patients to provide an example of a learned concept—for example, to interpret a food label—is useful in evaluating their understanding and ability to apply learned nutrition concepts.

What Is Active Listening?

Active listening is a manner of questioning and responding to a person that promotes full disclosure of opinions, feelings, emotions, and beliefs. This form of assessment can take time, but the information gathered allows for planning the most effective intervention methods. A few key questions can result in a wealth of information. Active listening is nonjudgmental and uses open-ended questions that elicit feelings and thoughts rather than yes or no responses. The following are examples of effective active listening questions:

Good Interviewing Questions

How do you feel about _____?
Can you tell me what you know about _____?
How is _____ a problem for your family?
Can you tell me more about _____?

How Can "I" Versus "You" Statements Help in the Nursing Process?

"I" statements versus "You" statements complement active listening techniques. "You" statements can sound judgmental and authoritarian, which can cause the patient or client to react defensively. Rephrasing "you" statements to "I" statements will promote patient interaction and communication.

An example of a "you" statement changed to an "I" statement is as follows: "You have a problem with fat intake" changed to "I am concerned about what appears to be a high-fat diet." Using the term *concerned* indicates empathy or concern for the patient. Follow this comment with an active listening questioning such as "How do you feel about your diet?" for a very effective communication strategy.

An "I" statement is your opinion, which makes the statement less threatening and final. Your position as an authority figure can prevent many patients from questioning statements that sound official, even if they feel that your statements are in error. A defensive reaction by the patient will essentially end your effectiveness in bringing about health changes. If patients feel that their opinions are being listened to, through the use of active listening techniques, they also will be more likely to listen to your opinions.

Does Choice Help in Patient Compliance?

Chronic illness often is best controlled or managed through ongoing support services. Developing goals and small achievable objectives is important. It is also important for the patient or client to have a feeling of choice in making health care decisions. This is often observed through a patient's acceptance of hospital food. If patients are given choices over their meal selections in the hospital, they often are more accepting of their therapeutic diet. A verbal commitment (action) from a patient can further increase the likelihood that the patient will believe in and adopt the agreed upon health change.

TEACHING
P•E•A•R•L

Choice is important for people of all ages. Even 2-year olds are more likely to eat vegetables if given a structured choice such as "Which do you want to eat tonight, carrots or broccoli?" This same principle can be applied to an adult situation, such as saying, "One salty food can be worked into your low-salt meal plan. Which would you prefer?" Or the choice might be between having the saturated fat of cheese one day and that of red meat the next in order to keep the total amount of saturated fat down.

What Is the Importance of Honesty and Respect in Patient Care and Education?

It is okay to admit lack of knowledge when questioned by a patient. There is a lot to know regarding how food and nutrition affect one's health. It is much better to admit you do not know an answer than to be caught giving inaccurate information, which could forever damage your credibility as a patient educator. Instead, you might say, "That's an interesting question. Perhaps we can find the answer in this brochure."

The most important aspect of patient communication is respect. Without respect, all attempts at effective communication will be lost. For example, if you have to leave the room, tell the patient. Do not assume the patient knows you will return. If the patient makes a comment unrelated to his or her health care needs, respond anyway. Showing respect for a patient's feelings and thoughts will greatly enhance the nutrition care process.

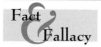

Fallacy: Doctors are always the best source for nutrition information.

Fact: Most doctors receive little nutrition information in medical school, especially in the area of nutrition education. Physicians who receive nutrition education are more likely to discuss nutrition and recommend diets with their patients (Lazarus, 1997). Physicians, other health care professionals, and even patients and their families should use the unique services of a registered dietitian when the health need arises, even if only to make a phone call and ask a question.

WHAT IS THE NURSE'S ROLE IN NUTRITION COUNSELING?

Nurses frequently find themselves involved in counseling individuals and families of varying cultural and economic status. To be successful in helping an individual accept a certain dietary regimen, the nurse must display warmth and understanding, establish a rapport, and be positive in approaching the patient. The nurse should stress the strengths in the person's diet history. For example, if the patient consumes breakfast routinely and eats a variety of foods from the food groups of the Food Guide Pyramid (see Chapter 6), the nurse can build on those important features in the meal pattern and compliment the individual's efforts in making good food choices. Effective communication is extremely important, and therefore the nurse should make use of all available tools, such as the mealtime tray, food models, posters, and food intake records. Specific problems can then be focused on, making it easier to attain realistic goals. Repeated counseling sessions are a must if continuity is to be maintained and if any behavioral modification is to become a permanent way of life. Nutrition counseling is a challenge, but it can be a rewarding experience to the nurse. Because the nurse spends more time with the patient than any other health care professional, it is critical that the nurse be well informed on how to provide appropriate nutritional guidance.

Critical Thinking

Case Study

The doctor sat in her office and thought about the young man who was planning to get married. She wondered whether his diagnosis of hypertriglyceridemia was genetic and decided to look again at his medical chart. Excess alcohol as a cause seemed to be ruled out. She looked down her notes until she read the following details in the patient's record:

Family History: Father with central obesity and family history of hypertension and cardiovascular disease; mother with central obesity and family history of diabetes, renal disease, and Native American heritage. Sibling with history of cerebral vascular accident.
   Anthropometrics: Height: 5'11"   Weight: 210 lb   BP: 130/85   PR: 70
WAIST/HIP: 1.3
   Labs: CHOL: 230 mg/dL   TRIG: 400 mg/dL

She decided the elevated triglycerides must be genetic and ordered a total lipid profile, including HDL cholesterol. She thought about her advice to the patient that he should give up red meat, which seemed to be prudent. Afterall, she herself followed a vegetarian diet. She finally decided to have her office assistant contact the managed care organization to arrange for preauthorization for referral to a registered dietitian. The doctor knew the RD could develop an individualized meal plan for this man that would still allow some meat. After all, he did not seem interested in giving it up completely.

Applications

1. How might the food habits of health professionals affect the care of their patients or clients?
2. How have managed care organizations affected your own ability to seek medical care?
3. Why did the doctor want to make the referral to the dietitian? Are there any other health care professionals she should have made referrals to?
4. Discuss a nursing diagnosis and expected nutrition outcome with referral to a registered dietitian.
5. After studying Chapter 9, return to this case study; identify the risk factors for the insulin resistance syndrome. What type of fat might be beneficial for this man's health?

Study Questions and Classroom Activities

1. Have a class role-play with one student serving as a nurse or other health care professional attempting to use the health belief model in assessing the needs of a volunteer patient. The "patient" should be from another ethnic background (refer to class activity in Chapter 1 regarding differences in ethnic cultures and food choices). Other class members should critique the role-play for good communication techniques and to determine how successfully the nutrition care process was put into practice. The role-play might be repeated to cover a number of different ethnic backgrounds.
2. List positive communication messages that promote honest answers to assessment questions.

References

Lazarus K: Nutrition practices of family physicians after education by a physician nutrition specialist. Am J Clin Nutr. June 1997; 65(6 Suppl):2007S–2009S.

Narayan MC: Cultural assessment in home healthcare. Home Health Nurse. October 1997; 15(10):663–670.

Schiavenato M: The Hispanic elderly: Implications for nursing care. J Gerontol Nurs. June 1997; 23(6):10–15.

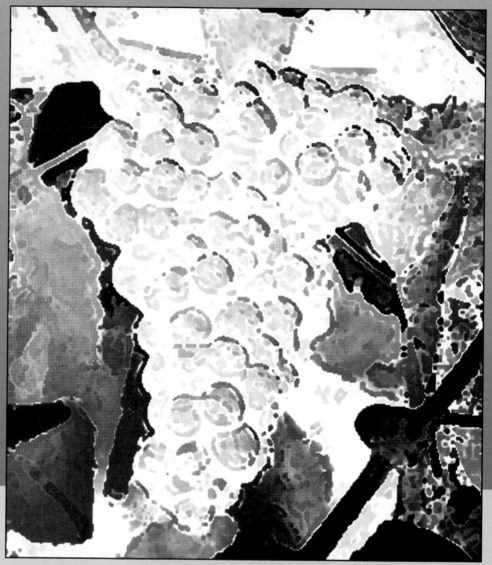

The Science and Application of Nutrition

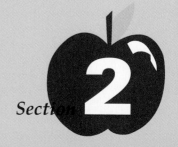

Section 2

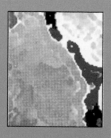

3
Carbohydrate, Protein, and Fat

The Energy Macronutrients of Balanced Meals

Objectives

After completing this chapter, you should be able to:

- Describe the macronutrient content of various foods and meal items.
- Describe the function and general recommendations for carbohydrate, protein, and fat in health prevention and disease management.
- Describe the role of the nurse or other health care professional in promoting an appropriate intake of carbohydrate, protein, and fat in a meal context.

Terms to Identify

Biological value	Ketosis	Omega-3 fatty acid
Complete protein	Kilocalories	Phospholipids
Diglycerides	Kwashiorkor	Polysaccharides
Disaccharides	Linoleic acid	Prostaglandins
Essential amino acids	Marasmus	Protein-energy
Essential fatty acids	Monoglycerides	malnutrition
Glycerol	Monosaccharides	Sterols
Hydrogenated fat	Monounsaturated fat	Sugar alcohols
Incomplete protein	Nitrogen balance	Trans fatty acid

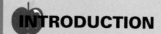 **INTRODUCTION**

The **kilocalories** (energy, abbreviated kcal) in the food we eat are the macronutrients carbohydrate, protein, and fat (see Fig. 3–1). Balanced meals contain all three macronutrients or ideally at least one serving from each of the three lower levels of the Food Guide Pyramid (see the inside front cover and Chapter 6). The macronutrients provide the fuel for body functioning (although of the three, protein serves this function least well). All three macronutrients contain the elements carbon, hydrogen, and oxygen. Protein is different from carbohydrate and fat in

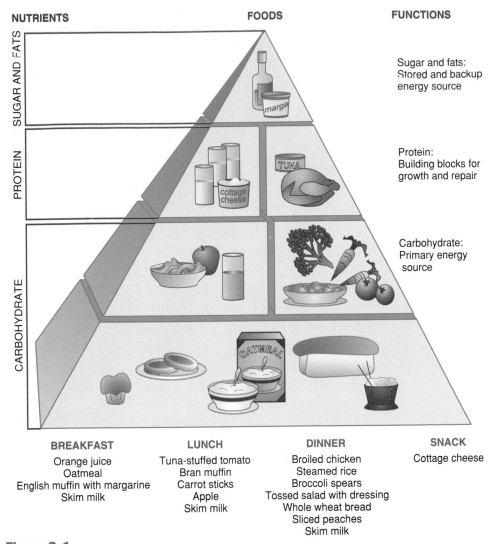

NUTRIENTS   FOODS   FUNCTIONS

SUGAR AND FATS

Sugar and fats:
Stored and backup
energy source

PROTEIN

Protein:
Building blocks for
growth and repair

CARBOHYDRATE

Carbohydrate:
Primary energy
source

BREAKFAST	LUNCH	DINNER	SNACK
Orange juice	Tuna-stuffed tomato	Broiled chicken	Cottage cheese
Oatmeal	Bran muffin	Steamed rice	
English muffin with margarine	Carrot sticks	Broccoli spears	
Skim milk	Apple	Tossed salad with dressing	
	Skim milk	Whole wheat bread	
		Sliced peaches	
		Skim milk	

Figure 3–1
Carbohydrate, protein, and fat content of the Food Guide Pyramid.

that protein contains nitrogen. Carbohydrate and protein provide 4 kilocalories per gram and fat provides 9 kilocalories, as noted on many food labels (see Fig. 6–1). Alcohol provides 7 kilocalories per gram, and although carbohydrate in origin, once carbohydrate is fermented into alcohol the body uses alcohol more like fats (see Chapter 4).

WHERE ARE THE THREE MACRONUTRIENTS FOUND?

Carbohydrate is made through the process of photosynthesis (when the sun's energy allows plant leaves to take in carbon dioxide [CO_2] from the air and water [H_2O] through the roots). The carbon (carbo) and water (hydrate) are formed into carbohydrate, and oxygen is given off by the plant. Hence, carbohydrate is mainly found in food of plant origin. Although we don't think of sugar as growing out of the ground, it is plant in origin. The carbohydrate found in table sugar is, however, in a very concentrated amount (½ cup of sugar contains 95 grams of carbohydrate—without any other nutritional value—whereas ½ cup of most plant foods contains only 15 grams of carbohydrate or less and is concentrated in the micronutrients vitamins and minerals). The only nonplant source of carbohydrate is milk, which makes sense if you think about it, because baby animals need a source of carbohydrate before they are able to eat solid foods (see Chapter 17). When cheese is made, enzymes are added to coagulate the protein and the liquid whey, which contains the carbohydrate lactose, is drained off. The trace amounts of lactose that are left are further converted to lactic acid during fermentation.

Protein is found in muscle, and thus all forms of meat (red, white, and fish) are mostly protein. Legumes (beans) and nuts are plant in origin, and thus contain carbohydrate (all plant based foods contain carbohydrate), but legumes also have the ability to draw nitrogen from the air making them high in protein. This is why legumes and nuts were included in the meat group of the Food Guide Pyramid (see Chapter 6). Other sources of protein are eggs, milk, and cheese. Whole grains and vegetables supply small amounts of protein but can add up to a significant quantity depending on the amount consumed. Grains (except quinoa) and vegetables do not contain complete protein as do meat, milk, and eggs. Fruits are very low in protein, which is why they have fewer kilocalories than bread even though they have the same amount of carbohydrate on a per-volume basis.

Fats are found in many protein foods and are added through cooking or to flavor foods. The amount of fat found in grains, vegetables, and most fruits is insignificant. Fats extracted from vegetable souces (corn, safflower, soybean, olive) are usually found in liquid form and generally are not harmful to health unless they are hydrogenated (turned into solid fats). Fats that are solid (mostly of animal origin such as butter and found in red meat) need to be limited to help prevent or manage a variety of health conditions.

CARBOHYDRATE: FUNCTIONS AND RECOMMENDATIONS FOR APPROPRIATE INTAKE

What Is the Function of Carbohydrate?

The carbon part of carbohydrate is the source of energy that humans burn, similar to the carbon found in coal. In fact, the human body is made up of millions of microscopic body cells that act as mini-furnances to burn our food energy. Thus, the primary function of carbohydrates is to meet the body's specific needs for energy (see Table 3–1). Carbohydrates are readily converted to energy. One gram of carbohydrate yields 4 kilocalories. Other functions of carbohydrate include the following:

1. It *spares* the burning of protein for energy (protein has more important functions, such as building and repairing body structures).
2. It *aids* in the more efficient and complete oxidation (burning) of fats for energy.

Table 3–1
Types and Sources of Carbohydrates

Type	Description	Sources
Monosaccharides (simple sugars)		
Glucose (blood sugar)	The end product of most carbohydrate digestion. The form in which carbohydrates are absorbed, resulting from its being the only fuel the central nervous system can use.	Found in fruits, certain roots, corn, and honey. Also found in blood as the product of starch digestion.
Fructose (fruit sugar)	Gives honey its characteristic flavor. Combined with glucose in table sugar.	Found in fruit, honey, and vegetables.
Galactose	A by-product of lactose digestion.	Naturally found only in mammary glands.
Disaccharides (double sugars)		
Sucrose (table sugar)	Composed of glucose and fructose. Commonly known as table sugar, which is made from sugar cane.	Found in sugar cane, sugar beets, molasses, maple sugar, maple syrup, many fruits and vegetables, and added to foods as table sugar.
Lactose (milk sugar)	Produced only by mammals. It is less soluble and less sweet than cane sugar and is digested more slowly. Composed of glucose and galactose.	Found in milk and unfermented milk products.
Maltose (malt sugar)	Formed when starch is changed to sugar during digestion. Composed of two glucose molecules.	Found in malt and malt products; not free in nature.
Polysaccharides (starch, complex carbohydrates)		
Complex carbohydrate (starch)	The reserve store of carbohydrates in plants; changed to glucose during digestion (through intermediate steps of dextrin and maltose).	Found in grains and grain products, seeds, roots, potatoes, green bananas, and other plants.
Dextrin	Formed from starch breakdown.	Cooked starch (toast).
Dietary fiber	Indigestible; provides bulk and stimulation for the intestines and helps prevent or manage many chronic illnesses.	Insoluble found in skins and seeds of fruits, vegetables, and grains. Soluble found in large amounts in legumes, greens, citrus fruits, oatmeal, and barley.
Glycogen	The reserve store of carbohydrates in animals; changed to glucose as needed.	Stored small amounts in the liver and muscles.

3. As *sugar*, it produces energy quickly.
4. As *starch*, it provides an economical and abundant source of energy after it is changed to glucose. Sugar and starch are both digested quickly in less than one hour.
5. As *lactose*, it has a certain laxative action (remains in the intestines longer and encourages desirable bacterial growth) and aids in the absorption of calcium.
6. As *dietary fiber* (insoluble and indigestible), it aids in the normal functioning of the intestines. Soluble forms, in significant amounts, lowers serum cholesterol levels (see Chapter 8) and lessens the post-prandial (after meal) rise in blood glucose. Recently, soluble fiber via oats (3 grams of fiber per 1-ounce serving) has been shown to enhance the body's use of insulin among persons with insulin resistance (Pick et al., 1996). Fiber slows down the time of digestion, which helps promote satiety (the feeling of fullness or being satisfied after eating) and allows for more stable blood sugar levels (see Chapter 9).

What Are the Three Basic Forms of Carbohydrate?

1. Simple carbohydrates, or sugars, are single or double units ($C_6H_{12}O_6$) and may also be referred to as **monosaccharides** (single units) and **disaccharides** (double units or double sugars). These double sugars are found in food and must break apart into single sugars before they can be absorbed into the bloodstream.
2. Complex carbohydrates, or starch, consist of several units of sugar linked together in a long chain—also referred to as **polysaccharides** (multiple units) or, more simply, starch.
3. Dietary fiber is like a twisted gold-chain necklace, on which the links are made up of sugar units that cannot be digested (broken apart into single units of sugar) by humans. Fiber thus does not raise blood glucose levels, because it cannot be broken down into single sugar units (see Chapter 9). Two types of fiber exist: soluble and insoluble based on whether the fiber dissolves in water. Insoluble fiber tends to be crunchy (e.g., celery and apple skins), whereas soluble fiber tends to be gummy (e.g., oatmeal, baked beans, applesauce, or the white of the apple). Insoluble fibers include cellulose and hemicelluose; soluble fibers include gums, lignins, and pectins (see Table 3–2).

What Are the Recommendations for Carbohydrate Intake?

The amount of carbohydrate recommended ranges from a low of 40 percent of total kilocalories or a minimum of 100 grams to prevent **ketosis** (rapid breakdown of body fat leading to a lowered pH or increased acidity level of the blood). Guidelines found on food labels promote 60 percent of kilocalories or 300 grams carbohydrate for a 2000-kilocalorie diet. The food groups in the Food Guide Pyramid (not including added sugars) is a low of about 150 grams of carbohydrate to 300 grams (using the range of minimum to maximum recommended number of servings for each food group—see the inside front cover and Chapter 6). Persons with syndrome X, also referred to as the insulin resistance syndrome (a condition whereby the body's cells resist the action of insulin; see Chapter 9), should avoid a high-carbohydrate/low-fat diet (Reaven, 1997).

Table 3–2
Food Sources of Various Fiber Components

Cellulose	Hemicellulose	Pectin
Whole-wheat flour	Bran	Apples
Bran	Cereals	Citrus fruits
Cabbage family	Whole grains	Strawberries
Peas and beans	**Gums**	**Lignin**
Apples	Oatmeal	Mature vegetables
Root vegetables	Dried beans	Wheat
	Brown rice	
	Barley	

Sugar is now considered appropriate as part of total carbohydrate as long as the minimum micronutrient needs are being met (consumption of the minimum number of food servings in the Food Guide Pyramid) and weight and level of health allow for added sugar. For example, some persons benefit by limiting carbohydrate to 200 grams per day, which equates to the minimum Food Guide Pyramid servings (150 grams carbohydrate). This could allow for the addition of ¼ cup of sugar (50 grams carbohydrate, which is approximately the equivalent of one can of soda, which contains 40 grams of carbohydrate or 10 teaspoons of sugar). Foods that are high in sugar but low in fiber, protein, and fat are digested rapidly—especially if in liquid form such as soda or fruit juice. This can be a problem for people with reactive hypoglycemia (the body overreacts to excess carbohydrates by producing too much insulin, referred to as hyperinsulinemia). This can cause symptoms of hypoglycemia such as weakness and shakiness (see Chapter 9) and can contribute to high levels of triglycerides.

The recommended amount of fiber (20 to 30 grams) can be met by including in the daily diet the recommended number of food servings of the Food Guide Pyramid (with 2 grams of fiber on average for each serving of whole grain, vegetable, and fruit. Legumes provide up to 10 grams of fiber per ½ cup serving). The fiber in grains is found in the germ and the bran layer, where most of the nutritional value is found in whole grains (see Fig. 3–2). With any increase in fiber intake, an increase in water intake is needed to prevent fecal impaction.

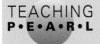

TEACHING
P•E•A•R•L

To describe the difference between soluble and insoluble fiber, say to the patient, "If you put the peel of an apple in a glass of water, it will sit there day after day. That is insoluble fiber, or roughage. But if you put the white part of the apple into water, it will dissolve into little particles. This is soluble fiber, known as pectin, which is used to thicken fruit juice into jam. Soluble fiber dissolves in the digestive tract and helps to thicken and slow the movement of food through the intestinal tract, which is particularly helpful in controlling blood sugar levels and cholesterol. Legumes have at least twice the amount of soluble fiber than fruit has, but they have the same amount of total carbohydrate."

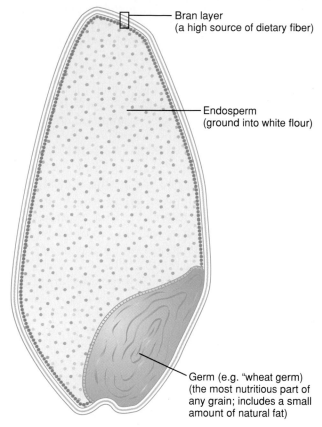

Bran layer (a high source of dietary fiber)

Endosperm (ground into white flour)

Germ (e.g. "wheat germ) (the most nutritious part of any grain; includes a small amount of natural fat)

Figure 3–2
Anatomy of a grain. Whole grains include all three portions of the grain.

What Is Carbohydrate Counting?

Carbohydrate counting is the newest tool in diabetes self-management. By focusing on the chief factor of elevated blood glucose—carbohydrate—meal choices become simpler and thus one can be more effective in managing blood glucose (see Chapter 9).

What Quantities of Food Are Needed to Meet the Carbohydrate Recommendations?

To help translate carbohydrate grams into real food recommendations either the Dietary Exchange System or the Food Guide Pyramid may be used (see Chapter 6). Carbohydrate content of plant foods can be determined by assessing three factors: water content, level of sweetness, and density (see Table 9–3). Generally speaking, there are approximately 15 grams of carbohydrate for every ½ cup of grain or fruit or 1 cup of milk or plain yogurt. Most vegetables provide 5 grams of carbohydrate for ½ cup cooked or 1 cup raw serving (see Fig. 3–3).

Dry plant material such as potatoes and bread products contain on average 15 grams of carbohydrate for ½ cup. Sweet potatoes (yams) are dry like white potatoes, so they have to contain at least 15 grams of carbohydrate for ½ cup; but the fact that they are also sweet doubles the carbohydrate (30 grams of carbohydrate for ½ cup of sweet potato). Grains that have a lot of air allow a larger volume for the same amount of carbohydrate (for example, 3 cups of popcorn or 1 cup of puffed cereals). A slice of bread provides a good size analogy for estimating carbohydrate—for example, a piece of pizza that is the size of a slice of bread contains one serving of starch (about 15 grams of carbohydrate).

Although most fruits are not dry, like grains, they are sweet. Generally there are 15 grams of carbohydrate for every ½ cup serving of fruit, which is why fruit has a kilocalorie content closer to bread than to most vegetables. Fruits that are very high in water content (such as watermelon or cantaloupe) contain 15 grams of carbohydrate in one cup, whereas only ¼ cup of dry fruit or ⅛ cup of dry sweet fruit (e.g., raisins) contains the 15 grams of carbohydrate (see Table 9–3).

Because vegetables grow out of the ground, they are also a source of carbohydrate due to the process of photosynthesis. However, most vegetables are high in water content and low in sugar and thus have the lowest carbohydrate content (see Fig. 3–3). High-carbohydrate vegetables are the dry potato, legumes, sweet corn, and sweet peas, which is why they are often referred to as starchy vegetables (they have the same 15 grams of carbohydrate for a ½-cup serving as starches have). Examples of low-carbohydrate vegetables are those that sound odd when the word *sweet* is used with them. It sounds odd to say sweet spinach, sweet broccoli, or sweet cabbage, all of which are low in carbohydrate (5 grams of carbohydrate for a ½-cup cooked serving), whereas carrots, which are sweet, contain 10 grams of carbohydrate, because the high water content replaces some of the carbohydrate.

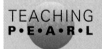

TEACHING
P•E•A•R•L

To clarify carbohydrate content during patient education you could say, "You can almost feel the water content of green beans when you eat them and you would never say 'sweet green beans.' You also wouldn't say 'sweet asparagus' or 'sweet celery.' These are all examples of low-carbohydrate (and thus low-calorie) vegetables because they are high in water content and are not sweet." Or you might say, "The number of prunes can be determined by the number of plums that fit into ½ cup measure (about three small plums), which means three prunes equals one fruit exchange or 15 grams of carbohydrate."

It is now recognized that fiber may be "subtracted" from the total carbohydrate listed on food labels, because the human body cannot digest fiber. The carbohydrate found in many nuts and seeds is mainly fiber, therefore they do not provide significant amounts of carbohydrate that can be counted as kilocalories or that can have an effect on blood glucose (see Chapter 9). A minimal amount of fiber is digested through bacterial fermentation in the colon, which allows for some kilocalorie contribution from fiber but which is generally considered insignificant.

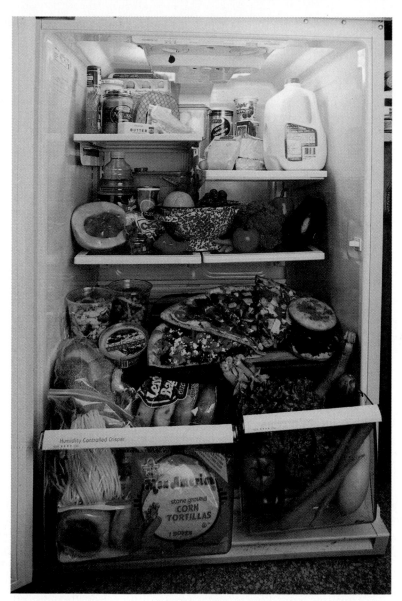

Figure 3–3

Vegetables low in carbohydrate are those that are high in water content and relatively low in sweetness as shown in the lower drawer of the refrigerator. Grains are found in a variety of forms such as in the lower bread drawer (tortillas [corn tortillas may serve as a grain substitute due to carbohydrate content], bagels, english muffins, pasta, and bread; on the lower shelf, grain is also found in pizza crust). Mixed dishes like pizza and the five-bean salad, as shown on the lower shelf, provide carbohydrate, protein, and some fat. Fruits and vegetables are generally fat-free as shown on the upper shelf. On the top shelf, the dairy foods, meat, peanut butter, and eggs are all protein foods that contain variable amounts of fat. (Egg should be stored either in a leak-proof container—as shown in the plastic container—or on the bottom shelf to prevent cross-contamination of salmonella in case eggs crack.) Solid fats, such as butter, contain mostly saturated fat, whereas mayonnaise and liquid salad dressing contain mostly unsaturated fats.

Ordinary table sugar, molasses, maple syrup, corn syrup, and honey are concentrated sources of carbohydrates but mainly provide empty calories, meaning they contain carbohydrates but few vitamins or minerals. Molasses (especially blackstrap) is the one exception, as it is relatively high in some nutrients such as iron, calcium, and potassium, and it also contributes some B vitamins. Sugar can be noted on food labels as sugar, syrup, or any word that ends in -*ose* (except cellulose, which is a type of fiber). Fruit sugar is called fructose, milk sugar is lactose, and table sugar is sucrose. Honey is a combination of fructose and glucose (glucose is also known as blood sugar). One teaspoon of sugar contains 4 grams of carbohydrate (and 16 kilocalories as 1 gram of carbohydrate is equivalent to 4 kilocalories). In carbohydrate counting, sugar may be included as part of the known need or tolerance for carbohydrate (determined by self-monitoring of blood glucose—see Chapter 9).

No significant animal sources of carbohydrate exist except for lactose found in milk. Cheese does not contain carbohydrate due to the fact that the liquid whey is drained off during production and what lactose remains is converted into lactic acid during fermentation. This is why the food exchanges count cheese as a meat equivalent—because there is equal protein to meat but no carbohydrate like milk. Yogurt contains simple carbohydrate but minimal lactose, as the double sugar is converted into simple sugars by the bacterial culture used to make yogurt. About 15 grams of carbohydrate are contained in 1 cup of milk or yogurt (officially milk has 12 grams of carbohydrate and plain yogurt has 17 grams, but it is easier for the consumer to remember 15 grams).

Sugar substitutes come in two main forms: nutritive (providing a carbohydrate source) and nonnutritive (containing insignificant amounts of carbohydrate). **Sugar alcohols** are nutritive and are easy to recognize by their names, which all end in -*ol* and sound like *alcohol*. The main sugar alcohols are sorbitol, mannitol, and xylitol. Sugar alcohols do not contribute to dental decay but otherwise have little advantage over sugar. Saccharin, aspartame, and acesulfame-K are all nonnutritive sweeteners that are useful for the management of diabetes.

What Problems Are Caused by Excess Carbohydrate Intake?

Obesity is the primary concern whenever one consumes an excess of kilocalories for his or her needs. This is true for any of the macronutrients but generally carbohydrates (and fats) are the chief kilocalorie sources leading to obesity.

Persons who "graze" on carbohydrate foods throughout the day are more prone to dental caries. Good oral hygiene can help compensate for a person who chooses to eat in this manner (see Chapter 19). Both sugars and starches are cariogenic (promoting dental cavities).

A high-serum triglyceride level (hypertriglyceridemia—also referred to as hyperlipidemia when total serum cholesterol is also elevated; see Chapter 8) will improve if one avoids an excessive intake of carbohydrate. Avoiding excess sugar intake is important for persons who are being treated for hypertriglyceridemia, in part because sugar is a concentrated form of carbohydrate.

Some individuals with diabetes need a moderate or low-intake of carbohydrate in order to maintain normal blood glucose levels. Persons with diabetes can monitor their blood glucose levels to determine the ideal amount of carbohydrate for their personal needs (see Chapter 9).

Although it is still in research stage, there is growing evidence that persons with insulin resistance and the consequent hyperinsulinemia (excess insulin in the blood) associated with a high-carbohydrate diet will benefit from a moderate intake of carbohydrates (about 50 percent of kilocalories or 250 grams of carbohydrate for 2000 kilocalories). Because carbohydrate is the primary cause of postprandial blood glucose excursions, carbohydrate induces insulin production. A decrease of carbohydrate intake will lower production of insulin, which may help to lower heart disease (see Chapter 8).

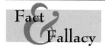

Fact & Fallacy

Fallacy: Only fats are fattening.

Fact: Starches and sugars (complex and simple carbohydrates) are comparable to protein in energy value, as both contribute 4 kilocalories per gram. In excess, both can cause excess kilocalorie intake and lead to weight gain. Fat, which provides 9 kilocalories per gram, is the most concentrated source of food energy supplying at least 1000 kilocalories for ½ cup. High-sugar foods, however, are also high in kilocalories because they are a concentrated carbohydrate source (½ cup sugar equates to almost 100 grams of carbohydrate) and thus provide 400 kilocalories for a ½-cup serving, such as a handful of jelly beans.

PROTEIN: FUNCTIONS AND RECOMMENDATIONS FOR APPROPRIATE INTAKE

What Are the Functions of Protein?

The nitrogen found in protein is what sets protein apart from the other macronutrients. Nitrogen gives protein its unique function of building and repairing all of the various body tissues, allows for the production of hormones and digestive enzymes, and is needed for a strong immune system. Although this is protein's primary role, it can also be broken down and stripped of its nitrogen so that it can be used as an energy source. Unless adequate carbohydrates and fats are provided for energy needs, some of the protein ingested will be used for kilocalorie needs rather than for building and repairing body tissues. Protein is composed of amino acids, often called the building blocks of protein. The functions of protein are as follows:

1. It is essential for life, supplying material to repair or replace worn-out tissues.
2. It is essential for growth, supplying material for tissue building.
3. It supplies some energy (4 kilocalories per gram) but is not as well equipped for this purpose as are carbohydrate and fat.
4. It supplies certain essential substances for the construction and proper functioning of important body compounds (enzymes, hormones, hemoglobin, antibodies, other blood proteins, and glandular secretions).

What Are Types of Protein?

The term **biological value** describes how well a particular protein food approximates the amount and combination of **essential amino acids** in the body. Essential amino acids cannot be produced by the body and hence need to be included through one's diet. A **complete protein,** or one high in biological value, is said to contain all of the eight essential amino acids, whereas an **incomplete protein** has some of the essential amino acids but is lacking others. Incomplete protein foods provided over the course of the day can provide adequate quantities of all the eight essential amino acids.

Generally speaking, animal sources of protein such as meat, fish, poultry, and dairy products (see Fig. 3–3) contain complete proteins of high biological value. Incomplete yet good sources of protein foods that are lacking one or more of the essential amino acids include whole grains, legumes, nuts, and seeds. Combining incomplete protein foods over the course of the day can give the body all of the essential amino acids needed for adequate protein status. Therefore, vegetarians can receive adequate protein without eating meat if food choices are made wisely (see Chapter 1).

What Are Amino Acids?

Twenty-two amino acids are known to be necessary for building and repairing body tissue in humans and for the formation of enzymes. Amino acids can be found in varying amounts and combinations in the food we eat, and most of them can be synthesized by the human body. However, essential amino acids cannot be synthesized and must be obtained from the diet. These essential amino acids are as follows:

Valine	Phenylalanine	Isoleucine
Lysine	Threonine	Leucine
Methionine	Tryptophan	Histidine (required for children)

The 13 nonessential amino acids that can be synthesized by the body in adequate amounts are the following:

Alanine	Cystine	Hydroxyproline
Arginine	Glutamic acid	Proline
Asparagine	Glutamine	Serine
Aspartic acid	Glycine	Tyrosine
Cysteine		

What Are the Recommendations for Protein Intake?

The protein allowance is based on the amount of protein necessary to maintain nitrogen balance. Generally, 45 to 60 grams of protein will meet the health needs of most adults. **Nitrogen balance** refers to a condition in which the nitrogen consumed in the form of protein is equal to the nitrogen lost daily in the urine and other body secretions. At this point, intake is considered to be meeting the body's needs. The requirement is then increased to account for the mixed protein diet (protein from a variety of foods). The allowance is 0.8 grams of protein for each kilogram of body weight (the kilogram weight is calculated by dividing weight in pounds by 2.2). This translates into 63 grams of protein for a man weighing 79 kilograms and 50 grams of protein for a woman weighing 63 kilograms. (See the inside front cover of this textbook for the recommended dietary allowance [RDA] for protein for different ages and genders.)

For infants, the allowances are based on the amount of protein provided by the quantity of milk required to ensure a satisfactory rate of growth. This is estimated to be 2.24 grams/kilograms/day during the first month of life and falls gradually to about 1.5 grams/kilograms/day by the sixth month of life. The protein requirement during growth is higher than that in adulthood, because nitrogen must be provided for the formation of new tissue. The allowances for children and adolescents are calculated from information on growth rates and body composition. The allowances decrease gradually from 1.5 grams/kilograms/day at 6 months to 1 year, to 0.8 grams/kilograms/day by age 18 years.

During pregnancy, at least 60 grams of protein daily is recommended. This is based on nitrogen retention of 16 milligrams/kilograms/day and on 50 percent utilization of dietary protein. The dietary protein allowance for a lactating woman is about the same as that for a pregnant woman.

The protein requirement is increased for any condition in which the body protein is broken down, such as hemorrhage, burns, poor protein nutrition, previous surgery, wounds, and long convalescence. Protein deficiency over a long period results in muscle loss, reduced resistance to disease, skin and blood changes, slow wound healing, and a condition known as nutritional edema.

What Quantities of Food Are Needed to Meet the Protein Recommendations?

In reference to food amounts, the minimum number of food servings in the Food Guide Pyramid provides 60 grams of protein, which is an appropriate amount for most people. Every serving of grains provides 2 to 3 grams of protein, vegetables provide 2 grams, milk provides 8 grams, and 1 ounce (¼ cup) of meat or cheese provides 7 grams (1 egg, ½ cup of beans, or ¼ cup of nuts equates to 1 ounce of meat).

WHAT PROBLEMS ARE ASSOCIATED WITH INADEQUATE PROTEIN INTAKE?

The term **kwashiorkor** refers to a condition in which the individual may have an adequate caloric intake but lacks adequate dietary protein. However, protein deficiency is frequently associated with a deficiency in calories as well. When the diet is low in calories, protein is used as a source of energy, leaving little of this nutrient to build and repair tissues and maintain immune function. Such a condition is termed **protein-energy malnutrition** (also called **marasmus**) and is prevalent in most developing countries (see Chapter 22). This condition occurs often during physiological stress (see Chapter 14) and is also seen in hospitalized patients.

What Problems Are Associated with Excess Protein Intake?

Excess protein is generally a problem for persons with renal insufficiency (see Chapter 10) and end-stage liver disease (see Chapter 11). Excess nitrogen from protein foods that must be excreted through the kidneys can place a burden on these organs. Excess protein also limits the body's ability to use calcium. Also, as most protein foods contain fat (see Fig. 3–3), excess protein can lead to an excess intake of fat, which promotes obesity, cardiovascular disease, and cancer.

Protein intake should be about 10 to 15 percent, up to a maximum of 20 percent, of the total daily kilocalories. (See later section on calculating grams of protein into percentages of total kilocalories.) The protein content of the recommended servings in the Food Guide Pyramid ranges from a minimum of 60 grams to a maximum of 115 grams of protein (see the inside cover and Chapter 6).

FATS: FUNCTION AND RECOMMENDATIONS FOR APPROPRIATE INTAKE

What Are the Functions of Dietary Fats?

The primary function of fat is to serve as a concentrated source of heat and energy. About one-third to one-half of the kilocalories in the current average American diet come from fat. The body cells, with the exception of the cells of the nervous system and erythrocytes, can use fatty acids directly as a source of energy. In addition, fats perform the following functions:

1. *Furnish* essential fatty acids (see Table 3–3).
2. *Spare* burning of protein for energy.
3. *Add* flavor and palatability to the diet.
4. *Give satiety* value to the diet (fats slow the digestive process and retard the development of hunger).
5. *Promote* absorption of fat-soluble vitamins.
6. *Provide* a structural component of cell membranes, digestive secretions, and hormones.
7. *Insulate* and control body temperature in the form of body fat.
8. *Protect* body organs.

Animal fats and fortified margarines not only contain some of the fat-soluble vitamins (A, D, E, and K) but also aid in their absorption. They also play a role in the absorption of fatty acids. Excess fat stored in the body as adipose tissue insulates and protects organs and nerves. Fats also lubricate the intestinal tract. Fat-like substances that have important roles in the body include **phospholipids** (fat plus the mineral phosphorus) and **sterols** (ergosterol in plants and cholesterol in animal fat).

Table 3–3
Fatty Acids and Their Common Food Sources

Fatty Acids	Common Food Sources
Saturated	
Lauric	Coconut, palm kernel oil
Myristic	Coconut
Palmitic	Palm oil, beef
Stearic	Cocoa butter, beef
Monounsaturated Fatty Acid	
Oleic	Olive oil, rapeseed (canola) oil, beef
Polyunsaturated Fatty Acids	
Linoleic	Corn oil, cottonseed oil, safflower oil, sunflower oil
Linolenic acid	Green leafy vegetables, soybean oil, soybean products (tofu), canola oil
Eicosapentaenoic acid	Mackerel, sardines, lake trout
Docosahexaenoic acid	Salmon, tuna, bluefish, halibut

Increasingly, **monounsaturated fats** are being favored over both saturated and polyunsaturated fats, because monounsaturated fats help prevent the lowering of the HDL or "good" cholesterol and are not associated with cancer as are high intakes of polyunsaturated fats (see Chapter 12). Tables 3–3 and 3–4 show how food fats break down in saturated, monounsaturated, and polyunsaturated fat percentages—note how you can visually determine this based on degree of solidity versus liquidity at cold temperatures (Fig. 3–3).

What Are the Functions of Essential Fatty Acids?

Essential fatty acids are necessary for the nutritional well-being of all animals and must be supplied in the diet. The principal essential fatty acid for humans is called **linoleic acid** and is found in vegetable oils. Two others, arachidonic acid and linolenic acid, are essential, but the body generally can produce them if adequate linoleic acid is consumed.

These essential fatty acids have multiple purposes, including (1) maintenance of the functioning and integrity of cellular and subcellular membranes, (2) cholesterol metabolism regulation, and (3) acting as the precursor of a group of hormonelike compounds (**prostaglandins**).

What Are the Functions of Cholesterol?

Cholesterol has an essential role in the structure of adrenal and sex hormones and in increasing the body's production of vitamin D through the action of ultraviolet light on the skin. It is made and stored in the liver and also occurs in the form of a lipoprotein in the blood. Excess cholesterol intake contributes to fatty deposits, in susceptible individuals, in blood vessels and arteries, which in turn contributes to

Table 3–4
Degree of Saturation in Common Foods (in percentages)*

#	Food	Saturated	Monounsaturated	Polyunsaturated
1	Walnuts	6%	24%	70%
2	Canola oil	8%	61%	31%
3	Almonds	8%	69%	23%
4	Pecans	8%	66%	26%
5	Filberts/Hazelnuts	8%	82%	10%
6	Pistachio nuts	13%	71%	16%
7	Corn oil	13%	26%	61%
8	Macadamia nuts	13%	84%	3%
9	Olive oil	14%	77%	9%
10	Soybean oil	15%	25%	60%
11	Avocados	16%	71%	13%
12	Peanut oil	19%	50%	31%
13	Cashews	20%	62%	18%
14	Tuna fish	30%	30%	40%
15	Poultry	31%	42%	27%
16	Eggs	37%	47%	16%
17	Red meat	48%	48%	4%
18	Milk chocolate	62%	34%	4%
19	Butter	66%	30%	4%
20	Coconut oil	94%		5%

*Percentages are based on the total amount of saturated, monounsaturated, and polyunsaturated fats. Purple = saturated fat; green = monounsaturated fat; orange = polyunsaturated fat.
Reference for fat content modified from Jean AT Pennington, Bowes & Church Food Values of Portions Commonly Used, 17th ed., Philadelphia, JB Lippincott, 1997.

cardiovascular disease. There is, however, growing evidence that cholesterol in food is not as harmful to our health as was once thought (see Chapter 8).

What Is the Difference between Fat and Cholesterol?

Fats are similar to carbohydrate in that they are composed of carbon, hydrogen, and oxygen. However, they differ from carbohydrate in that they contain a greater concentration of carbon, which leads to higher energy values (at least 9 kilocalories/gram versus 4 kilocalories/gram for carbohydrate). Saturated fats contain more hydrogen than unsaturated fats. Fats are listed on food labels as "total fat" and are broken down on the label as saturated, monounsaturated, and polyunsaturated fats (often the unsaturated fats are added together on the food label). If saturated acids predominate, the fat is called a saturated fat; if unsaturated acids predominate, the fat is called an unsaturated fat or more specifically either a polyunsaturated fat or a monounsaturated fat. Oleic acid, which is found in nuts, seeds, olives, canola oil, and avocados, is the main type of monounsaturated fat (olives and avocados also contain carbohydrate but are higher in fat content than in carbohydrate).

Polyunsaturated fats are generally referred to as linoleic and linolenic acids and are found in corn oil, safflower oil, and sunflower oil (Table 3–3). Saturated fats (e.g., stearic acid and butyric acid) typically are found in animal fat, such as milk fat, butter, and red meat. It is important to note that mineral oil is not a food fat, as it cannot be digested and used by the body. When used as a laxative, if at all, it should never be taken near mealtime as its use can negatively impact on fat-soluble vitamin absorption.

Lipids is a general term that includes all types of fats and fat-related compounds. Cholesterol is a fat-related compound that contains no kilocalories. It is found only in animal fats because it is made in the liver of animals. Fats from plant sources do not contain cholesterol.

TEACHING P•E•A•R•L

In patient education, you might explain that peanuts are cholesterol-free because they grow in the ground. You can add to this by saying that cholesterol is found only in animal fats. Most nuts can be safely eaten when a higher intake of monounsaturated fat is acceptable, such as in the treatment of hyperlipidemia when HDL cholesterol levels are low (see Chapter 8). Nuts that contain mainly monounsaturated fats are those from the temperate climate zone (tropical nuts such as brazil nuts and cashews contain relatively high amounts of saturated fat, whereas the nut of the most northern climate (walnuts) contain mainly polyunsaturated fat (see Table 3–4).

Fats that are of a liquid consistency at room temperature are referred to as oils, whereas those that are solid may be called fats. Liquid oils are composed predominantly of the unsaturated fatty acids; the solid fats are the saturated forms. The most unsaturated form of fat is called **omega-3 fatty acid.** Fish from cold-water areas are high in this kind of unsaturated fat. Polyunsaturated fats also will stay in liquid form if placed in the refrigerator; monounsaturated fats will become viscous; and saturated fats will become so hard that you have to cut them.

TEACHING P•E•A•R•L

The fat in cold-water fish is mainly of the most unsaturated form, called omega-3 fatty acids, which does not solidify in the cold arctic waters (imagine for a moment what would happen to these fish if their body fat was in the form of saturated fat—they would solidify and sink). Thus, fish from cold arctic waters have to be high in omega-3 fatty acids in order to survive.

The difference in degree of saturation relates to the amount of hydrogen in the fat molecule. Hydrogen atoms can be added to unsaturated liquid oils to make them more solid. By adding hydrogen the oil becomes a spread, or margarine. These are called **hydrogenated fats.** This form of fat is also now referred to as **trans fatty acid.** Solid stick margarines have the most hydrogen added, with tub margarines having less, and liquid margarines having the least amount. All liquid oils in moderation are heart healthy and can lower a person's cholesterol level as long as no weight gain occurs.

Both fats and oils are composed principally of triglycerides and various fatty acids in various proportions. These differences contribute to food flavor and other properties and have health implications. Triglycerides consist of a base of glycerol with three fatty acids and they compose the main type of circulating fat in the bloodstream; **diglycerides** have two fatty acids, and **monoglycerides** have one.

Fats are insoluble in water. **Glycerol** is a small, water-soluble carbohydrate. The addition of glycerol to fats in the body allows transport through the blood but contributes insignificant amounts of carbohydrate.

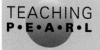

TEACHING P•E•A•R•L   A tip for patient education to explain hydrogenation is by saying, "Hydrogen is found in water (hydrogen and water). When clothes are hanging on the clothesline soaking wet, we could say they are saturated with water (or hydrogen). Thus, the more hydrogen in a fat, the more saturated it is."

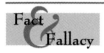

Fact & Fallacy

Fallacy: It is better to use butter, because we now know margarine also contributes to heart disease.

Fact: Although margarine does contain trans fatty acids, which promote cardiovascular disease, butter is no better. Butter contains both saturated fat and cholesterol, increasing the risk of heart disease. Liquid margarines contain insignificant amounts of hydrogen when compared to the harder margarines and therefore contain less trans fatty acids. We might adopt the approach of Italians, who dip their bread in olive oil thereby avoiding saturated and hydrogenated fats. Traditional Italian restaurants and many restaurants in California offer olive oil on the table for use with bread.

What Are the Recommendations for Intake of Fats and Cholesterol?

There are no specific requirements for fat other than the body's need for the essential fatty acids, which is usually met through a diet that contains appropriate food fats. A minimum of 20 grams of fat can meet the body's need for essential fatty acids, if the appropriate fats are consumed. The recommended intake of essential fatty acids for a population with a high fat intake, as is currently found in the United States, is 7 percent of dietary calories (National Academy of Sciences, National Research Council, 1989). The Committee on Diet and Health of the Food and Nutrition Board has recently recommended that individual intakes not exceed 10 percent of kilocalories for either polyunsaturated or saturated fats. The balance of fat should come from monounsaturated fats, with many advocates promoting that these fats should account for up to 20 percent of kilocalories. A reduction in the total kilocalorie intake from fat to a maximum of 30 percent fat, with equal distribution of polyunsaturated fats, monounsaturated fats, and saturated fats, is recommended by most authorities. Some individuals may benefit from a higher intake of fat (up to 40 percent) as long as monounsaturated or omega-3 fatty acids predominate. The Step One Diet of the National Cholesterol Education Program (NCEP) recommends less than 10 percent saturated fat and less than 300 mg cholesterol per day, whereas the Step Two diet recommends lowering intake of saturated fat to 6 to 7 percent of total kilocalories (see Chapter 8) and cholesterol intake to less than 200 mg per day. A diet low in both saturated fatty acids and trans fatty acids should be promoted (Aro et al., 1997).

What Quantities of Food Are Needed to Meet the Fat Recommendations?

In regard to food quantities, the fat content of the recommended servings in the Food Guide Pyramid ranges from a low of about 20 grams of fat (if the minimum number of food servings is consumed using skim milk, lean meat, and unprocessed grain products) to 80 grams of fat if whole milk and high-fat meats are used. It is not unusual for Americans to consume 100 to 150 grams of fat per day.

There are 5 grams of fat in each teaspoon of added fat or oils and on average 5 grams for every 1 ounce of red meat (but only 1 to 2 grams for white meat, fish, and legumes; see Fig. 6–1). Steak contains 8 grams of fat per ounce (which is why it is so tender and juicy), whereas stew beef has only 3 grams of fat per ounce (which is why you have to cook it in liquid for a long time in order to tenderize the meat). Thus, a person eating a pound of white-meat chicken (without the skin) will consume only 16 grams of fat (with about 5 grams of saturated fat—about 30 percent total fat—see Table 3–4), whereas someone eating the same amount of steak will consume 128 grams of fat—literally ½ cup of lard (and 64 grams of saturated fat or about 50 percent of the total fat—3 days worth of saturated fat!). A food containing 3 grams of fat or less per serving is considered a low-fat food. This includes grains that do not have significant amounts of fat added such as sliced bread used to make sandwiches, pasta, and most cereals, all vegetables, and most fruits (except coconut, avocado, and olives). One percent milk is also low-fat as it contains less than 3 grams of fat per cup.

What Are the Recommendations for Fat Substitutes?

Simplesse consists of very small particles of protein, generally of milk origin. These microparticles of protein provide a creamy consistency like fat. Simplesse is all-natural and fat-free, although it is not kilocalorie-free because it contains protein. Simplesse will increasingly be found in food products because of its acceptability. It is generally safe to use Simplesse, even in large quantities, except for the person with milk allergy since Simplesse contains milk protein (see Chapter 15).

Olestra is another fat substitute that still has some unresolved problems because it is not digestible. The consequence is that excess intake can cause unpleasant gastrointestinal problems, such as diarrhea, and many experts feel it may contribute to inadequate absorption of food nutrients, such as fat-soluble vitamins. Olestra has received approval by the FDA and is now being used in food products such as potato chips.

HOW ARE PERCENTAGES OF THE MACRONUTRIENTS CALCULATED?

The percentage of protein as total kilocalories is calculated by first multiplying the number of grams of protein in the diet by 4 kilocalories and then dividing that number by the total caloric intake from all foods consumed in one day. For example, a 2000-kilocalorie diet containing both animal and vegetable sources of protein in the form of 3 cups of milk (24 g protein), 6 slices of bread (18 g protein), 3 vegetables (6 g protein), and 4 ounces of meat (28 g protein) for a total of 76 grams of protein would be calculated as follows:

$$76 \times 4 = 304 \text{ kilocalories}$$
$$304 \div \text{ by 2000 calories} = 0.15 = 15\% \text{ protein}$$

The same calculation can be used to find carbohydrate percentage (excluding fiber content, as fiber is not digestible and therefore provides no kilocalories). For calculating the fat percentage, the number of grams of fat should be multiplied by 9 because fats yield 9 kilocalories per gram.

WHAT IS THE ROLE OF THE NURSE OR OTHER HEALTH CARE PROFESSIONAL IN EDUCATING THE PUBLIC ABOUT CARBOHYDRATE, PROTEIN, AND FAT INTAKE?

The goal of a nurse or other health care professional should be to educate patients about the positive role of carbohydrate, protein, and fat in their diets and to promote proper consumption of different sorts of foods, as based on the Food Guide Pyramid. The health care professional should use good interviewing skills in determining a patient's current dietary habits and the reasons such practices are being followed (for example, adherence to physician advice, which may have been given years ago, dental problems, health beliefs). Some patients, when given a rationale, may be receptive to dietary change, whereas others may strongly resist change. The nurse should never argue or give an impression of arguing but rather indicate respect for a patient's food choices and health beliefs while introducing new ideas about healthy diets.

Promoting consumption of complex carbohydrates and dietary fiber food sources (along with adequate fluid), and providing information on current thinking related to fiber, is an appropriate role for the health care professional. The minimum number of food servings portrayed at the base of the Food Guide Pyramid provide adequate carbohydrate and fiber. Sugar, while a source of carbohydrate, should be promoted as the Food Guide Pyramid portrays: as the tip of one's diet, not something to "fill up on."

The health care professional can help re-educate the public about how much protein in the daily diet the body really needs. The amount of protein we consume can generally be safely decreased, but an assessment of a patient's usual dietary intake should be determined before automatically recommending a reduced amount. In the past, the emphasis in meal planning was to have meat as the main part of the meal with side dishes such as starch and vegetables. It is now recommended that we view meat as the side dish with emphasis on vegetables and grains.

Many individuals are now aware that controlling the fat content of their diet plays a key role in the prevention and management of chronic diseases such as obesity, cardiovascular disease, and cancer. However, the health care professionals can help the public recognize that not all fats are bad and going too low in fat intake can have adverse health implications. Beyond this awareness, individuals need to learn what foods are low in saturated fat and cholesterol; these foods should be promoted in a way that makes them practical to consume as well as appealing. Meat alternatives such as legumes, for example, can be promoted simply by indicating verbally that they can be a delicious part of a meal (such as bean burritos or baked beans).

Finally, the health care professional should recognize when referral to a qualified nutritionist or registered dietitian is appropriate for highly motivated individuals or those at risk for obesity, cardiovascular disease, diabetes, cancer, or those who have not had success on a low-fat diet.

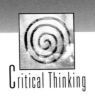

Case Study

Nellie was talking with her son when she began to feel a physical tremor in her body. Then she noticed her hands shaking.

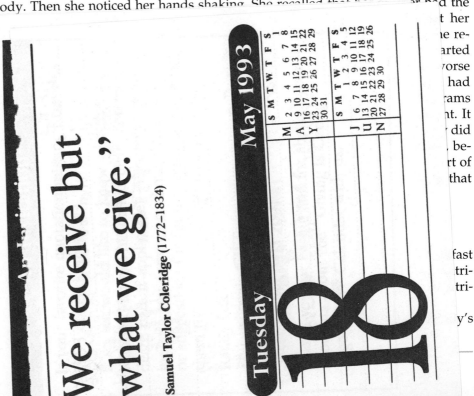

"We receive but what we give."

Samuel Taylor Coleridge (1772–1834)

May 1993

Tuesday 18

Study Questions and Classroom Activities

1. Discuss as a class how much belief is accorded to the experiences of family and friends in following good health care practices. How might belief in family advice affect advice provided by a health care professional? How might discrepancies be addressed?
2. What are the three different kinds of carbohydrates?
3. What is the difference between soluble and insoluble fiber?
4. Write a healthy day's menu that provides 20 to 30 grams of fiber.
5. How do proteins differ from carbohydrates and fats?
6. What is the difference between a complete and an incomplete protein?
7. What are some of the nutritional problems associated with an overconsumption of protein and those associated with too little protein?
8. Describe the texture of saturated versus unsaturated fats.
9. *Class activity.* Students are to bring in a sample of crackers and their respective food labels. In class, students will estimate how many crackers would take up the same amount of space as a slice of bread. Compare this estimate to the food label (how many crackers does it take to equal 15 grams of carbohydrate?). Then compare fat content and texture (hard or crumbly) for the different types of crackers for one serving of starch.
10. If a food label states that one bagel contains 60 grams of carbohydrate, how many servings of grain would it contain?

References

Aro A, Jauhiainen M, Partanen R, Salminen I, Mutanen M: Stearic acid, trans fatty acids, and dairy fat: Effects on serum and lipoprotein lipids, apolipoproteins, lipoprotein(a), and lipid transfer proteins in healthy subjects. Am J Clin Nutr. May 1997; 65(5): 1419–1426.

National Academy of Sciences, National Research Council: Recommended Dietary Allowances, 10th ed. Washington DC, National Academy Press, 1989.

Pick ME, Hawrysh ZJ, Gee MI, Toth E, Garg ML, Hardin RT: Oat bran concentrate bread products improve long-term control of diabetes: A pilot study. J Am Diet Assoc. December 1996; 96(12):1254–1261.

Reaven GM: Do high carbohydrate diets prevent the development or attenuate the manifestations (or both) of syndrome X? A viewpoint strongly against. Curr Opin Lipidol. February 1997; 8(1):23–27.

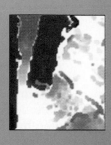

4

Digestion, Absorption, and Metabolism of the Energy Macronutrients

Objectives

After completing this chapter, you should be able to:

- Describe the mechanical and chemical processes of digestion, absorption, and metabolism of foods.
- Describe the digestion and metabolism of carbohydrates, proteins, and fats.
- Summarize the role of the mouth, stomach, and intestines in the digestive process.
- Describe the role of the endocrine system on metabolism.
- Describe the impact of alcohol on digestion, absorption, and metabolism of food nutrients.
- Describe the role of the nurse or other health care professional in aiding the digestive process.

Terms to Identify

Absorption	Duodenum	Krebs cycle
Albumin	Endocrine system	Metabolism
Anabolism	Enzymes	Oxidation
Basal metabolism	Glycogen	Peristalsis
Bile	Homeostasis	Specific dynamic action
Capillaries	Hormones	Villi
Catabolism	Hydrolysis	Wernicke-Korsakoff
Chyme	Ileum	syndrome
Digestion	Jejunum	

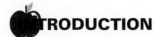

INTRODUCTION

Good nutrition goes beyond obtaining and consuming appropriate foods in a positive meal environment. Without adequate digestion and absorption, foods cannot be used for their intended biological functions. The process of digestion and cellular nutrition can affect health more than food choices can. Health care professionals need to be aware of the digestive and metabolic impact on food use.

WHAT IS MEANT BY THE DIGESTION, ABSORPTION, AND METABOLISM OF FOODS?

Digestion is the change of food from a complex to a simpler form and from an insoluble to a soluble state in the digestive tract. These changes facilitate absorption through the intestinal walls into the circulation for eventual use by the body (Fig. 4–1). The processes of digestion occur simultaneously:

1. *Physical (mechanical)*: During the physical, or mechanical, process, food is broken into small particles in the mouth, then mixed with digestive juices by a churning action in the stomach, and then propelled through the digestive tract in rhythmic movements known as **peristalsis.**
2. *Chemical*: During the chemical process, enzymes in digestive juices change food nutrients into simple soluble forms that can be absorbed: carbohydrates to simple sugars, fats to fatty acids and glycerol, and protein to amino acids. This chemical breakdown is called **hydrolysis** and involves the addition of water to molecules. Water, simple sugars, salts, vitamins, and minerals require no digestion.

Each digestive **enzyme** (chemicals produced by the body to break food down in preparation for absorption in the intestinal tract) has a specific action and optimal conditions under which it acts. The name of each group of enzymes ends in *ase:* amylases act on starch, lipases act on fat, and proteases act on protein. Other enzymes include lactase (to digest lactose) and sucrase (to digest sucrose). Other chemical substances assist in the physical and chemical processes, such as hydrochloric acid and mucin in the gastric secretion, **bile** (which promotes the digestion of fat) excreted from the liver into the duodenum, and certain **hormones** (chemicals produced by the body that in part affect how the body uses nutrients in food).

Digestibility of food refers to the rapidity and ease of digestion as well as to its completeness. Liquid foods and thoroughly masticated solid foods are more rapidly digested than are foods left in large pieces. The well-masticated food begins to leave the stomach 15 to 30 minutes after ingestion. Forms of liquid sugar such as fruit juice leave an empty stomach almost immediately.

Foods that stay in the stomach longer have a higher satiety value. Small meals move out of the stomach faster than larger ones do. Solid foods stay in the stomach longer than liquids. The amount and type of food eaten at one time also affect

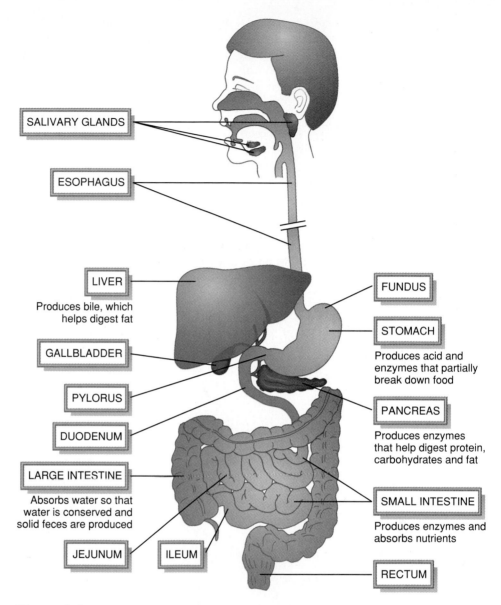

SALIVARY GLANDS

ESOPHAGUS

LIVER
Produces bile, which
helps digest fat

GALLBLADDER

PYLORUS

DUODENUM

LARGE INTESTINE
Absorbs water so that
water is conserved and
solid feces are produced

JEJUNUM   ILEUM

FUNDUS

STOMACH
Produces acid and
enzymes that partially
break down food

PANCREAS
Produces enzymes
that help digest protein,
carbohydrates and fat

SMALL INTESTINE
Produces enzymes and
absorbs nutrients

RECTUM

Figure 4–1
The digestive system.

the rapidity of digestion. Of the three macronutrients, carbohydrates are digested and leave the stomach most rapidly (about 1 hour), proteins are digested and leave less rapidly (about 2 hours), and fats require the longest time for digestion (about 4 hours). Thus, a balanced meal stays in the stomach longer than a meal of only carbohydrate foods. Foods containing a large amount of dietary fiber are digested more slowly than are low-fiber foods.

Absorption is the passage of soluble digested food materials through the intestinal walls into the blood, either directly or through osmosis by way of the lymphatic system. The greater part of absorption takes place in the small intestine, lower duodenum, and upper jejunum. Tiny fingerlike projections called **villi,** which contain small **capillaries** (tiny blood vessels), line the intestinal wall. The villi are in constant motion and trap the tiny nutrients, which are then taken in by the adjacent cells and transported through the circulatory and lymphatic systems to every body cell. Microvilli are even smaller projections on the surface of the villi (Fig. 4–2).

Simple sugars, amino acids, a few fatty acids, minerals, and water-soluble vitamins reach the general circulation through the capillaries. Water is also absorbed from the large intestine. Absorbed materials are carried by the blood to various organs and tissues to be used as needed. The body is able to digest and absorb about 90 to 98 percent of an average mixed diet.

Metabolism is a general term covering all physical and chemical changes that food nutrients undergo after their absorption from the gastrointestinal tract. It also covers the use of simple sugars, amino acids, fatty acids, and glycerol by the body cells. If the change is of a constructive nature, resulting in the building up of

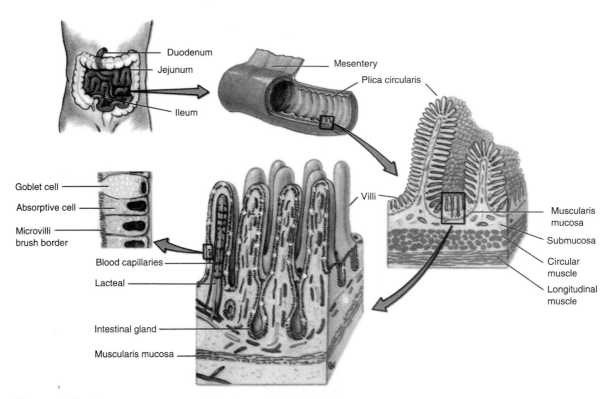

Figure 4–2

Wall of the small intestine. (From Applegate EJ: The Anatomy and Physiology Learning System. Philadelphia, WB Saunders, 1995, Fig. 16–9, p. 337.)

new substances, it is called **anabolism;** if it is of a destructive or oxidative nature, resulting in the release of energy, it is called **catabolism.** Energy metabolism refers to the oxidation of nutrients (carbohydrate, protein, and fat) within the body resulting in the release of heat and energy. All metabolism happens at the cell level with the human body cells acting like mini-furnaces to burn food energy (catabolism) as well as allow for anabolism. It is at the cell level that very complex biochemical reactions take place. Food nutrients must enter the body cells in order for the body to utilize these nutrients.

What Is Basal Metabolism?

The body needs energy for the internal, involuntary activities of organs and tissues and oxidation within the tissues as well as for circulation, respiration, digestion, elimination, and maintenance of muscle tone, heartbeat, and so on. All internal activities continue 24 hours a day, while a person is asleep and awake. The amount of energy required to sustain these processes alone is known as the **basal metabolism.** The basal metabolic rate is influenced by body composition, body size, and age. The more muscle tissue a person has, the more calories are needed. The basal metabolic rate varies from person to person, but on the average it amounts to approximately 1200 to 1400 kilocalories daily for women and 1600 to 1800 kilocalories daily for men. Total energy requirements and weight management are discussed in Chapter 20.

A simple and relatively accurate method of estimating basal metabolic rate is to multiply one's weight in kilograms by 0.9 for women and 1 for men, and then by 24 (which represents the number of hours in a day). This estimate is generally accurate enough, except during times of physiological stress (see Chapter 14). In large institutions, what are referred to as metabolic carts are used to measure a person's oxygen intake and carbon dioxide output. This technique can precisely measure the basal metabolic kilocalorie needs. Various measurements of oxygen use and carbon dioxide output have been used over the years to determine basal metabolic rate (Fig. 4–3).

The body also needs energy for the stimulating effect **(specific dynamic action)** that each food exerts on basal metabolism after digestion and absorption. This action raises the total energy needs about 10 percent for a person who eats a mixed diet.

HOW ARE THE MACRONUTRIENTS DIGESTED AND ABSORBED?

Carbohydrates

Carbohydrates (except for fiber) are easily digested, and the degree of absorption is high. Digestion of starch starts in the mouth with ptyalin and is completed in the small intestine. Glucose, which is normally formed from carbohydrate eaten in food, is absorbed into the bloodstream through the walls of the small intestine and is metabolized as shown in Figure 4–4.

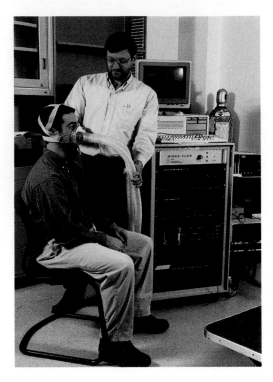

Figure 4–3
Measuring metabolic rate.

Simple sugars such as glucose and fructose are ready for absorption in the digestive tract without digestion. Double sugars such as sucrose must be changed to simple sugars for absorption, which is a quick process when there is adequate enzyme production. Double sugars are digested in the small intestine (see Fig. 4–4). Complex carbohydrates such as starch require two digestive steps to be changed to simple sugar (glucose) for absorption in the intestinal tract. Cooking starch facilitates digestion, as it breaks down the cell walls, which makes the action of the digestive enzymes easier. Dietary fiber is indigestible and passes through the intestinal tract virtually unchanged. Because most unprocessed plant foods contain fiber, the process of digestion is slower for them than for sugar and low-fiber plant food products such as white bread.

The carbon part of carbohydrate is burned as energy in animal cells, similar to the burning of carbon in coal and wood in actual furnaces. The black substance formed in burnt toast is carbon.

Protein

The protein in the daily diet must be broken down by digestion into the component parts, the amino acids and small peptides, before the body can absorb them into the blood from the small intestine and use them. Digestion of protein is started in the stomach by enzymes in the gastric juice and is continued and

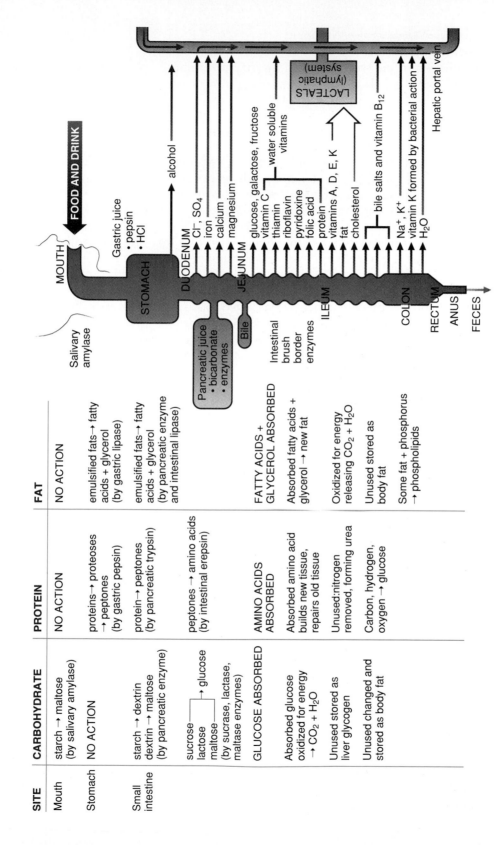

Figure 4–4

Digestive process of carbohydrate, protein, and fat. (*Key:* Cl = chloride; CO_2 = carbon dioxide; HCl = hydrochloric acid; H_2O = water; K^+ = potassium; Na^+ = sodium; SO_4 = sulfur.) (Modified from Mahan LK, Escott-Stump S: Krause's Food, Nutrition, and Diet Therapy, 9th ed. Philadelphia, WB Saunders, 1996, Fig. 1–7, p. 13.)

completed in the small intestine by enzymes from the pancreatic and intestinal juices (see Fig. 4–4).

Fat

Fats, because they are insoluble in water, require special treatment in the gastrointestinal tract so that their end products can be absorbed through the intestinal wall. No digestion of fat takes place in the mouth. Only finely emulsified fats, such as those found in butter, cream, and egg yolk, can start to be digested in the stomach. For the most part, fats must be emulsified by bile and bile salts before they are digested in the small intestine by enzymes from the pancreatic juice. Fats are changed to glycerol and fatty acids during digestion (see Fig. 4–4).

Fatty foods are generally digested without difficulty, but they require a longer time for digestion than carbohydrates do. Softer fats are more completely digested and absorbed than harder fats. Fried foods are not necessarily indigestible but are more slowly digested. The presence of carbohydrates in the diet is necessary for the complete **oxidation** of fats (the chemical step in releasing energy from fat) in the tissues; otherwise, acetone bodies accumulate and ketosis results.

How Are Macronutrients Converted to Energy?

When the body needs energy, a series of metabolic reactions occurs called the **Krebs cycle** (see Fig. 4–5, which shows the central pathways of energy metabolism). Oxygen is necessary for the release of energy by the cells in the body. The process of combining oxygen with a molecule is called oxidation. A person needs hemoglobin to supply oxygen to the cells, and a low level of hemoglobin means oxygen is not available for energy production, which results in a tired feeling. An increased intake of air into the body, such as that achieved with aerobic exercise, tends to raise the body's rate of metabolism through the process of oxidation (see Chapter 20).

WHAT ROLE IS PLAYED BY EACH PART OF THE DIGESTIVE TRACT?

The Mouth

The teeth provide the first mechanical function of chewing, with the cutting action with the anterior teeth (incisors) and the grinding action of the posterior teeth (molars). Chewing is important for digestion of all foods, but it is especially important for most fruits and raw vegetables because these have undigestible cellulose membranes around their nutrient portions, which must be broken before the food can be utilized. Chewing aids the digestion of food for a simple reason: Because the digestive enzymes act only on the surface of food particles, thorough chewing increases the amount of food surface area available to these enzymes.

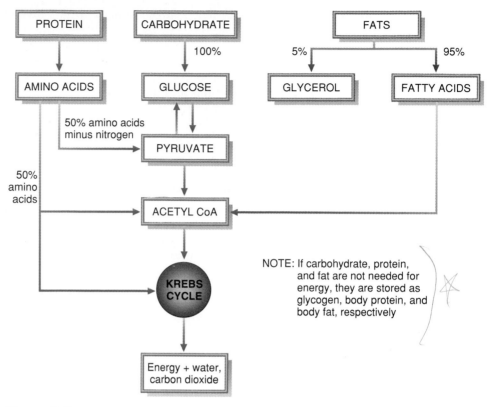

Figure 4–5
Metabolic pathways.

Another mechanical function is performed by saliva, which moistens food and prepares it for swallowing. The chemical function of the mouth is to change cooked starch to dextrin and then to maltose by the salivary enzyme ptyalin (amylase).

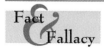

Fallacy: Washing food down with water is a good habit.

Fact: Food must be chewed thoroughly so that it can be mixed with saliva, which aids digestion. However, a glass of water at mealtime is beneficial to the digestive process, as long as it does not take the place of mastication.

Esophagus

In general, swallowing can be divided into three stages: (1) the voluntary stage, which initiates the swallowing process, or *mechanical function*; (2) the pharyngeal stage, which is involuntary and involves the passage of food through the pharynx to the esophagus; and (3) the esophageal stage, which involves passage of food from the pharynx to the stomach through peristaltic wave contractions (Fig. 4–6).

Respiration is generally only minimally stopped during the act of swallowing. Poorly chewed food, however, increases the risk of obstruction of the airway, especially for persons with an impaired swallowing reflex, in whom oxygen deprivation can occur as breathing and swallowing cannot be done simultaneously (Rogers et al., 1993).

The Stomach

The presence of food in the stomach stimulates functioning of the digestive tract. Food is kept in motion by the muscular walls of the stomach, which bring it into contact with the gastric juice secreted by stomach cells. The fundus of the stomach acts as a temporary storage place for food.

Various gastric juice enzymes work in the stomach to digest the different macronutrients. Complex proteins are partially digested by pepsin (protease); milk protein is coagulated by renin and then is partially digested by pepsin. Emulsified fats are digested to fatty acids and glycerol by lipase. Hydrochloric acid aids these digestive enzymes and increases the solubility of calcium and

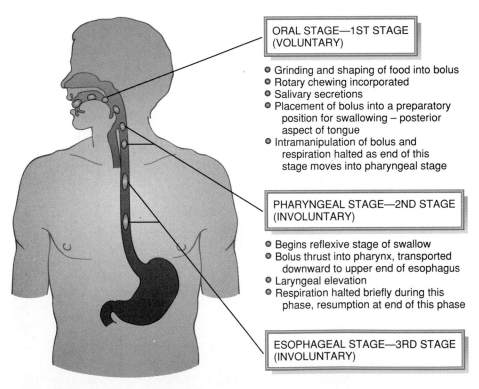

ORAL STAGE—1ST STAGE
(VOLUNTARY)

- Grinding and shaping of food into bolus
- Rotary chewing incorporated
- Salivary secretions
- Placement of bolus into a preparatory
  position for swallowing – posterior
  aspect of tongue
- Intramanipulation of bolus and
  respiration halted as end of this
  stage moves into pharyngeal stage

PHARYNGEAL STAGE—2ND STAGE
(INVOLUNTARY)

- Begins reflexive stage of swallow
- Bolus thrust into pharynx, transported
  downward to upper end of esophagus
- Laryngeal elevation
- Respiration halted briefly during this
  phase, resumption at end of this phase

ESOPHAGEAL STAGE—3RD STAGE
(INVOLUNTARY)

Figure 4–6
The stages of swallowing as they relate to appropriate food pathways.

iron. Mucus protects the lining of the stomach from the hydrochloric acid. Once solid food is reduced to a semiliquid state **(chyme),** it is passed from the stomach to the small intestine.

The Small Intestine

The small intestine is 20 feet long and is made up of the **duodenum** (the upper section), the **jejunum** (the middle section), and the **ileum** (the lower section). The food mass from a meal remains in the intestine for 3 to 8 hours, although liquids and pure carbohydrate foods pass more quickly.

Chyme mixes with the digestive juices of the small intestine, and with pancreatic juices and bile, both of which are excreted into the duodenum (bile is secreted by the liver and stored in the gallbladder). Alkaline juices from the small intestine neutralize chyme as it leaves the stomach. Bile prepares unemulsified fats for digestion. Pancreatic enzymes finish starch and fat digestion, and partially digest protein. The intestinal enzymes complete protein and carbohydrate digestion. Digested food moves with peristaltic waves through the small intestine where absorption of food nutrients occurs. Unused food, waste materials, and water move to the large intestine.

The Large Intestine

The large intestine consists of the cecum, the colon, the rectum, and the anal canal. Water is drawn out of the contents of the large intestine and absorbed, and solid feces are formed. Waste, including indigestible residue, undigested food particles, meat fibers, and decomposition products, is eliminated. Because no enzymes are produced in the large intestine, no digestion takes place there.

WHAT IS THE ROLE OF THE ENDOCRINE SYSTEM ON METABOLISM?

The **endocrine system** is a major control system of the body. More than a dozen hormones that the body produces regulate metabolism and the use of nutrients. Some hormones that have significance to nutrition and diet are as follows:

Insulin. This hormone is produced in the pancreas and allows carbohydrates to be metabolized for energy by facilitating the entry of blood sugar (glucose) into the cells where the Krebs cycle takes place. Insulin also affects the metabolism of fat. It is controversial whether excess insulin in the body leads to the gain of body fat, but excess insulin is correlated with obesity. Insulin does stimulate protein synthesis and decreases protein degradation. Insulin deficiency decreases the body's ability to metabolize carbohydrates and fats, and it contributes to weight loss.

Glucagon. This is the primary hormone produced when the body perceives the blood glucose level is dropping too far. Glucagon is one of several hormones that promotes the breakdown of **glycogen** (stored sugar) in the liver in order to raise blood glucose levels. Insulin and glucagon are the primary hormones involved in maintaining **homeostasis** (the regulation of body functions or processes) of blood glucose levels.

Epinephrine (also referred to as adrenalin). This hormone is produced mainly by the adrenal glands and helps release stored sugar in the liver in response to low blood sugar or stress. Energy metabolism is increased in response to epinephrine because of the resultant increased heart rate and oxygen intake. Excess epinephrine may raise the blood glucose too high if there is insufficient insulin for the metabolism of carbohydrates (see Chapter 9).

Cortisol. This hormone is also produced by the adrenal gland and also works in the opposite manner to insulin. It is often produced in increased amounts during the early morning hours. As a result, blood sugar levels tend to run higher first thing in the morning (this is referred to as the dawn phenomenon—see Chapter 9). An increased production of insulin may occur in the early morning hours to compensate for the dawn phenomenon, especially if large amounts of simple sugar are consumed. Steroid medications are similar to the cortisol hormone, as they tend to increase the appetite and their use is related to weight gain (see Chapter 20). They also raise blood glucose levels.

Growth Hormone. This hormone is produced by the pituitary gland. It raises the rate of metabolism and is associated with protein anabolism, which produces a positive nitrogen balance. It is also referred to as diabetogenic because it works against insulin in muscle tissue. Adolescents have an increased need for insulin because of increased levels of growth hormone. This hormone contributes to the dawn phenomenon as well.

Estrogen. This hormone is produced mainly in the ovaries and helps retain bone calcium, which results in a decreased risk of osteoporosis (see Chapter 21). Estrogen tends to cause blood glucose levels to rise because of its inhibiting effect on insulin. Premenstrual syndrome (PMS; see Chapter 16) may be caused in part by lowered levels of estrogen after ovulation. Without estrogen, insulin is able to lower the blood sugar level more effectively. Lowered blood sugar levels can result in the irritability, hunger, and headaches that often are associated with PMS.

Thyroxine. This is one of the hormones produced in the thyroid that raises the rate of metabolism. A high level of thyroxine increases the metabolic rate in part because it increases oxygen consumption. The thyroid hormones also help regulate lipid (fat) metabolism. Iodine binds to thyroxine, so measuring the amount of protein-bound iodine found in a blood sample is one technique for measuring the basal metabolic rate. The more iodine found bound to thyroxine, the more active the thyroid gland, therefore, the greater the metabolic rate.

HOW DOES ALCOHOL AFFECT DIGESTION, ABSORPTION, AND METABOLISM?

Alcohol is a source of kilocalories providing 7 kilocalories per gram. Alcohol is close to the kilocalorie content of fat, which provides 9 kilocalories per gram and carbohydrate and protein each provide 4 kilocalories per gram. Alcohol is made from a carbohydrate source, but once the carbohydrate is fermented into alcohol, it is no longer used like carbohydrate. This is why alcohol is found in the fat exchange group of the Dietary Exchange System (see Chapter 6). Alcohol is a fuel source for the human body since it is a source of kilocalories.

In moderation, alcohol is generally not harmful and may be beneficial. In moderation it is known to increase the sensitivity to insulin, thus it plays a role in carbohydrate metabolism (see Chapter 9). Persons who are not on diabetes medication may benefit with moderate amounts of alcohol due to the positive effects on insulin resistance, HDL cholesterol (also known as the "good" cholesterol or high-density lipoprotein), and blood clotting. Diabetes medication in combination with alcohol may allow serious hypoglycemia to develop with even moderate amounts of alcohol due to the increased insulin sensitivity (see Chapter 9). Moderate intake for men is two drinks or less per day, and for women is one drink or less. Persons with diabetes should seek individualized guidance from their physician.

Alcohol is toxic to the body when consumed in excess and thus impairs the entire process of digestion, absorption, and metabolism. This can affect nutritional status by interfering with normal use of food nutrients. Alcohol is widely known to harm the liver, which affects how protein is metabolized. Because protein is a vital component of all body cells, including digestive enzymes and hormones, alcohol toxicity directly impairs all normal body processes. A low-serum **albumin** (a form of protein found in the blood and a measure of protein status) will be found when there is inadequate protein intake for the body's needs or if the liver is too damaged to metabolize protein. Less well known problems with alcohol is its propensity to damage the pancreas, which can develop into secondary diabetes (see Chapter 9) due to the pancreas losing its ability to produce insulin. Alcohol also damages the villi in the intestinal system leading to poor absorption of nutrients. **Wernicke-Korsakoff syndrome** (also called Wernicke's encephalopathy) is a condition caused by alcoholism and compounded by a deficiency of vitamin B$_1$ (thiamine). This diagnosis should be considered in schizophrenic patients who are alcoholics or have diabetes (Casanova, 1996). Heavy alcohol use is associated with increased cancer, hypertension, cirrhosis of the liver, and symptomatic neuropathy (Bell, 1996).

Two principal enzymes involved in the metabolism of alcohol are alcohol dehydrogenase (ADH) and aldehyde dehydrogenase (ALDH). ADH is responsible for the metabolism of ethanol to acetaldehyde. ALDH catalyzes the conversion of acetaldehyde to acetate. The presence of an inactive form of ALDH2 is thought to be responsible for an increase in acetaldehyde levels in the body. Acetaldehyde is considered responsible for the facial flushing reactions often observed among Asians who have consumed alcohol. This may deter further consumption because of the unpleasant sensation.

What Are the Causes of Alcoholism?

It is for the concern of alcoholism that recommendations cannot be made to the public to start drinking moderate amounts of alcohol, unless the person is already drinking alcohol. As a better understanding of alcoholism develops, public health advice may change in the future. For now, individuals who already consume alcohol should be encouraged to drink moderate amounts for the best health outcomes.

Research into the causes of alcoholism is a relatively recent scientific endeavor. One area of study is the possibility of a genetic predisposition to alcoholism. Recent work has demonstrated that people have varying amounts of enzymes to metabolize alcohol. Findings suggest that a genetically controlled factor (deficiency in ALDH enzyme activity) might contribute to a decreased likelihood of alcohol intake and protection from alcoholism, because of an enhanced sensitivity to alcohol (Wall & Ehlers, 1995).

Although there is little research correlating the insulin resistance syndrome (see Chapter 9) with alcoholism, Hispanics and another group with a high rate of alcoholism, Native Americans (Lowe et al., 1997), are known to also experience high rates of diabetes. Alcoholism is associated with many rheumatic problems, including hyperuricemia with gouty arthritis (Jarallah, Shehab, Buchanan, 1992). Gout is a strong risk factor and correlate of the insulin resistance syndrome.

It is interesting to note that attention-deficit hyperactivity disorder (ADHD), which while generally a disorder of childhood and adolescence (see Chapters 15 and 17), is now increasingly recognized in adults who may have secondary depression with a tendency toward drug and alcohol abuse. One study found that a woman who began Ritalin (a medication used in ADHD) was able to reach an alcohol-free state (Durst & Rebaudengo-Rosca, 1997).

A multinational study is underway to aid in the development of biological screening tools (markers) that can identify problem drinkers. The second goal of the study is to begin to develop diagnostic *trait markers*, which provide biological information on genetically determined predisposing and protective factors in the development of alcoholism (Helander & Tabakoff, 1997).

What Are the Rates of Alcohol Abuse?

The French population has the highest average alcohol intake in the world (Zureik & Ducimetiere, 1996). In the United States the incidence of heavy drinking decreased among white men from 1984 to 1992 with the incidence now being 7 percent, with 10 percent among blacks and 17 percent among Hispanics (Caetano & Kaskutas, 1995). Hispanic groups, taken together, constitute nearly 9 percent of the U.S. population. Nationally, the rates for alcohol dependence among Hispanics and whites exceeded those for their black counterparts (Harford & Grant,1994). Alcohol use during pregnancy was pervasive among both immigrant and United States-born Latinas (7 percent) with little variation on risk factors. Increased general awareness of perinatal alcohol risk by medical providers and public health practitioners serving this population is needed (Vega et al., 1997).

There is agreement in the literature that women of the major ethnic groups in the United States have lower rates of alcohol use and suffer fewer alcohol-related problems than men. In adolescence, the highest rates of alcohol use are generally found among Native Americans (except those who live on reservations), followed in decreasing order by whites, Hispanics, African Americans, and Asian Americans (Edwards et al., 1995).

There has been a long-standing stereotype portraying Irish people as prone to excessive use of alcohol. The rates of abstinence from alcohol are higher in Ireland than in Britain, although of the Irish who use alcohol, they were more likely than their British counterparts to consume alcohol at levels greater than 14 to 21 drinks per week (Greenslade et al., 1995). One study showed that Jews had lower rates of alcohol abuse than Catholics and Protestants (Yeung & Greenwald, 1992).

As many as 15 percent of community-dwelling older persons are heavy drinkers, but their alcoholism is often hidden from their physicians. Depression, loneliness, and lack of social support are the most frequently cited antecedents to drinking for older alcoholics. Clinically, the same amount of alcohol once consumed safely may cause clinical symptoms in late life. Physiologic changes make older patients more susceptible to acute alcohol toxicity (Gambert, 1997).

What Is the Effect of Alcohol on Body Weight?

Some evidence suggests that consuming moderate amounts of alcohol is a risk factor for obesity, (Suter et al., 1997). However, another study showed that in free-living subjects over a 6-week period, the addition of two glasses of red wine to the evening meal did not adversely affect body weight or promote the development of obesity during this time period (Cordain et al., 1997).

WHAT IS THE ROLE OF THE NURSE OR OTHER HEALTH PROFESSIONAL IN PROMOTING POSITIVE NUTRITIONAL INTAKE AND METABOLISM?

The nurse or other health care professional in an institutional setting can indirectly promote the digestive process by providing a relaxed and unhurried atmosphere where patients can feel at ease to thoroughly chew their food. Direct intervention might include emphasizing the importance of thorough chewing.

The health care professional should be aware of possible issues of digestion in patients, such as swallowing problems and intestinal or gastric surgery, and should be alert to signs of malabsorption such as chronic diarrhea and unexplained weight loss. Patients with these types of problems should be referred to a registered dietitian once the attending physician makes a diagnosis. Digestive or intestinal problems, such as chronic constipation, may also be improved with medical nutrition therapy. See Chapter 11 for more information on gastrointestinal diseases and disorders.

Critical Thinking

Case Study

Bob looked up as the waitress came to his table with a tray of drink conconctions. He figured he was on vacation and these sounded like fun drinks to try. He chuckled as he thought back to when the nurse asked him if he drank often? He said no, he drank infrequently. Bob wasn't about to share with that young nurse that he drank like a fish on his days off from work—after all, he didn't think weekend drinking was frequent. He had figured out that occasional drinking didn't cause him to gain weight—which was a problem for some of his drinking buddies—especially if he skipped meals. He told himself he wasn't going to look like his friends and what would it hurt to drink excessively if it was only occasionally? He thought back to what the nurse had said about a low albumin level. He hadn't known what the nurse was talking about and he wasn't going to ask for an explanation.

Applications

1. What is the impact of alcoholism on our society and on individuals? How do class members feel about the suspected role of genetics in the development of alcoholism?
2. Was this man in denial of alcoholism?
3. What interviewing techniques might help elicit Bob's attitude toward alcohol? How might the nurse have explained the implications of low albumin in lay terms so that Bob understood it? Role-play this situation in class (one student to serve as Bob and another as the nurse).
4. How might alcohol interfere with the absorption and utilization of the food macronutrients, carbohydrate, protein, and fat?

Study Questions and Classroom Activities

1. What is the purpose of digestion?
2. What is absorption? In what part of the body does it take place?
3. In what form are all carbohydrates absorbed? All fats? All proteins?
4. How is the Krebs cycle involved in metabolism of energy?
5. Name the enzymes involved in the digestion of maltose and sucrose.

Practical Application

Trace the digestion of a meal composed of a ham sandwich on whole wheat bread, a glass of low-fat milk, and a fresh apple. Describe the mechanical and chemical processes that occur and name the enzymes involved.

References

Bell DS: Alcohol and the NIDDM patient. Diabetes Care. May 1996; 19(5): 509–513.

Caetano R, Kaskutas LA: Changes in drinking patterns among whites, blacks and Hispanics, 1984–1992. J Stud Alcohol. September 1995; 56(5):558–565.

Casanova MF: Wernicke's disease and schizophrenia: A case report and review of the literature. Int J Psychiatry Med. 1996, 26(3): 319–328.

Cordain L, Bryan ED, Melby CL, Smith MJ:Influence of moderate daily wine consumption on body weight regulation and metabolism in healthy free-living males. J Am Coll Nutr. April 1997; 16(2):134–139.

Durst R, Rebaudengo-Rosca P: Attention deficit hyperactivity disorder, facilitating alcohol and drug abuse in an adult. Harefuah. May 1, 1997; 132(9):618–622.

Edwards RW, Thurman PJ, Beauvais F: Patterns of alcohol use among ethnic minority adolescent women. Recent Dev Alcohol. 1995; 12:369–386.

Gambert SR: Alcohol abuse: Medical effects of heavy drinking in late life. Geriatrics. June 1997; 52(6):30–37.

Greenslade L, Pearson M, Madden M: A good man's fault: Alcohol and Irish people at home and abroad. Alcohol Alcohol. July 1995; 30(4):407–417.

Harford TC, Grant BF: Prevalence and population validity of DSM-III-R alcohol abuse and dependence: The 1989 National Longitudinal Survey on Youth. J Subst Abuse. 1994; 6(1):37–44.

Helander A, Tabakoff B: Biochemical markers of alcohol use and abuse: Experiences from the Pilot Study of the WHO/ISBRA Collaborative Project on state and trait markers of alcohol. International Society for Biomedical Research on Alcoholism. Alcohol Alcohol. March 1997; 32(2):133–144.

Jarallah KF, Shehab DK, Buchanan WW: Rheumatic complications of alcohol abuse. Semin Arthritis Rheum. December 1992; 22(3):162–171.

Lowe LP, Long CR, Wallace RB, Welty TK: Epidemiology of alcohol use in a group of older American Indians. Ann Epidemiol. May 1997; 7(4):241–248.

Rogers BT, et al.: Hypoxemia during oral feeding of children with severe cerebral palsy. Dev Med Child Neurol. 1993; 35:3–10.

Suter PM, Hasler E, Vetter W: Effects of alcohol on energy metabolism and body weight regulation: Is alcohol a risk factor for obesity? Nutr Rev. May 1997; 55(5):157–171.

Vega WA, Kolody B, Hwang J, Noble A, Porter PA: Perinatal drug use among immigrant and native-born Latinas. Subst Use Misuse. January 1997; 32(1):43–62.

Wall TL, Ehlers CL: Acute effects of alcohol on P300 in Asians with different ALDH2 genotypes. Alcohol Clin Exp Res. June 1995; 19(3):617–622.

Yeung PP, Greenwald S: Jewish Americans and mental health: Results of the NIMH Epidemiologic Catchment Area Study. Soc Psychiatry Psychiatr Epidemiol. November 1992; 27(6):292–297.

Zureik M, Ducimetiere P: High alcohol-related premature mortality in France: Concordant estimates from a prospective cohort study and national mortality statistics. Alcohol Clin Exp Res. May 1996; 20(3):428–433.

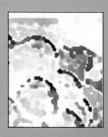

5

Food as the Source of Vitamins, Minerals, Phytochemicals, and Water

Objectives

After completing this chapter, you should be able to:

- Describe the main difference between the fat-soluble and water-soluble vitamins.
- Recognize at least one known function of each of the vitamins and minerals.
- List foods high in the various vitamins and minerals.
- Describe the function and common sources of electrolytes.
- Describe the importance of water and explain how to include appropriate amounts in the diet.
- Describe how the nurse or other health care professional can most appropriately promote the intake of vitamins, minerals, phytochemicals, electrolytes, and water.

Terms to Identify

Acid-base balance	Fat-soluble vitamins	Pernicious anemia
Anemia	Fortification	Phytochemicals
Arthralgias	Goiter	Precursor
Beriberi	Heme iron	Prothrombin
Cardiomyopathy	Hemoglobin	Rebound scurvy
Carotene	Hyperosmotic diarrhea	Recommended dietary
Chronic disease	Hypocalcemia	allowance (RDA)
Cirrhosis	Hypoparathyroidism	Retinol equivalent (RE)
Cretinism	International unit (IU)	Rickets
DNA	Intrinsic factor	Sickle cell disease
Electrolyte	Iron overload	Tetany
Elemental	Neuropathy	Vitamin B complex
Enrichment	Pellagra	

INTRODUCTION

As we become more knowledgeable about our vitamin and mineral needs, it is helpful to keep their history in perspective. Initially, food was recognized as the important element in health. One of the first major discoveries about the role of vitamins was that the use of lemons and limes offered protection against the dreaded scurvy that plagued ocean voyagers. Before this revelation, sailors often developed this severe vitamin C deficiency, which resulted in internal bleeding and death. The impact of toxic levels of vitamins was noted when Arctic explorers died from ingesting polar bear liver, which has a high level of vitamin A.

It was not until the 20th century that vitamins were chemically identified. This author had the rare opportunity of talking personally with a retired scientist who recalled being one of the first people asked to chemically isolate vitamin C during the 1920s. He and his colleagues laughed at the foolishness of this idea. We may no longer laugh about the importance of vitamins, but we cannot expect that in one person's lifetime all has been learned about the complexity of the body's need for vitamins.

Minerals, the seeming equivalent of vitamins in the consumer's eye, are elemental inorganic substances that have some similarities to vitamins but also have many differences. The most notable difference is that minerals are **elemental,** which means that they do not break down. This characteristic of minerals prevents their destruction by heat and air—destruction that vitamins are susceptible to. The elements found in the high school chemical periodic table are minerals. In the saying, "Ashes to ashes, dust to dust," the ashes are the minerals found in the body.

The roles and functions of vitamins and minerals in health are complex, and a body of knowledge is accumulating. The immune system, for example, is complicated and requires adequate protein and kilocalories without an excess (as obesity leads to poor immune response), while the minerals zinc, selenium, iron, and copper and vitamins A, C, E, and B$_6$, and folic acid all have important roles (Chandra, 1997). Excess of one vitamin or mineral can compete with another; for example, zinc competes with copper, and vitamin E can inhibit the activity of vitamin K. The most prudent approach for achieving an optimal vitamin and mineral nutritional status is a varied diet, with an emphasis on whole grains, legumes, dark green leafy vegetables, orange vegetables and fruits, and milk. If one is eating adequate amounts of legumes and protein, meat is not necessary for health.

Vitamin and mineral supplements, which generally are unnecessary, should be within 100 to 200 percent of the recommended dietary allowance (see the RDA table inside the front cover). Exceptions to this guideline should be made only with a warranted medical condition and the advice of a physician. Many health conditions, associated with the need for vitamins and minerals, are better resolved through the use of foods because the human body is extremely complex and the nutrient composition of foods best matches this need. This is the case with lung cancer, where only foods containing vitamins E and C and carotenoids, not the vitamin supplements, have been associated with reduced cancer risk

(Yong et al., 1997). The consumption of foods rich in antioxidant vitamins has been associated with reduced skin cancers (Gaziano & Hennekens, 1996). Although an estimated 40 percent of the U.S. population takes vitamin supplements, the efficacy of these supplements is not yet proven, and some have questioned their safety (Meyers et al., 1996). Currently the data seem insufficient to make recommendations for the use of vitamin supplements to prevent cancer. The results are certainly in line with the advice that a diet rich in fruits and vegetables will help reduce cancer risk (van Poppel & van den Berg, 1997).

Newly recognized substances in food, which are neither vitamins nor minerals, are referred to as **phytochemicals** and may be the cause of improved health with foods versus supplements. It is estimated that there are 100 or more yet-to-be identified phytochemicals available in food that contribute to health. Because the majority of these substances have not yet been identified, they are not available in supplements. There have already been a number of discoveries with phytochemicals and their correlation to health. It was shown that a high intake of one phytochemical, flavenoids, was inversely related to lung cancer risk when consuming foods, especially apples (Knekt et al., 1997). Lycopene, the carotenoid found in tomatoes, has been reported to offer protection against prostate cancer (Giles & Ireland, 1997). It appears that it is the phytochemicals found in plant-based diets that are associated with a reduced risk of many chronic diseases (Messina & Messina, 1996). Sulfur-containing phytochemicals present in cruciferous vegetables (cabbage, broccoli, cauliflower, and brussel sprouts) appear to possess anticarcinogenic properties (Stoewsand, 1995). Phytochemicals are found in tea, rosemary, and turmeric that are anti-inflammatory and cancer preventive (Chan, et al., 1995). Low-processed whole grains, legumes, vegetables, and fruits containing all the known vitamins and minerals will likely provide these phytochemicals in amounts beneficial to health.

Health care professionals are in a unique position of being able to positively influence a patient's nutrient intake. This chapter is aimed at increasing appreciation for the micronutrients in foods that our bodies require. The concept of adequate levels of nutrients for health has been reflected in the five food groups of the Food Guide Pyramid and in the **recommended dietary allowances (RDAs)**— *the levels of intake of essential nutrients that, on the basis of scientific knowledge, are judged to be adequate to meet known nutrient needs of practically all healthy persons.* The reference daily intakes (RDIs) are similar but developed for use on food labels (see Chapter 6). With the advent of fortification, many deficiency diseases such as **goiter** have been overcome in the United States although goiter is found in some areas of the world. (Goiter is a disease of the thyroid gland caused by lack of iodine; iodized salt helps prevent goiter.) There is concern about some minerals that are low in the U.S. population, specifically calcium, iron, zinc, and possibly copper and magnesium (Pennington, 1996).

The focus has now primarily shifted to setting maximum levels for prevention of **chronic disease** (any disease of long standing such as diabetes or hypertension); thus the advent of the Dietary Guidelines for Americans (see Chapter 6 for more information.) The principles of moderation, balance, and variety should be applied to food choices. All foods can be included when keeping this principle in mind. Even dietitians eat chocolate cake and in moderation, along with the minimum number of servings in the Food Guide Pyramid, health can be promoted and maintained.

HOW ARE VITAMINS AND MINERALS BEST INCLUDED IN ONE'S DIET?

Reliance on food sources for vitamins and minerals (Tables 5–1 through 5–4) offers little risk of ingesting toxic amounts and provides for a good balance and mix of vitamins and minerals. The base of the Food Guide Pyramid provides the B vitamins (especially thiamine and niacin), and whole grains provide a wide variety of minerals such as chromium and zinc. The second level of the pyramid, fruits and vegetables, supplies potassium and other minerals. The dark-green leafy vegetables are especially high in potassium and magnesium with high amounts of vitamins A (in the carotene form), C, and the B vitamin, folate. Deep orange fruits and vegetables such as sweet potatoes, carrots, and canteloupe are very high in carotene. Citrus fruits are very high in vitamin C. The third level of the pyramid shows the high-calcium milk group, which also provides the primary source of vitamin B_2. The addition of legumes, meat, or other protein foods further rounds out the nutritional needs providing B vitamins and many minerals, such as iron.

Many individuals do not realize that substances that are essential at one level can be harmful at higher doses. A number of trials currently underway are designed to prove that antioxidant vitamins prevent chronic diseases and to evaluate the long-term safety of the widespread use of supplements (Gaziano & Hennekens, 1996). The ability to consume toxic levels of micronutrients is far more likely to occur with the use of vitamin and mineral supplements. Because there are no long-term studies that establish the safety of large doses of vitamins, health-conscious consumers need to respect this. It would be much better if people took the 2.7 billion dollars, which is what the Food and Drug Administration (FDA) estimates is spent on vitamin and mineral supplements, and bought legumes, vegetables, fruits, and whole grains instead.

WHAT IS THE ROLE OF VITAMINS IN NUTRITION?

Vitamins are present in foods and are needed by the body in only minute amounts, but proper growth and development and optimal health are impossible without them. Some vitamins may be synthesized in the body, but for the most part they must be supplied in the daily diet of normal healthy persons. Early attention was paid to the clear-cut manifestations of diseases caused by vitamin deficiencies (Fig. 5–1).

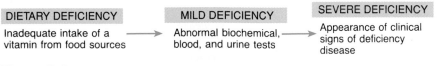

DIETARY DEFICIENCY
Inadequate intake of a vitamin from food sources

MILD DEFICIENCY
Abnormal biochemical, blood, and urine tests

SEVERE DEFICIENCY
Appearance of clinical signs of deficiency disease

Figure 5–1
The progression of the development of vitamin deficiencies.

Table 5–1
Fat-Soluble Vitamins

Functions	Good Sources	Symptoms of Deficiency	Symptoms of Toxicity
Vitamin A (Nomenclature: Preformed—retinol, retinal, retinoic acid; Precursor—carotene)			

Maintenance of epithelial cells and mucous membranes
Constituent of visual purple, important for night vision
Necessary for normal growth, development, and reproduction
Necessary for adequate immune response
	Preformed vitamin A:
	  liver
	Carotene (dark green leafy):
	  Spinach
	  Broccoli
	  Kale
	  Swiss chard
	  Turnip greens
	  Collard greens
	Carotene (deep orange):
	  Carrots
	  Sweet potatoes
	  Orange winter squash
	  Pumpkin
	  Tomatoes
	  Apricots
	  Watermelon
	  Cantaloupe
		Nyctalopia (night blindness)
		Keratinized skin (rough, dry skin)
		Dry mucous membranes
		Xerophthalmia (an eye disease)
			Appetite loss
			Hair loss
			Dry skin
			Bone and joint pain
			Enlarged liver and spleen
			Fetal malformations
			Headache
			Weakness
			Vomiting
			Irritability
			Hydrocephalus (children)
			Brittle nails
			Gingivitis
			Cheilosis
			Ascites

Vitamin E (Nomenclature: Tocopherol)			
Prevents oxidative destruction of vitamin A in the intestine Protects red blood cells from rupture (hemolysis) Helps maintain normal cell membranes by reducing the oxidation of polyunsaturated fatty acids	Wheat germ Vegetable oils Legumes Nuts Whole grains Fish Green leafy vegetables	Breakdown of red blood cells	Decreased thyroid hormone level Modest increases in triglycerides
Vitamin K (Nomenclature: Menadione [vitamin K_3], Phylloquinone [vitamin K_1])			
Necessary for formation of prothrombin and other factors necessary for blood clotting	Dark green leafy vegetables Cauliflower Soybean oil Green tea Synthesis of intestinal bacteria	Hemorrhage	No toxicity known

Table continued on following page

Table 5–1
Fat-Soluble Vitamins (*continued*)

Functions	Good Sources	Symptoms of Deficiency	Symptoms of Toxicity
Vitamin D (Nomenclature: Ergocalciferol [vitamin D$_2$], cholecalciferol [vitamin D$_3$]; Precursors—Ergosterol [plants], 7-dehydrocholesterol [in skin])			
Aids in absorption of calcium and phosphorus Regulates blood levels of calcium Promotes bone and teeth mineralization	Fortified milk Fish with bones (e.g., salmon, sardines) Cod liver oil	Rickets (children) Osteomalacia (adults)	Calcification of soft tissues Hypercalcemia Renal stones Appetite and weight loss Nausea and fatigue Growth failure in children

From the National Research Council: Diet and Health, Washington, DC, National Academy Press, 1989; Mahan KL, Escott-Stump S: Krause's Food, Nutrition, and Diet Therapy, 9th ed., Philadelphia, WB Saunders, 1996; and Davis J, Sherer K: Applied Nutrition and Diet Therapy for Nurses, 2nd ed., Philadelphia, WB Saunders, 1994.

Vitamins, although organic in nature, do not provide energy (kilocalories). But they do help in the metabolism of the macronutrients carbohydrate, protein, and fat. In this role vitamins are thought to act as catalysts.

Vitamins are classified as *body regulators* because of the following functions:

1. They regulate the synthesis of many body compounds (bones, skin, glands, nerves, brain, and blood).
2. They participate in the metabolism of protein, carbohydrates, and fats.
3. They prevent nutritional deficiency diseases and allow for optimal health at all ages.

What Is the Difference Between Fat-Soluble and Water-Soluble Vitamins?

Generally, vitamins are classified into two groups: fat-soluble (vitamins A, D, E, and K) and water-soluble (B-complex vitamins and vitamin C). Water-soluble vitamins are not stored in any significant amounts in the body, which means that they need to be included in the diet on a daily basis. In contrast are the **fat-soluble vitamins,** which are stored in body fat and can reach toxic levels. Deficiencies of fat-soluble vitamins in healthy individuals are less likely to occur than deficiencies of water-soluble vitamins.

The absorption of fat-soluble vitamins is enhanced by dietary fat (Table 5–5). Individuals afflicted with malabsorption of fat, or who are consuming an extremely low level of fat, are at higher risk for development of fat-soluble vitamin deficiencies. Fat-soluble vitamins are generally more stable than water-soluble vitamins and are less prone to destruction by heat, air, and light.

Text continued on page 91

Table 5–2
Water-Soluble Vitamins

Functions	Good Sources	Symptoms of Deficiency	Symptoms of Toxicity
Vitamin B₁ (Nomenclature: Thiamine)			
Plays a role in carbo-hydrate metabolism Helps the nervous system, heart, muscles, and tissue to function properly Promotes a good appetite and good functioning of the digestive tract	Whole grains Wheat germ Enriched white flour products Organ meats Pork Legumes Brewer's yeast	Polyneuritis Beriberi Fatigue Depression Poor appetite Poor functioning of intestinal tract Nervous instability Edema Spastic muscle contractions Wernicke's encephalopathy Korsakoff's psychosis	No toxicity known
Vitamin B₂ (Nomenclature: Riboflavin [formerly vitamin G])			

Essential for certain enzyme systems that aid in the metabolism of carbohydrate, protein, and fat	Milk and milk products
	Eggs
	Green leafy vegetables
	Organ meats
	  Liver
	  Kidney
	  Heart
	Dry yeast
	Peanuts
	Peanut butter
	Whole grains
		Tongue inflammation
		Scaling and burning skin
		Sensitive eyes
		Angular stomatitis and cheilosis
		Cataracts
			No toxicity known in humans

Vitamin B₃ (Nomenclature: Niacin, nicotinic acid)			
Part of two important enzymes that regulate energy metabolism Promotes good physical and mental health and helps maintain the health of the skin, tongue, and digestive system	Meats and organ meats Whole-grain flour products Enriched white flour products Legumes Brewer's yeast	Pellagra (rare) with skin and mouth manifestations Gastrointestinal disturbances Photosensitive dermatitis Depressive psychosis	Flushing caused by vasodilation Nausea and vomiting Abnormal glucose metabolism Abnormal plasma uric acid levels Abnormal liver function tests Gastric ulceration Anaphylaxis (swelling, pain, fever, or asthmatic symptoms caused by physical sensitivity) Circulatory collapse

Table continued on following page

Table 5–2
Water-Soluble Vitamins (*continued*)

Functions	Good Sources	Symptoms of Deficiency	Symptoms of Toxicity
Vitamin B₆ (Nomenclature: Pyridoxine, pyridoxal, pyridoxamine)			
Important in metabolism of protein and amino acids, carbohydrate, and fat Essential for proper growth and maintenance of body functions	Liver and red meats Whole grains Potatoes Green vegetables Corn	Not fully established but believed to lead to convulsions, peripheral neuropathy, secondary pellagra, possible depression, oral lesions	Sensory nerve damage Numbness of extremities Ataxia Bone pain Muscle weakness
Vitamin B₁₂ (Nomenclature: Cobalamin)			
Aids in hemoglobin synthesis Essential for normal functioning of all cells, especially nervous system, bone marrow, and gastrointestinal tract Important in energy metabolism, especially folic acid metabolism	Foods of animal origin Meats Organ meats Dry milk and milk products Whole egg and egg yolk Not found in significant amounts in plant sources	Pernicious (megaloblastic) anemia Subacute combined degeneration of the spinal cord Various psychiatric disorders May cause anorexia	No toxicity known
Folacin (Nomenclature: Folic Acid)			
Functions in the formation of red blood cells and in normal functioning of gastrointestinal tract Aids in metabolism of protein	Glandular meats Yeast Dark green leafy vegetables Legumes Whole grains	Impaired cell division Alterations of protein synthesis with possible neural tube defect Various psychiatric disorders Megaloblastic anemia Supplements mask the symptoms of pernicious anemia but not the neurological manifestations	No toxicity known
Choline			
A constituent of several compounds necessary for certain aspects of nerve function and lipid metabolism	Synthesized from methionine (an amino acid)	Occurs only when protein intake (methylamine) is low	No toxicity known in humans

Table 5-2
Water-Soluble Vitamins (*continued*)

Functions	Good Sources	Symptoms of Deficiency	Symptoms of Toxicity
Pantothenic Acid			
Essential part of complex enzymes involved in fatty acid metabolism	Animal products Liver Eggs Whole grains Legumes White potatoes Sweet potatoes	Nutritional melalgia (burning foot syndrome) Headache Fatigue Poor muscle coordination Nausea Cramps	Possible diarrhea
Biotin (Nomenclature: Once known as vitamin H)			
Essential for activity of many enzyme systems Plays a central role in fatty acid synthesis and in the metabolism of carbohydrates and protein	Liver Meats Milk Soy flour Brewer's yeast Egg yolk (raw egg white destroys biotin) Bacteria in the intestinal tract also produce biotin	Rare, but includes certain types of anemia, depression, insomnia, muscle pain, dermatitis	No toxicity known in humans
Vitamin C (Nomenclature: Ascorbic acid, dehydroascorbic acid)			
Helps protect the body against infections and in wound healing and recovery from operations Is important for tooth dentin, bones, cartilage, connective tissue, and blood vessels	Citrus fruits Tomatoes Strawberries Cantaloupe Currants Green leafy vegetables Green peppers Broccoli Cabbage Potatoes	Anemia Swollen and bleeding gums Loose teeth Ruptures of small blood vessels (bruises) Scurvy (rebound scurvy can occur when large doses, or megadoses, are suddenly stopped)	Urinary stones Diarrhea Hypoglycemia Interferes with tests for fecal and urinary occult blood Will provide a false positive test for glucosuria

From The National Research Council: Diet and Health, Washington, DC, National Academy Press, 1989; Mahan KL, Escott-Stump S: Krause's Food, Nutrition, and Diet Therapy, 9th ed., Philadelphia, WB Saunders, 1996; and Davis J, Sherer K: Applied Nutrition and Diet Therapy for Nurses, 2nd ed., Philadelphia, WB Saunders, 1994.

Table 5-3
Major Minerals (Macronutrients)

Functions	Sources	Deficiency Symptoms	Toxicity Symptoms
Mineral and Elemental Symbol: Calcium (Ca^{2+})			
Helps muscles to contract and relax, thereby helping to regulate heartbeat Plays a role in the normal functioning of the nervous system Aids in blood coagulation and the functioning of some enzymes Helps build strong bones and teeth May help prevent hypertension	Primarily found in milk and milk products; also found in dark green leafy vegetables, tofu and other soy products, sardines, salmon with bones, and hard water	Poor bone growth and tooth development, leading to stunted growth and increased risk of dental caries, rickets (bowing of legs) in children, osteomalacia (soft bones) and osteoporosis (brittle bones) in adults, poor blood clotting, and possible hypertension	Kidney stones in predisposed individuals
Mineral and Elemental Symbol: Chloride (Cl$^-$)			
Involved in the maintenance of fluid and acid-base balance Provides an acid medium, in the form of hydrochloric acid, for activation of gastric enzymes	Major source is table salt (sodium chloride); also found in fish and vegetables	Disturbances in acid-base balance, with possible growth retardation, psychomotor defects, and memory loss	No toxicity known
Mineral and Elemental Symbol: Magnesium (Mg^{2+})			
Helps build strong bones and teeth Activates many enzymes Participates in protein synthesis and lipid metabolism Helps regulate heartbeat	Raw dark green vegetables, nuts and soybeans, whole grains and wheat bran, bananas and apricots, seafoods, coffee, tea, cocoa, and hard water	Rare, but in disease states may lead to central nervous system problems (confusion, apathy, hallucinations, poor memory) and neuromuscular problems (muscle weakness, cramps, tremor, cardiac arrhythmia)	Increased calcium excretion
Mineral and Elemental Symbol: Phosphorus (P)			
Helps build strong bones and teeth Present in the nuclei of all cells Helps in the oxidation of fats and carbohydrates (energy metabolism) Aids in maintaining the body's acid-base balance	Milk and milk products, eggs, meats, legumes, whole grains, soft drinks (used to make the fizz)	Rare, but with malabsorption can cause anorexia, weakness, stiff joints, and fragile bones	Hypocalcemic tetany (muscle spasms)

Table 5–3
Major Minerals (Macronutrients) (*continued*)

Functions	Good Sources	Deficiency Symptoms	Toxicity Symptoms
Mineral and Elemental Symbol: Potassium (K⁺)			
Plays a key role in fluid and acid-base balance. Transmits nerve impulses and helps control muscle contractions and promotes regular heartbeat. Needed for enzyme reactions	Apricots, bananas, oranges, grapefruit, raisins, green beans, broccoli, carrots, greens, potatoes, meats, milk and milk products, peanut butter, legumes, molasses, coffee, tea, and cocoa	May cause impaired growth, hypertension, bone fragility, central nervous system changes, renal hypertrophy, diminished heart rate, and death	Hyperkalemia (excess potassium in the blood) with cardiac function disturbances
Mineral and Elemental Symbol: Sodium (Na⁺)			
Plays a key role in the maintenance of acid-base balance. Transmits nerve impulses and helps control muscle contractions	Salt (sodium chloride) is the major dietary source; minor sources occur naturally in foods such as milk and milk products and several vegetables	Hyponatremia (too little sodium in the blood)	May cause hypertension, which can lead to cardiovascular diseases and renal (kidney) disease; in the form of salt tablets, can cause gastric irritation
Mineral and Elemental Symbol: Sulfur (S)			
Part of three amino acids, and the B vitamins thiamine and biotin. Plays a role in oxidation-reduction reactions. Regulates cell membrane permeability	Protein-rich foods (meat, eggs, milk)	None documented in humans	Unlikely to cause significant symptoms

From The National Research Council: Diet and Health, Washington, DC, National Academy Press, 1989; Mahan LK, Escott-Stump S: Krause's Food, Nutrition, and Diet Therapy, 9th ed., Philadelphia, WB Saunders, 1996; and Davis J, Sherer K: Applied Nutrition and Diet Therapy for Nurses, 2nd ed., Philadelphia, WB Saunders, 1994.

What Are the Fat-Soluble Vitamins?

Vitamin A. Vitamin A can be obtained in two forms. The **precursor** form is **carotene,** which is found in abundance in dark green leafy vegetables and deep orange vegetables and fruits. The color of carotene is orange, which is why those foods high in carotene are of similar color and why a person's skin can change color when these foods are eaten in abundance. This is innocuous and fades away once carotene foods are decreased in the diet. Carotene is converted into vitamin A in the liver and is often simply referred to as vitamin A.

Preformed vitamin A, also called *retinol,* is found in animal products such as liver, milk fat, and egg yolks and is able to produce toxicity (see Table 5–1 and Fig. 5–2 for other specific food sources).

Table 5–4
Trace Minerals (Micronutrients)

Functions	Sources	Deficiency Symptoms	Toxicity Symptoms
Mineral and Elemental Symbol: Chromium (Cr^{3+})			
Activates several enzymes. Enhances the removal of glucose from the blood	Liver and other meats, whole grains, cheese, legumes, and brewer's yeast	Weight loss, abnormalities of the central nervous system, and possible aggravation of diabetes mellitus	Liver damage and lung cancer caused by industrial exposure
Mineral and Elemental Symbol: Cobalt (Co^{2+})			
An essential component of vitamin B_{12}. Activates enzymes	Figs, cabbage, beet greens, spinach, lettuce, watercress	Pernicious anemia	Polycythemia (excess number of red corpuscles in blood). Hyperplasia of bone marrow. Increased blood volume
Mineral and Elemental Symbol: Copper (Cu^{2+})			
Aids in the production and survival of red blood cells. Part of many enzymes involved in respiration. Plays a role in normal lipid metabolism	Shellfish—especially oysters—liver, nuts, and seeds, raisins, whole grains, chocolate, and legumes	Anemia, central nervous system problems, abnormal electrocardiograms, bone fragility, impaired immune response; may be a factor in failure to thrive in premature infants	In Wilson's disease, copper accumulation causes neuron and liver cell damage
Mineral and Elemental Symbol: Fluorine (F^-)			
Helps the formation of solid bones and teeth, thereby reducing incidence of dental caries (see Chapter 19) and may help prevent osteoporosis	Fluoridated water (and foods cooked in fluoridated water), fish, tea, gelatin	Increased susceptibility to dental caries	Fluorosis and mottling of teeth
Mineral and Elemental Symbol: Iodine (I^-)			
Helps regulate energy metabolism as a part of thyroid hormones. Essential for normal cell functioning, helping to keep skin, hair, and nails healthy	Primarily from iodized salt, also found in saltwater fish, seaweed products, vegetables grown in iodine-rich soils	Goiter, cretinism in infants born to iodine-deficient mothers, with accompanying mental retardation and diffuse central nervous system abnormalities	Little toxic effect in individuals with normal thyroid gland functioning. Goiter may also occur in toxic states
Mineral and Elemental Symbol: Iron (Fe^{3+})			
Essential to the formation of hemoglobin, which is important for tissue respiration and ultimately growth and development	Heme sources: organ meats—especially liver, red meats, and other meats. Nonheme sources: iron-fortified cereals, dark	Iron-deficiency anemia and possible alterations that impair behavior	Idiopathic hemochromatosis, which can lead to cirrhosis, diabetes mellitus, and cardiomyopathy

Table 5–4
Trace Minerals (Micronutrients) (*continued*)

Functions	Sources	Deficiency Symptoms	Toxicity Symptoms
Mineral and Elemental Symbol: Iron (Fe^{3+}) (*cont.*)			
Part of several enzymes and proteins in the body	green leafy vegetables, legumes, whole grains, blackstrap molasses, dried fruit, and foods cooked in iron pans		
Mineral and Elemental Symbol: Manganese (Mn^{2+})			
Need for normal bone structure, reproduction, normal functioning of cells, and the central nervous system A component of some enzymes	Nuts, whole grains, vegetables and fruits, coffee, tea, cocoa, and egg yolks	None observed in humans	Parkinson-like symptoms have been noted in miners
Mineral and Elemental Symbol: Molybdenum (Mo)			
A component of three enzymes Important for normal cell functioning	Organ meats, legumes, whole grains, dark green vegetables	Vomiting, tachypnea (fast breathing), tachycardia, coma, hypermethioninemia in premature infants (methionine is an amino acid)	No toxicity known
Mineral and Elemental Symbol: Selenium (Se)			
Part of an enzyme system Acts as an antioxidant with vitamin E to protect the cells from oxygen	Protein-rich foods (meat, eggs, milk), whole grains, seafood, liver and other meats, egg yolks, and garlic	Keshan's disease (a human cardiomyopathy) and Kashin-Beck disease (an endemic human osteoarthropathy)	Physical defects of the fingernails and toenails and hair loss Nausea Abdominal pain Diarrhea Peripheral neuropathy Fatigue Irritability
Mineral and Elemental Symbol: Zinc (Zn^{2+})			
Plays a role in protein synthesis Essential for normal growth and sexual development, wound healing, immune function, cell division and differentiation, and smell acuity	Whole grains, wheat germ, crabmeat, oysters, liver and other meats, brewer's yeast	Depressed immune function, poor growth, dwarfism, impaired skeletal growth and delayed sexual maturation, acrodermatitis	Severe anemia, nausea, vomiting, abdominal cramps, diarrhea, fever, hypocupremia (low blood serum copper), malaise, fatigue Impaired immunity also found in toxic states Renal damage

From The National Research Council: Diet and Health, Washington, DC, National Academy Press, 1989; Mahan KL, Escott-Stump S: Krause's Food, Nutrition, and Diet Therapy, 9th ed., Philadelphia, WB Saunders, 1996; and Davis J, Sherer K: Applied Nutrition and Diet Therapy for Nurses, 2nd ed., Philadelphia, WB Saunders, 1994.

Table 5–5
Some Nutrient Interactions with Vitamins and Minerals

Nutrient	Inhibiting Nutrient	Enhancing Nutrient
Vitamins		
Vitamin A (carotene)	Excess vitamin E, deficiency of protein, iron, and zinc	Dietary fat
Vitamin D		Dietary fat
Vitamin E		Dietary fat
Vitamin K	Excess vitamin E	Dietary fat
Vitamin B_1	Tannins (as found in coffee)	
Vitamin B_2	Excess vitamin B_1	
Vitamin B_3	Deficiency of vitamin B_6	
Vitamin B_6	Excess choline and leucine	Deficiency of vitamin C
Vitamin B_{12}	Excess vitamin C, deficiency of vitamin B_6	
Folacin	Thiamine hastens decomposition in supplements	
Choline	Excess inositol	
Vitamin C	Deficiency of vitamin B_6	
Minerals		
Calcium	Excess sodium, protein, phosphorus, oxalates	Vitamin D, lactose, and certain amino acids
Phosphorus	Excess iron	
Magnesium	Excess sodium, calcium, vitamin D, phosphate, protein, and alcohol	
Iron	Excess manganese	Vitamin C, copper, cobalt
Zinc	Excess iron, copper, tin, folic acid, tannins, and possibly calcium	Possible fluoride role
Copper	Excess zinc, molybdenum, and vitamin C	Possible fluoride role. Estrogen increases copper serum levels
Molybdenum	Excess sulfur	

Deficiency of vitamin A has long been known to increase the risk of infection and is associated with blindness in many countries (see Chapter 22). It is now known that a good intake of vitamin A helps with bone growth, a healthy immune system, reproduction, and improved vision.

Approximately 10 to 15 cases of vitamin A toxic reactions are reported per year in the United States, generally at doses greater than 100,000 international units (see the following section) per day (Meyers et al., 1996). The only known evidence of adverse effects from beta-carotene supplements is found among heavy smokers (Hathcock, 1997).

How is Vitamin A measured? **Retinol equivalents (REs)** and **international units (IUs)** are two different methods of describing the amount of vitamin A in foods. The use of IU indicates that both preformed vitamin A and carotenoids are measured; this is still a common method used in food composition tables and in diet planning. Because the biological activities of carotenoids and vitamin A are different, however, REs began to be used. Simply said, numbers used in the IU system are about five times those expressed in the RE system.

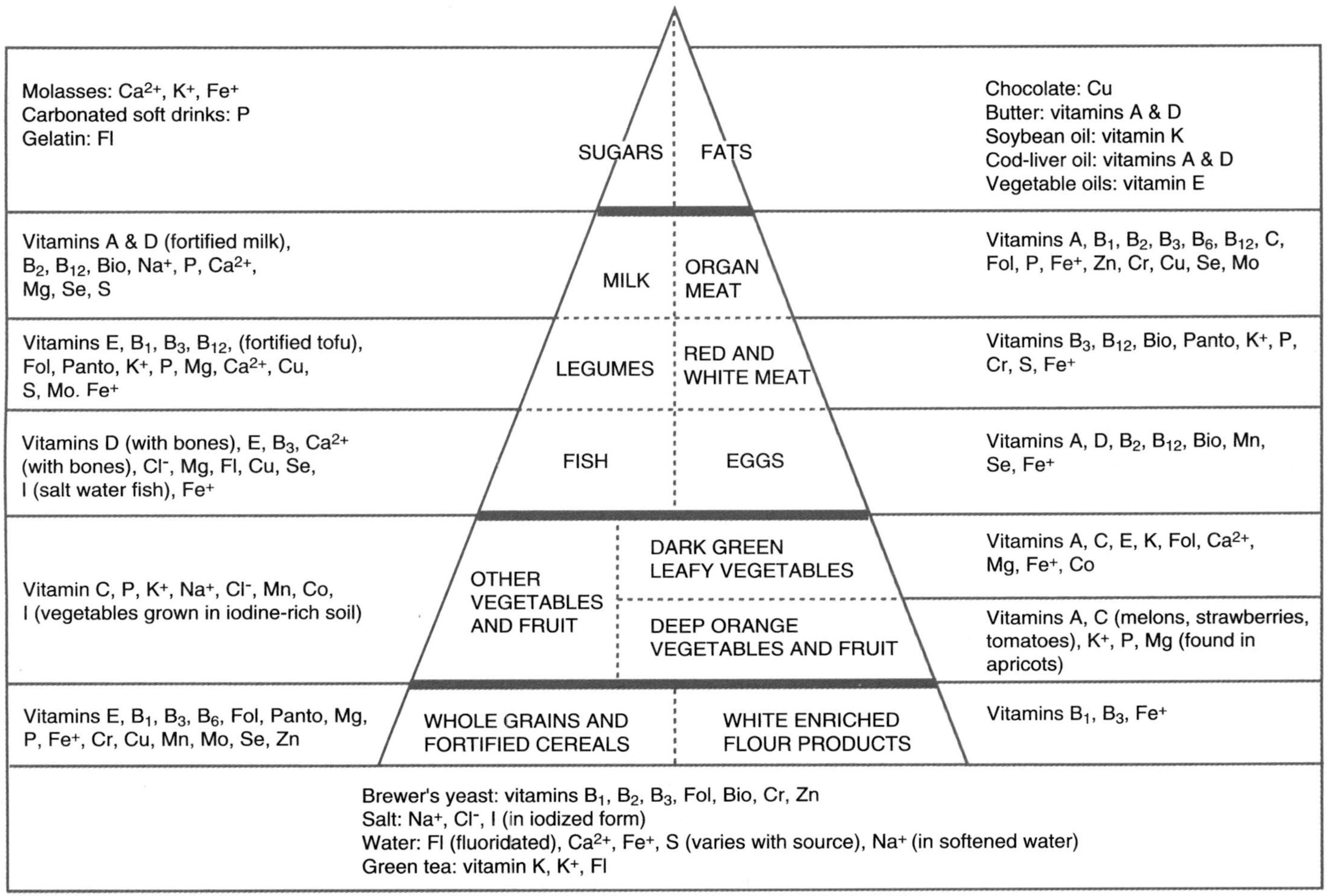

Figure 5–2

Vitamin and mineral content of the Food Guide Pyramid (listed in the following order: fat-soluble vitamins, water-soluble vitamins, major minerals, and trace minerals). (Key: Bio = biotin; Ca^{2+} = calcium; Cl^- = chloride; Co = cobalt; Cr = chromium; Cu = copper; Fe^+ = iron; Fl = fluorine; Fol = folate; I = iodine; K^+ = potassium; Mg = magnesium; Mn = manganese; Mo = molybdenum; Na^+ = sodium; P = phosphorus; Panto = pantothenic acid; S = sulfur; Se = selenium; Zn = zinc.)

Chocolate: Cu
Butter: vitamins A & D
Soybean oil: vitamin K
Cod-liver oil: vitamins A & D
Vegetable oils: vitamin E

Vitamins A, B_1, B_2, B_3, B_6, B_{12}, C, Fol, P, Fe^+, Zn, Cr, Cu, Se, Mo

Vitamins B_3, B_{12}, Bio, Panto, K^+, P, Cr, S, Fe^+

Vitamins A, D, B_2, B_{12}, Bio, Mn, Se, Fe^+

Vitamins A, C, E, K, Fol, Ca^{2+}, Mg, Fe^+, Co

Vitamins A, C (melons, strawberries, tomatoes), K^+, P, Mg (found in apricots)

Vitamins B_1, B_3, Fe^+

FATS — SUGARS
ORGAN MEAT — MILK
RED AND WHITE MEAT — LEGUMES
EGGS — FISH
DARK GREEN LEAFY VEGETABLES — OTHER VEGETABLES AND FRUIT
DEEP ORANGE VEGETABLES AND FRUIT
WHITE ENRICHED FLOUR PRODUCTS — WHOLE GRAINS AND FORTIFIED CEREALS

Brewer's yeast: vitamins B_1, B_2, B_3, Fol, Bio, Cr, Zn
Salt: Na^+, Cl^-, I (in iodized form)
Water: Fl (fluoridated), Ca^{2+}, Fe^+, S (varies with source), Na^+ (in softened water)
Green tea: vitamin K, K^+, Fl

Molasses: Ca^{2+}, K^+, Fe^+
Carbonated soft drinks: P
Gelatin: Fl

Vitamins A & D (fortified milk), B_2, B_{12}, Bio, Na^+, P, Ca^{2+}, Mg, Se, S

Vitamins E, B_1, B_3, B_{12}, (fortified tofu), Fol, Panto, K^+, P, Mg, Ca^{2+}, Cu, S, Mo. Fe^+

Vitamins D (with bones), E, B_3, Ca^{2+} (with bones), Cl^-, Mg, Fl, Cu, Se, I (salt water fish), Fe^+

Vitamin C, P, K^+, Na^+, Cl^-, Mn, Co, I (vegetables grown in iodine-rich soil)

Vitamins E, B_1, B_3, B_6, Fol, Panto, Mg, P, Fe^+, Cr, Cu, Mn, Mo, Se, Zn

Vitamin D. Vitamin D has been known since the early part of this century to prevent **rickets** (bowing of the legs caused by the increasing weight on the soft bones of growing children who do not receive enough vitamin D), although rickets in children had been recognized for centuries (Fig. 5–3). After vitamin D was chemically isolated in 1935, it was eventually added to milk, which ultimately replaced cod-liver oil as a means to prevent rickets (1 teaspoon of cod-liver oil provides about 100 percent of the RDA for vitamin D and vitamin A). Milk was an appropriate food to fortify with vitamin D because this vitamin greatly enhances the absorption of calcium, of which milk is the best source.

Sunlight also contributes to vitamin D status by converting a vitamin D precursor in the skin to an active form. This conversion varies according to the length and intensity of exposure and the color of the skin. Institutionalized el-

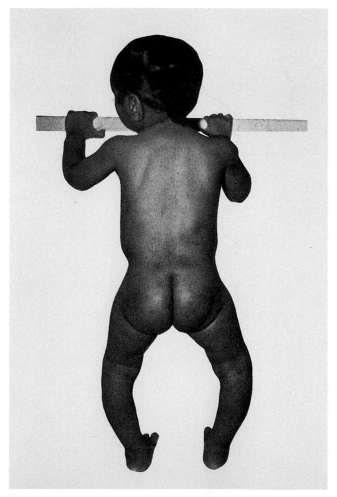

Figure 5–3
Rickets in young child. Chest and lower extremities are deformed.
(From Nutrition, A Scope Publication, Fourth Edition, Kalamazoo, Michigan, The Upjohn Company, 1980, Figure 56, page 82.)

derly persons are at high risk for vitamin D deficiency because of negligible exposure to the sun and may benefit with supplementation. Patients with renal (kidney) disease may also require supplementation because of impaired metabolism (see Chapter 10). As persons age, the ability of the body to produce vitamin D from sunlight exposure becomes impaired.

In France it was noted that low vitamin D status during puberty was normalized after a short-term use of 100,000 IU vitamin D3 supplementation, which showed the safety of this intermittent supplementation to adolescents during the winter season (Zeghoud et al., 1995). This may especially have implications for U.S. adolescents who follow vegan diets or others who do not consume vitamin D–fortified milk, especially during the winter months when there is inadequate sunlight exposure.

Vitamin E. Vitamin E was initially recognized as essential for reproduction in rats. Because the role of this vitamin is still not well defined, it has become the target of many unscientific claims. Vitamin E acts as an antioxidant and therefore may serve a role in preventing cell damage from oxidation. Although known toxic effects from excess ingestion of vitamin E are limited primarily to premature infants, persons receiving anticoagulant medications, such as coumadin, may have complications associated with megadoses of vitamin E because it inhibits the clotting action of vitamin K . At this time, there is not enough medical justification for the use of large doses of vitamin E, particularly as it is widely distributed in common foods. A mere ¼ cup of almonds provides 100 percent of the RDA for vitamin E. The frequency of vitamin E toxic reactions is not well delineated, but case reports are few at dosages less than 3200 mg/day (Meyers et al., 1996).

Vitamin K. Vitamin K was first recognized as an antihemorrhagic factor. Because vitamin K is essential for the formation of **prothrombin** (a clotting factor), defective coagulation of the blood is the main symptom of vitamin K deficiency. In addition to dietary sources (see Table 5–1), vitamin K is synthesized by bacteria in the jejunum and ileum.

Vitamin K deficiency is most likely to occur in individuals receiving antibiotics over an extended period who are not able to absorb fat and who have a low intake of foods containing vitamin K. Infants are also at risk because of their inability to adequately colonize the vitamin K–synthesizing bacteria. Vitamin K injections are recommended for newborn infants, and infant formulas are now routinely supplemented with this vitamin. Persons receiving antibiotic therapy should be considered for vitamin K supplementation. Persons who take coumadin to reduce the risk of blood clot formation need a consistent intake of vitamin K to maintain stable prothrombin rates.

Water-Soluble Vitamins

The **vitamin B complex** refers to all water-soluble vitamins except ascorbic acid (vitamin C). Vitamin B_1 was the first of this group to be discovered and was found to prevent **beriberi** (a condition involving inflammation of the nerves). With further study, vitamin B proved to be not a single substance but a combination of substances, each one of which was given a letter or a descriptive term, or later a chemical designation as its chemical nature became known.

Several factors in the vitamin B complex are recognized today. The RDAs have been established for six: thiamine (vitamin B_1), riboflavin (vitamin B_2), niacin (vitamin B_3), vitamin B_6 (pyrodoxine), vitamin B_{12} (cobalamin), and folacin (see the table on the inside front cover). Important functions in the body have been assigned to biotin, choline, and pantothenic acid, but no definite daily allowances have been established, although estimated safe and adequate intakes are now given.

A lack of B-complex vitamins is one of the widespread forms of malnutrition. Because of the similar distribution of the B vitamins in foods, a deficiency of several factors is observed more often than is a deficiency of a single factor. The interrelationship of many of these vitamins in life processes means that signs of dietary deficiency are often similar when the diet lacks any one of several factors (Fig. 5–4). Many physiological and pathological stresses influence the need for the B vitamins, but generally an adequate diet including whole grains will meet these needs.

Thiamine (vitamin B_1). The requirement for thiamine is small but important and is based on the kilocalorie requirement. Thiamine is needed in increased amounts during pregnancy and lactation, but these levels are easy to achieve through an increased intake of food. Deficiency of this vitamin does occur such as when unenriched processed white flour and white rice or sugar is consumed as a main staple of the diet. Deficiency characteristics include beriberi (muscle wasting or edema), mental confusion, anorexia, and enlarged heart. Alcoholics can also develop Wernicke-Korsakoff syndrome (see Chapter 4) and neuropathy, which is associated with deficiency of thiamine but also a genetic predisposition

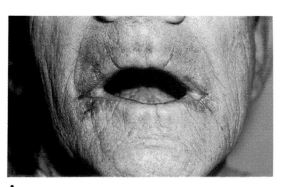

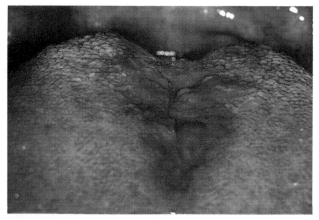

A   B

Figure 5–4

Vitamin B deficiencies. (A) Angular cheilosis due to vitamin B complex deficiency. (B) Depapillation of the tongue from the same cause. (Part A from Callen, Greer, Hood, Paller, & Swinyer: *Color Atlas of Dermatology*, Philadelphia, WB Saunders, 1993, Figure 20–27, p. 326; part B from Murphy GF, Herzberg AJ: *Atlas of Dermatopathology*, Philadelphia, WB Saunders, 1996, p. 322.)

to thiamine deficiency (Manzo et al., 1994). The only known toxicity is from intravenously administered thiamine. However, the potential exists for toxicity from extremely large doses in supplement form, for there is no research showing long-term safety.

Riboflavin (vitamin B$_2$). The requirement for riboflavin is also related to kilocalorie needs. Riboflavin is involved in many enzyme reactions that allow for energy use. It is important for healthy eyes, skin, lips, and tongue with deficiency symptoms associated with skin changes such as chelosis (see Fig. 5–4) and vulval and scrotal skin changes as well as general dermatitis. Without an adequate consumption of milk and milk products, riboflavin intake is likely to be impaired. There are no known toxic levels of this vitamin.

Niacin (nicotinic acid or vitamin B$_3$). Niacin requirements are related to kilocalorie intake and are essential for energy metabolism. Niacin needs are in part met by the conversion of the protein tryptophan, as found in milk and eggs, which can offset inadequate intakes of niacin. The niacin deficiency disease **pellagra** is a syndrome of various skin, digestive, and mental disturbances. Pellagra was once common in the southern United States and still is common in parts of Africa and Asia (National Research Council, 1989). Niacin is a general term but, more specifically, there are two forms: nicotinic acid and nicotinamide (niacinamide).

Vitamin B$_6$. Three interrelated substances—pyridoxine (from plants), pyridoxal, and pyridoxamine (from animal products)—are collectively known as vitamin B$_6$. The need for vitamin B$_6$ increases in conjunction with high-protein diets, pregnancy, certain tuberculosis therapies, certain medications, and some contraceptives. Vitamin B$_6$ functions primarily in protein and amino acid metabolism but is also important in energy metabolism. Vitamin B$_6$ may be of importance in red blood cell regeneration and normal nervous system functioning.

A magnesium deficiency impairs vitamin B$_6$ status (Planells et al., 1997). Excess pyridoxine can be related to neuropathy. Women who take 500 to 5000 mg of vitamin B$_6$ per day to treat PMS (premenstrual syndrome, see Chapter 16) have shown peripheral **neuropathy** (problems of the peripheral nervous system; also commonly found in persons with diabetes) within a few years. The use of vitamin B$_6$ at doses less than 100 mg per day appears safe for adults. Vitamin B$_6$ may be involved in a metabolic derangement, which is correlated with autism (Moreno-Fuenmayor et al., 1996). Renal patients may benefit from higher doses of B vitamins than is currently recommended (Robinson et al., 1996).

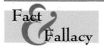

Fallacy: Women experiencing premenstrual syndrome (PMS) should be advised to take a vitamin B$_6$ supplement.

Fact: There is no scientific evidence to support this hypothesis. Women who are insistent on this approach would be better off increasing their vitamin B$_6$ intake through the use of whole grains, such as wheat germ or legumes. A balanced diet, evenly spaced throughout the day to help maintain blood glucose levels, may also be advisable.

Vitamin B$_{12}$ (cobalamin). Cobalt, a mineral, is an essential part of vitamin B$_{12}$. **Pernicious anemia** (a form of anemia that can lead to permanent neurological impairment and death) is caused by a lack of **intrinsic factor,** a glycoprotein secreted in the stomach that attaches to vitamin B$_{12}$ to aid its absorption. Vitamin B$_{12}$ is found bound to protein in foods of animal origin. There is relatively little in vegetables, which is why strict vegetarians (vegans) may need a vitamin B$_{12}$ supplement. Intestinal malabsorption can also cause a deficiency with the ileum being the main site of absorption of vitamin B$_{12}$.

Folate. The active form of folate is folic acid, which is formed from folate by vitamin C. Many forms of this water-soluble vitamin exist. Folate aids in the metabolism of protein and **DNA** (deoxyribonucleic acid, a basic structure of genes and therefore found in all cells). Folate helps prevent spina bifida (a condition that starts in the first few days of conception when the spinal cord is not fully enclosed—it is recommended that all women of child-bearing years consume adequate folate to prevent this condition). Grain products that are fortified with B vitamins now must also be fortified with folic acid.

High-risk groups that may benefit from a folate supplement, as recommended by the National Academy of Sciences, include pregnant women who smoke, use specific medications, abuse alcohol, lack the ability to purchase folate-dense foods, are adolescents, or are carrying multiple fetuses. In normal, healthy adults, supplemental folate can be considered nontoxic, but very large doses (100 times the RDA) may precipitate convulsions in epileptic patients.

Although folic acid is effective in preventing spina bifida in growing fetuses and may help prevent heart disease and some cancers, certain safety issues must be evaluated before the general population is encouraged to increase intake. These safety concerns include problems identifying a B$_{12}$ deficiency with resultant neurological damage, reduced zinc absorption, drug interactions that are designed to inhibit folate metabolism, hypersensitivity reactions, and increased susceptibility to malaria (Campbell, 1996).

Folate got its name from the word *foliage* and thus all dark green leafy vegetables are high in folate. Ideally, raw, fresh, dark green leafy vegetables such as spinach or broccoli should be consumed, because folate may be destroyed in cooking and lost in cooking water. Legumes and wheat germ are also high sources of folate.

Choline. Choline is a constituent of several compounds that are necessary for certain aspects of nerve function and lipid metabolism. No RDA has been established and no disease related to choline deficiency has been demonstrated in humans. Mixed diets are estimated to provide adults with 400 to 900 mg of choline daily, and such diets are evidently adequate. In addition, the body can synthesize choline from methionine (an amino acid).

Pantothenic Acid. Pantothenic acid is an essential constituent of complex enzymes involved in fatty acid metabolism and synthesis of certain products. It is widely distributed in foods and occurs abundantly in animal sources, whole-grain cereals, and legumes. The estimated safe and adequate intake is 4 to 7 mg daily; the higher level is suggested for pregnant and lactating women. Dietary deficiencies are unlikely, but marginal deficiencies may exist in generally malnourished individuals, along with deficiency of other B-complex vitamins. The usual dietary intake is between 5 and 20 mg daily.

Biotin. Biotin is a sulfur-containing vitamin that is essential for the activity of many enzyme systems. It is widely distributed in nature and is bound to protein in foods and tissues. It plays a central role in synthesis of fatty acid and participates in several metabolic reactions. The estimated safe, adequate intake is 30 to 100 µg daily for adults.

Biotin deficiency has been shown to be induced by excess intake of raw egg white or by long-term parenteral nutrition (see Chapter 14). Insufficient biotin content in the feeding regimen results in symptoms such as loss of appetite, nausea and vomiting, hair loss, dermatitis, and an increase in cholesterol. There is no known toxicity.

Vitamin C

Vitamin C (ascorbic acid) performs a variety of functions. Higher levels may be necessary during conditions of stress, with certain medications, or in persons who smoke. Inadequate vitamin C intake may eventually lead to swollen and bleeding gums, loose teeth, and ruptures of small blood vessels (Fig. 5–5), which are early forerunners of scorbutus, also known as scurvy. However, these increased needs can easily be met with an extra serving of a food high in vitamin C. Vitamin C aids in the formation and maintenance of the intracellular cement substance of body tissues thus being important for tooth dentin, bones, cartilage, connective tissue, and blood vessels. Through its role of promoting skin integrity it is thought to help protect the body against infections. Vitamin C helps heal wounds, which is critical for a patient recovering from a surgical operation.

Vitamin C is generally not toxic in doses less than 4 grams per day (Meyers et al., 1996). However, some individuals are at risk of toxicity. These include about one-eighth of the men with an African, Asian, Sephardic Jewish, or Mediterranean

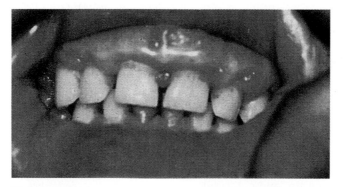

Figure 5–5
Scorbutic gingivitis. (From Nutrition, A Scope Publication, Fourth Edition, Kalamazoo, Michigan, The Upjohn Company, 1980, Figure 53, page 80.)

heritage who were born with glucose-6-phosphate dehydrogenase deficiency. In these individuals, megadoses of vitamin C will instantly affect red blood cells and can lead to death within hours. In addition, megadoses of vitamin C can precipitate an acute sickle cell crisis in those with **sickle cell disease** (a disease in which the red blood cells take on a sickle shape). Also, because megadoses of vitamin C cause **hyperosmotic diarrhea** (which occurs when excess substances attract water in the intestinal tract through the process of osmosis, resulting in watery stools), persons with preexisting diarrhea, such as 60 percent of AIDS patients, can go into hypovolemic shock. One study found safe doses of vitamin C were less than 1000 mg daily, as doses of 500 mg and higher have decreased bioavailability and the absorbed amount is excreted. Oxalate and urate excretion were elevated at 1000 mg of vitamin C daily, which can promote the development of renal stones (see Chapter 10). Daily doses of between 200 to 400 mg of vitamin C were found to be adequate and safe (Levine et al., 1996).

Rebound scurvy may occur if the body has become accustomed to high blood plasma levels of vitamin C and the dose is then discontinued. Instead, health professionals recommend that people in this category gradually decrease from high doses. Much more research is needed on the safety of high doses of vitamin C and other vitamins. A more prudent approach at the present time is to obtain vitamin C and other vitamins and minerals from food sources to help avoid toxicity problems.

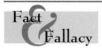

Fallacy: People who have colds should take megadoses of vitamin C (1 gram per day).

Fact: Although cold symptoms may lessen to a minor degree, the risks of large doses of vitamin C can outweigh any possible benefits. Since the RDA for vitamin C is less than 100 mg/day, a 1-gram dose is more than ten times the RDA. This quantity can result in rebound scurvy when the dosage is stopped. Also, a vitamin C supplement that is in chewable pill form promotes dental decay because the acidity of vitamin C is very destructive to dental enamel.

HOW DO MINERALS FUNCTION IN NUTRITION?

As Building Material

Minerals function as building material, as noted in the following:

Bony tissue: Calcium and phosphorus in bones and teeth, and fluoride in teeth
Soft body tissue (muscles, nerves, glands): All salts, especially phosphorus, potassium, sulfur, and chloride
Hair, nails, skin: Sulfur
Blood: All salts, especially iron for hemoglobin and copper for red blood cells
Glandular secretions: Chlorine in gastric juice, sodium in intestinal juice, iodine in thyroxine, manganese in endocrine secretions, and zinc in enzymes

As Regulators

Minerals also function as regulators, as noted in the following:

Fluid pressure: All salts, especially sodium and potassium
Muscle contraction and relaxation: Calcium, potassium, sodium, phosphorus, and chlorine
Nerve responses: All salts, with a balance between calcium and sodium
Blood clotting: Calcium
Oxidation in tissues and blood: Iron, iodine
Acid-base balance: Balance between acid compounds—chlorine, sulfur, and phosphorus—and base compounds—calcium, sodium, potassium, and magnesium

How Are Minerals Classified?

Minerals are usually classified into two groups: major minerals and trace minerals. The major minerals are those present in the human body in amounts greater than 5 grams. The trace minerals are found in the human body in amounts less than 5 grams. See Tables 5–3 and 5–4 for lists of the major and trace minerals, their functions and sources, and symptoms of deficiency and toxicity. The known RDA for minerals can be found inside the front cover. Other trace minerals are now thought to be essential but no RDA has been set for amounts needed for health. These minerals include aluminum, arsenic, bromine, cadmium, germanium, lead, lithium, nickel, rubidium, silicon, tin, and vanadium (Uthus & Seaborn , 1996). It is believed that an adequate diet will allow for safe levels of intake, especially if whole grain, legumes, and leafy green vegetables are consumed regularly.

Major Minerals

Calcium. As calcium phosphate, calcium is the major mineral constituent of the body. Ninety-nine percent of calcium is found in bones (giving rigidity) and teeth, with the remainder found in the blood, other body fluids, and soft tissues. In conjunction with the other minerals, calcium facilitates passage of materials into and out of cells. Vitamin D is required for proper absorption and utilization of dietary calcium. Inadequate calcium in the diet leads to poor bone growth and tooth development, stunted growth, rickets in children (Fig. 5–3), osteomalacia and osteoporosis in adults, thin and fragile bones, and poor blood clotting.

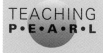 TEACHING P•E•A•R•L
An interesting experiment and useful teaching technique is to soak a chicken bone in vinegar, which leaches the calcium from the bone. This activity clearly demonstrates how calcium lends rigidity to the bone, as without it bone becomes extremely soft and pliable.

Milk, the best source for calcium, is also a major contributor of protein, vitamin D, riboflavin, potassium, and magnesium. For this reason, milk intake is vital for health. Calcium supplements cannot replace the nutritive value of milk. For persons who are weight-conscious or trying to control their fat intake, low-fat or skim milk can be used. Individuals who cannot tolerate milk can use alternatives such as low-lactose milk and soy milk. Figure 5–2 shows where calcium foods are found in the Food Guide Pyramid. Although dark green leafy vegetables are high in calcium, the calcium in chard, beet greens, spinach, and rhubarb generally is not available to the body. This is because an insoluble salt forms with the oxalic acid found in these foods. It is important to note that protein intake may affect calcium needs by increasing the acidity of urine. Vegetarians, with their lower meat and protein intake, generally have a less acidic urine, which helps the body retain calcium.

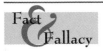

Fallacy: Butter and eggs are high in calcium because they are dairy products.

Fact: Butter comes from milk fat and does not contain significant amounts of calcium. (Margarine, which contains milk solids, has more calcium than butter does.) Eggs do not have any significant amounts of calcium either.

Magnesium. Deficiency of magnesium is rare because normal kidney functioning helps maintain appropriate levels of magnesium in the body. Magnesium deficiency can occur as a result of frequent urination, such as in uncontrolled diabetes, and with the use of diuretics. Conversely, renal insufficiency and reduced renal function in general in the elderly population increase the risk for toxicity symptoms as a result of excessive intake of magnesium. Antacids, laxatives, or other drugs containing magnesium should be used cautiously in such individuals. Along with the other minerals, magnesium is vital for the metabolism of adenosine triphosphate (ATP) and thus plays a role in metabolic processes and muscle contractions. The major food sources of magnesium are those containing chlorophyll (magnesium is a part of the chlorophyll molecule), such as the dark green leafy vegetables.

Phosphorus. The amount of phosphorus in the body is second only to the amount of calcium. The largest amount of phosphorus is found with calcium in the bones; the remainder is in soft tissues and fluids. A wide variation in the ratio of calcium to phosphorus is tolerated in the adult diet that includes adequate vitamin D. A ratio of 1.5:1 is recommended in early infancy to prevent tetany caused by **hypocalcemia** (low blood levels of calcium). Phosphorus helps enzymes act in energy metabolism. Rich sources of phosphorus include protein foods.

High-phosphorus, low-calcium consumption as found when carbonated soda replaces milk as a beverage has been shown to change the calcium-regulating hormones that inhibit peak bone mass in young women. Evidence that high phosphorus intakes may impair synthesis of the active metabolite of vitamin D and disrupt calcium balance, particularly in older women, is of concern (Calvo & Park, 1996).

Potassium. Potassium is an electrolyte. Serum potassium fluctuations can be fatal because potassium affects the heartbeat. This is one reason that taking potassium supplements (as found in salt substitutes [potassium chloride]) should be based on a physician's recommendation. It is imperative that individuals who are taking potassium-depleting diuretics receive additional potassium, preferably through food and again on the advice of a physician. Persons taking hypertensive medications called ACE inhibitors retain potassium and thus need to avoid use of salt substitutes containing potassium. Potassium is necessary for enzyme reactions intracellularly as well as for the synthesis of proteins.

There is no RDA for potassium; however, the recommended intake is about 1500 to 6000 mg, which is easily met by a variety of food sources.

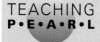

Based on kilocalories and carbohydrate content, leafy green vegetables contain far more potassium than the usually recommended bananas and orange juice for a person taking a potassium-depleting diuretic. One average banana contains 120 kilocalories and 30 grams of carbohydrate. For the same amount of potassium, ½ cup spinach or broccoli provides only 25 kilocalories and 5 grams carbohydrate.

Sodium. Sodium is an electrolyte and is naturally found in low levels in food, although rather significant levels are found in some foods such as milk and certain vegetables. The major dietary sources are table salt (sodium chloride) and foods that have added salt, such as processed meats, convenience foods, and canned vegetables and soups (canned fruit is low in sodium). One teaspoon of salt contains about 2000 mg of sodium.

There is no RDA for sodium, but the recommended range for healthy individuals is between 2000 and 4000 mg, a level lower than that generally consumed. The recommended intake of 2400 mg of sodium per day for the general public appears on food labels (see Fig. 6–1). See Chapter 8 for a more detailed discussion of sodium as relates to heart disease.

Trace Minerals

Iron. Populations at risk for iron deficiency include infants older than 6 months, children through the preschool years, adolescents, menstruating women, pregnant women, and vegetarians. These individuals need carefully planned diets to meet iron needs. Supplements may be necessary during pregnancy.

More than one-half of the 4 to 5 grams of iron in the body is in hemoglobin found in the bloodstream. **Hemoglobin** facilitates tissue respiration by carrying oxygen from the lungs to the tissue cells and by carrying the carbon dioxide formed in oxidation away from cells. Copper, protein, vitamin B_{12}, and folate are necessary for hemoglobin synthesis. Tests for levels of hemoglobin indicate whether **anemia** (a condition of reduced oxygen delivery to the body cells) is present.

Excess iron inhibits absorption of zinc (see Table 5–5), but true toxicity from food sources has been documented only from long-term ingestion of home brewed alcohol made in iron stills. However, toxic overdoses from iron supplements do occur in the United States. **Iron overload** (idiopathic hemochromatosis) has recently been estimated to be a common disorder affecting 1.5 million persons in the United States. Iron overload is highly prevalent among males of northern European descent but also has been found among Hispanics and African Americans, and 10 percent of persons serve as carriers of this genetic condition (MMWR Morb Mortal Wkly Rep, 1996). Various complications of iron overload, such as **cirrhosis** (a disease of the liver), diabetes mellitus, skin pigmentation, **arthralgias** (joint pain), cardiac disease, and fatigue (Adams et al., 1997), can be averted by early detection if those affected avoid excess iron intake with regular blood donation. One study attempted to quantify a hypothesized relationship of iron overload to psychiatric illness and noted that it may be associated with a small portion of treatment-resistant psychiatrict patients (Feifel & Young, 1997). To assess if a person has iron overload, health professionals are recommended to measure the transferrin index, which is the serum iron level divided by measured transferrin. Values greater than 1.0 are associated with this disorder (Beilby et al., 1992).

It is important to recognize that iron comes in two forms: heme, found in meat, and nonheme, found in plant products. **Heme iron**—which is found in high quantities in red meat and organ meats such as liver, kidney, and heart—is absorbed extremely well by the body. In contrast, nonheme iron found in plant foods such as blackstrap molasses, whole grains, iron-fortified cereals and enriched breads, dark green leafy vegetables, dried fruit, and legumes is poorly absorbed unless vitamin C foods or meat are consumed at the same meal. For example, orange juice or coleslaw, with its high vitamin C content, would enhance the iron absorption from a peanut butter sandwich or other nonheme iron source. The use of iron cooking pans is also known to increase the iron content of food greatly; the amount of increase is related to the length of cooking time and acidity of the food.

Iodine. Iodized salt and ocean or saltwater fish are the most common sources of iodine. Inadequate iodine intake leads to goiter (Fig. 5–6). **Cretinism,** or mental retardation, was once a relatively common phenomenon in infants born to mothers who had iodine deficiency during pregnancy. The present intake of iodine in the United States is considered adequate, although use of iodized salt is still important, especially in noncoastal regions where fish intake is limited.

Selenium. The RDA for selenium was first set in 1989 (see the table on the inside front cover). The selenium requirement for adults appears to be related to body weight. Selenium has a close metabolic relationship with the antioxidant vitamin E but other functions are likely to exist.

Selenium toxicity and deficiency have been noted mainly as a result of soil selenium content. Selenium deficiency was first noted in China where it was associated with **cardiomyopathy** (a form of heart disease). Hair loss and toxic defects in fingernails and toenails have been found in regions where there is a high content of selenium in the soil.

Zinc. Zinc is a component of more than 50 enzymes. Although zinc is stored primarily in bone, it is poorly mobilized, and therefore regular dietary intake is

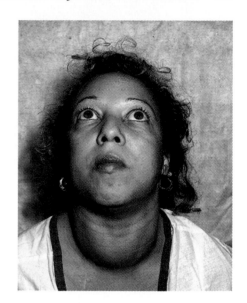

Figure 5–6
Goiter. (From Swartz MH: Textbook of Physical
Diagnosis, 3rd ed., Philadelphia, WB Saunders,
1997, Figure 7–6, p. 140.)

crucial. Individuals with malabsorption, such as those with chronic diarrhea,
chronic pancreatitis, celiac sprue (a condition involving the intestinal tract that is
caused by an allergy to gluten found in certain grains, see Chapters 11 and 15),
Crohn's disease (an inflammatory disease of the intestinal tract, see Chapter 11),
and the short bowel syndrome, are at particular risk for zinc deficiency. Zinc absorption is also impaired by excessive intake of iron, copper, tin, folic acid, and
possibly calcium. Persons who have polyuria from uncontrolled diabetes (see
Chapter 9) or who take diuretics may be predisposed to loss of zinc in the urine.
Zinc promotes cell division and differentiation, mainly because of its role in protein synthesis. It has been found to reduce the risk of retinal degeneration of the
eye among older adults (Flynn, 1993).

Other Trace Minerals

The following minerals do not have established RDAs at present but are essential
to the body. Human requirements for these minerals are not known, but estimated safe and adequate intakes have been suggested until further data are available (see Table 5–6 for copper, manganese, fluoride, chromium, and molybdenum).

Chloride. Chloride is found in extracellular fluids. It is an **electrolyte** (electrolytes conduct electrical flow through the body, as discussed later in this chapter) and is part of gastric juice. Deficiency is generally found only in association
with sodium depletion as occurs with excessive fluid loss as in diarrhea, vomiting, or excessive sweating. The only excess known to occur results from water-
deficiency dehydration.

Table 5–6
Trace Minerals: Estimated Safe and Adequate Daily Dietary Intakes

Category	Age (years)	Copper (mg)	Manganese (mg)	Fluoride (mg)	Chromium (µg)	Molybdenum (µg)
Infants	0–0.5	0.4–0.6	0.3–0.6	0.1–0.5	10–40	15–30
	0.5–1	0.6–0.7	0.6–1.0	0.2–1.0	20–60	20–40
Children and	1–3	0.7–1.0	1.0–1.5	0.5–1.5	20–80	25–50
adolescents	4–6	1.0–1.5	1.5–2.0	1.0–2.5	30–120	30–75
	7–10	1.0–2.0	2.0–3.0	1.5–2.5	50–200	50–150
	11+	1.5–2.5	2.0–5.0	1.5–2.5	50–200	75–250
Adults		1.5–3.0	2.0–5.0	1.5–4.0	50–200	75–250

From National Academy of Sciences, National Research Council: Recommended Dietary Allowances, 10th ed. Washington, DC, National Academy of Sciences, National Academy Press, 1989.

Chromium. This mineral activates several enzymes. It plays a role in carbohydrate metabolism as a component of glucose tolerance factor, which enhances the removal of glucose from the blood through its action on insulin. Good sources of chromium include brewer's yeast, liver, whole grains, meat, and cheese. Most of the chromium is removed from grains during the processing of white flour products and is not returned during the enrichment process.

"Chromium supplements have been purported to increase muscle mass and decrease body fat. However, the preponderance of evidence has not supported this claim. There is little information available on the long-term use of chromium supplements, but at present, supplements within the Estimated Safe and Adequate Daily Dietary Intake (ESADDI) level do not appear harmful" (Clarkson, 1997).

One study found highly significant age-related decreases in chromium levels in serum, hair, and sweat levels, which was associated with the consumption of refined carbohydrate foods (Davies et al.,1997).

Cobalt. This mineral is an essential component of vitamin B_{12}, which is found in animal protein foods such as meat, fish, eggs, and milk. Inadequate intake of cobalt may result in pernicious anemia along with a vitamin B_{12} deficiency. No other deficiency symptoms or toxicities are known.

Copper. This mineral aids in the absorption of iron from the intestinal tract and in the production and survival of red blood cells and is an essential part of many enzymes. There is also evidence that copper helps prevent heart disease.

Fluoride. This mineral helps in the formation of solid bones and teeth. It also helps reduce the incidence of dental caries (see Chapter 19). There is some evidence that it aids calcium in bone formation. The Food and Nutrition Board recommends fluoridation of public water supplies if natural fluoride levels are low.

The American Dental Association recommends fluoride supplements until about age 13 years or until the adult teeth are fully formed. Like other trace minerals, fluoride is toxic when consumed in excessive amounts.

Manganese. This mineral is essential for normal bone structure, normal reproduction, and normal functioning of the central nervous system. It is a component of some enzymes. In general, there is low risk of toxicity but since workers exposed to manganese dust or fumes developed central nervous system problems, it is prudent to limit daily intake to the safe and estimated 2 to 5 mg (see Table 5–6).

Molybdenum. This essential mineral is a component of an enzyme (xanthine oxidase). The role of molybdenum in humans is not well understood but may be implicated in certain neurological dysfunction due to its being an essential component of various enzymes. The foods known to be high in this mineral include legumes, milk, and whole grains (see Table 5–6 for suggested intake).

Sulfur. Sulfur is a component of skin, hair, nails, cartilage, and some organ tissue. It is a component of all body proteins, along with thiamine and biotin. Protein foods are the primary source of sulfur. Little is known about the impact on human health of a deficiency or toxicity.

Nickel, Tin, Vanadium, and Silicon. Findings produced in experimental animal feeding suggest that these elements are essential, but the implications for human nutrition are not well known. Vanadium may affect the activity of various intracellular enzyme systems and alter their physiological functions. There have been accounts of vanadium, in the form of vanadyl sulfate, having insulin-like properties or promoting insulin signaling in cells and therefore helping in blood glucose management (see Chapter 9). One study found that given in 50-mg doses twice daily, vanadyl sulfate was tolerated for 4 weeks with a 20 percent decrease in fasting glucose levels (Boden et al., 1996). Although this is very significant, it is unknown if there will be other side effects if the dose is continued for a longer period or at a higher dose.

When there is little research examining the safety of large doses of minerals, prudence needs to be the rule. This certainly applies to vanadium, in which two forms, vanadate and vanadyl, have been established as likely reproductive and developmental toxicants in mammals (Domingo, 1996). The same applies to arsenic, as high intakes found in drinking water has been associated with bladder cancer (Guo et al., 1997); however, low serum levels of arsenic found among hemodialysis (see Chapter 10) patients may contribute to increased death risk and arsenic supplementation may be appropriate (Mayer et al., 1993).

An assessment of the estimated daily dietary intake is as follows (Uthus & Seaborn, 1996):

Arsenic	12–50 µg
Nickel	100 µg
Silicon	20–50 mg (2–5 mg in dietary intake based on 10 percent bioavailability in natural diets)
Vanadium	10–20 µg

8. While cooking foods containing ascorbic acid, avoid stirring, as oxygen destroys vitamin C.
9. Cook vegetables quickly in a covered container until just fork-tender. Store leftovers covered.

WHAT IS FOOD FORTIFICATION?

The question sometimes posed in the war among cereal brands—"How many bowls of your cereal does it take to equal one of ours?"—is an example of food fortification, which differs from **enrichment,** a method to replace known nutrients lost in processing such as the B vitamins and iron in white flour products. In contrast, **fortification** means "to make stronger; to fortify" and involves either adding nutrients in higher amounts than naturally occur or adding nutrients that are generally not present, for example, adding calcium to orange juice. Food fortification does play an important role in the promotion of the health of our society. Examples are iodized salt, which helped eradicate goiter, and iron-fortified cereal and infant formula, which help prevent iron deficiency anemia. Grain products are now being fortified with folic acid in an attempt to reduce the birth defect spina bifida.

The food industry generally has a profit motive rather than society's health as its basis for food fortification. Advertisements that promote fortified food as the best alternative can mislead the public. To use the preceding example, calcium-fortified orange juice is not a replacement for milk, because milk offers many other nutrients. Also, because we know that overconsumption of vitamins and minerals can be harmful, if not toxic, indiscriminate use of and reliance on fortified foods is not a healthful practice, particularly if those foods are used as a replacement for a balanced, varied diet.

WHAT IS THE NUTRITIONAL FUNCTION OF WATER?

Water is the principal constituent of the body. One-half to three-quarters of body weight is water. Most water is in cells (intracellular), and the remainder is in blood, lymph, various secretions and excretions, and around cells (extracellular). The water requirement for adults is 1 mL per kilocalorie and for infants is 1.5 mL per kilocalorie. Fluid balance is essential, and intake must balance output. Fluid requirements are closely related to salt requirements; intake of increased amounts of water is needed under conditions of extreme heat or excessive sweating. Water is absorbed in the small intestine and colon with digested food. Because water is not stored, daily intake is necessary. Water requirements are increased for infants receiving high-protein formulas; comatose patients; those with fever, polyuria, or diarrhea; or those on high-protein diets. Water is normally lost through urine, in expired air, in feces, and through the skin. Water serves a number of functions in the body:

- Helps every organ to function properly
- Aids digestion, absorption, circulation, and excretion

- Serves as a solvent for body constituents and as a medium for all chemical changes in the body
- Carries nutrients to and waste products from cells as part of the blood
- Participates in the regulation of body temperature
- Is involved with the lubrication of the moving parts of the body

Water can be found in varying quantities in foods (foods contain from 10 to 98 percent water); it is formed in the body's metabolic processes and is an end product of oxidation. The average diet with milk (87 percent water) contains about 1000 mL water daily. With the addition of 1 quart of water (4 cups), the recommended 2000 mL of water can be met. Beverages containing caffeine or alcohol generally should not be counted as fluid because these substances promote diuresis and do not contribute to the body's need for fluid as much as water.

WHAT IS THE ROLE OF THE NURSE OR OTHER HEALTH CARE PROFESSIONAL IN EDUCATING THE PUBLIC ON VITAMINS AND MINERALS?

The nurse or other health care professional needs to be aware of how positive nutritional messages about food can be conveyed in informal settings, such as while a patient is eating a meal. Emphasis should be on positive messages such as "That cantaloupe looks really good. Did you know that one half of a cantaloupe has all the vitamin A and vitamin C that you need for the day?" or "No milk? Can I get you something else in the dairy group—pudding, yogurt, cheese?" These types of messages reinforce good nutritional practices.

It is a disservice to consumers to speak of minerals as if they alone can cure some of humankind's ills. Claims such as "Calcium prevents osteoporosis," "Selenium prevents cancer," or "Zinc promotes sexual performance" have an element of truth but are simplistic messages at best. Rather, a better approach would be to take facts, put them in their proper perspective, and apply them to the relevant food sources. For example, a nurse might say, "Milk and milk products help prevent osteoporosis," "Fruits and vegetables are known to reduce cancer risk," or "Wheat germ and legumes help promote sexual maturation." This approach promotes good nutritional status without placing undue emphasis on one mineral over another. This is particularly important in our pill-popping society in which interactions of one mineral with another or excess intake can lead to toxicity or imbalances.

The health care professional should also assess supplement usage. Are excessive amounts being taken, particularly of the fat-soluble vitamins? For persons concerned with their vitamin needs, a quick comparison of their diet to the foods in the Food Guide Pyramid can decrease fears of vitamin deficiency. People need to be reminded that nature supplies us with our needed vitamins, minerals, and other nutrients through foods; the vitamin pill industry is a profit-oriented one that does not have the experience of Mother Nature. It may be helpful to point out that an excess of one vitamin or mineral (in supplement form) can have a negative impact on the body's use of other vitamins or minerals. Also, it cannot be stressed enough that if a person chooses to take a supplement it should not exceed 100 to 200 percent of the RDA unless advised by a physician. Referral to a medical doctor or a registered dietitian is appropriate for high-risk individuals (persons with an impaired ability to excrete excess vitamins, such as persons with renal disease, elderly individuals, pregnant women, or younger children).

Critical Thinking

Case Study

Maria was surprised her son's iron level was so low. "Antonio Junior's hematocrit is 33 percent and his hemoglobin is 11 mg/dL, which shows he needs an iron supplement," the nurse practitioner told her. "We'll work toward the goal of a hematocrit of at least 37 percent and hemoglobin of 12." The nurse practitioner wrote a prescription for ferrous sulfate and provided a list of foods high in iron, explaining that vitamin C foods help the absorption of nonmeat sources of iron such as dried beans and peas. She further suggested cooking in an iron frying pan as the iron in the pan would increase the iron content of the food cooked in it.

Maria considered what the nurse practitioner had said. Although she had always thought her family ate well, she decided in fact that they did not eat meat often. As the nurse practitioner said also, Antonio was going through a growth spurt and his body simply needed more iron. Maria decided she would ask her sister to ship a case of Grandma Brown's™ baked beans, Antonio's favorite, which they couldn't get where they were now living.

Applications

1. List heme and nonheme sources of iron. Why would vitamin C foods help iron absorption?
2. What positive messages was this nurse practitioner relaying to this mother?
3. What are some signs and symptoms of iron-deficiency anemia?
4. How does food availability affect the ability to eat well? How might rural Americans eat differently than those living in an urban setting or in different regions of the country?

Study Questions and Classroom Activities

1. Bring vitamin bottles to class to identify the RDI percentage of various vitamins and minerals. Do amounts vary from one brand to another? Why might this be? Do any labels show megadoses (greater than 10 times the RDI)?
2. Why do minerals not break down when cooked, as some vitamins do?
3. Why must some foods containing vitamins be eaten daily? Which vitamins can be stored by the body? Which ones cannot be stored?
4. What is meant by the vitamin B complex? What foods need to be included in the diet to ensure an adequate amount of the B-complex vitamins?

5. List the foods in the Food Guide Pyramid, with the correct servings, that will help meet your vitamin and mineral requirements.
6. Calculate the calcium content of your diet. How could you meet the RDA for calcium without relying on supplements?
7. Name several procedures in food care, preparation, and cooking that will help retain the water-soluble vitamins and minerals.
8. Role-play in class, portraying each of three negative characteristics (lack of knowledge, food dislikes, or inadequate food habits), singly or in combination, in order to practice strategies to encourage an adequate intake of foods high in vitamin A.

References

Adams PC, Deugnier Y, Moirand R, Brissot P: The relationship between iron overload, clinical symptoms, and age in 410 patients with genetic hemochromatosis. Hepatology. January 1997; 25(1):162–166.

Beilby J, Olynyk J, Ching S, Prins A, Swanson N, Reed W, Harley H, Garcia-Webb P: Transferrin index: An alternative method for calculating the iron saturation of transferrin. Clin Chem. October 1992; 38(10):2078–2081.

Boden G, Chen X, Ruiz J, van Rossum GD, Turco S: Effects of vanadyl sulfate on carbohydrate and lipid metabolism in patients with non-insulin-dependent diabetes mellitus. Metabolism. September 1996; 45(9):1130–1135.

Calvo MS, Park YK: Changing phosphorus content of the U.S. diet: Potential for adverse effects on bone. J Nutr. April 1996; 126(4 Suppl):1168S-1180S.

Campbell NR: How safe are folic acid supplements? Arch Intern Med. August 12, 1996; 156(15):1638–1644.

Chan MM, Ho CT, Huang HI: Effects of three dietary phytochemicals from tea, rosemary and turmeric on inflammation-induced nitrite production. Cancer Lett. September 4, 1995; 96(1):23–29.

Chandra RK: Nutrition and the immune system: An introduction.Am J Clin Nutr, August 1997; 66(2):460S-463S.

Clarkson PM: Effects of exercise on chromium levels. Is supplementation required? Sports Med. June 1997; 23(6):341–349.

Davies S, McLaren Howard J, Hunnisett A, Howard M: Age-related decreases in chromium levels in 51,665 hair, sweat, and serum samples from 40,872 patients—Implications for the prevention of cardiovascular disease and type II diabetes mellitus. Metabolism. May 1997; 46(5):469–473.

Davis JR, Sherer K: Applied Nutrition and Diet Therapy for Nurses, 2nd ed. Philadelphia, WB Saunders, 1994; p. 227.

Domingo JL: Vanadium: A review of the reproductive and developmental toxicity. Reprod Toxicol. May 1996; 10(3):175–182.

Feifel D, Young CW: Iron overload among a psychiatric outpatient population. J Clin Psychiatry. February 1997; 58(2):74–78.

Flynn ME: Environmental Nutrition. March 1993; 16(3):5.

Gaziano JM, Hennekens CH: Update on dietary antioxidants and cancer. Pathol Biol (Paris). January 1996; 44(1):42–45.

Giles G, Ireland P: Diet, nutrition and prostate cancer. Int J Cancer. 1997; Suppl 10:13–17.

Guo HR, Chiang HS, Hu H, Lipsitz SR, Monson RR: Arsenic in drinking water and incidence of urinary cancers. Epidemiology, September 1997; 8(5):545–550.

Hathcock JN: Vitamins and minerals: Efficacy and safety. Am J Clin Nutr. August 1997; 66(2):427–437.

Knekt P, Jarvinen R, Seppanen R, Hellovaara M, Teppo L, Pukkala E, Aromaa A: Dietary flavonolds and the risk of lung cancer and other malignant neoplasms. Am J Epidemiol. August 1, 1997; 146(3):223–230.

Levine M, Conry-Cantilena C, Wang Y, Welch RW, Washko PW, Dhariwal KR, Park JB, Lazarev A, Graumlich JF, King J, Cantilena LR: Vitamin C pharmacokinetics in healthy volunteers: Evidence for a recommended dietary allowance. Proc Natl Acad Sci USA. April 16, 1996; 93(8):3704–3709.

Manzo L, Locatelli C, Candura SM, Costa LG: Nutrition and alcohol neurotoxicity. Neurotoxicology. 1994; 15(3):555–565.

Mayer DR, Kosmus W, Pogglitsch H, Mayer D, Beyer W: Essential trace elements in humans. Serum arsenic concentrations in hemodialysis patients in comparison to healthy controls. Biol Trace Elem Res. April 1993; 37(1):27–38.

Messina M, Messina V: Nutritional implications of dietary phytochemicals. Adv Exp Med Biol. 1996; 401:207–212.

Meyers DG, Maloley PA, Weeks D: Safety of antioxidant vitamins. Arch Intern Med. May 1,1996; 156(9):925–935.

MMWR Morb Mortal Wkly Rep: Iron overload disorders among Hispanics—San Diego, California, 1995. November 15, 1996; 45(45):991–993.

Moreno-Fuenmayor H, Borjas L, Arrieta A, Valera V, Socorro-Candanoza L: Plasma excitatory amino acids in autism. Invest Clin. June 1996; 37(2):113–128.

National Research Council: Recommended Dietary Allowances, 10th ed. Washington, DC, National Academy of Sciences, National Academy Press, 1989.

Pennington JA: Intakes of minerals from diets and foods: Is there a need for concern? J Nutr. September 1996; 126(9 Suppl):2304S-2308S.

Planells E, Lerma A, Sanchez-Morito N, Aranda P, Llopis J: Effect of magnesium deficiency on vitamin B2 and B6 status in the rat. J Am Coll Nutr. August 1997; 16(4):352–356.

Robinson K, Gupta A, Dennis V, Arheart K, Chaudhary D, Green R, Vigo P, Mayer EL, Selhub J, Kutner M, Jacobsen DW: Hyperhomocysteinemia confers an independent increased risk of atherosclerosis in end-stage renal disease and is closely linked to plasma folate and pyridoxine concentrations. Circulation. December 1, 1996; 94(11): 2743–2748.

Stoewsand GS: Bioactive organosulfur phytochemicals in Brassica oleracea vegetables—A review. Food Chem Toxicol. June 1995; 33(6):537–543.

Uthus EO, Seaborn CD: Deliberations and evaluations of the approaches, endpoints and paradigms for dietary recommendations of the other trace elements. J Nutr. September 1996; 126(9 Suppl):2452S-2459S.

van Poppel G, van den Berg H: Vitamins and cancer. Cancer Lett. March 19, 1997; 114(1–2): 195–202.

Yong LC, Brown CC, Schatzkin A, Dresser CM, Slesinski MJ, Cox CS, Taylor PR: Intake of vitamins E, C, and A and risk of lung cancer. The NHANES I epidemiologic followup study. First National Health and Nutrition Examination Survey. Am J Epidemiol. August 1, 1997; 146(3):231–243.

Zeghoud F, Delaveyne R, Rehel P, Chalas J, Garabedian M, Odievre M: Vitamin D and pubertal maturation. Value and tolerance of vitamin D supplementation during the winter season. [Article in French.] Arch Pediatr. March 1995; 2(3):221–226.

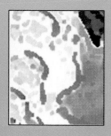

6

Guides for Good Food Choices

Objectives

After completing this chapter, you should be able to:

• Recognize and differentiate between the various food guides available.

• Evaluate a daily diet for moderation, variety, and balance.

• Explain the significance of nutrition labeling.

Terms to Identify

Daily reference values (DRVs)
Nutrition labeling

Recommended dietary allowances (RDAs)

Reference daily intakes (RDIs)

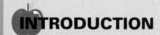

INTRODUCTION

The definition of healthy eating has changed over the years. In the 1940s, there were seven recommended food groups, and butter was one of them. In the 1920s, even sugar was considered a food group. It's no wonder that many older Americans find the new guidelines confusing. In the 1950s, the time the baby-boom generation was being born, the Basic Four Food Groups classification (meat, grains, dairy, and vegetables and fruits) was developed by the U.S. Department of Agriculture (USDA) to replace the older concept of seven food groups. In 1990, the USDA replaced the Basic Four with the Food Guide Pyramid (see inside front cover), only to be met with an uproar from the meat and dairy industries because consumption of less meat and milk was being advocated by their position in the smaller portion of the pyramid. The dried bean and lentil industry was not pleased either because legumes were placed in the upper portion of the pyramid rather than at the base along with other plant foods. Nutritionists also agree that legumes are a healthy substitute for meat and should be recommended for more use, not less. Nevertheless, the Food Guide Pyramid best represents healthy eating in the 1990s and is here to stay until at least the 21st century.

Ever since World War II, the formulation of national and international food and nutrition policies has been based on the **recommended dietary allowances (RDAs).** In the last decade, the USDA, the U.S. Department of Health and Human Services, the American Medical Association, the American Institute of Cancer Research, and governments of other countries including Canada (see inside back cover) have developed guidelines in which moderation, variety, and balance are the focus. The Food Guide Pyramid and the new food labels meet these goals.

Health professionals should understand how to use the new food labels, the Food Guide Pyramid, and other guides such as the RDAs to educate the general public in sound nutrition practices. These guidelines can also be used to evaluate your own dietary habits.

WHAT IS MEANT BY MODERATION, VARIETY, AND BALANCE?

Moderation means that any food can be worked into a healthy way of eating. There are no good foods and bad foods. Foods that are higher in fat and sugar should be eaten in smaller amounts or less frequently than foods that are nutrient dense. Variety refers to eating a number of different foods within each of the food groups of the Food Guide Pyramid—not just the same two or three types of vegetables, for example. Balance refers to the amount of macronutrients as well as the micronutrients in the diet. Selecting a variety of low-processed foods from each of the three lower levels of the Food Guide Pyramid will allow for a balanced diet (see inside front cover).

WHAT ARE THE RECOMMENDED DIETARY ALLOWANCES (RDAs)?

RDAs are the levels of intake of essential nutrients that are judged to be adequate to meet the known nutrient needs of practically all healthy persons. The RDA guide is revised every ten years with the tenth edition being published in 1989. It is shown inside the front cover of this text. Intakes amounting to less than the lower end of the range of the RDAs may lead to deficiency. Intakes amounting to more than the upper limit may give rise to toxic effects, especially involving trace minerals. Recommended dietary allowances should not be confused with *requirements* for a specific individual because requirements vary considerably. Most authorities believe that two-thirds of the RDA will meet the nutrient needs of healthy individuals. However, problems such as premature birth, inherited metabolic disorders, infections, chronic diseases, and the use of medications may require special dietary modifications. These special circumstances are not addressed in the RDAs.

The *allowance* refers to the amount of nutrient that must be consumed to ensure that the requirements of most people are met. Recommendations for dietary intake must make allowance for the portion of the ingested nutrient that is not absorbed or digested. The allowance is set above the average requirement and varies from nutrient to nutrient. For some nutrients, there is limited information about the variability of individual requirements, and judgments must be made. Thus the *R* in RDAs stands for *recommended*, not required.

The allowances for energy are treated differently from the allowances for specific nutrients. Recommended energy allowances for groups of people represent the average needs of individuals, whereas recommended allowances for nutrients are high enough to meet the upper level of requirement among individuals within the groups. Energy needs vary from person to person depending on physical activity and the characteristics of the individual, including age, sex, body size and composition, and genetic factors.

Scientists are now interested in the amount of the nutrient that it takes to prevent chronic diseases from occurring rather than to prevent deficiencies, and this will likely influence RDA numbers. A review of past and current data suggests that the current RDAs for the elderly are too low for riboflavin, vitamin B_6, folic acid, vitamin B_{12}, vitamin D, and calcium and are probably too high for vitamin A (Russell,1997).

HOW DOES NUTRITION LABELING AID THE CONSUMER?

Mandatory **nutrition labeling** went into effect in 1994 with the goal of helping consumers adhere to the Dietary Guidelines for Americans (see the following section). The change is aimed at reducing the prevalence and complications of chronic illnesses, such as heart disease, hypertension, and diabetes (see Chapters 8 and 9). Nutrition labeling is a valuable tool for learning to apply nutrition information in a practical way. A health-conscious shopper uses the percentages shown on the label to determine how well each serving of the food fulfills recommended nutritional requirements. For example, if one serving of a food contains 25 percent of the RDA of a particular nutrient, it means that each serving is good for one-fourth of a person's recommended daily requirement for that vitamin, mineral, or amount of fat.

Ingredients are still listed in order of quantity in a product. If sugar is listed as the first ingredient, the amount of sugar in the product is greater than the amount of any of the other ingredients. It is also easy now to quantify exactly how much is included in a serving of food. For example, one teaspoon of sugar equates to 4 grams on the food label; therefore, a can of soda pop containing 40 grams of sugar is equivalent to 10 teaspoons of sugar. Consumers need to learn how to interpret food labels (see Fig. 6–1).

To calculate the kilocalories in a given food, the food label on larger food packages also lists the conversion factor to change grams into kilocalories—that is, fat 9, carbohydrate 4, protein 4 (refer to Chapter 3). Thus, 1 teaspoon of sugar contains 16 kcalories (4 grams carbohydrate multiplied by 4).

If consumers use the food labels while making food purchases, they will be promoting their health through the inclusion of adequate nutrient intake (protein, carbohydrate, vitamins, and minerals) while reducing their risk of chronic illness through a reduction of fat, salt, and sugar and an increase in fiber. Food

Nutrition Facts

Serving Size: ½ cup whole grain
Servings Per Container: 4

Amount Per Serving

Calories 80   Calories from Fat 18

	% Daily Value*
Total Fat 2 g	**1** %
Saturated Fat 1 g	**<1** %
Unsaturated Fat 1 g	**<1** %
Cholesterol 5 mg	**2** %
Sodium 140 mg	**6** %
Total Carbohydrate 15 g	**3** %
Dietary Fiber 2 g	**8** %
Sugars 2 g	
Protein 3 g	

Vitamin A 0%	•	Vitamin C 0%
Calcium 2%	•	Iron 4%

* Percent Daily Values are based on a 2,000 calorie diet. Your daily values may be higher or lower depending on your calorie needs:

	Calories:	2,000	2,500
Total Fat	Less than	65 g	80 g
Sat Fat	Less than	20 g	25 g
Cholestrol	Less than	300 mg	300 mg
Sodium	Less than	2,400 mg	2,400 mg
Total Carbohydrate		300 g	375 g
Dietary Fiber		25 g	30 g

Calories per gram:
Fat 9 • Carbohydrate 4 • Protein 4

- 1 tsp fat/oil = 5 g fat

- count ½ total fat as saturated fat if hydrogenated

- 1 tsp sugar = 4 g sugar

- ¼ cup sugar = 50 g sugar
                = 50 g CHO

- If fiber >5 g, subtract from CHO

- 15 g CHO = 1 slice bread
            = ½ cup fruit
            = 1 cup milk

- ½ cup beans
  = ±8 g fiber + 7 g PRO

- ¼ cup meat (1 oz)/1 cup milk
  = 7 g PRO + 1–10 g fat
      chicken/fish = 1 g fat
      ½ cup beans = 1 g fat
      red meat = 5 g fat
      cheese = 10 g fat
      nuts = 20 g fat

Figure 6–1
Reading the food label.

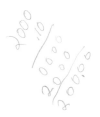

labels used in conjunction with the Food Guide Pyramid can be a highly effective and ultimately simple means to promote health.

The health claims that can be made on food labels under the new law are as follows:

1. Fiber: Foods high in fiber may reduce the risk of cancer and heart disease.
2. Fat: A low-fat diet may reduce the risk of cancer and heart disease.
3. Sodium: A low-sodium diet may help prevent high blood pressure.
4. Calcium: Foods high in calcium may help prevent osteoporosis.

Foods exempt from nutrition labeling include those sold in restaurants, cafeterias, and airplanes, unless a health claim is made. Coffee, tea, spices, and foods produced by small businesses or packaged in small containers are not required to carry a nutrition label.

What Are Daily Reference Values?

Daily reference values (DRVs) is a term developed for the new food labels. This term includes **reference daily intakes (RDIs),** which are essentially equivalent to the old U.S. RDAs. The main difference between U.S. RDAs and RDIs is that RDIs now reflect the *average* amounts of the updated 1989 RDAs. RDIs can be found on the new food labels for vitamins A and C and the minerals calcium and iron (Fig. 6–1).

Daily reference values also include the recommended amounts of fat, saturated fat, total carbohydrate, and dietary fiber based on preset kilocalorie levels of 2000 and 2500 (see Fig. 6–1) on food labels, as follows:

Fat is based on 30 percent of kilocalories.
Saturated fat is based on 10 percent of kilocalories.
Carbohydrate is based on 60 percent of kilocalories.
Fiber is based on 11.5 grams of fiber per 1000 kilocalories.

The reference quantity for sodium intake on the new food labels is 2400 mg/day. This amount will meet required sodium needs in all healthy Americans without providing an excess, although up to 3000 mg of sodium per day for most individuals is also reasonable. Medical conditions may necessitate a smaller or larger intake of sodium. Cholesterol is another DRV not based on kilocalorie intake (300 mg).

WHAT ARE THE DIETARY GUIDELINES FOR AMERICANS?

In 1980, the Public Health Service of the Department of Health and Human Services, together with the U.S. Department of Agriculture, published the first edition of *Dietary Guidelines for Americans*. This report, revised every five years, includes seven recommendations that address the relationship between diet and chronic diseases. The wording of these guidelines was subsequently modified in 1995 to reflect a more positive tone. Table 6–1 gives suggestions on how often

Table 6–1

Frequency of Use of Foods for Implementing Dietary Guidelines

Food Groups	Choose More Often	Choose Less Often	Major Contributions
Fats	Corn, cottonseed, olive, sesame, soybean, safflower, sunflower, peanut, canola oils Mayonnaise or salad dressing (made from above oils) Avocado Olives	Butter, lard Margarine made from hydrogenated or saturated fats Coconut or palm oil Hydrogenated vegetable shortening Bacon Meat fat/drippings, gravy, sauces	Vitamin A, calories, essential fatty acids
Soups	Lightly salted soups with fat skimmed Cream-style soups (with low-fat milk)	Commercially prepared soups and mixes	Fluid, calories (may contain a variety of vitamins, minerals, and protein, depending upon type)
Sweets and desserts	Desserts that have been sweetened lightly and/or contain only moderate fat, such as puddings made from skim milk, angel food cake, fruit-based desserts	Desserts high in sugar and/or fats, candy, pastries, cakes, pies, whole-milk puddings, cookies	Calories (fats, carbohydrates)
Beverages	Water Unsweetened soft drinks Decaffeinated drinks	Sweetened beverages Caffeine-containing beverages Alcoholic beverages	Fluid, calories (unless sugar-free)
Milk and milk products	Low-fat or skim milk Low-fat cheeses Low-fat yogurt	Whole-milk Whole-milk cheeses Whole-milk yogurt Ice cream	Calories, calcium, protein, phosphorus, vitamins A and D, riboflavin
Vegetables, including starchy vegetables	Fresh, frozen, or canned; potatoes—baked or boiled Include one dark green or deep orange vegetable daily	Deep-fat fried vegetables, chips Pickled vegetables Highly salted vegetables or juices	Calories, vitamins A and C, dietary fiber, potassium, zinc, cobalt, folic acid
Fruits	Unsweetened fruits or juices Include one citrus fruit/juice or one tomato/juice daily	Sweetened fruits or juices Coconut Avocado	Calories, dietary fiber, vitamins A and C

Table continued on following page

Table 6–1
Frequency of Use of Foods for Implementing Dietary Guidelines (*continued*)

Food Groups	Choose More Often	Choose Less Often	Major Contributions
Breads, starches, and cereals	Whole grain breads or cereals Muffins, bagels, tortillas Enriched pasta, rice, grits, or noodles	Snack chips or crackers Sweetened cereals Pancakes, doughnuts, biscuits	Calories, B-complex vitamins, magnesium, copper, iron, dietary fiber
Meats or substitutes	Lean meats, fish, shellfish, poultry without skin Low-fat cheeses (such as cottage cheese and part skimmed mozarella) Peanut butter Soybeans, tofu Dry beans and peas	Fried or fatty meats/fish Fried poultry or poultry with skin High-fat cheeses (such as cheddar and processed cheeses) Eggs Nuts	Calories, protein, iron, zinc, copper, B-complex vitamins
Miscellaneous	Herbs, spices, flavorings	Salt and salt/spice combinations	Sodium

foods should be consumed in order to meet these dietary guidelines. Table 6–2 shows the evaluation of an adequate diet for an adult. The seven Dietary Guidelines for Americans are as follows (USDA, 1995):

Eat a Variety of Foods

The greater the variety of foods in the diet, the less likely that either a deficiency or an excess of any single nutrient will occur. Variety also reduces the likelihood of exposure to excessive amounts of contaminants in any single food item. One way to assure variety, and with it a well-balanced diet, is to select foods each day from each of the five major groups of the Food Guide Pyramid (see inside front cover).

Balance the Food You Eat with Physical Activity—Maintain or Improve Your Weight

People who need to reduce their weight should aim to lose a maximum of 1 to 2 pounds per week until they reach their goal. The process of losing weight successfully depends on good eating habits, which include eating slowly, preparing smaller portions, and avoiding second helpings. It is also important to increase physical activity. Emphasis should be on foods with high nutrient density that are low in fat and sugar. Alcohol should be avoided because of its low nutrient density.

Table 6-2
Evaluation of the Foundation of an Adequate Diet for an Adult

Food	Average Serving		Kilo-calories	Protein (g)	Fat (g)	Carbo-hydrate (g)	Minerals			Ascorbic Acid (mg)	Vitamins		
	Household Measure	Weight (g)					Calcium (mg)	Iron (mg)	A (RE)		Thiamine (mg)	Riboflavin (mg)	Niacin (mg)
Milk (whole or equivalent)	1pt	488	300	16	16	22	582	0.2	152	4	0.18	0.8	0.4
Meat group													
Eggs	1	50	80	6	6	1	28	1	78	0	0.04	0.15	trace
Meat, poultry, fish[1]	3 oz (cooked)	85	322	19	26	0	9	2	trace	—	0.09	0.19	4.6
Vegetable and fruit group													
Vegetables:													
Deep green or orange[2]	1 salad or cooked	50 raw or cooked	23	0.9	trace	5	20	0.5	2644	9	0.03	0.06	0.3
Other cooked[3]	½ cup	85	52	2.5	trace	13	19	1.1	54	4.8	0.04	0.26	0.4
Potato, peeled and boiled	1 medium	122	90	3	trace	20	8	0.7	trace	22	0.12	0.05	1.6
Fruits:													
Citrus[4]	1 serving	125	50	0.3	trace	13.5	23	0.4	28	50	0.07	0.03	0.31
Other (fresh and canned)[5]	1 serving	135	99	0.4	trace	25	8	0.6	23	6	0.03	0.04	0.36

Bread and cereal group													
Cereal (whole-grain and enriched)[6]	½ cup cooked	25 (dry)	80	2.2	1	16	6	0.65	379	0.20	0.18	1.5	4.5
Bread (whole grain and enriched)	3 slices 1 whole wheat 2 white	78	170	7	3	40	90	2	trace	0.29	0.15	2.4	trace
Totals[7]			1266	57.3	52	180.5	793	9.61	3358[8]	1.09[9]	1.9	11.9[10,11]	100.3
Recommended Daily Dietary Allowances*													
Man (age 25–50 years: wt, 174 lb; ht, 70 in.)			2900	63			800	10	1000 RE	1.5	1.7	19	60
Woman (age 25–50 years: wt, 138 lb; ht, 64 in.)			2200	50			800	15	800 RE	1.1	1.3	15	60

Data from Nutritive Value of Foods, Home and Garden Bulletin No. 72, US Department of Agriculture.

[1]Evaluation based on figures for cooked (lean and fat) beef, lamb, and veal.
[2]Evaluation based on lettuce, cooked carrots, green beans, winter squash, and broccoli.
[3]Evaluation based on average for cooked peas and beets.
[4]Evaluation based on Florida oranges and white and pink grapefruit—whole and juice.
[5]Evaluation based on canned peaches, applesauce, raw pears, apples, and bananas.
[6]Evaluation based on oatmeal and corn flakes.
[7]With the addition of more of the same foods, or other foods, to meet calorie requirement, the totals will be increased.
[8]With the use of liver, this figure will be markedly increased.
[9]With the use of pork, legumes, and liver, this figure will be markedly increased.
[10]The average diet in the United States, which contains a generous amount of protein, provides enough tryptophan to increase the niacin value by about one-third.
[11]These figures are expressed as niacin equivalents, which include dietary sources of the preformed vitamin and the precursor, tryptophan.
*From National Academy of Sciences, National Research Council: Recommended Dietary Allowances, 10th ed., Washington, DC, National Academy of Sciences, National Academy Press, 1989.

Choose a Diet Low in Fat, Saturated Fat, and Cholesterol

To avoid consumption of too much fat, especially saturated fat and cholesterol, lean meat, fish, poultry, and legumes are recommended as protein sources. Eggs and organ meats, such as liver, should be eaten in moderation. Low-fat or nonfat milk is encouraged. The maximum amount of fat in the diet generally should be 30 percent of total daily kilocalories. Of this amount, an equal breakdown of saturated, monounsaturated, and polyunsaturated fats (10 percent each) is recommended for the general public.

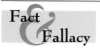

Fallacy: Eggs are high in cholesterol and should be avoided.

Fact: The egg is one of nature's most nutritious foods; it has a low to moderate fat content and provides a good source of vitamins A, D, and B_{12} and iron. Even though eggs contain about 250 mg of cholesterol, researchers now suggest that the amount of total and saturated fat in the diet is more important in lowering serum cholesterol than the amount of cholesterol. Up to four whole eggs per week is considered appropriate although research is beginning to show this may be unnecessarily strict since egg yolks are low in saturated fat. Egg whites are fat-free and thus cholesterol-free.

Choose a Diet with Plenty of Grain Products, Vegetables, and Fruits

Eating complex carbohydrates (starches) is recommended. This can be achieved by selecting foods that are good sources of fiber. For most Americans, a moderate increase in dietary fiber is desirable, although it is not clear exactly how much and what type of fiber we need in our daily diet. There is no need to take fiber supplements unless medically indicated. The use of whole grains and legumes along with the recommended amounts of vegetables and fruits will provide adequate fiber (20 to 30 g daily). Dark green leafy and orange vegetables and most orange fruits will provide more beta-carotene, which is associated with a lower cancer risk. Vitamin C is also associated with reduced cancer risk and is found in vegetables and fruits.

Choose a Diet Moderate in Sugars

Using added sugar in moderation (1 tablespoon daily can be safely included for all persons) and using processed foods low in sugar such as fresh fruits or fruits canned without sugar or those in light syrup will allow for good health. Food labels now indicate sugar content. Sugar in most recipes can be reduced by one-third or more, and spices such as cinnamon, nutmeg, ginger, and vanilla can enhance the natural sweetness of foods.

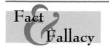

Fallacy: Juice contains less sugar than soda pop.

Fact: Juice contains as much total sugar as does soda pop. The sugar in juice is primarily fructose, whereas the sugar in soda pop is sucrose or high-fructose corn syrup, but they all are simple sugars and will raise blood sugar for persons with impaired glucose tolerance (see Chapter 9). Juice, however, does contain vitamins and minerals, which soda pop does not.

Choose a Diet Moderate in Salt and Sodium

Fresh fruits, vegetables, meats, and unprocessed grains are generally low in sodium. Most convenience foods contain added sodium compounds, and "fast foods" are often high in sodium. Consumption of salted potato chips, pretzels, nuts, and popcorn; condiments such as soy sauce, steak sauce, and garlic salt; cheese; pickled foods; and cured meats and cold cuts should be limited. It is important to read food labels carefully to determine the amounts of sodium in processed foods and snack items. The recommended daily amount as listed on the new food labels is 2400 mg per day.

To avoid too much sodium, only a small amount of salt should be used in cooking, and only a little salt, if any, should be added at the table. In most recipes, the salt content can be reduced by one-half or eliminated entirely. It is good to experiment with spices and herbs for seasoning instead of salt and to learn to enjoy the flavor of foods without salt. Salt substitutes containing potassium should be used only on the advice of a physician, as excess potassium can be harmful for some persons.

If You Drink Alcoholic Beverages, Do So in Moderation

Alcoholic beverages tend to be high in kilocalories and low in nutrients. For persons who drink alcohol, a maximum of one to two drinks per day is recommended. Vitamin and mineral deficiencies occur commonly in heavy drinkers, in part because of poor intake but also because alcohol alters the absorption and use of some essential nutrients such as fat- and water-soluble vitamins.

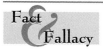

Fallacy: Following the *Dietary Guidelines for Americans* will guarantee well-being.

Fact: Even though good eating habits are basic to good health and vitality, it is important to remember that lifestyle, heredity, and environment also play important roles. Moderate exercise, for example, is a primary factor in controlling hypertension, weight, osteoporosis, and other chronic health conditions.

HOW DOES THE FOOD GUIDE PYRAMID RELATE TO THE RDAs AND THE DIETARY GUIDELINES?

The U.S. Department of Agriculture's Food Guide Pyramid, which was released in the 1990s, portrays the Dietary Guidelines for Americans by emphasizing maximum amounts of foods (see inside front cover). The RDAs can also be applied to the five food group system of the pyramid. Nutritional adequacy can be met by meeting the RDAs through the minimum number of recommended food servings in the Food Guide Pyramid. Choosing a wide assortment of foods from the two lower levels of the pyramid (foods that are high in carbohydrate and fiber and low in fat), moderate amounts of foods from the third level (the protein foods, which generally contribute fat as well), and minimal amounts from the upper tip of the pyramid (added fats and sugars) is advised. Selecting foods in this manner will allow adherence to the Dietary Guidelines for Americans while meeting the RDAs. Other countries have similar guides that vary with cultural food habits and the availability of foods. Canada's new food guide is represented as a rainbow and is shown on the inside back cover. The *Guide to Good Eating* by the National Dairy Council (Fig. 6–2) uses the five food groups and can be used in conjunction with the Food Guide Pyramid.

Similar guides have been developed around the world, including the Mediterranean and Asian Pyramids, which emphasize legumes and oils as being a basic part of a healthy diet, with the Greek Columns food guide specifically recommending legumes six days a week.

How Do the Food Pyramid Groups Supply Needed Nutrients?

As shown in Figures 3–1 and 5–2, all of the needed nutrients can be found in the lower three levels of the Food Guide Pyramid. Complete analytical data regarding food supply and human needs are available for key nutrients (see Appendix 5 for food composition tables).

Foods within the five food groups can also be identified for their macronutrient and vitamin and mineral content. For example, animal products in the milk and meat groups (third level of the pyramid) have more protein and fat than foods found in the fruit, vegetable, bread, and grain groups. Foods in the second level (vegetables and fruits) provide the main source of vitamins A, C, and folic acid, whereas the foods in the base of the pyramid are the main source of carbohydrate and the B vitamins.

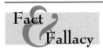

Fallacy: Children instinctively know how to make food choices to stay healthy.

Fact: Children need the guidance of adults in selecting foods. Many chronic diseases such as cancer, heart disease, and high blood pressure may start developing in childhood as a result of poor food choices. Using the Food Guide Pyramid to teach children to eat more plant foods is appropriate.

GUIDE TO GOOD EATING

Anyone can eat for good health.
Just follow these 2 simple steps:

1. **Eat foods from all Five Food Groups every day.**
Each food group provides you with different nutrients.

2. **Eat _different_ foods from each food group every day.**
Some foods in a food group are better sources of a nutrient than others. By eating several foods from each food group, you increase your chance of getting all the nutrients you need.

Every day eat:

Suggested Serving Sizes

MILK
Group for calcium

2-4 servings*

| Milk 1 cup | Yogurt 1 cup | Cheese 1½ – 2 oz | Cottage cheese ½ cup | Ice cream, ice milk, frozen yogurt ½ cup |

MEAT
Group for iron

2-3 servings

| Cooked, lean meat 2-3 oz | Cooked, lean poultry, fish 2-3 oz | Egg 1 | Peanut butter 2 tbsp | Cooked, dried peas, dried beans ½ cup |

VEGETABLE
Group for vitamin A

3-5 servings

| Juice ¾ cup | Raw vegetable ½ cup | Raw leafy vegetable 1 cup | Cooked vegetable ½ cup | Potato 1 medium |

FRUIT
Group for vitamin C

2-4 servings

| Juice ¾ cup | Raw, canned, or cooked fruit ½ cup | Apple, banana, orange, pear 1 medium | Grapefruit ½ | Cantaloupe ¼ |

GRAIN
Group for fiber

6-11 servings

| Bread 1 slice | English muffin, hamburger bun ½ | Ready-to-eat cereal 1 oz | Pasta, rice, grits, cooked cereal ½ cup | Tortilla, roll, muffin 1 |

Some foods don't have enough nutrients to fit in any of the Five Food Groups. These foods are called "Others." These foods are okay to eat in moderation. They should not replace foods from the Five Food Groups.

*USDA recommends 2–3 servings of Milk Group foods. Four servings are recommended on the Guide to Good Eating for teens, adults under 25 years of age, and pregnant and lactating women due to their higher needs for calcium.

"OTHERS"
Category

Fats and oils, sweets, salty snacks, alcohol, other beverages, and condiments

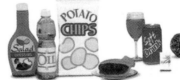

REVIEWED FAVORABLY BY THE AMERICAN ACADEMY OF FAMILY PHYSICIANS FOUNDATION

Figure 6–2
Guide to good eating. (From the National Dairy Council, Rosemont, IL, 1994.)

WHAT IS THE EXCHANGE SYSTEM AND HOW DOES IT COMPARE WITH THE FOOD GUIDE PYRAMID?

The Exchange System for Meal Planning, developed by the American Dietetic Association and the American Diabetes Association, is a food guide aimed at managing diabetes and weight (see Chapter 9 for more information and Appendix 9 for the complete Dietary Exchange System). The Dietary Exchange System groups foods according to the amounts of the macronutrients carbohydrate, protein, and fat that they contain. The Food Guide Pyramid puts less emphasis on amounts of carbohydrate and fat in foods.

The Exchange System for Meal Planning counts cheese in the meat group based on the similar protein content but in recognition of the higher fat content. Cheese is not included in the milk group in the Dietary Exchange System because it does not contain carbohydrate as does milk. The Food Guide Pyramid counts equivalent amounts of milk and cheese based on calcium content.

The Exchange System for Meal Planning counts legumes in the starch/bread group based on the comparable carbohydrate content (½ cup of legumes contains about 15 grams of available carbohydrate). Because of the high protein content of legumes (about 5 grams per ½-cup serving), the Food Guide Pyramid includes legumes in the meat group.

Carbohydrate content of the fruit group is not considered in the Food Guide Pyramid. It counts one whole banana as a serving, whereas the Dietary Exchange System counts only one-half of a banana as a serving. The Dietary Exchange System calculates 15 grams of carbohydrate for one serving of fruit.

The Dietary Exchange System counts a fat serving as 5 grams of fat, which is equivalent to 1 teaspoon of added fat. The Food Guide Pyramid does not specifically state portion sizes for fats.

WHAT IS THE ROLE OF THE NURSE OR OTHER HEALTH PROFESSIONAL IN THE USE OF FOOD GUIDES?

The nurse or other health professional should be aware of nutritional inadequacies or excesses as represented in the Food Guide Pyramid. For persons who require a higher kilocalorie intake, the addition of more foods from the base of the Food Guide Pyramid (whole grains and fruits) would be the wisest choice, although added sugars and liquid unsaturated fats may also be appropriate as a kilocalorie source. Many patients will require dietary modification for various conditions, such as cardiovascular disease, which requires a lower sodium intake. Foods needed for long-term health, however, should still fall within the parameters of the Food Guide Pyramid. In the case of limiting sodium intake, it would be appropriate for a nurse to advise reading labels for sodium content. Emphasis should be placed on the food groups needed for health but with specific guidelines provided, such as fresh and frozen vegetables are low in sodium, whereas canned vegetables are high in sodium. Problems with patient adherence to the goals of nutrition or multiple therapeutic diets beyond normal nutrition should be documented and the patient should be referred to a registered dietitian.

Critical Thinking

Case Study

The young couple was at the caterer's deciding what to serve for their wedding reception. Anna was concerned that they have kosher foods available for her best friend and maid of honor, but she also needed to offer something her dad could eat with his diabetes. They decided that because their friend did eat fish, salmon steaks would likely be enjoyed by all. They also wanted to have shrimp jambalaya for the Cajun side of the family, potatoes with cabbage (which was one of the new groom's favorite foods), and stuffed artichokes (a favorite on the bride's side). The caterer said he would use a small amount of butter in cooking, but would use mostly olive oil because it would be better for Anna's dad's cholesterol level but still had a nice flavor.

Applications

1. Bring food labels to class that show that a type of food is kosher.
2. If this were a wedding where the menu included steak, baked potatoes with sour cream, and broccoli with cheese sauce, what might be done to maintain a diet low in saturated fat?

Study Questions and Classroom Activities

1. How do the Dietary Guidelines for Americans fit into the Food Guide Pyramid?
2. Why should the RDAs not be used to evaluate the adequacy of an individual's diet?
3. Name some of the factors that affect an individual's nutrient requirements.
4. On the table of RDAs printed on the inside front cover of this text, underline in red pencil the figures that indicate the requirements for calories and each of the nutrients for a person of your age, and jot them down on the chart below. You will be referring to these figures throughout the course.

My RDA:

Protein	_____ IU	Folate	_____	g
Vitamin A	_____ IU	Vitamin B$_{12}$	_____	µg
Vitamin D	_____ IU	Calcium	_____	mg
Vitamin E	_____ IU	Phosphorus	_____	mg
Vitamin C	_____ mg	Magnesium	_____	mg
Vitamin K	_____ µg	Iron	_____	mg
Thiamine	_____ mg	Zinc	_____	mg
Riboflavin	_____ mg	Iodine	_____	µg
Niacin	_____ mg	Selenium	_____	µg
Vitamin B$_6$	_____ mg			

5. Bring some sample nutrition labels to class to discuss how you would use the percentage values on the label in planning a day's menu for yourself.
6. Referring to a food label, determine how much protein is needed to meet the 2000 kilocalorie guidelines of 65 grams of fat and 300 grams of carbohydrate.
7. Plan a day's menu using the maximum recommended number of servings in the Food Guide Pyramid for a total intake of about 2000 kilocalories.
8. Assess the following menu for the questions below:

Breakfast	**Lunch**	**Dinner**
Banana	Hot dog on roll	Cheeseburger
Corn flakes	Mustard and relish	French fries
Whole milk	Chocolate chip cookies	Coleslaw
Sugar	Coke	Milkshake
Toast, butter, and jelly		

- Judge the meals according to the Food Guide Pyramid.
- List the foods and amounts lacking for a teenage girl.
- Is a teenage girl likely to lose weight eating this way? Why or why not?
- What suggestions would you make to this menu to have it meet the Dietary Guidelines for Americans?

WHAT HAS HAPPENED TO YOUR FOOD HABITS AND NUTRITIONAL ATTITUDES AS YOU HAVE STUDIED ABOUT NUTRIENTS AND FOODS FOR GOOD NUTRITION?

Now is a good time for you to check your food habits.

1. Keep a record of your food intake (at meals and between meals) for 1 week.
2. Score your diet for each day, using the accompanying Food Selection Score Card, and determine your average score for the week. Repeat this activity later in the semester and compare the scores to see if you have improved your eating habits.
3. Analyze and comment on your last food selection score in the space provided.

Food Groups	Perfect Score	My Score	Comments
Milk group			
Meat group			
Vegetable group			
Fruit group			
Bread and cereal group			
Water	_____	_____	

100

Food Selection Score Card

Score your diet for each day and determine your average score for the week. If your final score is between 85 and 100, your food selection standard has been good. A score of 75 to 85 indicates a fair standard. A score lower than 75 indicates a low standard.

Maximum Score for Each Food Group	Credits	Columns for Daily Check
20	Milk Group: Milk (including foods prepared with low-fat milk, part skim cheese and yogurt) Adults: 1 glass, 10; 1½ glasses, 15; 2 glasses, 20 Children: 1 glass, 5; 1½ glasses, 10; 2 glasses, 15; 4 glasses, 20*	
25	Meat Group: Eggs, meat, cheese, fish, poultry, dry peas, dry beans, and nuts 1 serving of any one of above, 10 1 serving of any two of above, 20	
35	Vegetable and Fruit Group: Vegetables: 1 serving, 5; 2 servings, 10; 3 servings, 15 Potatoes may be included as one of the preceding servings If dark green or orange vegetable is included, extra credit, 5 Fruits: 1 serving, 5; 2 servings, 10 If citrus fruit, raw vegetable, or canned tomatoes are included, extra credit, 5†	
15	Bread and Cereal Group: Bread—dark whole grain, enriched or restored Cereals—dark whole grain, enriched or restored 2 servings of either, 10; 4 servings of either, 15	
5	Water (total liquid including milk, decaffeinated coffee and tea, or other beverage): Adults: 6 glasses, 2½; 8 glasses, 5 Children: 4 glasses, 2; 6 glasses, 5	
100	Final Score	

*Count ½ cup milk in creamy soups, puddings, cream pies.
†Count ½ serving vegetables in soups or fruit in salad
Deductions from final score: Each meal omitted, 10; excessive consumption of soft drinks, 10.

- What improvements have you made in your food selection habits thus far?
- What further improvements do you desire to make?
- What thought have you given to the principles of meal planning as you have selected the necessary foods for your various meals?

Note to Instructor: Each student should keep and score a week's food intake at least once more (preferably twice) before the end of the course.

4. Why are good food habits important? How are they formed? How can they be improved?
5. What are five good food habits for *you* to acquire and follow daily?

References

Russell RM: New views on the RDAs for older adults. J Am Diet Assoc. May 1997; 97:(5):515–518.

US Department of Agriculture, Agriculture Research Service, Dietary Guidelines Advisory Committee. *Report of the Dietary Guidelines Advisory Committee on the Dietary Guidelines for Americans.* Report to the Secretary of Health and Human Services and the Secretary of Agriculture, 1995.

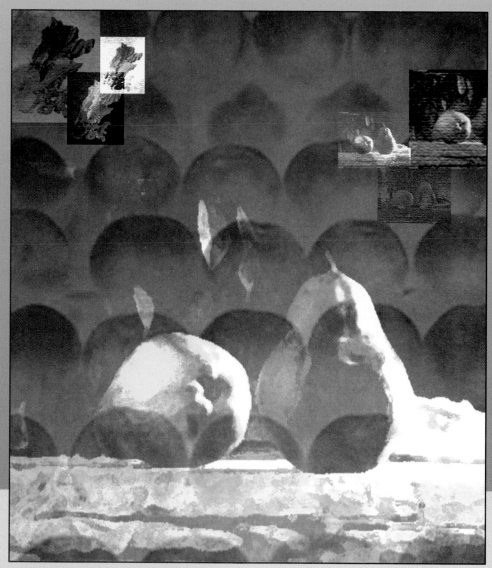

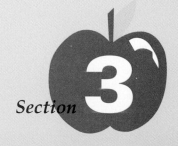

Chronic and Acute Illness

Section **3**

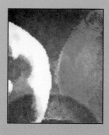

7

Nutrition in the Institutional Setting

Objectives

After completing this chapter, you should be able to:

- Describe strategies used to modify the normal diet during illness.
- Discuss meal service considerations in institutional settings.
- Identify patient risk factors for poor nutritional status.
- Recognize potential drug and nutrient interactions.
- Discuss nutrition discharge planning.

Terms to Identify

Addison's disease	Gout	Polyneuritis
Albumin	Ketogenic diet	Purines
Anthropometry	Megaloblastic anemia	Tetany
Ascites	Midarm circumference	Therapeutic diet
Diuretics	Nephrosis	Triceps skin fold
Dumping syndrome	Osteomalacia	Wilson's disease
Elbow breadth	Pernicious anemia	Xerophthalmia
Gastrostomy	Phenylalanines	
Gluten-sensitive enteropathy		

INTRODUCTION

In the previous two sections, the relationship of good nutrition to health was discussed in terms of the following:

1. Nutrients: their functions, recommended dietary allowances, food sources, and use by the body
2. Foods: nutritional contributions, selection and care, and daily requirements
3. The application of basic nutritional principles to family feeding
4. The nutrition care planning process

The purpose of this chapter is to alert the health care professional to the many types of therapeutic diets used in institutional settings and their interplay with preexisting health conditions such as malnutrition. Specific guidelines on medical nutrition therapy should be provided by a registered dietitian who will look at the total nutritional needs in relation to therapeutic needs. Food can make an important contribution to recovery from illness, through the provision of macro- and micronutrients. Malnourished elderly patients are of particular concern as they experience 2 to 20 times more complications, have up to 100 percent longer hospital stays, and have hospital costs ranging from $2000 to $10,000 more than for younger patients (Wellman et al., 1997). Patients with significant weight loss prior to surgery are at a greater risk of major postsurgical complications. Medical nutrition therapy is a fundamental aspect of total health care. Good nutritional status should be maintained and poor nutritional status must be improved during treatment of illness or injury. More specific dietary intervention guidelines can be found in other chapters throughout this textbook. You may also want to refer to a diet manual such as the one used by your local hospital or by the American Dietetic Association (see Appendix 1).

WHAT IS THE ROLE OF THERAPEUTIC NUTRITION?

Therapeutic nutrition is simply the role of food and nutrition in the treatment of various diseases and disorders. Also referred to as medical nutrition therapy or a **therapeutic diet,** it involves the modification or adaptation of the normal or basic diet according to the needs of the individual.

Medical nutrition therapy may be necessary for one or more of the following reasons:

1. To maintain or improve nutritional status
2. To improve clinical or subclinical nutritional deficiencies
3. To maintain, decrease, or increase body weight
4. To rest certain organs of the body
5. To eliminate particular food constituents to which the individual may be allergic
6. To adjust the composition of the normal diet to meet the ability of the body to adjust, metabolize, and excrete certain nutrients and other substances

WHAT IS A BASIC HOSPITAL DIET?

For reasons of economy, efficiency, convenience, and uniformity of service, a basic routine diet is a necessity in hospitals and other types of institutions that care for the sick. Such a routine diet must be nutritionally adequate to maintain good nutrition or improve nutritional status. The Food Guide Pyramid continues to be the basis for any therapeutic diet.

The basic routine diet, variously referred to from hospital to hospital as the *house, general, regular, standard, full diet,* or *diet as tolerated (DAT),* is served to patients who do not require a therapeutic diet. Many factors affect the choice of foods to be served on this basic diet. For example, the type of hospital (e.g., private or state), budget, food preferences of patients, adaptability to large-quantity preparation, and so forth are taken into consideration with institutional menus.

The consistency of the basic diet may be modified in progressive steps from a liquid diet to a regular diet for a variety of health conditions. Liquid diets are often ordered on a patient's admission to the hospital or after surgery. The most restrictive form of liquid diets is the clear liquid diet, which generally includes gelatin, some clear fruit juices, and fat-free broth. As a patient becomes able to handle milk products, he or she may make a transition to a full liquid diet including cream-based soups and ice cream. The next transition may be to the soft diet, which is moderately low in roughage and fatty foods.

Table 7–1 lists information about each of the basic hospital diets. Some differences exist from hospital to hospital in the foods allowed in each category, as well as in the number of kinds of diets. When a patient is admitted to the hospital, the physician will select the type of diet, often with input from a staff dietitian. In some hospitals, the dietitians are responsible for ordering hospital diets. Diets may be changed if and when the patient's condition makes it desirable. The nursing staff often identifies and communicates needed changes in the patient's diet.

The method of feeding and the time for feeding may also vary. For example, tube or intravenous feedings may be necessary to meet an individual's needs. Sometimes hourly feedings or several meals a day are preferred to three meals daily (see the following section on meal service considerations).

How Are Hospital Diets Modified for Therapeutic Purposes?

The basic diet becomes therapeutic when it is modified in the following ways:

1. The energy value (kilocalories) may be increased or decreased.
2. Fiber (bulk, roughage) may be increased or decreased.
3. Specific nutrients (one or more) may be increased or decreased.
4. Specific foods or types of foods (such as allergens for persons with allergies, fried foods, or gas-forming foods) may be decreased.
5. Any one of these modified diets may be further altered to become a soft or liquid diet.
6. Condiments and any specific foods that the individual cannot tolerate may be eliminated from the diet.

Table 7–1
Progressive Basic Hospital Diets

Clear Liquid Diet	Full Liquid Diet	Soft Diet*	Regular, House, General, or Full Diet
Characteristics			
Temporary diet of clear liquids without residue; nonstimulating, non-gas-forming, nonirritating; 400–500 kilocalories	Foods liquid at room temperature or liquefying at body temperature	Normal diet modified in consistency to have limited fiber. Liquids and semisolid food; easily digested	Practically all foods. Simple, easy-to-digest foods, simply prepared, palatably seasoned; a wide variety of foods and various methods of preparation; individual intolerances, food habits, ethnic values, and food preferences considered
Adequacy			
Inadequate; deficient in protein, minerals, vitamins, and kilocalories	Can be adequate with careful planning; adequacy depends on liquids used. If used longer than 48 hours, high-protein, high-calorie supplements to be considered	Entirely adequate liberal diet	Adequate and well balanced
Use			
Acute illness and infections. Postoperatively. Temporary food intolerance. To relieve thirst. To reduce colonic fecal matter. 1- to 2-hour feeding intervals. Prior to certain tests	Transition between clear liquid and soft diets. Postoperatively. Acute gastritis and infections. Febrile conditions. Intolerance for solid food. 2- to 4-hour feeding intervals	Between full liquid and light or regular diet. Between acute illness and convalescence. Acute infections. Chewing difficulties. Gastrointestinal disorders. Three meals with or without between-meal feedings	For uniformity and convenience in serving hospital patients. Ambulatory patients. Bed patients not requiring therapeutic diets
Foods			
Water, tea, coffee, coffee substitutes. Fat-free broth. Carbonated beverages. Synthetic fruit juices. Ginger ale. Plain gelatin	All liquids on clear liquid diet plus: All forms of milk. Soups, strained. Fruit and vegetable juices. Eggnog (pasteurized)	All liquids. Fine and strained cereals. Cooked tender and puréed vegetables. Cooked fruits without skin and seeds	All foods from the Food Guide Pyramid

Table 7-1

Progressive Basic Hospital Diets (*continued*)

Clear Liquid Diet	Full Liquid Diet	Soft Diet*	Regular, House, General, or Full Diet
Sugar No milk or fats Orange juice may cause distention Salt, plain hard candy, fruit ices, all fruit juices without pulp	Plain ice cream and sherbets Junket and plain gelatin dishes Soft custard Cereal gruels	Ripe bananas Ground or tender meat, fish, and poultry Eggs and mild cheeses Plain cake and puddings Moderately seasoned foods Enriched white, refined whole-wheat bread (no seeds)	
	Puréed meat and meat substitutes only; for use in soups only Butter, cream, margarine, sugar, honey, hard candy, syrup; salt, pepper, cinnamon, nutmeg, and flavorings; puréed vegetables for use in soups only		
Modification			
Liberal clear liquid diet includes fruit juices, egg white, whole egg, thin gruels	Consistency for tube feedings: foods that will pass through tube easily	Low residue—no fiber or tough connective tissue; traditional bland—no chemical, thermal, physical stimulants; cold soft—tonsillectomy; mechanical or "dental" soft—requiring no mastication (diced, chopped, mashed foods in place of puréed); light or convalescent diet—intermediate between soft and regular	For a light or convalescent diet, fried foods, rich pastries, foods rich in fats, coarse vegetables, possibly raw fruits and vegetables, and gas-forming vegetables may be omitted

*Because of trend toward more liberal interpretation of diets and foods, in some hospitals the soft diet may be combined with the light diet, with cooked low-fiber vegetables allowed in place of purées.

Table 7–2 shows how the food groups of the Food Guide Pyramid are included in the modified menus.

How Are Therapeutic Diets Named and Described?

Therapeutic diets are usually named in terms of the diet modification; they are generally not based on the name of the disease, or its symptoms, or the name of the person or persons who originated or modified the diet. This makes possible a universal understanding of terms and also reduces the number of therapeutic diets.

Adaptations are sometimes classified as *qualitative* when they are in types of foods or consistency and *quantitative* when they consist of increases or decreases of certain nutrients or calories. Preferably, every therapeutic diet is planned for the particular patient for whom it is ordered. It is the ultimate responsibility of the staff dietitians to assess the appropriateness of diets ordered by physicians and to document in the patient's chart any further recommendations for modifications to the physician's diet order.

The diet prescription is ideally written in terms of energy requirements based on the individual's weight and activity, and in terms of requirements for protein, fat, carbohydrate, minerals, vitamins, and fiber, with regard for the increased or decreased needs for each because of the patient's illness. The dietitian translates this prescription into foods and meals for hospital meal planning. If the patient needs to adhere to the diet after hospital discharge, the dietitian then instructs the patient regarding the diet. The dietitian reviews with the patient the importance of the diet and offers guidance on how to follow the meal plan at home. The dietitian also communicates with the nurses on staff so that they can reinforce the meal plan with the patient and the patient's family.

What Are Examples of Therapeutic Diets and Indications for Use?

Qualitative Modifications

Mechanical Soft Diet. This type of diet is used for the individual who has difficulty chewing because of a lack of dentures or teeth or because of inflammation of the oral cavity. Severe dental decay may cause pain upon chewing.

Tube Feeding. This type of feeding is used for patients with an esophageal obstruction or severe burns or those who have undergone gastric surgery or who, for some other reason, have an inability to chew or swallow without aspirating. It is also sometimes necessary for patients with anorexia nervosa (see Chapter 15). Tube feeding is appropriate only when the gastrointestinal system is functioning. The site of placement needs to be considered as well. For example, a **gastrostomy** (a surgical opening into the stomach) feeding site may be indicated in the case of esophageal obstruction.

Bland Diet. The bland diet has evolved over time from the sippy diet, which emphasized a high cream and milk intake (with the goal of coating the stomach),

Table 7-2
Menu Modification of Food Groups of the Food Guide Pyramid for Therapeutic Diets

Food Group	Regular	Soft	Liberal Bland	Sodium Restricted	Low Fat	Kilocalorie Restricted
Breads and cereals	All breads and cereals allowed	All breads and cereals allowed Modify in consistency as needed (milk, toast, rice pudding, and so on)	Allowed as tolerated	Avoid instant hot cereals, breads with salted toppings, salted crackers Salt-free products may be used, depending on level of sodium restriction	Avoid products with added fat	Avoid products with added fat
Fruits and vegetables	All fruits and vegetables allowed	Use juices, soft, canned, or cooked vegetables and fruits; chop and mash as needed	Allowed as tolerated	Avoid dried fruits with sodium preservatives Avoid high-sodium canned vegetables and juices	Avoid vegetables in cream or cheese sauces	Avoid vegetables in cream or cheese sauces, fruits packed in syrup Limit to amounts prescribed in diet
Milk	All milk and dairy products allowed	All milk and dairy products allowed	Allowed as tolerated	Milk may be limited depending on level of sodium restriction	Use skim milk and low-fat cheeses	Use skim milk and low-fat cheeses unless calorie level allows use of higher-fat products
Meat	All meat and alternates allowed	Use soft, tender, or ground meats plain or in casseroles and soups	Avoid spicy meats and high-fat meats if not well tolerated	Avoid all processed and cured meats	Use lean meats	Use lean meats, limit to amounts prescribed in diet
Fats, sugars and miscellaneous	Condiments and seasonings as desired Fats, sugar, and alcohol in moderation	Condiments and seasonings as desired Fats, sugar, and alcohol in moderation	*Omit:* Black pepper, chili powder, alcohol, and caffeine-containing beverages	Avoid salt and salt seasonings, salted snack foods, commercially canned soups	Limit use of fats and oils	Limit use of fats, oils, alcohol, and foods high in sugar

143

to a more recent bland diet that eliminates the known gastrointestinal (GI) irritants—caffeine, alcohol, and black pepper—while promoting small frequent meals aimed at diminishing the effects of stomach acid. The bland diet currently is being prescribed less routinely due to the awareness that some forms of ulcers are caused by a bacterium called Helicobacter pylori and are thus best controlled with appropriate antibiotic treatment (Pohle et al., 1997). If this diet is used, it should be individualized so that only known food irritants are eliminated, temporarily, until the gastric ulcer has healed. Moderate amounts of caffeine, alcohol, and seasonings may be tolerated, especially if consumed as part of a balanced meal. Patients who have had chronic gastric ulcers may be avoiding certain foods under the belief they should be eliminated (such as acidic fruits), but this may not be helpful in treatment and may contribute to poor nutritional status if continued long term.

Restricted-Residue Diet. This diet may be used for patients after gastrointestinal surgery or for those with gastritis, Crohn's disease (Matsui et al., 1995), severe diarrhea, ulcerative colitis, diverticulitis (an inflammatory condition of the intestines, see Chapter 11), typhoid fever, or partial intestinal obstructions.

High-Residue or High-Fiber Diet. This type of diet may be prescribed for atonic constipation (intestinal stasis) or for diverticulosis (a noninflammatory condition of outpouchings in the intestinal tract). It is also being promoted for the prevention or therapy of gastric ulcers, cancer of the colon, hypercholesterolemia, diabetes (a condition of elevated blood sugar, see Chapter 9), and obesity. An intake of about 20 to 30 grams of fiber per day is recommended (see Chapter 3 for the average fiber content of foods listed on the Food Guide Pyramid; emphasis is on soluble fiber for treatment of diabetes and its associated dyslipidemia—see Chapters 8 and 9).

Modifications in Carbohydrate

Lactose-Free Diet. Patients who have a total or partial inability to metabolize this milk sugar must avoid lactose in their diet in order to avoid gastrointestinal problems of abdominal bloating and diarrhea. Milk is now available in which 100 percent of the lactose content has been converted to simple sugars for easy absorption by those persons with lactose intolerance.

Diabetic Diet. This diet is carefully calculated for each patient to minimize the occurrence of hyperglycemia (elevated blood sugar), hypoglycemia (low blood sugar), and to attain or maintain ideal body weight and promote good health. Traditional diabetic diets were ordered as a kilocalorie level followed by the acronym ADA, which stands for American Diabetes Association. For example, the diet might read 1200 ADA or 2000 ADA. The ADA acronym is increasingly being described "As Dietitian Advises," because the traditional ADA diet is less effective than individualized medical nutrition therapy as provided by a registered dietitian. Carbohydrate counting is increasingly being used as an effective and easy method of establishing a diabetic diet that is based on individual blood glucose readings (see Chapter 9). In the hospital setting carbohydrate counting may be used with consistent provision of meal carbohydrate (with the option of including sugar into the total meal carbohydrate content), which can allow for improved meal intake while controlling blood glucose. Fat intake may also be modified based on lipid levels, obesity, or for achieving blood glucose goals (see Chapter 9).

Dumping-Syndrome Diet. Patients who have had a partial gastrectomy or gastric bypass surgery may require this special diet. This diet is low in concentrated sweets and limits fluids at mealtimes to avoid "dumping" of the stomach contents into the small intestines, which results in diarrhea. This diet is generally followed temporarily until normal stomach function returns after surgery.

Low-Sugar, High-Protein Diet. This diet is used for patients with reactive hypoglycemia (a condition related to inappropriate insulin secretion, see Chapter 9) and includes six small meals. Emphasis is on complex carbohydrates with protein at each meal although between meal snacks are often well tolerated without inclusion of protein. By spreading the carbohydrate out over the day, in five to six meals, hyperglycemia can better be controlled as well as hypoglycemia, which occurs in individuals who produce excess insulin in relation to carbohydrate intake.

Modifications in Fat

Low-Kilocalorie Diet. This diet is used to achieve weight loss and usually is aimed at lowering fat intake. The ideal proportion of fat and carbohydrate is still unknown although the majority of Americans will likely benefit with a low-fat diet. Other than fat, carbohydrate is the main kilocalorie source that can prevent weight loss if consumed in excess. Persons with insulin resistance (see Chapters 8 and 9) may lose weight better if a more moderate-fat, moderate-carbohydrate diet is consumed. Total kilocalories still best predicts weight loss.

Restricted-Fat Diet. Fat is restricted for patients with diseases of the liver, gallbladder, or pancreas, in which disturbances of digestion and absorption of fat may occur. Generally 40 to 50 grams of fat per day is an adequate and realistic restriction.

Fat-Controlled Low-Cholesterol Diet. This diet is often recommended for individuals with elevated blood cholesterol levels and for those with atherosclerosis (a form of heart disease with plaque buildup inside blood vessels and arteries, see Chapter 8). Individual differences in outcomes of fat restriction in the diet does occur. Those with elevated triglycerides and low HDL-cholesterol (see Chapters 8 and 9) may have better lipid and atherosclerosis outcomes if they maintain a moderate fat intake with emphasis on low-saturated fat, moderate amounts of monounsaturated fats, and moderate carbohydrate restriction.

High-Fat Diet. This diet may be indicated for purposes of weight gain. The type of fat ideally should be monounsaturated fat, to help prevent cardiovascular disease and cancer. The maximum fat intake is generally 35 to 40 percent of kilocalories.

Ketogenic Diet. In some cases, a **ketogenic diet** is used to control a type of epilepsy. This diet is extremely high in fat (85 percent) with protein (10 percent) and carbohydrate (5 percent). Close medical supervision is required to ensure individual tolerance and achievement of treatment goals (reduced seizure activity).

Modifications in Protein

Restricted-Protein Diet. This diet is used for patients in hepatic coma or with chronic uremia (a condition of severe kidney disease, see Chapter 10), renal disease (kidney disease), or liver disease. Generally the lowest protein intake recommended is 0.8 grams of protein per kilogram of body weight. Adequate kilocalorie intake is also important.

Gluten-Free Diet. Gluten is the protein found in grains. Individuals with celiac disease (often referred to as nontropical sprue in children and also known as **gluten-sensitive enteropathy,** see Chapter 11) have gluten intolerance and must be on a gluten-free diet. Foods omitted are those that contain even trace amounts of wheat, oats, rye, barley, and triticale (a hybrid grain). This is a very difficult diet to follow due to the use of wheat in manufacturing a wide variety of foods. A medical diagnosis via intestinal biopsy is advised prior to initiation of a gluten-free diet due to the difficulty in adhering to it.

Restricted-Phenylalanine Diet. This diet is used in confirmed cases of phenylketonuria (PKU) (an inborn error of metabolism, see Chapter 18), in which **phenylalanines** (a type of amino acid) cannot be processed by the body. All babies have a PKU test at birth; those without PKU need not worry about phenylalanine in the diet.

Restricted-Purine Diet. A decrease in **purines** (a form of protein) may be useful in lowering the blood uric acid level in **gout** (an inflammatory condition of the joints). There is new evidence, however, that gout is a very strong marker for insulin resistance (see Chapter 9). We may learn that medical nutrition therapy used to treat insulin resistance (low saturated fat with high soluble fiber and moderate carbohydrate intake) will also have a favorable impact on gout.

Low-Tyramine Diet. This diet is designed to restrict foods containing tyramine and related compounds. It is used for patients who are taking medications known as monoamine oxidase (MAO) inhibitors for clinical depression. The diet helps to prevent adverse reactions such as palpitation, severe headache, and hypertension. Table 7–3 lists foods excluded on a low-tyramine diet.

High-Protein Diet. A high-protein diet is used to correct a protein inadequacy for any reason such as pre- and postoperative nutritional needs, high fever, burns, injuries, increased metabolism, **nephrosis** (a form of kidney disease found in children that may or may not be treated with a high-protein diet), chronic nephritis (unless there is nitrogen retention), **pernicious anemia** (a form of megaloblastic anemia characterized by lack of vitamin B_{12}, a vitamin found in animal protein foods such as meat and milk), ulcerative colitis, hepatitis (inflammation of the liver, see Chapter 11), celiac disease and cystic fibrosis, tuberculosis and other wasting diseases, wounds, or nutritional anemia. A low serum **albumin** level (a lab value that indicates protein status) may indicate a need for a high-protein diet.

Modifications in Minerals and Electrolytes

Restricted-Sodium Diet. This type of diet is very common and is prescribed for patients with congestive heart failure, hypertension, renal disease with edema, cirrhosis of the liver with **ascites** (a buildup of abdominal fluid often associated with liver disease), and possibly for toxemia, also referred to as preg-

Table 7-3
Foods Excluded on a Low-Tyramine Diet

Aged cheese—All cheeses except cottage, cream, and other unripened cheeses
Fermented sausage—Bologna, salami, pepperoni, and liver sausage
Pickled herring and salted dried fish
Broad beans and pods—Lima and Italian beans, lentils, snow peas, dried beans and
    peas, and soybeans
Fruits—Bananas, avocados, canned figs, and raisins
Cultured dairy products—Buttermilk, yogurt, and sour cream
Chocolate and products made with chocolate
Caffeine—Coffee, tea, and cola drinks
Beer and ale
Wines (especially Chianti)
Yeast extracts
Licorice
Soy sauce and any food product that is made with soy sauce

nancy-induced hypertension (see Chapter 16 for further discussion). The level of sodium restriction most often ranges between 2000 and 3000 mg sodium per day. More restrictive sodium levels, such as 1000 mg, are generally reserved for congestive heart failure.

Increased-Sodium Diet. This type of diet may be useful in treating **Addison's disease** (in which the body loses excess salt). A high level of sodium (4000 to 6000 mg) is easily included in a day's diet.

Restricted-Potassium Diet. If potassium is not excreted from the body properly, a restricted diet may be necessary. This commonly occurs in people with renal disease (see Table 10–3 for food items low in potassium).

Increased-Potassium Diet. Persons on potassium-depleting medications, such as diuretics, need to have a high-potassium diet. Table 7–4 lists high-potassium foods.

Restricted-Copper Diet. Wilson's disease (in which the body stores excess amounts of copper), oliguria, and anuria (see Chapter 10) all call for a restriction of copper intake. High-copper foods such as shellfish, liver, legumes, and whole grains should be avoided (see Table 5–4 and Fig. 5–2).

High-Calcium and High-Phosphorus Diet. An increase in calcium and phosphorus intake is desirable in a person with rickets, **osteomalacia** (a condition in which the bones become soft unless the condition is due to renal disease—see Chapter 10), **tetany** (a condition that comprises muscle spasms generally related to low blood levels of calcium), dental caries due to poor calcification of teeth, and acute lead poisoning.

High-Iron Diet. Nutritional or hemorrhagic anemia calls for a high intake of dietary iron. Only iron-deficient forms of anemia are treated with iron.

High-Vitamin Diet. If a specific vitamin deficiency is diagnosed, an increased intake of vitamins may be necessary. An increase in vitamin A is necessary to combat night blindness and **xerophthalmia** (an eye disease); increased intake of vitamin D is recommended for rickets and osteomalacia; increased vitamin K is

Table 7–4
Foods High in Potassium

Very High Potassium Sources (>300 mg potassium)	Moderately High Potassium Sources (>200 mg potassium)
Milk, 1 c	Grapefruit, 1 whole
Yogurt, 1 c	Oranges, 1 whole or 4 oz juice
Apricots, 3 whole or 6 halves	Green beans, 1 c
Banana, 1 small	Tomato, 1 whole or ½ c juice
Broccoli, 1 stalk or 1 c cooked	Peanut butter, 2 tbsp
Cantaloupe, 1 quarter	Molasses, 1 tsp blackstrap or 4 tsp "green label"
Carrots, 1 c cooked	
Potatoes, ½ c	
Spinach, ½ c cooked	
Turnips, 1 c cooked	
Winter squash, ½ baked	
Legumes (dried beans and peas), ½ c cooked	

needed in persons receiving long-term antibiotics who have fat malabsorption; increased thiamine (vitamin B_1) is necessary to avoid beriberi and **polyneuritis** (inflammation of nerves); increased niacin (vitamin B_3) is needed to combat pellagra; and increased ascorbic acid (vitamin C) may improve wound healing and fight scurvy. Increasingly, antioxidant vitamin supplements (vitamins A, C, and E) are being recommended, although the ideal amounts are not known for individual safety and efficacy needs. Foods remain the medium of choice for increased vitamin intake due to the naturally occuring phytochemicals found in food that are not found in supplements.

WHAT ARE SOME COMMON TEST DIETS?

A variety of diets have been established to aid in the assessment of certain disorders or as part of diagnostic tests. The following are among the most common.

Fecal Fat Determination Diet. It is necessary to measure fecal fat for one step in the diagnosis of cystic fibrosis or malabsorption syndromes. The test diet includes a minimum of 100 g of fat per day for 2 to 3 days prior to the test.

Glucose Tolerance Test Diet. This is a test done in the fasting state, which is used to diagnose gestational diabetes (see Chapter 9). It is also used in the diagnosis of reactive hypoglycemia, although there is some controversy as to duration of test (3 hours versus 6 hours) and interpretation of results.

Meat-Free Test Diet. Meat, poultry, and fish contain hemoglobin, myoglobin, and enzymes that may give a false positive result in tests for gastrointestinal bleeding. Therefore, patients scheduled for these tests must sometimes eat a meat-free diet for as many as 4 days before the tests.

Calcium Test Diet. This test determines urinary calcium excretion, as for the diagnosis of hypercalciuria. A diet of 1000 mg of calcium is necessary and may be supplied with a combination of dietary and supplemental intake. Three cups of milk or its equivalent will provide almost 1000 mg of calcium.

WHAT ARE IMPORTANT CONSIDERATIONS IN MEAL SERVICE?

Attractive food service plays an important role in stimulating the appetite and enjoyment of food. A good appetite is necessary to ensure adequate nutritional intake. Mealtime is often the major event of the day for the patient, and every effort must be made to prepare the room and the patient to receive the meal. Some patients eat better if arrangements can be made for the use of china dishware. Holidays are often a time of sadness for patients in an institutional setting. Using colorful napkins and tray decorations at these times can stimulate the appetite.

The patient's attitude toward food may reflect a more general attitude toward illness, as it may be the one area about which a patient feels free to vent negative feelings. The nurse needs to listen to what the patient is really saying (the underlying message). Any complaints of meal service should be taken seriously, especially if the patient's food intake is poor. A request for a staff dietitian consultation is appropriate when the complaints are severe enough that the patient is at nutritional risk. Food from home can be calculated into the diet when a cooperative plan is made. Health professionals need to exert caution to ensure food poisoning does not result. Poor food handling at home or failure to keep hot foods hot while they are being transported to the hospital can cause food poisoning (see Chapter 22).

What Are Some Suggestions for Assisting a Patient During Mealtimes?

The patient's room should be adjusted for adequate but not glaring light and a comfortable temperature. If the patient wears glasses, make sure that they are on and are clean. If the patient is blind, the foods should be described before eating begins. Medication for pain or nausea is sometimes indicated for improved meal intake.

It is important that you, as the person assisting the patient, be relaxed and seated in a comfortable position. You should engage in pleasant neutral conversation, avoiding discussion of the patient's illness or any criticism of the meal or the patient. This is a good time to teach the patient. Explain the reasons for the various foods offered, especially if the patient does not understand the diet well.

If the patient must be fed, you should alternate one food with another and offer liquids frequently. Offer liquids also whenever they are requested. Open containers, cut meat, and apply condiments if necessary to ensure an adequate intake. If the patient cannot eat a meal or a portion of the meal for valid reasons, such as the meat being too tough, offer to get substitute food (providing the patient's condition warrants it).

How Can the Hospital Diet Be Modified for the Patient Who Cannot Eat Enough at Mealtimes?

A referral to a staff dietitian should be made for a patient who is losing weight or not gaining weight adequately. The person may be a candidate for the following:

- Between-meal nourishments such as sandwiches, puddings, or milkshakes
- Addition of high kilocalorie items on meal trays such as extra margarine, mayonnaise, gravy, or desserts
- Liquid nutritional supplements with meal trays or between meals
- Tube feedings or total parenteral nutrition (the provision of a special liquid nutrition mixture through an artery, see Chapter 14)

WHAT IS LONG-TERM CARE?

Long-term care consists of a whole group of medical and psychosocial activities and services designed to keep a person as independent as possible for as long as possible. Acute care is undertaken in a hospital setting, whereas long-term care is provided in a variety of settings. Currently, long-term care generally involves placing the patient in a nursing home. As the cost of health care continues to rise, the setting is increasingly changing to the home or small group homes. Services brought to the patient such as meals, home-health aide assistance, and public health nursing can help maintain a person's independence.

One approach used in long-term care is characterized by staff performing *for* the resident, resulting in a lack of progress on the part of the patient. In respect to nutrition, the resident who is wheelchair bound may not be allowed independence in wheeling to the dining room or may be fed instead of assisted, even though encouragement, adaptive feeding utensils, and transfer to a regular chair may promote independence. The preferred approach is characterized by allowing the resident to do things for himself or herself, such as ambulating independently to the dining area and self-feeding. The focus is on consumption of a balanced meal, appropriate food consistency, and where and how the meal is consumed. The dining atmosphere, quality of food, and the service provided are all conducive to rehabilitation.

HOW DOES THE HEALTH CARE TEAM FUNCTION IN THE INSTITUTIONAL SETTING?

The institutional setting is the ideal place for implementing the total health care team philosophy. Most, if not all, of the respective health care professionals are available for consultation by each team member. Recommendations for input by the various health care professionals should be documented in the patient charts and personal or verbal contact should be made. This form of communication will help ensure that patients receive the best care possible and do not accidentally "slip through the cracks." The nurse is in the ideal position to make sure all necessary health care professionals are consulted. Regular team meetings can help ensure effective coordination of patient care.

Various activities or interventions are needed to carry out plans to meet patient-centered nutritional goals. They include diet prescription, any necessary modification of food consistency, nutritional supplements, nutritional support, assistance and encouragement at mealtime, counseling, and advice about meeting the individual's nutritional needs after discharge. Implementation includes ongoing monitoring of laboratory data, weight records, and food and fluid intake.

Each member of the health care team has an opportunity to aid in implementing the nutrition care plan, whether it be in the form of encouraging the patient to eat, providing adaptive eating equipment, or encouraging the patient to exercise and socialize.

HOW IS NUTRITIONAL STATUS ASSESSED?

As soon as the patient arrives at the institution, members of the health team proceed to gather pertinent and accurate information. Professionally standardized techniques are used in assessing three main areas: (1) dietary history, (2) anthropometry, and (3) biochemical and clinical data. The patient is ideally weighed at admission and several body measurements, including height, are taken. The nurse inquires about food intolerances and allergies. If family members are present, they may also contribute to the assessment by revealing the individual's past health and eating habits. The social worker writes the social history, which the dietitian uses in gathering dietary information. The physician's report of the physical examination; results of blood, urine, and skin tests; anthropometric measurements; and the diet history are equally important in assessing nutritional status, which is the first step in nutritional care planning.

The data obtained are recorded and analyzed so that the health care professional can identify those individuals who may need prompt nutritional support and those who may need only a modified diet and counseling. Very often a person looks well nourished but through proper assessment is found to be in a high-risk state. Table 7–5 gives indicators of good and poor nutritional status.

Dietary History

Many factors influence a person's nutritional status, and they should be taken into account in a dietary history. Asking what types of foods the individual eats and how often—over at least a 24-hour period or ideally for an average of 3 to 7 days—will help the dietitian determine if the patient is in the habit of consuming the basic five food groups regularly. Appetite and weight changes may be significant and should be analyzed. There may also be a recent change in eating habits as a result of illness. Recent versus usual dietary intake should be noted. It is important to note if the patient has unintentionally lost more than 10 pounds within the last 6 months, and it is especially important to note if there has been a more rapid weight loss. Chewing and swallowing difficulties can hamper the individual's intake of food and may thus be detrimental to nutritional status. A sore mouth and ill-fitting dentures are potential problems to be noted in the dietary history. Medications and illnesses, especially those involving the gastrointestinal tract, are noted because they may affect the appetite, nutrient utilization, or both. Elimination practices may indicate the need for additional roughage and liquids.

Cultural and religious food habits, food preferences, the impact of food and drug interactions, meal patterns, and lifestyle cannot be overlooked in planning

Table 7–5
Physical Signs Indicative or Suggestive of Malnutrition

	Normal Appearance	Signs Associated with Malnutrition	Possible Disorder or Nutrient Deficiency	Possible Nonnutritional Problem
Hair	Shiny; firm; not easily plucked	Lack of natural shine; dull and dry Thin and sparse Dyspigmented Flag sign Easily plucked (no pain)	Kwashiorkor and, less commonly, marasmus	Excessive bleaching of hair Alopecia
Face	Skin color uniform; smooth, healthy appearance; not swollen	Nasolabial seborrhea (scaling of skin around nostrils) Swollen face (moon face) Paleness	Riboflavin Kwashiorkor	Acne vulgaris
Eyes	Bright, clear, shiny; no sores at corners of eyelids; membranes a healthy pink and moist; no prominent blood vessels or mound of tissue or sclera	Pale conjunctiva Bitot's spots Conjunctival xerosis (dryness) Corneal xerosis (dullness) Keratomalacia (softening of cornea) Redness and fissuring of eyelid corners Corneal arcus (white ring around eye) Xanthelasma (small yellowish lumps around eyes)	Anemia (e.g., iron) Vitamin A Riboflavin, pyridoxine Hyperlipidemia	Bloodshot eyes from exposure to weather, lack of sleep, smoke, or alcohol
Lips	Smooth, not chapped or swollen	Angular cheilosis (white or pink lesions at corners of mouth)	Riboflavin	Excessive salivation from improper fitting dentures
Tongue	Deep red in appearance; not swollen or smooth	Magenta tongue (purplish) Filiform papillae atrophy or hypertrophy —red tongue	Riboflavin Folic acid Niacin	Leukoplakia
Teeth	No cavities; no pain; bright	Mottled enamel Caries (cavities) Missing teeth	Fluorosis Excessive sugar	Malocclusion Periodontal disease Health habits
Gums	Healthy; red; do not bleed; not swollen	Spongy, bleeding Receding gums	Vitamin C	Periodontal disease

Table 7–5
Physical Signs Indicative or Suggestive of Malnutrition (*continued*)

	Normal Appearance	Signs Associated with Malnutrition	Possible Disorder or Nutrient Deficiency	Possible Nonnutritional Problem
Glands	Face not swollen	Thyroid enlargement (front of neck swollen)	Iodine	Allergic or inflammatory enlargement of thyroid
		Parotid enlargement (cheeks become swollen)	Starvation Bulimia	
Nervous system	Psychological stability; normal reflexes	Psychomotor changes	Kwashiorkor	
		Mental confusion	Thiamine	
		Sensory loss		
		Motor weakness		
		Loss of position sense		
		Loss of vibration	Thiamine	
		Loss of ankle and knee jerks		
		Burning and tingling of hands and feet (paresthesia)		
		Dementia	Niacin, vitamin B_{12}	

From Mahan CK, Escott-Stump S: Krause's Food, Nutrition and Diet Therapy, 9th ed. Philadelphia, WB Saunders, 1996, p. 380.

nutritional care for an individual. The psychological significance of food needs to be considered. Food may have been used as a reward or withheld during punishment, which can affect why a person chooses specific foods to eat or to avoid. The fact that food tastes and habits cannot be changed overnight—or, in some cases, ever—must be understood by the health care professional. Minor modification of the diet may be the best goal in many situations.

No nutrition care plan, including the therapeutic diet, will be effective if the meals are not eaten. The patient's own acceptance of the plan is as important a factor in recovery (or more important in some cases) as medication or physical treatment. Timing of medications in relation to mealtimes may need to be considered in order to promote better nutritional intake. Scheduling of tests in consideration of mealtime is also important. The nurse can be very helpful in arranging logistics of patient care while ensuring that the patient has adequate time and opportunity to eat meals. Some attention to food preferences, as much as is possible with the necessary dietary restrictions and limited hospital personnel facilities, needs to be made. Attention to the appearance and service of the food and the attitude of the person who serves it also contribute to the acceptance of the diet and the success of treatment.

Anthropometry

The science that deals with body measurements, such as size, weight, and proportions, is called **anthropometry.** It is especially useful in screening hospitalized patients who may have varying degrees of protein-energy malnutrition (kwashiorkor and marasmus are two forms, see Chapter 3). This condition is most likely to develop when the patient is under the stress of an acute illness or major surgery, at which time the desire or ability to eat is impaired. Risk of infection and complications may easily develop. Hospitalized patients are at high risk for malnutrition upon arrival but vigilence is required to prevent its development or worsening in the hospital. This condition has been referred to as the "skeleton in the closet," because malnourished hospitalized patients have often gone unrecognized in the past. The nurse is in the ideal position to note patient dietary intake and changes in anthropometric or biochemical data in order to alert the physician or clinical dietitian to the need for more aggressive nutritional support.

Who Should Be Assessing Anthropometry?

The nurse is in the best position to monitor patient weight status. It is especially important to regularly monitor weights of children (Fig. 7–1), and any undesirable changes should be reported to the staff dietitian. Weight monitoring should be done on a weekly basis. High-risk patients can benefit from daily weight monitoring, which can give health professionals the information they need to aggressively treat fluid problems. Hospitalized patients may be weighed using a bed scale (Fig. 7–2).

The dietitian is the professional trained in anthropometry; he or she takes measurements of elbow breadth, skin-fold thickness, and mid-upper arm circum-

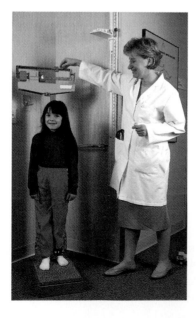

Figure 7–1

Monitoring patient weight. (From Jarvis C: Physical Examination and Health Assessment. Philadelphia, WB Saunders, 1996, p. 881.)

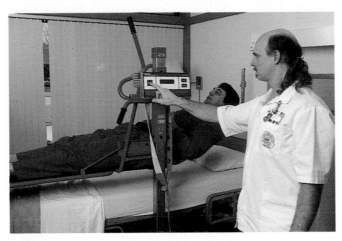

Figure 7–2
Using a bed scale to assess body weight. (From Lindeman C,
McAthie M: Fundamentals of Contemporary Nursing Practice,
Philadelphia, WB Saunders, 1999.)

ference to help determine the extent of the body's fat and protein stores in relation to body frame size and height. A discussion of various anthropometric measurements follows.

Triceps Skin Fold. Triceps skin fold is an index of the body's fat or energy stores. A low skin-fold thickness measurement may indicate malnutrition. Figure 7–3 shows how the measurement is taken. This technique is used for both men and women. The most common site for measuring skin-fold thickness is the posterior side of the upper arm at the midpoint. Accuracy and consistency of measurement are paramount.

Midarm Circumference. Midarm circumference indicates the level of the body's protein stores, which are found mainly in the muscles. The nondominant arm is flexed at a 90-degree angle, and the circumference is measured with a nonstretchable measuring tape after the midpoint of the upper arm is determined (see Fig. 7–3).

Elbow Breadth. Elbow breadth determines body frame size. It is a reliable measurement that changes little with age and is not affected by body fat stores. The elbow breadth measurement is helpful in determining desirable weight ranges, because body frame size reflects factors that influence weight, such as bone thickness, muscularity, and length of trunk in relation to total height. Calipers are applied to either side of the two prominent bones of the elbow while the forearm is bent upward at a 90-degree angle. The fingers are straight and the inside of the wrist is turned toward the body. See Appendix 11 for frame size measurements.

Body Weight. This measurement is often expressed as relative weight, desirable weight, or as a percentage of usual weight. Any assessment of body weight can be misleading if the patient is retaining fluid or is dehydrated. Weight loss is best expressed in terms of percentage of weight change:

$$\text{Usual weight} - \text{present weight} \div \text{usual weight} \times 100$$

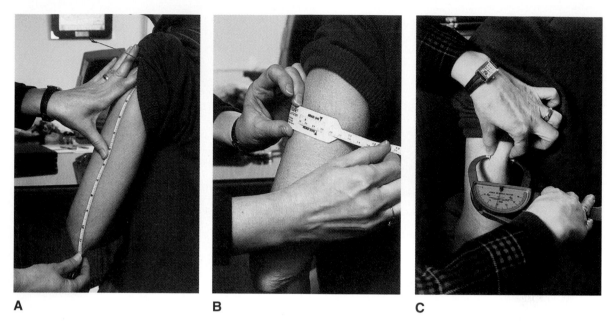

Figure 7–3
(A) and (B) Measuring midarm circumference. (C) Triceps skin-fold thickness.

or

$$\text{Loss of weight in kilograms} \div \text{usual weight in kilograms} \times 100$$

Anthropometric measurements are not as precise as biochemical methods for assessing nutritional status, but they are inexpensive, noninvasive, and easily obtained. According to some clinical researchers, accurate body composition measurements are more difficult to obtain for obese people than for thin people because of the compression factor involving the use of the calipers. However, anthropometric measurements are very useful because they can help justify the use of special nutritional support when a patient is shown to be at risk for development of protein-energy malnutrition.

Biochemical and Clinical Data

Several lab tests of the blood, urine, and skin are used in assessing nutritional status. Protein-energy malnutrition in its various forms can be detected by monitoring the blood serum levels of albumin, transferrin, and lymphocytes. These elements are all associated with body protein status. A person's level of immunity is discovered with skin antigen tests.

A nitrogen balance study can also be helpful in determining nutritional status. A negative nitrogen balance signifies that the body is using some of its protein reserves for energy. Nitrogen balance is determined from the urinary urea nitrogen content of a 24-hour urine collection. Clinical dietitians can calculate nitrogen bal-

Table 7–6
Summary of the Nutritional Assessment Process

Area of Screening	Method	Information Gathered
Diet history	Patient family interview	Food preferences and intolerances; taste, appetite, and recent weight changes; desired weight and usual weight; estimation of typical kilocalorie and nutrient intake
Clinical	Physical examination	Indicators of malnutrition: appearance of hair, skin, oral cavity, fingernails, presence of edema
	Radiography	Skeletal condition
	Anthropometry	Level of protein and fat reserves in the body, body frame size, weight, and height
Biochemical	Laboratory tests of blood and urine	Composition of blood to compare with normal ranges for hemoglobin, albumin, transferrin, total plasma protein, and so on; nitrogen content in 24-hour urinary output
	Skin tests	Immunity to certain diseases, response to antigens; possible identification of vitamin and mineral deficiencies

ance with this information and determine patient protein needs to promote healing or preserve lean muscle mass. Certain vitamin and mineral deficiencies may also be detected with lab tests when the tests are evaluated in conjunction with physical findings and dietary assessment of usual intake.

A summary of the nutrition assessment process is shown in Table 7–6. A nutrition assessment form is found in Figure 7–4.

HOW IS THE NUTRITION CARE PLAN IMPLEMENTED AND EVALUATED?

To carry out plans to meet patient-centered nutritional goals, various activities or interventions are needed. These activities include the diet prescription, any necessary modification of food consistency, nutritional supplements, nutritional support, assistance and encouragement at mealtime, and nutrition counseling in preparation for discharge.

Evaluation is achieved through observation of the individual's condition and acceptance of dietary changes. Weight status and improvements in lab values must also be evaluated. New methods for achieving a nutritional goal can then be tried and evaluated. Progress should be written in the medical record. Figure 7–4 shows a sample nutrition assessment and planning form that may be used.

WHY ARE FOOD AND DRUG INTERACTIONS CONSIDERED IN THE NUTRITIONAL CARE PLANNING PROCESS?

The health care team must be aware of the many factors that can adversely affect a person's nutritional status, including the effects of drugs on nutrient absorption, excretion, and metabolism, especially when long-term and multiple-drug therapy is necessary (Tables 7–7 and 7–8). Children, elderly persons, chronically

Text continued on page 165

NUTRITIONAL ASSESSMENT AND CARE PLAN

Name: _____ Date: _____
D.O.B.: _____ Age: _____ Diagnoses: _____

SUBJECTIVE DATA

Food habits: _____
_____
Fluid intake: _____
Activity level: _____

OBJECTIVE DATA

Diet order: _____ Meal pattern: _____
Consistency: _____   Breakfast   Lunch   Supper
Medications: _____

Supplements: _____ Male/Female: _____
Bowel/bladder functions: _____ Weight HX: _____

Laboratory values: _____ Weight: _____ Height: _____
_____ Physical indicators: _____
_____

Meal observations: _____

Medical factors affecting nutritional status: _____
_____

Physical limitations: _____
_____

PROBLEM	GOAL	INTERVENTION

Recommendations: _____
_____

Signature: _____

Figure 7–4

Sample nutrition assessment and care plan.

Table 7–7
Drug-Nutrient Interactions*

Drugs	Vitamins/Minerals Depleted	Suggested Foods to Eat	Foods to Avoid
Analgesics			
Aspirin	Folic Acid	Yeast, wheat germ, whole grains, enriched breads, corn, cornmeal, egg yolk, legumes, nuts, organ meats, lean pork, almonds, milk and dairy products, leafy vegetables, oysters	Crackers, jellies, syrups, other processed high-carbohydrate foods
	Iron	Liver, fortified cocoa, lentils, lean roast beef, nuts, molasses, apricots, enriched breads and cereals, dark green leafy vegetables, pork	
	Vitamin C	Black currants, broccoli, Brussels sprouts, raw green cabbage, cauliflower, leafy green vegetables, paprika, pimentos, strawberries, citrus fruits	
Antacids			
Aluminum hydroxide (Amphojel)	Phosphorus, thiamine	Poultry, fish, meats, enriched breads, cereals, nuts, legumes, milk and milk products	Alcoholic beverages
Bicarbonate (Tums)	Iron, thiamine	Same as Analgesics	Alcoholic beverages; for sodium bicarbonate, anything high in sodium
Antibiotics			
Penicillins	Iron, potassium	Same as Analgesics; banana, citrus, and other high-potassium foods	*Note:* Avoid foods high in iron for at least 2 hours after taking any antibiotic
Tetracyclines	Vitamin C; B vitamins	Same as Analgesics	Do not take with food or any dairy products
Neomycins	Vitamin B$_{12}$	Liver, kidney, milk, muscle meats, fish	Alcoholic beverages
	Vitamin A and D, iron	Fish-liver oils, leafy green vegetables, apricots, beet tops, butter, deep orange vegetables, cheese, egg yolk, deep orange fruits (peaches, mangos, papayas), milk	

Table continued on following page

Table 7–7
Drug-Nutrient Interactions (*continued*)

Drugs	Vitamins/Minerals Depleted	Suggested Foods to Eat	Foods to Avoid
Anticoagulants			
Coumadin, Dicumarol			Alcoholic beverages, caffeine, fried or boiled onions, leafy green vegetables, liver
Antidiabetic Drugs			
			Excessive sugar, alcohol
Antihypertensive Drugs			
	Vitamin K	Leafy vegetables	Excessive imported licorice
Digitalis			
Cardiovascular	Vitamin K, potassium	Same as Antihypertensive Drugs; foods high in potassium (see Diuretics)	Foods high in sodium, high-fiber foods, prune juice, herbal teas
	Magnesium	Nuts, legumes, whole grains, leafy vegetables, water	
Diuretics			
Potassium-wasting	Potassium	Apricots, molasses, dates, bananas, milk, nuts, bamboo shoots, prunes, mushrooms, grapefruit, oranges	Alcoholic beverages
Triamterene (potassium-sparing)	Folic acid	Same as Analgesics	Foods high in potassium
Gantrisin			
(Anti-infective)	Folic acid, vitamin K, other B vitamins	Same as Analgesics	Alcoholic beverages
Laxatives			
Mineral oil (not currently recommended as a laxative but included because of its depletion effect on nutrients)	Vitamin A	Same as Antibiotics	Fried greasy foods, fatty foods
	Vitamin D	Yeast, milk and milk products, fish-liver oils, salmon, sardines, egg yolk, butter	
	Vitamin K	See Antihypertensive Drugs	
	Calcium	Milk, cheese, ice cream, leafy green vegetables, Brazil nuts, legumes, clams, oysters, tofu, whole grains, water	

Table 7–7
Drug-Nutrient Interactions (*continued*)

Drugs	Vitamins/Minerals Depleted	Suggested Foods to Eat	Foods to Avoid
Phenolphthalein	Phosphorus; vitamins A, D, and K	Same as Antacids and Laxatives	
Dioctyl sodium sulfosuccinate (stool softener)	Vitamin A	Same as Antacids and Laxatives	
Bisacodyl	Potassium	Same as Diuretics	Fried, greasy food, fatty foods, do not take *with* milk and milk products
Levodopa	Vitamin C, Vitamin B$_{12}$	Same as most foods under Analgesics; note those to avoid	Coffee, dry skim milk, beans, oatmeal, wheat germ, beef liver, pork, tuna, sweet potatoes, peas, bacon, avocado, malted milk, cheese, wine
Oral Contraceptives			
Estrogen-containing	Thiamine, folic acid, riboflavin	See Analgesics (folic acid)	
	Vitamin B$_6$	Wheat germ, corn, soybeans, liver, meat, whole grains, peanuts	
	Vitamin B$_{12}$	See Antibiotics, Analgesics	
Thyroxine			Excessive soy-protein products, kale, cabbage, carrots, cauliflower, spinach, pears, peaches, Brussels sprouts, turnips
Tranquilizers			
Barbiturates	Folic acid	See Analgesics	Alcoholic beverages

*Perhaps vitamins or minerals in foods will be adversely affected by prescribed drugs. Check with the physician—a vitamin/mineral supplement may be necessary.

From Resource Kit for Modified Diets—Nutrition Education Materials published by the American Dietetic Association, Chicago, Illinois.

Table 7–8
Drugs That Interact with Vitamins and Minerals

	Clinical Consequences	Nursing Considerations
Anticoagulants Interact with		
Vitamin C	Large doses of ascorbic acid—3 g or more—may inhibit absorption of warfarin (Coumadin, Panwarfin, Sofarin), lowering plasma levels of the drug. That in turn can reduce the drug's anticoagulant effect.	If prothrombin time decreases in patients taking warfarin and vitamin C, the vitamin may have to be discontinued or the vitamin dose lowered.
Vitamin E	Very large doses of vitamin E—1200 IU a day—may increase warfarin's anticoagulant effects and the risk of bleeding.	Advise patients taking warfarin to avoid vitamin E supplements, unless a doctor prescribes them.
Vitamin K	If patients taking warfarin or dicumarol increase their intake of green, leafy vegetables or other foods rich in vitamin K, prothrombin time may decrease. A diet that's low in the vitamin, on the other hand, may prolong PT and increase the risk of hemorrhage.	Caution patients on anticoagulant therapy not to significantly increase or decrease their intake of foods rich in vitamin K, particularly spinach, kale, cabbage, cauliflower, and liver.
Anticonvulsants Interact with		
Folic acid	Prolonged use of phenytoin (Dilantin), phenobarbital, or primidone (Myidone, Mysoline) may cause folic acid deficiency, bringing on megaloblastic anemia, depression, apathy, and, on rare occasions, dementia. However, folate supplements may interfere with the drugs' effects, increasing the risk of seizures.	Check serum and RBC folic acid levels periodically. If folate supplements are needed to correct anemia, the daily dose should not exceed 1 mg. The doctor may increase the anticonvulsant dosage accordingly.
Vitamin D	Long-term therapy with phenytoin (Dilantin) or phenobarbital can cause vitamin D deficiency by inactivating the vitamin in the liver and increasing its biliary excretion.	Because vitamin D deficiency inhibits calcium absorption, serum calcium levels should be monitored. Also watch for signs and symptoms of osteomalacia: increased serum alkaline phosphatase, bone pain in the back, thighs, shoulders, and ribs, and muscle weakness in the legs. Patients on phenytoin or phenobarbital should take 400 to 800 IU of vitamin D daily and maintain a diet rich in calcium.
Antipsychotics Interact with		
Vitamin B_2	Chlorpromazine (Thoradol, Thor-Prom, Thorazine), fluphenazine (Permitil, Prolixin), and thioridazine (Mellaril) may cause a mild vitamin B_2 deficiency by interfering with the vitamin's metabolism.	Encourage a diet rich in B vitamins, including milk, cheese, and green, leafy vegetables. Watch for early signs of B_2 deficiency, including sore, burning lips, tongue, and mouth; photophobia; and blurred vision. Administer vitamin B_2 supplements, as ordered, if a deficit develops. Severe depletion can bring on angular stomatitis—cracks at the corners of the mouth—and seborrheic dermatitis in the nasolabial folds.

Table 7–8
Drugs That Interact with Vitamins and Minerals (*continued*)

	Clinical Consequences	Nursing Considerations
Bile Acid Sequestrants Interact with		
Beta carotene	The cholesterol-lowering agents cholestyramine (Questran) and colestipol (Colestid) can cause deficiencies in beta carotene, a vitamin A precursor, and other fat-soluble vitamins, by binding bile acids, which in turn interferes with the bile-dependent absorption of fat-soluble vitamins.	Patients may need beta carotene supplements if signs and symptoms of a vitamin A deficiency—night blindness, and dry, scaly, rough skin—develop.
Iron	Patients taking the cholesterol-lowering agents cholestyramine and colestipol may not respond to iron supplements because the drugs bind to iron in the gastrointestinal tract, inhibiting its absorption.	Advise patients to take iron supplements at least 1 hour before or 4 to 6 hours after taking cholestyramine or colestipol.
Cephalosporins Interact with		
Vitamin K	Cefamandole (Mandol), cefotetan (Cefotan), cefoperazone (Cefobid), and moxalactam (Moxam) can cause vitamin K deficiency and subsequent bleeding by destroying the intestinal flora that make the vitamin.	Monitor prothrombin time. If bleeding occurs, stop the drug and administer vitamin K IM, as ordered. Elderly patients and those with malnutrition, renal impairment, or hepatic impairment are at high risk for bleeding and may require prophylactic vitamin K.
Chloramphenicol (Chlormycetin) Interacts with		
Vitamin B_{12}	Patients who take this antibiotic and parenteral B_{12} (cyanocobalamin) for pernicious anemia may not respond to the vitamin because the drug inhibits maturation of RBC precursors in the bone marrow.	Monitor reticulocyte count closely. If it doesn't improve during vitamin B_{12} therapy, the doctor may have to switch to another antibiotic.
Iron	Patients with iron-deficiency anemia may not respond to iron supplements if they're taking chloramphenicol.	If the patient cannot be switched to another antibiotic, higher doses of iron may be needed.
Cisplatin (Platinol) Interacts with		
Magnesium	This antineoplastic agent can cause magnesium deficiency by increasing the urinary excretion of the mineral.	Monitor serum Mg levels, and watch for signs and symptoms of a deficiency—muscle spasms, depression, premature ventricular beats, and tachycardia. Encourage a Mg-rich diet including nuts, fish, whole-grain breads and cereals, and green, leafy vegetables. If cisplatin-induced nausea makes that impossible, Mg supplements—the usual daily dose is 350 mg—may be needed.

Table continued on following page

Table 7–8
Drugs That Interact with Vitamins and Minerals (*continued*)

	Clinical Consequences	Nursing Considerations
Digoxin (Lanoxin, Lanoxicaps) Interacts with		
Magnesium	By increasing urinary excretion of watch magnesium, digoxin can cause Mg deficiency, which in turn increases the drug's toxicity.	Monitor serum Mg levels and for signs of a deficiency. Instruct patients on digoxin to avoid alcohol, which increases Mg excretion.
Diuretics Interact with		
Vitamin B$_1$	Loop diuretics such as furosemide (Lasix) can cause a B$_1$ deficiency by increasing urinary excretion of the vitamin.	Patients may need vitamin B$_1$ supplements if signs of a deficiency develop; monitor blood vitamin levels for a therapeutic response. A mild deficit can cause confusion, muscle weakness and tenderness, fatigue, and depression. More severe depletion causes paralysis and edema in the legs and congestive heart failure.
Isoniazid (INH, Laniazid, others) Interacts with		
Vitamin B$_6$	Patients taking this drug may develop vitamin B$_6$ deficiency because it blocks the vitamin's conversion to its active form and increases its urinary excretion.	Monitor closely for convulsions and peripheral neuropathy, a particular risk for diabetics and alcoholics. Administer 25 mg/day of vitamin B$_6$, as ordered, as prophylaxis.
Isotretinoin (Accutane) Interacts with		
Vitamin A	Combining isotretinoin—used to treat severe cystic acne—and vitamin A supplements can cause vitamin A and drug toxicity. Both the drug and the vitamin are members of the retinoid family, so the combination increases the risk of retinoid overload.	Advise patients taking the drug to avoid vitamin A and multivitamin supplements. Report signs and symptoms of retinoid toxicity: headache, nausea, vomiting, elevated liver enzymes, hair loss, hepatomegaly, and dry, fissured skin.
Levodopa (Larodopa, Dopar) Interacts with		
Vitamin B$_6$	B$_6$ supplements can diminish the therapeutic effects of this anti-Parkinsonian drug by accelerating its metabolic breakdown, reducing the amount that reaches the brain.	Advise patients on levodopa not to take vitamin B$_6$ supplements. Patients who take Sinemet, a combination of carbidopa and levodopa that isn't affected by the vitamin, may take the supplements.
Lithium (Eskalith, Lithane, others) Interacts with		
Sodium	The risk of lithium toxicity increases when a patient goes on a low-sodium regimen, while a sudden increase in salt may blunt drug action.	Advise patients on lithium to maintain their normal sodium intake. If restrictions are required, watch for and report early signs of lithium toxicity—nausea, abdominal pain, diarrhea, vomiting, sedation, and mild tremor. More severe reactions include extreme thirst, frequent urination, an enlarged thyroid gland, hypotension, and seizures.

Table 7–8
Drugs That Interact with Vitamins and Minerals (*continued*)

Clinical Consequences		Nursing Considerations
Methotrexate (Folex, Mexate, others) Interacts with		
Folic acid	The drug can cause folic acid depletion, leading to megaloblastic anemia.	Monitor patients for evidence of mega-loblastic anemia: pallor, irritability, dyspnea, glossitis, low RBC count, and increased mean corpuscular volume (MCV). Patients on long-term therapy with large doses of methotrexate will probably need leucovorin (Well-covorin), an activated form of folic acid.
Pentamidine (Pentam 300, NebuPent) Interacts with		
Folic acid	The drug, taken by HIV-positive patients for the prevention and treatment of *Pneumocystis carinii* pneumonia (PCP), can cause folic acid deficiency and subsequent megaloblastic anemia.	Monitor patients for signs of megaloblastic anemia. Patients may need folic acid supplements if they're on long-term pentamidine therapy.
Pyrimethamine (Daraprim) Interacts with		
Folic acid	This anti-parasitic agent, which is used to treat toxoplasmosis, can cause folic acid deficiency and subsequent megaloblastic anemia.	Monitor patients for megaloblastic anemia. The doctor may order 3 to 9 mg IM of leucovorin daily to be administered with pyrimethamine as prophylaxis.
Trimethoprim (Proloprim, Trimpex, and contained in Bactrim and Septra) Interacts with		
Folic acid	Prolonged use of trimethoprim, an antibiotic used to treat PCP and urinary tract infection, may cause mild folate depletion by blocking an enzyme that activates folic acid.	The drug is contraindicated in patients with folic-acid deficiency anemia. Patients on long-term trimethoprim therapy should receive folate supplements.
Verapamil (Calan, Isoptin) Interacts with		
Calcium	Calcium supplements may reduce the drug's therapeutic effect.	If the patient must take IV or oral calcium, monitor closely for elevated BP and arrhythmias.

From Cerrato PL, Vitamins and Minerals. RN, June 1993, pp. 29–32. © Medical Economics Publishing, Montvale, NJ. Reprinted by permission.

ill persons, and those with a marginal or inadequate nutrient intake are most susceptible to drug-induced nutritional deficiencies. A good nutritional status and a nutritious diet can reduce this risk. A proper diet can also reduce the risk of any altered effectiveness of drugs. The success of a patient's treatment often depends on the effectiveness of medications. The registered dietitian can provide specific dietary instructions to the patient as to when to take medications in relation to meals and which foods, if any, must be avoided. The staff pharmacist may also need to be consulted for multiple medication regimens.

How Do Drugs Affect Nutrient Absorption?

Drugs may affect absorption of nutrients by damaging the intestinal mucosa, by binding with nutrients, or by decreasing the availability of bile acid, which would inhibit the absorption of the fat-soluble vitamins. Folate absorption is decreased by the use of the anti-inflammatory agent sulfasalazine, but rather than the use of folate supplements, a varied and adequate diet should be encouraged.

How Do Food and Nutrients Affect Drug Action?

Food and some beverages, such as coffee or cola drinks, as well as specific nutrients can adversely affect drug action. For example, natural licorice in large quantities can complicate treatment in patients receiving antihypertensive agents because licorice can cause sodium retention, which could result in edema and hypertension.

How Do Food and Vitamin Supplements Affect Drug Action?

Some patients benefit from nutritional supplements, but the health professional needs to be aware of potential interaction with medications (Table 7–8). Large amounts of vitamin K in a supplement, for example, can reduce the effectiveness of anticoagulants. Tetracycline should not be administered at the same time as a mineral supplement (e.g., calcium), since the absorption of the minerals would be inhibited.

How Do Drugs Affect Nutrient Excretion?

Certain drugs such as **diuretics** (medications that cause fluid loss) can deplete potassium (e.g., furosemide or lasix, and thiazides). A sodium-restricted diet and potassium-rich foods (see Table 7–4) are often prescribed. Potassium-depleting medications often induce hyperglycemia with a resultant need to follow a moderate carbohydrate diet. When a diuretic and digitalis are given together, two conditions may result—hypokalemia and hypomagnesemia—and digitalis toxicity must be guarded against. It must be remembered, however, that other diuretics such as spironolactone and the newer ACE inhibitors (a type of blood pressure medication) are potassium-conserving, in which case extra dietary potassium is not necessary and may even create a problem; salt substitutes containing potassium should be avoided when these medications are used.

How Do Drugs Affect Nutrient Metabolism?

Certain drugs bind with enzymes and affect the metabolism of some nutrients. For example, long-term ingestion of pyrimethamine, an antimalarial drug, will likely produce **megaloblastic anemia** (a form of anemia often associated with

nduce severe
consultation
to the oral

or folic acid or folacin), because it antagonizes folacin. Pheno-
toin, which are used in the treatment of epilepsy, can increase
tion. Ingestion of adequate dietary vitamin D should be en-
te the absorption of calcium.

eight loss.
he desire for

utes or more

iated with the use of medications such as steroidal, antihyper-
nflammatory agents occurs frequently because of sodium and
Other medications, such as some antipsychotic medications,
appetite with associated weight gain.

(a sense of

calorie foods

ns to Aid in the Relief

atient regarding factors contributing to appetite loss such as

GI irritation)

tient about the importance of an adequate, well-balanced diet.
ant environment for eating. If possible, eliminate distractions
ure.

contribute to
, colas, pep-

occurs or meals are not well tolerated, offer small, frequent, at-
or snacks.
y in color, texture, taste, and temperature.

nvironment.

rs by using seasonings. Requests can be made from the dietary
r small containers of spices to be kept at the patient's bedside.
akened patients to select easy-to-chew menu items.

ay stimulate

cription of calorie-dense nutritional supplements between meals.

secretion).
by milk

ysfunction

arless gum or candy, water, or lemon juice as mouth rinses.
ge good oral hygiene before and after meals.

app
at

re Mouth

with

ease dry, acidic, spicy, or salty foods. Moisten (dunk) foods in beverages
wallow with liquid (milk, gravy).

fore

er moist, soft foods such as custards, casseroles, or mashed potatoes.
void spicy, rough textured or highly acidic foods.
uggest that the patient lick or suck ice chips. Add cold foods such as ice
cream, sherbet, or popsicles to menu selections.
Offer warm water rinses or saliva substitutes (e.g., Optimoist).

6. Stress good oral hygiene. Lack of saliva production can quickly i
   dental caries. If dry mouth persists for 2 weeks or longer, a denta
   is needed. Perform dental care cautiously to minimize traum
   mucosa.

Appetite Stimulation or Weight Gain

1. Assess weight gain as a possible reversal of depression-induced v
2. Educate the patient that certain drugs may increase appetite and
   sweets.
3. Encourage a slow rate of eating with increased chewing (20 min
   for first portions).
4. Encourage low-calorie foods and beverages.
5. Encourage adequate fiber intake, which may help induce satiet
   fullness).
6. Instruct patient or food provider to control access to specific high-
   and beverages.

Good Advice!

Epigastric Distress (Stomach discomfort, heartburn, or indigestion)

1. After drug administration (particularly medications that cause
   remain upright for 15 to 30 minutes.
2. Evaluate dietary habits for specific foods or beverages that may
   epigastric distress such as alcohol, caffeine, decaffeninated coffe
   permint, chocolate, pepper, chili powder, and spicy foods.
3. Offer small quantities of food at frequent intervals in a relaxed e
   Avoid overeating.
4. Avoid extremely hot or extremely cold foods or liquids (which m
   acid secretion).
5. Limit citrus juices, tomato products, and other highly acidic foods
6. Avoid greasy, fried, or fatty foods (may delay gastric emptying).
7. Evaluate the intake of milk or dairy products (may stimulate acid
8. Avoid eating at least one hour before bedtime.

?
By how much?
we use so

Nausea

1. Respect patients' food preferences. If a food item does not sound
   a patient, it should not be forced. Often what patients think wil
   their system is well tolerated.
2. Offer small quantities of easily digestible foods at frequent i
   slowly.
3. Reduce food volume at meals. Serve liquids after meals or limit
   meals.
4. Suggest intake of bread, crackers, or cereals early in the mor
   rising.
5. Cold foods may be better tolerated than hot foods. Avoid luke

or b
warm food

6. Emphasize low-fat foods, which will leave the stomach earlier than greasy foods.
7. Collaborate with the physician to prescribe antiemetics ½ hour before meals.

Diarrhea

1. Focus on fluid and electrolyte replacement by providing potassium-rich fruit juices and sodium through broths or other foods. Pedialyte is often used with children. Sports drinks such as Gatorade may be appropriate for adults.
2. A clear liquid diet may be necessary for 24 hours or longer to provide bowel rest. Low-residue, lactose-free liquid supplements may be tolerated and needed for extended bowel rest.
3. Intake of frequent small amounts of bland foods (grain products) are allowed as tolerated.
4. Return to normal diet gradually, being careful of high-roughage foods (soluble fiber may be helpful).
5. In the case of antibiotic-induced diarrhea, the addition of plain or lemon/vanilla yogurt with active bacterial cultures may be well tolerated and promote the treatment of diarrhea.

Gastrointestinal Gas (Flatulence and/or belching)

1. Evaluate possible causes of ingested air such as eating fast, chewing gum, drinking through a straw, or talking while chewing.
2. Avoid vegetables and fruits known to cause gas such as beans, cabbage, cauliflower, and broccoli. Consider offering an enzyme product known as Beano to help digestion and thereby reduce gas production. Fiber intake may be tolerated when it is slowly increased in the diet to allow for thorough digestion; adequate water intake is important with an increased fiber intake.
3. Evaluate for lactose intolerance and provide a low-lactose diet as warranted.
4. Limit consumption of carbonated beverages.

Constipation

1. Evaluate if prolonged reliance on chemical laxatives has led to poor bowel reflexes.
2. Patient may need education concerning misconceptions about constipation.
3. Evaluate the diet for fiber and water content.
4. Encourage adequate intake of fiber or other nonlaxative bulking agents and water. Promote regular exercise and recognition of need for defecation—usually after meals, especially breakfast (Smith, 1997).

WHAT IS DISCHARGE PLANNING?

The last step in the nutrition care planning process, called discharge planning, begins as soon as the patient is admitted to the health care facility. By the time the patient is ready to leave, needs have already been assessed and nutritional status evaluated, and changes have been made in the nutrition care plan in response to the patient's progress. Before developing a final meal plan, it is important to gain input from the patient so that goals are mutually determined. This helps in promoting dietary compliance after discharge. Recommendations should also be in line with the needs of other family members. Dietary instruction should include counseling on weight control, diet in relation to the patient's medications and physical condition, and a review of the foods allowed and avoided on a modified dietary regime. It needs to be stressed to the patient that one dietary instruction may not be sufficient for long-term dietary modification. Identification of an ongoing support system for change should be made whether it is referral to an outpatient dietitian or other community program.

WHAT IS THE ROLE OF THE NURSE OR OTHER HEALTH CARE PROFESSIONAL IN INSTITUTIONAL SETTINGS?

The role of the nurse is to be positive and supportive in the context of the total health care team, helping to assess patients at high nutritional risk. Nurses are often at the front line in patient care and can assist the registered dietitian in providing nutritional care They do this by recognizing high-risk patients and referring them to the proper health care professional and by contributing to the primary care process by ensuring that the meal service received is appropriate to individual needs. Long-term positive nutritional messages can be reinforced, which is especially important for those persons who will be discharged to their homes.

Critical Thinking

Case Study

After barely surviving a two-car accident, Royce was hooked to a ventilator with his head nearly completely bandaged due to a severe head injury. Surrounded by his family, Royce seemed to recognize his wife's voice and tried to open his eyes. Later he tried to speak but no words came out. Royce had an NPO sign above his head and a dextrose and saline IV line in his arm. As his family members sat quietly by his bedside and prayed that he would be okay, the doctor discussed the options to increase the possibility for a successful recovery.

Applications

1. Why should health care professionals be careful with what they say around a seemingly comatose person?
2. What does NPO mean?

Study Questions and Classroom Activities

1. Name six ways the basic normal diet is modified for therapeutic purposes.
2. Name six considerations to remember in meal service.
3. What are some characteristics of good and poor nutritional status that may be noted in the clinical area of assessment.
4. Why should food and drug interactions be considered in the assessment process?
5. List appropriate reasons to request medical nutrition therapy by a dietitian for a patient.
6. What is the percentage of weight change for an individual who currently weighs 110 pounds and whose usual weight is 130 pounds?
7. If a man who is 5'10" has an elbow breadth of 2.5 inches, what is his body frame size? (Refer to Appendix 11.)
8. How is protein-energy malnutrition detected in a hospital patient?
9. If a patient is placed on a low-protein diet, what groups of the Food Guide Pyramid will be affected? What advice could be given to help a person follow a low-protein diet without jeopardizing nutritional intake?

References

Matsui T, Ueki M, Yamada M, Sakurai T, Yao T: Indications and options of nutritional treatment of Crohn's disease: A comparison of elemental and polymeric diets. J Gastroenterol. November 1995; 8(30 Suppl):95–97.

Pohle T, Hilker E, Domschke W: Development of duodenal ulcer concomitant with successful Helicobacter pylori eradication. Gastroenterol. July 1997; 35(7):563–565.

Smith CH, in Powers and Moore's Food Medication Interactions, 10th ed., edited by Pronsky ZM. Published and distributed by Food-Medication Interactions, Pottstown, PA, 1997; pp. 14–17.

Wellman NS, Weddle DO, Kranz S, Brain CT: Elder insecurities: Poverty, hunger, and malnutrition. JADA, October 1997; 10(Suppl 2): S120–S122.

8

Cardiovascular Disease

Objectives

After completing this chapter, you should be able to:

- Identify risk factors related to the development of cardiovascular disease.
- Describe medical nutrition therapy for cardiovascular disease and hypertension.
- Describe how the management of the dyslipidemia found in conjunction with the insulin resistance syndrome differs from management of LDL-cholesterol.
- Describe appropriate foods to prevent or manage cardiovascular disease.
- Describe the role of the nurse or other health care professional in the prevention and management of cardiovascular disease.

Terms to Identify

Antioxidants	Dyslipidemia	Mortality
Arteriosclerosis	Edema	Myocardial infarction (MI)
Atherosclerosis	Endocardium	Myocardium
Cardiovascular disease (CVD)	Homocysteine	National Cholesterol Education Program (NCEP)
Cerebrovascular accident (CVA)	Hypercholesterolemia	Pericardium
Congestive heart failure (CHF)	Hyperinsulinemia	Sodium
Coronary thrombosis	Hypertension	Trans fatty acids
	Hypertriglyceridemia	Triglycerides
	Lipids	
	Morbidity	

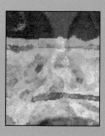**INTRODUCTION**

If you are like most people, you probably do not worry about heart disease. Men have traditionally been viewed as the population at risk for heart disease. However, heart disease is the most serious health problem facing women, even though this may not be widely known. **Cardiovascular disease (CVD),** otherwise referred to as coronary heart disease (CHD) or more simply heart disease, kills more people than all forms of cancer combined and is still the leading cause of death for Americans. The good news is that there has been progress in preventing the **mortality** (death) and **morbidity** (effects of disease) of heart disease. The proportion of Americans with high cholesterol has continued to drop, in part due to better screening and interventions.

Although it is true that some individuals are not prone to CVD, the general population will benefit from dietary changes that lower the total fat content to 30 percent, especially those that lower saturated fat to less than 10 percent. Factors in the environment as related to food choices and genetic heritage play a role in CVD risk. For example, stroke mortality is higher in the Southeast compared with other regions of the United States, and the prevalence of hypertension is also high (black men = 35 percent, black women = 37.7 percent, white men = 26.5 percent, white women = 21.5 percent). Dietary sodium and saturated fat intake are also high in the Southeast; dietary potassium intake appears to be relatively low, although at similar levels to other areas of the United States (Hall et al., 1997). There may be a genetic predispostion to coronary heart disease in the southeastern part of the United States, which is where early Scottish immigrants often settled. Scotland is known to have a very high rate of coronary heart disease (Bolton-Smith et al., 1996).

Individual guidance should complement the general guidelines to allow for specific needs; for example, guidelines can be adjusted to suit frail, elderly persons or terminally ill patients who may need to rely on high-fat foods for adequate kilocalorie intake. For everyone, attempts to lower the risk of CVD should not take precedence over sound nutritional intake. Meat, milk, and cheese are still important to one's diet; however, moderation and an emphasis on low-fat and low-sodium alternatives can result in a healthy balance. Figure 8–1 shows the eating plan tips of the American Heart Association.

Altering the eating habits of the public in the most appropriate manner remains a major challenge, however. Unfortunately, some individuals have interpreted the low-fat message as meaning extremely low-fat or no-fat diets, which can also be harmful to one's health, while others continue to consume a very high-fat diet. Specific guidance on medical nutrition therapy is best provided by a registered dietitian who will look at individuals subfractions of cholesterol (LDL, HDL, and triglycerides–see the following sections) and modify percentages of fat and carbohydrate based on the specific abnormal lipid values as appropriate for an individual's particular food habits and food preferences.

WHAT ARE THE TYPES AND CAUSES OF CARDIOVASCULAR DISEASE?

Cardiovascular disease relates to the heart and the entire vascular system. Thus, **hypertension** (high blood pressure), **cerebrovascular accident** (**CVA** or, more commonly, stroke), and **arteriosclerosis** (hardening of the arteries) are all examples of cardiovascular disease. In diseases of the heart, one or several parts may be damaged. The affected part may be the muscle (**myocardium**), the outer covering (**pericardium**), the lining (**endocardium**), the blood vessels, or the valves. Risk factors that have been found to be associated with risk of strokes include

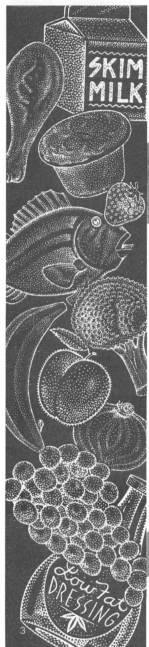

EATING PLAN TIPS

TO CONTROL THE AMOUNT AND KIND OF FAT, SATURATED FATTY ACIDS, AND DIETARY CHOLESTEROL YOU EAT:

- Eat up to 6 ounces (cooked) per day of lean meat, fish and skinless poultry.
- Try main dishes featuring pasta, rice, beans and/or vegetables. Or create "low-meat" dishes by mixing these foods with small amounts of lean meat, poultry or fish.
- The approximately 5 to 8 teaspoon servings of fats and oils per day may be used for cooking and baking, and in salad dressings and spreads.
- Use cooking methods that require little or no fat — boil, broil, bake, roast, poach, steam, sauté, stir-fry or microwave.
- Trim off the fat you can see before cooking meat and poultry. Drain off all fat after browning. Chill soups and stews after cooking so you can remove the hardened fat from the top.
- The 3 to 4 egg yolks per week included in your eating plan may be used alone or in cooking and baking (including store-bought products).
- Limit your use of organ meats such as liver, brains, chitterlings, kidney, heart, gizzard, sweetbreads and pork maws.
- Choose skim or 1% fat milk and nonfat or low-fat yogurt and cheeses.

TO ROUND OUT THE REST OF YOUR EATING PLAN:

- Eat 5 or more servings of fruits or vegetables per day.
- Eat 6 or more servings of breads, cereals or grains per day.

4

Figure 8–1

The American Heart Association Diet: An eating plan for healthy Americans. (From the American Heart Association, National Center, Dallas, Texas, Copyright 1991–1996; used with permission.)

age, diabetes, diastolic blood pressure greater than 114, and left ventricular hypertrophy as noted with an electrocardiogram (Rocha et al., 1997).

What Is Atherosclerosis?

Atherosclerosis is a complex disease of the arteries; it is a form of arteriosclerosis. The passageways through the arteries become roughened and clogged with fatty deposits so that blood cannot flow freely, like clogged sink pipes that are full of "gunk" (Fig. 8–2). Atherosclerosis is thought to be a cause of heart attack (**coronary thrombosis** or **myocardial infarction [MI]**, or plain "coronary") and CVA.

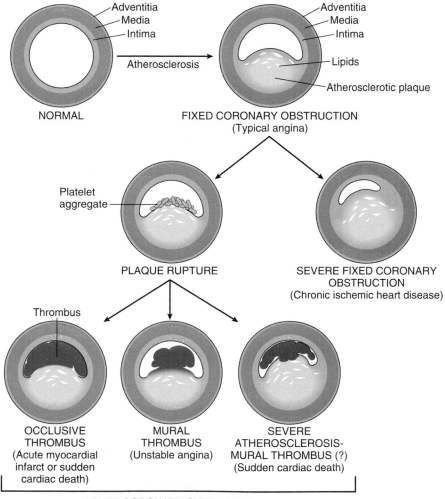

Figure 8–2

The atherosclerosis process. (From Kumar V, Cotarn RS, & Robbins SL: Basic Physiology, 6th ed. Philadelphia, WB Saunders, 1997, p. 319.)

WHAT ARE RISK FACTORS FOR CARDIOVASCULAR DISEASE?

New guidelines were developed by the Adult Treatment Panel (ATP) of the National Cholesterol Education Program (NCEP). These risk factors include the following:

Positive Risk Factors for Coronary Heart Disease

1. Elevated total blood cholesterol at or above 240 mg/dL
2. Increased low-density lipoprotein cholesterol at or above 160 mg/dL
3. Male, 45 years or older
4. Female, 55 years or older or with premature menopause and no estrogen replacement therapy
5. Decreased high-density lipoprotein cholesterol less than 35 mg/dL
6. Hypertension
7. Cigarette smoking
8. Diabetes mellitus
9. Family history of premature coronary heart disease

Negative Risk Factor for Coronary Heart Disease (subtract one risk factor)

1. High HDL-cholesterol (greater than 60 mg/dL)

The guidelines of the National Cholesterol Education Program now recommend that adults aged 20 years and older have their total and HDL-cholesterol measured. This is in part due to the recognition that atherosclerosis begins early in life and cholesterol levels in young adults predict CHD risk 30 to 40 years later (Cleeman, 1997).

What Is the Insulin Resistance Syndrome and Its Association with Cardiovascular Disease?

The insulin resistance syndrome, also known as syndrome X and the metabolic syndrome, has only recently been given credence as it is estimated to occur in at least one out of four Americans according to the researchers (O'Neill, 1995). It is a diagnosis made by correlates. The four primary correlates include hypertension, central obesity, elevated triglycerides with a low HDL-cholesterol level, and may or may not also include Type 2 diabetes (see Chapter 9). Gout and polycystic ovary syndrome are the latest correlates of the insulin resistance syndrome.

Insulin resistance means the individual body cells resist the action of insulin. Because insulin is required to keep blood sugar at normal levels, persons with insulin resistance tend to produce large amounts of insulin in relation to the amount of carbohydrate consumed (as carbohydrate is the main cause of increased meal-related blood glucose levels). **Hyperinsulinemia** (excess insulin in the blood) is gaining acceptance as a cause of atherosclerosis, and it is believed to alter the lining of the blood vessels promoting increased plaque deposition. Although more research is needed to confirm the role of hyperinsulinemia, this theory does help explain why cardiovascular disease often precedes the diagnosis of diabetes (which is generally related to insulin resistance—refer to Chapter 9). One study did find that both non-diabetic African Americans and Hispanics have increased insulin resistance and higher insulin responses associated with a glucose tolerance test (Haffner et al., 1996). Other explanations of how insulin resistance promotes CVD is its association with hypertension and **dyslipidemia** (elevated triglycerides with low HDL-C—see the following sections). It has only recently been realized that **hypertriglyceridemia** (excess triglycerides in the blood) has a role in CHD (Fruchart & Packard, 1997).

Treatment for hypercholesterolemia differs between individuals with insulin resistance and individuals who only have elevated LDL-cholesterol. Persons with dyslipidemia (high triglycerides and low HDL-C) associated with insulin resistance usually benefit from a moderate fat intake (30 to 35 percent) and moderate carbohydrate intake (50 percent) (Coulston, 1997). Persons who only have elevated LDL-cholesterol will most likely benefit from a low-fat, high-carbohydrate diet (fat 20 to 25 percent of kilocalories; carbohydrate > 60 percent of kilocalories). The National Cholesterol Education Program advises individualized diet planning (such as from a registered dietitian) before inititiating lipid-lowering drugs. This recommendation is not routinely being done, as noted in one study which found that a low-fat, high-complex-carbohydrate diet with daily aerobic exercise lowered total cholesteol 19 percent and triglycerides 29 percent. The study also found that 51 percent of the primary care physicians had not used medical nutrition therapy before initiating lipid-lowering drugs and 29 percent did not use medical nutrition therapy along with the medication as recommended by the National Cholesterol Education Program (Barnard et al., 1997).

Are There Other Risk Factors for Coronary Heart Disease?

Levels of **homocysteine,** a new risk factor associated with CHD and a type of protein, may contribute to atherogenesis through the promotion of platelet coagulability, increased smooth muscle cell proliferation, and stimulation of LDL oxidation. Homocysteine can be reduced with pharmacologic doses of folic acid, pyridoxine, vitamin B_{12}, or betaine, but further research is required (Duell & Malinow, 1997).

What Are Safe Blood Cholesterol Levels?

Although controversy exists in the medical community regarding safe and ideal blood values for total cholesterol and low-density lipoprotein cholesterol, there is growing recognition that low-to-moderate levels are best. The levels set by the **National Cholesterol Education Program (NCEP)** coordinating committee indicate that total cholesterol should be less than 200 mg/dL; levels between 200 and 239 mg/dL are defined as borderline high blood cholesterol, and those greater than 240 mg/dL are defined as high-risk levels. The NCEP also indicates that low-density lipoprotein cholesterol should be less than 130 mg/dL, borderline levels should be 130 to 159 mg/dL, and high-risk levels should be greater than 160 mg/dL (see Tables 8–1 and 8–2). Cholesterol levels that are very low (less than 150 mg/dL) are controversial as being a risk factor to health.

Table 8–1
Cholesterol (Lipid) Goals

Every adult, age 20 and older, should have his or her blood cholesterol checked at least once every five years. Here's a quick look at the numbers and what they mean.

Total Cholesterol

Desirable blood cholesterol	Less than 200 mg/dL
Borderline-high blood cholesterol	200–239 mg/dL
High blood cholesterol	240 mg/dL and above

HDL-Cholesterol*

Low HDL-Cholesterol	Less than 35 mg/dL

Triglycerides†

Normal triglycerides	Less than 200 mg/dL
Borderline high triglycerides	200 to 400 mg/dL
High triglycerides	400 to 1000 mg/dL
Very high triglycerides	Greater than 1000 mg/dL

*These levels are for anyone 20 years of age or older.
†These are based on fasting plasma triglyceride levels.
From National Heart, Lung, and Blood Institute and the American Heart Association.

Table 8–2
Treatment Decisions Based on LDL-Cholesterol

Dietary Therapy

	Initiation Level	LDL Goal
Without CHD and with fewer than 2 risk factors	≥160 mg/dL	<160 mg/dL
Without CHD and with 2 or more risk factors	≥130 mg/dL	<130 mg/dL
With CHD	>100 mg/dL	≤100 mg/dL

Drug Treatment

	Consideration Level	LDL Goal
Without CHD and with fewer than 2 risk factors	≥190 mg/dL*	<160 mg/dL
Without CHD and with 2 or more risk factors	≥160 mg/dL	<130 mg/dL
With CHD	≥130 mg/dL†	≤100 mg/dL

*In men under 35 years old and premenopausal women with LDL-cholesterol levels 190–219 mg/dL, drug therapy should be delayed except in high-risk patients like those with diabetes.
†In CHD patients with LDL-cholesterol levels 100–129 mg/dL, the physician should exercise clinical judgment in deciding whether to initiate drug treatment.
From The 2nd Report of the expert panel on Detection, Evaluation, and Treatment of High Blood Cholesterol in Adults, by the NIH, National Heart, Lung, and Blood Institute, July 1993.

What Are Lipoproteins and the Different Forms?

High-density lipoprotein (HDL), low-density lipoprotein (LDL), and very low density lipoprotein (VLDL) are all forms of cholesterol found in the blood. **Lipids** is a term used to describe all forms of fat found in the blood. Chylomicrons are another form of lipoprotein. VLDL is the main carrier of **triglycerides** (a type of blood fat) synthesized in the body. It is believed that HDL, which has more protein than does LDL or VLDL, allows more cholesterol to be taken from the body's cells, resulting in greater transport and removal of cholesterol through the liver. HDLs have been termed the "good" lipoproteins or fats, and in fact research has shown that individuals with more HDLs have less heart disease. An easy way to remember the role of HDL is to think *H* for *housecleaner*, as a high level of HDL seems to keep blood vessels and arteries clean. The total cholesterol number is the mathematical sum of the HDL-C, plus the LDL-C, plus one-fifth of the triglyceride level (if triglycerides are less than 400).

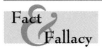

Fact & Fallacy

Fallacy: My grandfather lived to be 100 and ate eggs and bacon daily; therefore I do not have to worry about heart disease.

Fact: Individuals who subscribe to the preceding idea need to be reminded that one's heredity also comes from the grandmother's side of the family as well as from both parents. Careful questioning often reveals some form of CVD risk in the family's history, even if it is not heart disease specifically. A person might also be exposed to other risk factors that did not affect previous generations of his or her family, such as cigarette smoking, diabetes, or low levels of physical activity.

HOW IS CARDIOVASCULAR DISEASE PREVENTED AND TREATED BY DIET CHANGES?

Medical nutrition therapy is often the preferred choice prior to the initiation of medication (see Table 8–2). The American Heart Association (AHA) advises that the nature of coronary heart disease is such that prevention is the primary means by which a reduction in morbidity and mortality will be accomplished. Therefore it appears prudent to follow a diet aimed at lowering serum lipid concentrations. Many persons in the United States and the world have consumed diets similar to those recommended by the National Cholesterol Education Program (NCEP's Step One Diet—see Table 8–3) for many years. Both Step One and Step Two diets promote less than 30 percent fat kilocalories, but Step One promotes a maximum of 10 percent saturated fat and 300 mg cholesterol and Step Two promotes 7 percent saturated fat and 200 mg cholesterol.

Studies have shown that there is a low incidence of coronary disease in populations who habitually subsist on a low-fat and low-cholesterol diet or on a diet

Table 8–3
Recommended Diet Modifications to Lower Blood Cholesterol: The Step One Diet

Food Group	Choose	Decrease
Fish, chicken, turkey, and lean meats	Fish; white-meat poultry without skin; lean cuts of beef, lamb, pork, or veal; shellfish	Fatty cuts of beef, lamb, pork; spare ribs; organ meats; regular cold cuts; sausage; hot dogs; bacon; sardines; roe
Skim and low-fat milk, cheese, yogurt, and dairy substitutes	Skim or 1% fat milk (liquid, powdered, evaporated); buttermilk; substitute 1 cup skim milk alone or with up to 1 cup nonfat dry-milk powder added instead of whole milk (for consistency in cooking);	Whole milk (4% fat): regular, evaporated, condensed; cream; half and half; 2% milk; imitation milk products; most nondairy creamers; whipped toppings
	For acceptable whipped topping; combine ⅓ cup ice water, 1 tbsp lemon juice, ¾ tsp vanilla, and ⅓ cup nonfat dry-milk powder; beat 10 minutes or until stiff; add 2 tbsp sugar	
	Nonfat (0% fat) or low-fat yogurt	Whole-milk yogurt
	Low-fat cottage cheese (1% or 2% fat)	Whole-milk cottage cheese (4% fat)
	Low-fat cheeses, farmer, or pot cheeses (all of these should be labeled no more than 2–6 g fat/oz)	All-natural cheeses (e.g., blue, Roquefort, Camembert, Cheddar, Swiss)
		Low-fat or "diet" cream cheese, low-fat or "diet" sour cream
		Cream cheese, sour cream
	Sherbet, sorbet	Ice cream
Eggs	Egg whites (2 whites = 1 whole egg in recipes), or mix together 1 egg white, 2 tsp nonfat milk powder, and 2 tsp acceptable oil*; cholesterol-free egg substitutes	Egg yolks
Fruits and vegetables	Fresh, frozen, canned, or dried fruits and vegetables	Vegetables prepared in butter, cream, or other sauces
Breads and cereals	Homemade baked goods using unsaturated oils sparingly, angel food cake, low-fat crackers, low-fat cookies	Commercial baked goods: pies, cakes, doughnuts, croissants, pastries, muffins, biscuits, high-fat cookies
	Rice, pasta, barley, bulgur, legumes	Egg noodles
	Whole-grain breads and cereals (oatmeal, whole wheat, rye, bran, multigrain, etc.)	Breads in which eggs are a major ingredient, cereals with coconut oil or palm oil or palm kernel oil
Fats and oils	Acceptable unsaturated vegetable oils*	Butter, coconut oil, palm oil, kernel oil, bacon fat, hydrogenated vegetable shortening
	Margarine or shortening made from one of the acceptable unsaturated oils	
	Reduced-fat margarine	
	Mayonnaise, salad dressings made with acceptable unsaturated oils	Dressings made with egg yolk
	Low-fat dressings	
	Seeds and nuts, nonhydrogenated, old-fashioned-style peanut butter (100% peanuts)	Coconut, hydrogenated peanut butter

*Acceptable oils include canola, corn, cottonseed, olive, safflower, sesame, soybean, and sunflower.
From National Cholesterol Education Program Expert Panel. Report on detection, evaluation, and treatment of high blood cholesterol in adults. Arch Intern Med. 1994; 148:36.

that is low in saturated fats and cholesterol. For example, people in Italy have a low incidence of heart disease. This is felt to be related to a low intake of saturated fat, even though total fat intake is high because of the use of olives and olive oil. To be maximally effective in the prevention of atherosclerosis, a diet that reduces serum lipids will need to be consumed throughout one's life. It should be palatable, effective, economically feasible, and nutritionally adequate to allow for long-term use. Table 8–4 shows amounts of fat to equal 30 percent at a variety of kilocalorie levels and how to calculate amounts of fat for different percentages.

The use of antioxidant vitamin supplements is sometimes advocated to reduce CHD risk; however, receiving these vitamins via foods will also increase one's intake of fiber and naturally occuring phytochemicals, which may be important as well. Increasing vegetables and fruits rich in carotenoids appears useful in decreasing risk of CHD but "the pharmacological use of supplemental

Table 8–4
Recommended Total Fat for Various Kilocalorie Levels

Kilocalorie Level	Total Recommended Fat (30%)
1200	40 g
1500	50 g
1800	60 g
2100	70 g
2400	80 g
2700	90 g
3000	100 g

To calculate percentage of fat of total kilocalories:

1. Multiply total kilocalories by percentage of fat (0.30 used above), which yields the number of kilocalories to be contributed by fat.
2. Divide the number of kilocalories of fat by 9 to determine the total grams of fat.

To calculate the percentage of total kilocalories of a given amount of fat:

1. Multiply grams of fat by 9 to equal kilocalories contributed by fat.
2. Divide kilocalories from fat by total kilocalories to determine the percentage.

An easier way to calculate the recommended number of grams of fat is to divide the total kilocalories by 30. For example:

$$\frac{1800 \text{ kilocalories}}{30} = 60 \text{ g of fat}$$

Use the exchange list system (see Appendix 9) for an easy method to calculate fat content from a given menu. Foods not listed in the exchange list will generally be listed in a food composition table from which fat content can be determined (see Appendix 5).

What Are the American Heart Association Dietary Guidelines?

1. Total fat intake should be 30 percent or less of total kilocalories (Table 8–4 shows total recommended fat for various kilocalorie levels).
2. Saturated fatty acid intake should be 8 to 10 percent of total kilocalories.
3. Polyunsaturated fatty acid intake should be up to 10 percent of total kilocalories.
4. Monounsaturated fatty acids make up the rest of total fat intake, about 10 to 15 percent of total kilocalories.
5. Cholesterol intake should be less than 300 mg per day.
6. Sodium intake should be no more than 2400 mg (2.4 g) per day (American Heart Association, 1991–1996).

beta-carotene for the prevention of cardiovascular disease can no longer be recommended" (Mayne, 1996). The elements selenium, copper, zinc, chromium, and manganese seem to counteract the development of cardiovascular diseases, but since trace elements and human health have been scarcely studied, supplements of these minerals cannot yet be advocated (Houtman, 1996). Foods high in antioxidants, trace minerals, and naturally occuring phytochemicals and fiber continue to be the first line approach to prevent and treat CHD along with reduced saturated fat and moderate cholesterol intake.

What Advice Is Appropriate for Children's Needs?

Because atherosclerosis, or the accumulation of plaque in the arteries, begins in childhood, it is believed that adult nutrition guidelines may be helpful for healthy children older than 2 years of age. In one pediatric setting, children identified with high levels of cholesterol (>185 mg/dL) were placed on a Step One diet and found to have lower serum cholesterol levels of at least 8 percent (Fitch et al., 1997). Because of a child's growth needs, however, as well as a need to develop positive associations with eating, a punitive, overly restrictive diet is not in a child's best interest. Parents may be advised to limit fatty foods but to do so with an attitude of moderation, not total elimination. Parents can place positive emphasis on low-fat foods such as fruits, vegetables, low-fat milk products, and low-fat, whole-grain products and thereby help promote a healthy attitude toward eating. If a low-fat diet is undertaken with too much zeal, a child may experience undesirable weight loss or stunting of growth. An increased intake of monounsaturated fats would be appropriate in such situations. Foods such as natural peanut butter, olives, avocados, and most nuts (if the child is old enough to avoid choking) can provide adequate kilocalorie intake without increasing saturated fats.

How Can Dietary Intake of Saturated Fat and Cholesterol Be Controlled?

1. Eat no more than four egg yolks a week.
2. Moderate the use of shrimp and limit organ meats.
3. Use fish, skinless chicken and turkey, and veal in most of the meat meals for the week; use moderate-sized portions (3 oz of meat equals the size of a deck of cards) of beef, lamb, pork, and ham less frequently. Substitute low-fat protein foods such as legumes for meat occasionally (e.g., red beans and rice or tofu and vegetable stir-fry).
4. Choose lean cuts of meat, trim visible fat, and discard the fat that cooks out of the meat. Removing the skin from a piece of chicken eliminates about 1 tsp of fat.
5. Avoid deep-fat frying and use an oil that is low in saturated fats (corn, safflower, sunflower, peanut, or canola) when frying is done.
6. Restrict the use of fatty luncheon and variety meats such as sausage and salami.
7. Instead of butter and cooking fats that are solid or completely hydrogenated, emphasize liquid vegetable oils, such as olive oil or sesame seed oil, and soft or liquid margarines. Cooking with other liquids such as wine, water, broth, or fruit juice will help reduce the fat content of meals.
8. Instead of whole milk and cheeses made from whole milk and cream, use skim milk and skim or part-skim milk cheeses.
9. Use more plant foods in place of animal foods. For example, fill up on whole-grain breads and vegetables rather than meat. Think of meat as a side dish rather than as the main dish.
10. When shopping, look for food labels with less than 15 g of fat for a meal and less than 2 g of fat for a snack. The level of saturated fat should be no more than one third of the total amount of fat. An acceptable level of sodium per meal is 800 mg; snack foods should have less than 200 mg of sodium per serving.

Where Are Saturated Fats Found?

Saturated fat is generally the hard or solid fats in the diet. Saturated fat is the prinicipal fat in butter and in red meat (see Table 3–4). Tropical oils (which do become solid at cold refrigerator temperatures) are also high in saturated fat content. Vegetable shortenings or hydrogentated fats are vegetable oils that have added hydrogen, turning them into solid fats called **trans fatty acids.** These types of fats are not yet specifically found on food labels, although the labels will state what kind of fat was used—whether it was animal fat or vegetable oil and if the vegetable oil was left in its liquid state or was hydrogenated (saturated). You can determine if the vegetable oil used is saturated (palm oil and coconut oil), polyunsaturated (liquid corn, safflower, or sunflower oil), or monounsaturated (peanut oil, olive oil, canola oil, and the form of fat found in avocados). Food labels state total fat grams and amounts of saturated fat per serving of food but does not always break down the two forms of unsaturated fat.

It is easy to determine if a fat is saturated from its texture. If it is hard at cold temperatures it contains saturated fats. For example, when you take butter out of the refrigerator it is so hard you cannot cut it. Fat on red meat is saturated, which you can tell as you cut it off. But you have never cut a layer of fat off fish because the fat found in fish is primarily unsaturated (in liquid form). The same applies to chicken, in which the fat is soft; in other words, chicken has less saturated fat than red meat does.

Where Is Cholesterol Found?

There are two main sources of cholesterol. One is the body's natural production of cholesterol in the liver, in the gastrointestinal tract, and in almost all body cells that have a nucleus. This natural cholesterol production is affected by diet. Saturated fats tend to increase the production of cholesterol, and unsaturated fats tend to have the opposite effect. Intake of cholesterol in the diet has little impact on the body's own natural cholesterol production, although it may impair the ability of the body to clear LDL-cholesterol from the blood.

The second source of cholesterol is the foods we eat. It is important to remember that cholesterol is found only in animal products and specifically in animal fat. Skim milk and egg whites, although both animal products, have no measurable fat and therefore no significant amount of cholesterol. Plant fats such as peanut butter do not contain any cholesterol. It now appears that reducing saturated fat in the diet is more important than reducing cholesterol intake.

What Is the Role of Unsaturated Fats in the Prevention and Control of CVD?

As discussed in Chapter 3, unsaturated fats are known to reduce the body's own natural production of cholesterol. Foods with a high P:S ratio (the amount of polyunsaturated versus saturated fat) are generally helpful in preventing and controlling CVD, although persons with low levels of HDL-cholesterol are best to emphasize the monounsaturated fats (see Table 3–4).

The general recommendation is to consume equal amounts (10 percent each of total kilocalories) of saturated, monounsaturated, and polyunsaturated fats, composing a total of 30 percent of fat in the diet. For individuals with elevated total cholesterol and LDL cholesterol who do not respond to this dietary pattern, even less saturated fat should be consumed, as found in the Step Two diets of the NCEP.

What Are Omega-3 Fatty Acids?

The most unsaturated form of fat found in foods is referred to as omega-3 fatty acids. This form of fat is prevalent in cold-water fish and other foods such as dark-green leafy vegetables. Mother Nature made fish living in cold water regions with unsaturated fats that can stay soft at cold temperatures.

Omega-3 fats are known to reduce blood levels of triglycerides and thus are recommended in the control of cardiovascular disease. These fats also reduce the inflammation process of the body and tend to reduce the clotting time of the blood. One study found that patients with elevated lipids associated with kidney transplants were able to reduce their hyperlipidemia, after an earlier trial on an American Heart Association Step Two diet, through either low-dose simvistatin or with 6 g (just over 1 tsp) of fish oil (Castro et al., 1997). As little as 5.5 g of fish oil per week was associated with a 50 percent reduction in the risk of primary cardiac arrest and decreased ventricular fibrillation associated with a myocardial infarction, or heart attack (Stone, 1997).

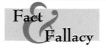

Fallacy: Fish oil capsules should be recommended for management of CVD.

Fact: Fish from the cold northern oceans contain more omega-3 fatty acids than do fish from temperate southern seas. Greenland Eskimos, who have a low incidence of atherosclerosis, have a high intake of the omega-3 type of fat through consumption of almost 1 pound of fish daily, and this finding opens an area of promise. However, because the optimal dose of these omega-3 fatty acids has not been established, recommending their widespread use is not advocated. In addition, it is not known if it is the EPA (a form of omega-3 fatty acids) or other substances in the fish that cause the lower incidence of cardiovascular disease among the Greenland Eskimos. Advice to eat more tuna fish is generally well accepted. One half teaspoon of cod liver oil per day is also safe.

What Is the Connection between CVD and Fiber?

There is growing evidence that dietary fiber may play a role in preventing and controlling CVD. As noted in Chapter 3, the water-soluble fibers—pectins from fruits, gums from legumes, and the water-soluble fiber in oat grain—appear to be effective in reducing serum cholesterol levels. The benefits of soluble fiber are so impressive that daily consumption has been advised, whether it comes from oat bran, brown rice, legumes, barley, or other sources. (See Appendix 6 for fiber content of foods.)

What Are Antioxidants and What Is Their Role in CVD?

The main **antioxidants** are vitamins C, E, and beta-carotene (the precursor to vitamin A). These nutrients are believed to help prevent harm from oxygen in the blood vessels, thereby reducing the plaquing process on artery walls. Foods containing these antioxidants are known to reduce CVD (see Chapter 5).

It is hypothesized that dietary antioxidants may help prevent the development and progression of atherosclerosis. The available evidence helps substanti-

One-Day Sample Menu for a Step One Diet (approximately 2000 kilocalories)

Breakfast

grapefruit half
1 c oatmeal
1 slice whole-wheat toast
2 tsp natural peanut butter

8 oz skim milk
coffee
2 tsp brown sugar or jelly

Lunch

turkey sandwich:
   3 oz turkey (no skin)
   2 slices bread
   tomato slices

½ c cole slaw made with 1 tsp
   mayonnaise dressing
small apple
iced tea with lemon

Afternoon Snack

8 oz low-fat Yogurt

¼ c almonds

Supper

3 oz pork tenderloin
1 c brown rice
½ c spinach sauteed in 2 tsp
   olive oil and garlic

½ c carrots with lemon juice
1 c tossed salad with 1 tbsp Italian
   dressing
8 oz skim milk

Evening Snack

3 c low-fat popcorn

ate this hypothesis but is not yet conclusive. The results of several ongoing large randomized intervention trials will provide valuable information about the efficacy and safety of supplemental dietary antioxidants in prevention of atherosclerosis (Duell, 1996).

Can Excess Iron in the Diet Cause CVD?

Some researchers have hypothesized that women are at decreased risk of heart disease when compared to men because menstruation lowers iron stores, which may limit the oxidation of lipids. One study showed that nonsmoking men who donated blood once or twice in the previous three-year period had a reduced risk of cardiovascular events such as myocardial infarcts, angina, and stroke as well as procedures such as angioplasty and bypass surgery, thus lending further support to the iron hypothesis (Meyers et al., 1997). Women after menopause do have an increased rate of heart disease. The role of iron in heart disease is still, however, in the theory stage. As iron-deficiency anemia is a health problem, caution should be exercised. Individuals at risk of high serum iron levels, such as those with hemochromatosis (see Chapter 5) should be advised to avoid iron. For the general public, avoidance of iron is not yet recommended.

WHAT IS THE ROLE OF EXERCISE IN THE MANAGEMENT OF CARDIOVASCULAR DISEASE?

Exercise is a well-known component of weight control, and because obesity is a risk factor associated with the development of CVD, it should be an integral aspect in both the prevention and the treatment of CVD. However, exercise should be practiced as appropriately determined by a physician, particularly for the person at high risk for CVD.

In addition, regular aerobic exercise (any exercise that makes a person take in more air, such as a brisk walk) is associated with increased levels of HDL cholesterol and decreased levels of LDL cholesterol, and it has been recommended that patients with low HDL levels (see Table 8–1) be encouraged to exercise. Again, aerobic exercise should be appropriate for the person's condition, and consultation with a physician is always prudent.

WHAT IS HYPERTENSION AND WHAT IS ITS ROLE IN THE TREATMENT OF CARDIOVASCULAR DISEASE?

Hypertension is an elevation of the blood pressure to greater than normal levels, which is generally considered to be more than 140/90 mmHg (the top number is the systolic pressure and the bottom number is the diastolic pressure; the diastolic pressure is the more significant number). Hypertension is often associated with CVD, diabetes, and renal disease. It is one of the most important risk factors associated with the development of CVD. The underlying insulin resistance with hyperinsulinemia (see Chapter 9) of diabetes found in adults is generally believed to increase sodium retention. Thus diabetes, hypertension, and CVD are often found together. One study supports the notion that reduced hyperinsulinemia reduces blood pressure as demonstrated by the study of the mineral vanadium, which caused significant decreases in both plasma insulin concentration and blood pressure (Bhanot et al., 1995). Reducing insulin production via reduced carbohydrate intake may thus reduce the incidence of hypertension for those individuals with insulin resistance.

What Dietary Treatments Are Used for the Control of Hypertension?

Because obesity is a predisposing factor in hypertension, a low-kilocalorie diet is often prescribed to reduce weight. Although this is the ideal solution—weight loss is known to reduce insulin resistance and reduce LDL-cholesterol levels—it can be difficult to achieve. However, stabilizing the weight of one who has been experiencing a steady weight gain may achieve the desired outcomes of an improved lipid profile and reduced blood pressure. Sodium restriction is often recommended. Further adjustments in protein and fluids as well as sodium intake are made if there is concurrent kidney disease. Sodium restriction improves the effectiveness of diuretic therapy. Patients who take potassium-depleting diuretics are advised to increase their potassium intake to replenish what is lost in the increased urine volume. Bananas and orange juice are frequently recommended for their potassium content, but many foods are high in potassium. Most fresh vegetables (especially dark green leafy ones), most fruits, legumes, milk, and fresh meats are good sources of potassium (see Table 7–4) and add only a small amount of sodium to the diet. Physicians should be consulted before using a potassium substitute for salt; individuals on ACE inhibitors should not use salt substitutes containing potassium.

Salt is often linked to hypertension simply because the **sodium** in salt causes the body to accumulate fluid. Any excess fluid puts greater pressure on the walls of the blood vessels, creating higher blood pressure. Many people with high blood pressure find that reducing salt in the diet will often bring their pressure within the normal range.

Excess alcohol may also raise blood pressure. A moderate intake of alcohol is generally considered safe unless there are contraindications to its use. A low-saturated fat and high-soluble fiber intake may also lower blood pressure, probably through reduced insulin resistance.

What Are the Purposes and Indications for Sodium-Controlled Diets?

There are several reasons for restricting sodium intake (see Chapter 5 to review information on sodium). The indications for restricting sodium intake include the following:

1. Hypertension (to relieve elevated or high blood pressure)
2. **Congestive heart failure (CHF)** (a condition in which the heart cannot pump blood adequately)
3. **Edema,** (a condition of fluid build-up, which can be treated by helping the body to eliminate sodium and fluids)
4. Renal disorders with edema
5. Adrenocorticotropic hormone and cortisone therapy
6. Cirrhosis of the liver with ascites (a disease often caused by alcoholism but also derived from other causes)
7. To meet the Dietary Guidelines for Americans of 2400 mg of sodium per day

What Is a Sodium-Restricted Diet?

A sodium-restricted diet is a normal adequate diet with a modified sodium content, from a very low amount of 1000 mg to 3000 mg.

An average diet prepared in the kitchen with some commercially prepared foods, foods salted during cooking, and some salt added at the table provides about 3000 to 7000 mg of sodium daily. (These numbers should not be confused with salt intake—sodium composes 40 percent of salt. One teaspoon of salt

Table 8–5
Sodium Restricted Diets

Foods	2–4 g Sodium	1 g Sodium
Milk	3 c milk or yogurt, no processed cheese; natural cheese (1 oz) can replace 1 c milk; free use of low-sodium cheese	2 c milk or yogurt; up to 1 oz natural cheese can be substituted for 1 c milk; free use of low-sodium cheese
Meat and meat substitutes	Limited use of processed meats; free use of fresh meat	No processed meat; use salt-free canned tuna; limited use of regular peanut butter; free use of low-sodium peanut butter
Breads and cereals	Avoid breads and crackers with salt topping; regular bread may be used in normal amounts; free use of low-sodium bread and cereal products; avoid canned soups and vegetables and cereals with added salt	Up to 2 slices regular bread may be used or 1 serving regular processed cereal; free use of low-sodium breads and cereals
Vegetables and fruits	All fresh, frozen, and dried; all canned fruit but limited use of canned vegetables; free use of low-sodium canned vegetables; no salted products such as potato chips or french fries	Use only low-sodium canned vegetables; limited use of naturally high-sodium vegetables (beets, carrots, celery, spinach); free use of all others
Condiments		
Sweets		
Brown sugar	Free use	Free use
Table sugar	Free use	Free use
Honey	Free use	Free use
Jams and jellies	Free use	Free use
Maple syrup	Free use	Free use
Molasses	Free use	Free use
Sauces		
Catsup	Limited use	Use low-sodium
Mayonnaise	Limited use	Use low-sodium
Mustard	Limited use	Use low-sodium
Soy sauce	Limited use	Use low-sodium
Worcestershire sauce	Limited use	Not allowed
Butter/margarine	Limited use	Use low-sodium
Other		
Cooking oil	Free use	Free use
Vinegar	Free use	Free use
Spices		
Natural	Free use	Free use
Salt-based	Limited use	Not allowed
Lemon	Free use	Free use
Horseradish	Free use	Limited use
Salt	Very limited use (few sprinkles)	Use salt substitute (physician approval)

contains about 2000 mg of sodium.) For therapeutic purposes, sodium intake may vary from 1000 mg daily to 2000 mg or more. Diets in which sodium is limited were formerly called low-salt diets, when salt was omitted only in the preparation of food, and salt-free diets, when it was not allowed either in cooking or at the table. Such diets are now named in terms of the level of sodium restriction, the most usual being the 2000 to 4000 mg sodium diet (mild restriction), the 1000 mg sodium diet (moderate), and the 500 mg sodium diet (very strict and seldomly used nowadays). Table 8–5 shows the differences among sodium-restricted diets for different sodium levels. See Chapter 5 for more information on sodium.

Although the initial elimination of salt from the diet is very difficult for a person used to its taste, the taste for salt can be unlearned. Use of spices, herbs, lemon juice, or vinegar can help enhance the taste appeal of food while the preference for salt is changing.

Is Calcium Related to Hypertension?

There is growing evidence that a nutritionally adequate amount of calcium in the diet plays a role in the control of hypertension. However, the situation appears to be more complex with other nutrients, such as sodium, potassium, and magnesium. Milk contains calcium, potassium, and magnesium. Vegetarians generally have lower blood pressure, and one explanation is that the lower protein and sodium content of their diets allows more efficient use of dietary calcium. Weight control, sodium restriction, and an adequate intake of calcium and potassium food sources (milk, fruit, and vegetables) along with reduced saturated fat and increased soluble fiber all contribute to the control of hypertension.

WHAT IS THE ROLE OF DRUG THERAPY IN THE MANAGEMENT OF CARDIOVASCULAR DISEASE?

Drug therapy has a place in the management of CVD. However, as all drugs have potential negative side effects, medical nutrition therapy, such as the AHA Step One Diet, should be the first step in CVD management. If **hypercholesterolemia** (high serum cholesterol levels) does not respond to medical nutrition therapy as provided by a registered dietitian, several medications may be prescribed in addition to medical nutrition therapy. The level of elevated lipids also dictates the drug of choice, as some medications lower total cholesterol and LDL cholesterol whereas others lower triglyceride levels.

In the management of hypertension, beta-blockers such as the thiazide medications are the drug of last resort for the person who has diabetes, although they are effective in nondiabetics. Other antihyperensive medications, ACE inhibitors, calcium channel blockers, alpha-agonists, and low-dose diuretics may be more appropriate for the person with diabetes or the insulin resistance syndrome (Lapuz, 1997).

WHAT IS THE ROLE OF THE NURSE OR OTHER HEALTH CARE PROFESSIONAL IN THE PREVENTION AND CONTROL OF CARDIOVASCULAR DISEASE?

The nurse and other health care professionals are important team members in the fight against CVD. A large body of evidence reinforces the belief that nutritional changes can lower the risk of CVD. Yet many individuals either are not aware of how to make appropriate dietary changes to help prevent CVD or believe that the cost of change is greater than the results accrued. The nurse has the opportunity through direct patient contact to assess the reasons that various individuals may not be following the general CVD reduction guidelines.

A health care professional can assess whether lack of knowledge is the reason for poor dietary compliance by saying, "You probably have heard about cholesterol and saturated fat in television commercials, but are you aware of which foods contain high amounts?" Sometimes a negative attitude or belief may be the reason for not making dietary changes. To assess this, a good question would be, "How do you feel about all the talk concerning cholesterol?"

Through positive reinforcement of steps taken, no matter how small, and referral to appropriate services, the nurse and other health care professionals can play a key role in reducing this society's primary health risk.

Critical Thinking

Case Study

Allan was at his family gathering eating Haggis. His grandmother used to fix it and now his mother continued to prepare it during holidays. He wondered if it was okay to eat Haggis since he found out he had high cholesterol. He wasn't surprised at this diagnosis because his grandfather had died of a heart attack while only in his fifties. Actually, Allan thought to himself, he'd rather go with a quick heart attack than to linger like his older sister who had become paralyzed after her stroke. He didn't want to linger in a nursing home.

Applications

1. How do heritage and cultural food habits interrelate in chronic health conditions? How might your ethnic heritage dictate the foods you should include to maintain cardiovascular health?
2. Find out what Haggis is and what country it is associated with. What changes in the American food availability and choices may have influenced cardiovascular disease risk for various populations in the United States, such as persons with Native American, African, Hispanic, Asian, Greek, Italian, Irish, French, German, or Scottish heritage? What foods did these population groups subsist on over the centuries? What are some heart-healthy foods that these populations may still eat today that are not commonly found in U.S. restaurants?

Each student in the class might choose a different ethnic heritage to research and present to the class.

3. What risk factors does Allan have for cardiovascular disease?

Study Questions and Classroom Activities

1. Interview family members regarding personal family history of CVD and hypertension. Use Figure 8–3 to determine your personal risk factors for heart disease.
2. List traditional ethnic foods from your family's meals (those your grandparents ate or those that are currently consumed); which foods do you like to eat that are low in saturated fat and high in soluble fiber?
3. Collect samples of vegetable oils, including at least one that is predominantly a saturated fat, one that is a monounsaturated, and one that is a polyunsaturated fat, and refrigerate all of them. Compare textures to determine the degree of solidity.
4. Taste-test low-sodium food products. Compare these foods with different seasonings, such as spices, herbs, lemon, and jelly.

H E A R T

Everyone plays the game of health whether he wants to or not. What is your score? Add up the numbers in each category that most nearly describe you.

Heredity	1 No known history of heart disease	2 One relative with heart disease over 60 years	3 Two relatives with heart disease over 60 years	4 One relative with heart disease under 60 years	6 Two relatives with heart disease under 60 years
Exercise	1 Intensive exercise, work and recreation	2 Moderate exercise, work and recreation	3 Sedentary work & intensive recreational exercise	5 Sedentary work & moderate recreational exercise	6 Sedentary work & light recreational exercise
Age	1 10–20	2 21–30	3 31–40	4 41–50	6 51–65
Lb	0 More than 5 lb below standard weight	1 ± 5 lb standard weight	2 6–20 lb overweight	4 21–35 lb overweight	6 36–50 lb overweight
Tobacco	0 Nonuser	1 Cigar or pipe	2 10 cigarettes or fewer per day	4 20 cigarettes or more per day	6 30 cigarettes or more per day
Habits of eating Fat	1 0% No animal or solid fats	2 10% Very little animal or solid fats	3 20% Little animal or solid fats	4 30% Much animal or solid fats	5 40% Very much animal or solid fats

Your risk of heart attack:

 4–9 Very remote 16–20 Average 26–30 Dangerous
 10–15 Below average 21–25 Moderate 31–35 Urgent danger — reduce score!

Other conditions — such as stress, high blood pressure, and increased blood cholesterol — detract from health and should be evaluated by your physician.

Figure 8–3

Risk factors in heart disease. (Courtesy of the School of Public Health, Loma Linda University, Loma Linda, CA.)

5. List 20 everyday foods and then read food labels of these foods to determine fat and sodium content.
6. Evaluate your family's saturated fat intake per food labels.
7. Class role-play: One volunteer will play Allan in the case study; another will serve as a health care professional describing the different types of blood fats and food fats and how they interact. The health care professional should assess Allan's health belief values toward cardiovascular disease and offer options for dietary changes to decrease his risk of CVD.
8. If your client has been placed on a low saturated fat diet, what could you recommend he take for lunch to his construction work site? What could you recommend for a dessert if his triglyceride level is normal or if it is elevated?
9. Bring some family recipes to class. Assess whether these recipes contribute to heart disease because they are high in saturated fat, or sodium, or both. How could the recipes be modified to lower the fat and sodium content?

References

American Heart Association: The American Heart Association Diet, An Eating Plan for Healthy Americans, 1991–1996, Dallas, TX.

Barnard RJ, DiLauro SC, Inkeles SB: Effects of intensive diet and exercise intervention in patients taking cholesterol-lowering drugs. Am J Cardiol. April 15, 1997; 79(8): 1112–1114.

Bhanot S, Michoulas A, McNeill JH: Antihypertensive effects of vanadium compounds in hyperinsulinemic, hypertensive rats. Mol Cell Biochem. December 1995; 153(1–2): 205–209.

Bolton-Smith C, Woodward M, Fenton S, Brown CA: Does dietary trans fatty acid intake relate to the prevalence of coronary heart disease in Scotland? Eur Heart J. June 1996; 17(6):837–845.

Castro R, Queiros J, Fonseca I, Pimentel JP, Henriques AC, Sarmento AM, Guimaraes S, Pereira MC: Therapy of post-renal transplantation hyperlipidaemia: Comparative study with simvastatin and fish oil. Nephrol Dial Transplant. October 1997; 12(10):2140–2143.

Cleeman JI: Adults aged 20 and older should have their cholesterol measured. Am J Med. February 17, 1997; 102(2A):31–36.

Coulston A: Insulin resistance: Its role in health and disease and implications for nutrition management. Topics in Nutrition. Issue no 6, p. 10, 1997.

Duell PB: Prevention of atherosclerosis with dietary antioxidants: Fact or fiction? J Nutr. April 1996; 126(4 Suppl):1067S–1071S.

Duell PB, Malinow MR: Homocyst(e)ine: An important risk factor for atherosclerotic vascular disease. Curr Opin Lipidol. February 1997; 8(1):28–34.

Fitch J, Garcia RE, Moodie DS, Secic M: Influence of cholesterol screening and nutritional counseling in reducing cholesterol levels in children. Clin Pediatr (Phila). May 1997; 36(5):267–272.

Fruchart JC, Packard CJ: Is cholesterol the major lipoprotein risk factor in coronary heart disease?—A Franco-Scottish overview. Curr Med Res Opin. 1997; 13(10):603–616.

Haffner SM, D'Agostino R, Saad MF, Rewers M, Mykkanen L, Selby J, Howard G, Savage PJ, Hamman RF, Wagenknecht LE, et al.: Increased insulin resistance and insulin secretion in nondiabetic African-Americans and Hispanics compared with non-Hispanic whites. The Insulin Resistance Atherosclerosis Study. Diabetes. June 1996;45(6): 742–748.

Hall WD, Ferrario CM, Moore MA, Hall JE, Flack JM, Cooper W, Simmons JD, Egan BM, Lackland DT, Perry M Jr, Roccella EJ: Hypertension-related morbidity and mortality in the southeastern United States. Am J Med Sci. April 1997; 313(4):195–209.

Houtman JP: Trace elements and cardiovascular diseases. J Cardiovasc Risk. February 1996; 3(1):18–25.

Lapuz MH: Diabetic nephropathy. Med Clin North Am. May 1997; 81(3):679–688.

Mayne ST: Beta-carotene, carotenoids, and disease prevention in humans. FASEB J. May 1996; 10(7):690–701.

Meyers DG, Strickland D, Maloley PA, Seburg JK, Wilson JE, McManus BF: Possible association of a reduction in cardiovascular events with blood donation. Heart. August 1997; 78(2):188–193.

O'Neill, M.: New York Times, February 8, 1995 pp. 1 + C6.

Rocha E, Gouveia-Oliveira A, Cotter A, Laranjeiro A, Sousa A, Mendes F, Teixeira H, Galvao J, Miguel JM: Risk factors for cerebrovascular stroke in a cohort of hypertensive patients. Rev Port Cardiol. June 1997; 16(6):543–556. [Article in Portugese.]

Stone NJ: Fish consumption, fish oil, lipids, and coronary heart disease. Am J Clin Nutr. 1997; 65:1083–1086.

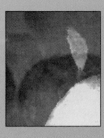

9

Diabetes Mellitus

Objectives

After completing this chapter, you should be able to:

- Describe the different types of diabetes mellitus.
- Describe the symptoms and clinical findings of diabetes mellitus.
- Relate the nutritional management of diabetes mellitus to the Dietary Guidelines for Americans and the Food Guide Pyramid.
- Explain differences in the nutritional management of the different forms of diabetes.
- Describe the importance of the self-monitoring of blood glucose.
- Explain the role and special concerns of exercise in diabetes management.
- Describe the role of health care professionals in facilitating the nutritional aspects of diabetes management.

Terms to Identify

Albuminuria
Autonomic neuropathy
Beta cells
Carbohydrate counting
Common gene therapy
Counter-regulatory hormones
Dawn phenomenon
Diabetes mellitus
Diabetic coma
Diabetic retinopathy
15:15 rule
1500 rule

Food exchange lists
Gastroparesis
Gestational diabetes mellitus (GDM)
Glucagon
Glucose
Glycated
Glycemic index
Glycogenolysis
Glycosuria
Hemoglobin
Honeymoon period
Hormones
Hyperglycemia

Hyperglycemic hyperosmolar nonketotic syndrome (HHNK)
Hyperinsulinemia
Hypoglycemic unawareness
Insulin-dependent diabetes mellitus (IDDM)
Insulin reaction
Insulin resistance syndrome
Insulin-to-carbohydrate ratio

Islets of Langerhans
Ketoacidosis
Ketonuria
MODY
Non-insulin-dependent
   diabetes mellitus
   (NIDDM)
Oral hypoglycemic agents

Pancreas
Pattern management
Peripheral neuropathy
Podiatrist
Polydipsia
Polyphagia
Polyuria
Post-prandially

Reactive hypoglycemia
Renal threshold
Self-monitoring of blood
   glucose (SMBG)
Somogyi effect
Waist-to-hip ratio
   (WHR)

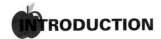INTRODUCTION

Insulin resistance is frequently the underlying cause of Type 2 diabetes, the most prevalent form of diabetes (a condition related to blood glucose levels). Insulin resistance means that the body cells resist the action of insulin. An estimated one out of four Americans have insulin resistance. One theory of why insulin resistance is so common is that historically many of our ancestors faced periods of famine. It is believed that our biological heritage—acquired when people had to survive in a hunter-gatherer culture, before modern agriculture and food preservation were widely available—has not yet adapted to a westernized lifestyle with abundant food supplies and little physical activity.

The varying levels of insulin resistance and insulin production require individualized medical nutrition therapy. Some individuals produce large amounts of insulin in relation to the carbohydrate consumed in their diet. This is referred to as hyperinsulinemia. The Food Guide Pyramid and the Dietary Guidelines for Americans, appropriate for the general public, are specific management strategies for the control of diabetes. Maintaining desirable body weight, emphasizing complex carbohydrate foods high in soluble fiber, with lowering one's intake of sugar, saturated fat, and sodium all help the person with diabetes live a full and productive life.

The changing demographics of this country will result in an increased number of persons with diabetes because of an increased proportion of elderly persons and of persons of color in the population: both groups are at high risk for diabetes. Caribbean Latinos, for example, are two to three times more likely than non-Hispanic whites to develop diabetes, but a study in the Boston area found that this group had little understanding of the long-term consequences of diabetes, fatalism regarding the course of the disease, multiple barriers to diet and exercise interventions, skepticism regarding the value of preventive health behaviors, and prevalent use of traditional nonmedical remedies (Quatromoni et al., 1994). There is also a growing recognition that a higher than normal blood sugar level that is not actually diabetes is linked to heart disease. All health care professionals, especially nurses, should become thoroughly versed in the management of diabetes. Very few people know that diabetes is related to heart disease, stroke, kidney disease, hypertension, blindness, and nerve damage with circulation problems. Health care professionals can play a vital role in educating the public about diabetes and helping to sort out known versus perceived methods to manage the disease.

WHAT IS THE INSULIN RESISTANCE SYNDROME?

Insulin resistance is sometimes referred to as the **common gene theory.** This is because it is commonly found and is the common cause of many chronic health conditions. The **insulin resistance syndrome,** originally referred to as Syndrome X in 1988 by Dr. Gerald Reaven and also called the metabolic syndrome, is a condition diagnosed by correlates. The correlates include the following:

- Hypertension: blood pressure (BP) > 140/90; lower BP goals are set with the diagnosis of diabetes or renal disease
- High-levels of triglycerides: >200 mg/dL, with low-levels of HDL-cholesterol (<35 mg/dL)
- Central obesity: waist-to-hip ratio (WHR) > 0.8 in women or 1.0 in men, or waist in inches > 35 in women or > 40 in men (Bjorntorp, 1997)
- Diabetes: fasting blood glucose (FBG) > 126 mg/dL on two occasions
- Gout: uric acid > 7
- Polycystic ovary syndrome: Lack of ovulation and hirsutism (excessive body hair)

Persons with insulin resistance usually have hyperinsulinemia as well. Research continues on the "chicken versus egg" concept. The growing belief is that insulin resistance is a genetically inherited condition that is worsened by obesity and lack of activity, which leads to the hyperinsulinemia. There is some evidence that hyperinsulinemia exacerbates insulin resistance. Further, some limited evidence but much anecdotal evidence indicate that carbohydrates cause an increase in central obesity, which supports the theory that hyperinsulinemia promotes weight gain, causing a vicious cycle of obesity, diabetes, and the other correlates of the insulin resistance syndrome (see also Chapter 20). Much more will be learned in the future on the cause and treatment of insulin resistance and its associated correlates.

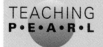

TEACHING P•E•A•R•L To explain insulin resistance, health care professionals can use the analogy of a coal stove. Each of the millions of microscopic body cells can be considered microscopic coal stoves—thus we are made up of millions of furnaces waiting to burn the carbon found in our carbohydrate foods. The insulin acts as the shovel to put the carbon (coal) into the body cells (coal stoves) so that it can be burned for energy. When the door on the stove (receptor sites on body cells) resists opening (insulin resistance), the coal pile (blood glucose caused by consuming excess carbohydrate) begins to pile up. Small shovels full of coal (small carbohydrate meals) are more efficiently burned without promoting after-meal hyperglycemia (too much sugar in the blood).

WHAT ARE THE BASIC FACTS ABOUT DIABETES MELLITUS?

Diabetes mellitus, commonly referred to by the public as "having sugar," is a serious metabolic disorder related to the utilization of carbohydrate and its end product **glucose** (blood sugar). The metabolism of protein and fat is affected as well. According to the American Diabetes Association, diabetes affects approximately 16 million individuals in the United States, or 5 percent of the total population and 10 to 15 percent of Medicare beneficiaries (that is, the elderly population). Of the 1 in 20 Americans who have diabetes, only about half know they have it. Mortality statistics of diabetes are underrated because most people with diabetes die from related causes such as heart disease.

Etiology

Type 1 diabetes mellitus usually results from a destruction of the beta cells in the pancreas, causing a complete lack of insulin production **(insulin-dependent diabetes mellitus [IDDM]).** Type 1 diabetes was previously referred to as juvenile-onset diabetes because the peak age of onset is during puberty. It is again being called Type 1 diabetes (in arabic numeral form versus the roman numeral). This is due to the IDDM (Type 1) classification being confused when a person with Type 2 diabetes used insulin to control blood glucose levels. In this other form of diabetes, formerly called adult-onset, Type II, or **non-insulin-dependent diabetes mellitus (NIDDM),** the chief cause of **hyperglycemia** (excess insulin in the blood) is insulin resistance at the cell level. There are varying amounts of insulin production in Type 2 diabetes: high, normal, or low. Figure 9–1 shows the differences between Type 1 and Type 2 diabetes.

Heredity is a risk factor for the development of diabetes. Persons with Type 1 tend to have few relatives with diabetes but do have the genetic predisposition for its development. It is believed that some stressor, such as a viral illness, allows the body's immune system to go "haywire" and attack the beta cells where insulin is produced. Higher rates of Type 1 diabetes are generally found among people with family heritage from northern latitudes. Exceptions to this are Liguria and Sardinia in Italy, which rival the rates of Type 1 diabetes found in northern European countries (Mazzella et al., 1994).

Heredity plays a critical role in the development of Type 2 diabetes. The propensity to insulin resistance is inherited and is exacerbated by obesity and excess saturated fat intake. Individuals with insulin resistance often produce two to three times more insulin than is normally expected. Persons with this form of diabetes generally have many family members with a history of diabetes, high blood pressure, heart disease, and obesity. The genetic predisposition and incidence of Type 2 diabetes increase in people whose ancestors are from regions nearer the equator, with the highest prevalence being among persons of African, Native American, Asian, Pacific Island, and Southern European heritage such as the Hispanic population. In these populations, Type 2 diabetes may be present in 10 percent to as much as 50 percent of the adult population, with impaired glucose tolerance (IGT) being even more prevalent (Florez, 1997). Persons of northern

	INSULIN-DEPENDENT	NON–INSULIN-DEPENDENT
GENDER:	Males and females.	Increased rate among females.
ETHNICITY:	Increased rates among persons with Northern European heritage.	Increased rates among persons with heritage from equatorial countries (highest rates found with Native American, Hispanic, African American, Asian, Pacific Islander, Mediterranean).
AGE OF ONSET:	Generally under 30 years with peak onset prior to puberty.	Generally over 40 years, although the genetic predisposition is inherited and onset may be seen at younger ages.
WEIGHT:	Usually normal or underweight; unintentional weight loss often precedes diagnosis.	Usually overweight but may be of normal weight.
TREATMENT:	Insulin injections necessary to prevent death. Food and exercise have to be balanced with insulin injections.	Weight loss is usually the first goal. Reduction of sugar and fat, and increase of fiber (soluble) helpful. Oral hypoglycemic agents or insulin or both may be necessary for good blood sugar management but are not necessary to prevent imminent death. Exercise important.
BETA CELL* FUNCTIONING:	Totally absent (no insulin is produced) after the "honeymoon period": residual insulin is produced for about 1 year after diagnosis.	Excess insulin production usually evident (hyperinsulinemia) but due to insulin resistance at the cell level, there is relative insulin insufficiency. Insulin production may also be normal or below normal.

* Beta cells are found in the pancreas.

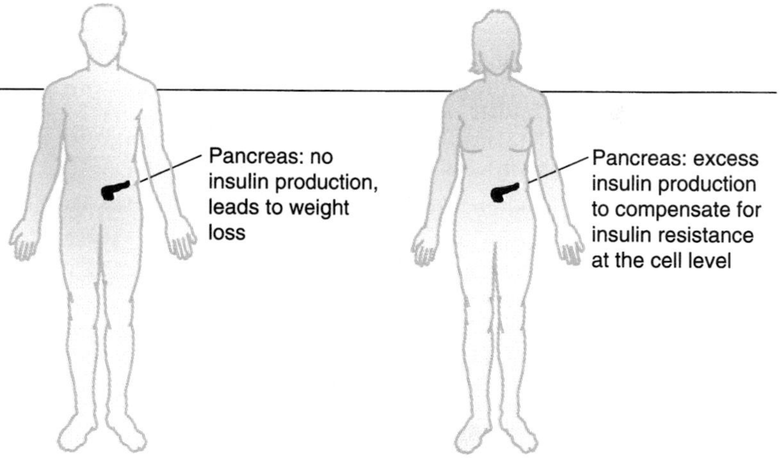

Pancreas: no insulin production, leads to weight loss

Pancreas: excess insulin production to compensate for insulin resistance at the cell level

Figure 9–1
Differences between Type 1 and Type 2.

European heritage tend to have a lower incidence of Type 2 diabetes. Asian Indians have a high rate of diabetes but low rates of obesity. They do, however, have high **waist-to-hip ratios** (**WHR:** waist measurement divided by hip measurement) with high levels of insulin resistance and hyperinsulinemia (Snehalatha, 1997).

There is a great deal of evidence that links a more Westernized lifestyle (a low-fiber, high-fat, and high-sugar diet with low levels of physical activity) with the development of Type 2 diabetes. This has been noted most recently in China, where the incidence of diabetes has increased three times in a 10-year period as economic development has brought about changes from a traditional to a modernized lifestyle (Pan et al., 1997). But the genetic predisposition toward diabetes must be present before diet and obesity can cause diabetes. Part of the change in diet to more processed foods means lowered intake of trace minerals. Trace minerals are removed in the processing of grains, which may promote increased insulin resistance. Zinc and chromium, as found in brewer's yeast, are known cofactors for insulin production. It is very likely that manganese, vanadium, and selenium have a favorable effect on carbohydrate metabolism as well (Kimura, 1996). Emphasizing legumes and whole grains in the diet will allow for high intakes of trace minerals.

Type 1 Diabetes

Because insulin production is minimal or completely lacking in Type 1 diabetes, insulin is required in the form of daily injections (Fig. 9–2 shows standard two-injection results and three-injection results; three injections are now recommended so that the nighttime peak action of NPH [a form of long-lasting insulin] occurs closer to morning). Without insulin, ketoacidosis sets in quickly and makes a person very ill. **Ketoacidosis** is an acidic state caused by a rapid breakdown of body fat. The onset of this type of diabetes is usually sudden and severe. The person with Type 1 diabetes has most, if not all, of the clinical signs and symptoms at the time of diagnosis that will be discussed in following sections.

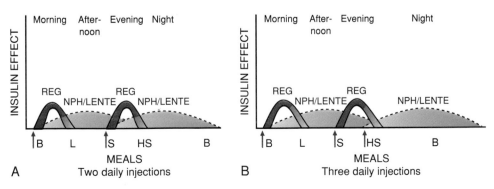

Figure 9–2
Peak action and Insulin injection times.

Control is accomplished only through insulin injection along with structured meals and exercise. During the first year after diagnosis of this form of diabetes, there may be a temporary period of insulin production before the beta cells completely exhaust their insulin production. This is referred to as the **honeymoon period.** Thus, a person with Type 1 diabetes may find that she or he needs little or no insulin after early treatment of hyperglycemia. Patients should be forewarned that this situation will change as the honeymoon period comes to an end.

Because onset typically begins in childhood, management issues become complex. The complete lack of natural insulin production makes the balancing of food and exercise with insulin injection a challenge. Regular blood sugar monitoring is required to prevent and compensate for high and low blood sugar readings. There is great stress on the family to care for a child with diabetes. Sibling relationships can suffer. Diabetes summer camp programs, in which acceptance of the disease and control strategies are emphasized, can be very helpful for families. Approximately 5 to 10 percent of all cases of diabetes are Type 1 diabetes.

Type 2 Diabetes

Insulin resistance at receptor sites is the underlying mechanism in Type 2 diabetes. Elevated production of insulin usually occurs in the body's attempt to regulate blood glucose levels. The onset of this type of diabetes is slow and gradual and is often asymptomatic. Hyperglycemia is usually evident, but ketoacidosis is frequently not a problem at the time of diagnosis, as it is with Type 1 diabetes. If the body has an inadequate amount of insulin for its needs, oral hypoglycemic drug therapy, insulin, or both may be required. Because most persons with Type 2 diabetes have hyperinsulinemia, changes in the diet often are adequate for blood glucose control. Obese individuals may need to reduce their weight if treatment is to be successful. Often however, weight loss can be difficult to achieve as, at least for some individuals, the body will adjust its kilocalorie needs for weight maintanence even in the presence of reduced kilocalories (Leibel et al., 1995). Fortunately for most persons with diabetes who eat less than is needed, the blood glucose level will be reduced even if weight loss is minimal. A person with Type 2 diabetes who requires insulin for good blood glucose management may be able to decrease or discontinue insulin treatment eventually if he or she maintains good dietary and exercise management. Reduction of stressors such as infection, burns, and surgery is also important for blood glucose management without insulin. Thus, a person with Type 2 diabetes may need temporary use of insulin while hospitalized for surgery or during times of illness. Most persons with diabetes have Type 2 diabetes, and most of these persons are overweight.

Maturity Onset Diabetes of Youth (MODY)

This form of diabetes is just now beginning to be understood. **Maturity onset diabetes of youth (MODY)** is a form of diabetes that develops in younger adults but is more similar to Type 2 diabetes. It may or may not require insulin therapy.

Impaired Fasting Glucose (Impaired Glucose Tolerance)

Impaired glucose tolerance (IGT) has been referred to in the past as borderline diabetes. A newer term is now advised: *impaired fasting glucose (IFG),* which is diagnosed when fasting plasma glucose is greater than 110 mg/dL (diabetes being two FBG greater than 126 mg/dL). (The Expert Committee on the Diagnosis and Classification of Diabetes Mellitus, 1997). Impaired glucose tolerance is associated with an increased risk of macrovascular disease (Florez, 1997). Treatment remains the same as that for Type 2 diabetes (see the following sections).

Gestational Diabetes

Gestational diabetes mellitus (GDM) is a temporary form of diabetes that occurs during the latter part of pregnancy. It is often found in women with a family history of Type 2 diabetes and thus is generally related to the genetic predisposition to insulin resistance. Because it occurs after fetal development (see Chapter 16), the risk for birth defects is different than for a woman who has Type 1 or preexisting Type 2 diabetes. There is virtually no difference in pregnancy outcomes for a woman who has GDM or for a woman with Type 1 or Type 2 diabetes if near normal blood glucose is achieved prior to conception and maintained at near normal levels throughout the pregnancy (as compared to a woman without diabetes). Increased placental hormones produced during the latter stages of pregnancy, which work counter to insulin (see the section on counter-regulatory hormones), are the primary cause of GDM.

Weight loss is not an appropriate goal for the woman with gestational diabetes because of the growth needs of the developing fetus. Diet control focuses on slow but steady weight gain, avoidance of concentrated sugar sources (as they are high in carbohydrate content), and frequent, small, balanced meals. A prescribed kilocalorie-restricted diet is generally unnecessary and can even be harmful unless the patient understands that the kilocalorie restriction is for control of weight gain, not for weight loss.

The blood sugar goals during pregnancy are very strict (the goal for all blood glucose levels, including post-prandial, are less than 120 mg/dL). Self-monitoring of blood glucose is essential, as is checking for morning urine ketones. Occasionally a woman with GDM will require insulin to maintain good control of blood sugar levels. The detection of ketones may signal the need for more carbohydrate (such as when a woman with GDM tries too aggressively to lower carbohydrate in an attempt to avoid the use of insulin). If the need for carbohydrate to prevent ketone formation results in hyperglycemia, insulin will be required until the time of delivery. See Chapter 16 for more information on diabetes and pregnancy.

Reactive Hypoglycemia

In **reactive hypoglycemia,** excess carbohydrates cause the body to produce too much insulin. However, because the overproduction of insulin is delayed, the blood glucose level first rises too high and then falls too quickly (Fig. 9–3 shows

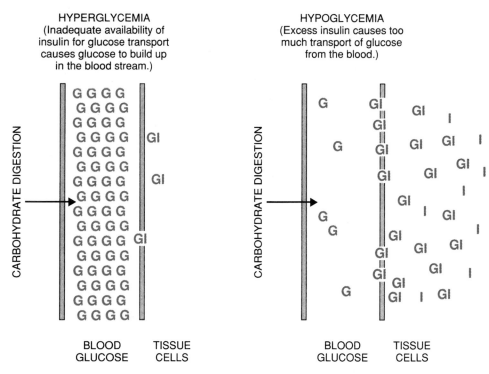

Figure 9-3
Hyperglycemia and hypoglycemia.

the difference between hyper- and hypoglycemia). This form of glucose intolerance may be a precursor to the development of diabetes.

Reactive hypoglycemia is characterized by serum glucose levels that fall in the range of 50 to 60 mg/dL, with symptoms of hypoglycemia (Table 9–1) that are relieved by eating. The symptoms progress as the blood glucose level falls or when it reaches a low level. Persons with uncontrolled diabetes may experience feelings of hypoglycemia at normal levels of blood glucose until their body has time to adjust to a lower, more normal level of blood glucose.

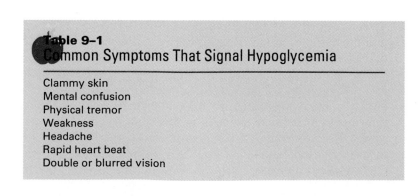

Table 9–1
Common Symptoms That Signal Hypoglycemia

Clammy skin
Mental confusion
Physical tremor
Weakness
Headache
Rapid heart beat
Double or blurred vision

Table 9–2
High-Protein Snack Ideas for Reactive Hypoglycemia*

Graham cracker with peanut butter
Apple or banana slices with peanut butter
Celery with peanut butter
Cheese and crackers
Nuts and raisins (small amount of raisins)
Cottage cheese and fruit
Unsweetened fruit juice and cheese
Half sandwich (meat, peanut butter, or cheese)
Hard-cooked egg and small glass of milk
Hot cereal with melted peanut butter
Cold cereal with bite-sized chunks of peanut butter
Bagel and cream cheese
Parmesan muffin (English muffin with margarine and parmesan
  cheese)
Half a cantaloupe stuffed with cottage cheese

*Regular meals should be reduced in portion sizes to compensate for the added kilocalories consumed through snacks. Regular meals also need to be balanced, including a protein source and excluding large quantities of concentrated sweets. Snacks should be consumed about 2 to 3 hours after regular meals.

The person with reactive hypoglycemia needs to eat small amounts of carbohydrate (about 30 to 50 grams) frequently (every 3 hours). Including a protein source with meals and snacks helps to maintain appropriate blood glucose levels because it slows carbohydrate digestion, causing only minimal stimulation of insulin secretion (Table 9–2 lists high-protein snack ideas). The need for protein to be included with the carbohydrate is based on individual symptoms. Caffeine and alcohol may exacerbate the symptoms of hypoglycemia owing to their effect on liver glycogen and **glycogenolysis** (the breakdown of glycogen into glucose).

WHAT ARE MEASURES OF GOOD DIABETES MANAGEMENT?

Self-Monitoring of Blood Glucose

Self-monitoring of blood glucose (SMBG) is a form of treatment in the sense that the patient can take responsibility for diabetes management. Because control of the blood glucose level is the chief goal of diabetes management, knowledge of its level is a valuable guide. Self-monitoring consists of taking a drop of blood and placing it on a strip that is inserted into a blood glucose meter. Several types of meters are available, as are automatic lancet devices. Patients should be given information on available meters so that they can select the one that best suits their needs. Recommended times to test blood glucose (BG) levels include before meals and 1 to 2 hours post-prandially in order to identify responses to carbohydrate content and other meal factors such as time of day (breakfast will often raise blood glucose more than meals consumed at other times of the day due to the dawn phenomenon, discussed later). This is referred to as **pattern management** as "patterns" may be noted when hyperglycemia or hypoglycemia may be predicted based on SMBG and food and activity records.

Typically, a meal can be expected to raise the blood sugar by 40 to 50 points. With a fasting blood sugar level of 100 mg/dL, an ideal meal should keep the blood sugar level to about 150 mg/dL. If the blood sugar level goes higher than this, it is due to either excess carbohydrate in the meal, per individual needs, or a need for medication.

The advantage of SMBG is the knowledge and flexibility it affords in diabetes management. Less guesswork is involved, and SMBG allows the diabetic patient greater objectivity in decision making to prevent both hyper- and hypoglycemia.

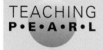 TEACHING **P•E•A•R•L**

Questions such as "How do I adjust my diet and insulin for exercise?" or "Can I eat a piece of birthday cake safely?" can be addressed through self-monitoring of blood glucose. For example, a person might find that a half piece of birthday cake with his or her evening meal may raise blood sugar to an acceptable level. If blood sugar goes above 200 mg/dL two hours after eating the cake, the person might consider not eating more.

The carbohydrate content of a piece of cake can be determined by looking at the food label of the cake and frosting container based on the portion consumed. A homemade cake can be estimated for carbohydrate content knowing that ½ cup of flour contains 45 grams of carbohydrate and ½ cup of sugar contains 95 grams of carbohydrate (see Table 9–3). The amount of carbohydrate found in a given recipe can thus be calculated for the portion consumed.

Ketone Checks

All persons with diabetes should know about ketones. Ketones form from the breakdown of body fat when there is inadequate insulin, inadequate carbohydrate, or both. For persons with GDM, ketones should be checked daily if they are restricting carbohydrate content and for individuals with Type 1 diabetes whenever their blood sugar is over 240 mg/dL on two or more occasions or when they are ill. Ketones are particularly important to assess during illness, when the likelihood of elevated blood glucose and dehydration occurs. Symptoms of nausea, vomiting, and deep labored breathing may be signs of impending ketoacidosis. **Ketonuria** (ketones in the urine) is treated with insulin (medical guidance needs to be sought) and increased water intake with moderate amounts of carbohydrate. If ketone production is severe, hospitalization will be required.

What Is Hemoglobin A_{1C} and What Is Its Role in Diabetes Management?

Most people know that hemoglobin is a component of the red blood cells used to carry oxygen throughout the body. The amount of **hemoglobin A_{1C} (HbA$_{1C}$)**, a

Table 9–3
Carbohydrate (CHO) Counting

Grains and Starchy Vegetables (15 g Carbohydrate)

3 c popcorn
1 c puffed cereals
½ c pasta, *dry vegetable* (potato, beans) or *sweet vegetable* (corn, peas, winter squash)
1 slice bread or 1 ounce equivalent (½ c)
⅓ c rice
¼ c *dry/sweet vegetable* (yams or "sweet potato")

Fruits (15 g Carbohydrate)

1 c high water-content fruits (melon and berries)
½ *c most fruits*
¼ c most dried fruits
½ banana
⅛ c dry/sweet fruits (raisins or dried banana chips)

Milk (~15 g Carbohydrate)

1 c milk or yogurt (unsweetened)

Low-Carbohydrate Vegetables (5 g Carbohydrate)

1 c raw vegetables (*high in water/low in sweetness*)
½ c cooked vegetables (*high water/low sweetness*)
(Do not count CHO unless = 15 g or more)

Concentrated Carbohydrate Sources

1 tsp sugar = 4 g carbohydrate
½ c sugar = 95 g carbohydrate
1 tbsp flour = 5 g carbohydrate
½ c flour = 45 g carbohydrate

subfraction of hemoglobin, measures the attachment of glucose to hemoglobin (see Fig. 9–4 for correlations between HbA_{1C} and average blood glucose). It is the glycated proteins (body proteins attached permanently to glucose) that are believed to be a major cause of complications of diabetes. Frequent daily blood glucose measurement, using a blood glucose meter, is still important both to mea-

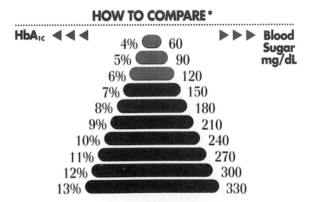

HOW TO COMPARE*

HbA_{1c} ◀◀◀   ▶▶▶ **Blood Sugar mg/dL**

4%	60
5%	90
6%	120
7%	150
8%	180
9%	210
10%	240
11%	270
12%	300
13%	330

Figure 9–4

Hemoglobin A_{1C} and average blood glucose goals. (From Diabetes Control and Complications Trial (DCCT): Results of Feasability Study, Diabetes Care, Vol. 10, 1987, pp. 1–19.)

sure hypoglycemia and to assess the amount of carbohydrate per meal or per insulin unit that is appropriate for good BG management. Testing for HbA_{1c} is recommended every 3 months, because the hemoglobin molecule lives for about 3 months time. The goal is to see improvement, or lowering, in HbA_{1C} levels as well as to maintain a normal level of HbA_{1C} (<6–7 percent), thereby reducing long-term diabetic complications. Persons with retinopathy (a form of eye disease, discussed later) are advised to attain a reduction of no more than 2 percentage points per year in HbA_{1C} due to concerns that the retinopathy may worsen and possibly result in blindness if BG levels are treated too rapidly.

Lipid Screening

Lipid (blood fat) abnormalities go hand in hand with poor control of diabetes. Coronary heart disease (CHD) is found to be consistently higher among the population with Type 2 diabetes and is also found to precede diabetes, which may be due to metabolic disturbances associated with the insulin resistance syndrome (Morici et al., 1997). An increased level of blood glucose is believed to contribute to these abnormalities, along with insulin resistance. A high level of triglycerides (>200 mg/dL) with an associated low level of high-density lipoprotein cholesterol (<35 mg/dL) is generally found in persons with uncontrolled Type 2 diabetes. The cholesterol and low-density lipoprotein cholesterol may or may not be elevated. There is usually improvement in the blood lipids as diet, weight, and blood glucose levels are improved. Medication is sometimes needed as well.

Albuminuria Screening

All patients with diabetes mellitus should have their urine tested for albumin. Persons who have had Type 1 diabetes for more than 5 years and all persons with Type 2 diabetes should be tested annually, as the person may have had diabetes for many years prior to the diagnosis. **Albuminuria** (albumin in the urine) is associated with advancing kidney disease and should be treated aggressively with ACE inhibitors. Once macroalbuminuria (very large amounts of albumin in the urine) occurs, a moderate protein intake of 0.8 gram of protein per kilogram of body weight is advised, along with reduction in sodium intake (2 grams of sodium are generally adequate) if the person has concomitant hypertension (see Chapter 10).

WHAT IS INTENSIVE INSULIN MANAGEMENT?

This term was coined during the DCCT (Diabetes Control and Complications Trial) in 1993 when it was first proven and reported that achieving near normal blood glucose reduced diabetes complications by upwards of 75 percent in persons with Type 1 diabetes. These results were found by achieving average blood glucose levels of less than 155 mg/dL. To achieve this level of BG control safely, without increased risk for severe hypoglycemia or hyperglycemia, the study participants were taught to give insulin in three daily injections (to more closely mimic how Mother Nature provides insulin) or give insulin by insulin pump. It is now recommended that insulin injection be more frequent in an attempt to better mimic how insulin is normally produced. Normally the body produces small amounts around the clock with increased amounts each time we eat a meal containing carbohydrate. The goal of intensive insulin therapy is normalization of blood sugar. All patients who use insulin should know when the peak time of action for their insulin is likely to occur. This knowledge will allow them to plan a meal or snack and avoid exercise at these times (see Fig. 9–2).

By additionally altering insulin dose based on the carbohydrate content of meals, more stable and desirable blood glucose levels can be achieved. **Carbohydrate counting** is a form of medical nutrition therapy whereby a person with diabetes can learn how to adjust short-acting insulin (called "Regular" or "R" or Humalog insulin) based on the person's varying intake of carbohydrate. To safely apply carbohydrate counting, it is critical to know what insulin is and how it acts.

What Is Insulin and How Is It Produced?

Insulin is a hormone that is produced in the **beta cells** of the **islets of Langerhans** found in the **pancreas;** it is produced in response to hyperglycemia. Because insulin is composed of protein, oral intake of insulin is not possible, as it would be digested before being used. Thus, persons taking oral diabetes medication are not taking insulin, but rather are using the medication to help their own natural insulin production work more effectively (such people are diagnosed as having Type 2 diabetes because they are producing insulin).

Insulin allows blood glucose into body cells where it can be burned for energy. The body will normally produce small amounts of insulin at all times as it is needed to metabolize carbohydrate for the continual energy necessary to sustain life. This type of "background" insulin as used in Type 1 diabetes management will be referred to as either the "basal rate" with insulin pumps or the "long-acting" insulin types used with injections such as NPH insulin. Larger amounts of meal-related insulin are normally produced in the pancreas in relation to carbohydrate consumption. Thus, "meal bolus insulin" using short-acting insulins is now being used in relation to the carbohydrate content of the meals in both the insulin pump and by injection with a syringe. This is referred to as the **insulin-to-carbohydrate ratio,** which is usually 1:15—1 unit short-acting "regular" insulin is given for each 15 grams of carbohydrate. Individuals using this approach need to work closely with certified diabetes educators and registered dietitians to verify their individual ratio (which can range from a low of 1:3 to a high of 1:20) before they start adjusting their insulin dose on their own.

Previously, insulin was obtained only from beef or pork pancreas, which first became available for human use in the 1920s. Prior to this time, persons with

Type 1 diabetes did not survive. Now human insulin is the main form of insulin used, and it responds quicker than the old animal forms. This form of insulin is made either by genetic manipulation or by enzymatic manipulation of pork insulin so that it contains the same protein structure as human insulin. It does not come from humans.

The newest form of insulin is marketed under the name Humalog and generically is referred to as Lispro because the amino acids lysine and proline are switched in the insulin molecule. This newest form of insulin works very rapidly as the insulin tends not to form hexamer crystals and is able to get into the bloodstream more quickly. The result is that Lispro (Humalog) insulin enters the bloodstream in 5 to 15 minutes (versus 30 minutes with all other forms of insulin), has a peak action time of 2 hours (versus 3 hours with regular short-acting insulin), and is totally cleared from the body in about 3 to 5 hours (Fineberg, 1997). Persons using Humalog insulin thus need to be alerted to different peak action times and to symptoms of ketonuria.

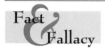

Fallacy: A person can get AIDS from human insulin.

Fact: Since human insulin is made genetically, it is not possible to contract AIDS or any other disease from it. Insulin needles, including blood lancets, should not be shared as disease can spread through contaminated needles.

How Is Insulin Prescribed?

Only health care professionals licensed to prescribe can alter insulin doses. Other health care professionals can advise a person with diabetes to seek medical opinion on dose changes as noted by review of SMBG records. Dosage changes might also be considered if specific guidelines have been reviewed with the person's physician such as when a dietitian might advise a particular insulin dose based on verified insulin to carbohydrate ratios. Generally a long-acting insulin (such as NPH or "N" insulin) is given in the morning and at bedtime, and short-acting, regular or "R" insulin is given at breakfast and dinner. The person with Type 2 diabetes who is not able to produce enough insulin to compensate for the cell's insulin resistance may be given a long-acting insulin in one to two injections.

Insulin pumps only use the short-acting "R" insulin, although they increasingly will be using the new Lispro insulin, Humalog. Persons transferring to a pump will likely need about 75 percent of their usual dose of insulin, which is generally divided with half for the basal rate and half for the meal bolus needs. For example, a person on 60 units of insulin by injection will need about 45 units on the pump (75 percent). About half of this dosage is given in the basal rate (22 units divided by 24 hours or 0.9 units given per hour via the insulin pump). The other half of the calculated insulin needs is used to "cover" mealtime carbohydrate.

The amount of hourly basal insulin needed in insulin pumps is tested to verify that the BG level remains stable. The basal rate can be slowly increased or decreased by about 0.1 unit per hour based on individual needs. Often an increased basal rate is needed to cover the dawn phenomenon (discussed later) with lower basal rates for other times of the day. A temporary increase in basal rate may be needed during times of illness. Once basal rates are set correctly, the person using the pump can safely have a great deal of flexibility in timing of meals and amounts eaten if the insulin-to-carbohydrate ratio is accurately determined and applied.

How Is the Insulin to Carbohydrate Ratio Determined?

By using SMBG records, the effect of a given amount of carbohydrate consumed for the number of units of short-acting or regular insulin given can be determined. The goal is for the blood glucose to rise no higher than about 50 "points" (mg/dL) after meals (generally 1 to 2 hours after meals will be the highest BG level, except if Humalog insulin is used, in which case the peak BG is noted in about 45 minutes after meals). If the blood glucose level ends up 4 to 5 hours later from where it started before the meal (give or take 20 to 30 "points"), simple math tells you the outcome. For example, if these BG goals are achieved (an increase of 50 points 1½ hours after the meal with return to the pre-meal number 4 to 5 hours later) and 45 grams of carbohydrate were consumed in a meal with 3 units regular insulin given, the ratio is 1:15 or 1 unit of insulin for every 15 grams of carbohydrate. This needs to be repeated more than once to verify it is correct as many variables will affect BG levels.

Persons with Type 2 diabetes generally look at the total amount of carbohydrate consumed per meal that allows for these same goals. By reducing post-prandial hyperglycemia, HbA$_{1C}$ goals can be better achieved with complications of diabetes being reduced. Controlling post-prandial BG excursions may further allow for decreased use of insulin or oral diabetes medications.

What Is the 1500 Rule?

The **1500 rule** is an estimate that is used to determine expected "point" drop of BG per unit of insulin. It is used by counting up total units of insulin used (including both long-acting and short-acting insulins) and dividing total units of insulin into the number 1500. For example, a person who takes 100 units of insulin will have an expected BG point drop of 15 points per 1 unit of regular insulin. This can be applied to correct hyperglycemia but needs to be done with medical guidance in order to assess the cause of the hyperglycemia. If a person only takes 30 units of insulin, it becomes obvious that a more dramatic reduction (a 50-point drop in BG per unit of insulin) and a potentially fatal result can occur unless the person understands the impact of insulin for his or her individual needs.

What Other Hormones Are Involved in Diabetes Management?

Several **hormones** (chemicals produced by the body that regulate body functioning) act in concert to regulate blood glucose levels. Insulin, produced in the pancreas, is the only hormone that lowers blood glucose levels. Many hormones act to raise glucose levels, chief among them being glucagon, epinephrine (also called adrenalin), cortisol, and growth hormone. These are called **counter-regulatory hormones** because they work in an opposite manner to insulin. Any deviation in the balance of these hormones will cause fluctuations in blood glucose levels. The **Somogyi effect** may be noted with an increased production of the counter-regulatory hormones in response to hypoglycemia. The implication is that hyperglycemia often follows hypoglycemia. In this example, a decreased insulin dose may correct hyperglycemia because the underlying cause of hypoglycemia is being corrected.

The **dawn phenomenon** occurs commonly for both types of diabetes and is related to increased production of cortisol and growth hormone (both counter-regulatory hormones) in the early morning hours. A person with Type 2 diabetes or GDM thus may require a smaller amount of carbohydrate at breakfast to prevent hyperglycemia post-prandially. The person with Type 1 diabetes may require a different insulin-to-carbohydrate ratio at breakfast than at other meals, or those on insulin pumps may require a higher basal rate of insulin in the early morning hours.

Persons taking insulin should be prescribed a glucagon kit that a family member or coworker can be taught to use if the person with diabetes becomes unconscious from severe hypoglycemia. Glucagon is normally produced by the body in response to hypoglycemia, but a person who is receiving insulin by injection may also need glucagon by injection. When a person is unconscious or unable to swallow because his or her nerves have lost their energy source, oral intake of carbohydrate or sugar is not recommended. The glucagon kit contains a syringe with sterile water that is mixed in a vial with a glucagon tablet and injected after being dissolved. The person receiving the medication should be rolled on his or her side in case of vomiting.

WHAT ARE THE SYMPTOMS AND CLINICAL FINDINGS OF DIABETES?

The warning signs of diabetes are unusual thirst; frequent urination; abnormal hunger; sudden weight loss (which usually indicates Type 1 diabetes, but can also occur in Type 2 diabetes with severe hyperglycemia); skin disorders, infections such as vaginal yeast infection, and delayed wound healing; blurred vision; and unexplained weakness and fatigue.

Hyperglycemia. Hyperglycemia is associated with the complications of diabetes. It also causes many of the symptoms of diabetes. Hyperglycemia needs to be monitored using the 3-month hemoglobin A_{1C} test. Renal disease is felt to be worsened when albumin, a body protein, is **glycated**—when blood glucose connects to the body proteins (Mangrum et al., 1997). Blurred vision can be caused when excess sugar in the eye changes the shape of the lens. Infections increase with hyperglycemia as the body's immune system does not work as efficiently. There are conditions under which the body's blood glucose levels rise normally, such as stress of infection, illness, or surgery. Sometimes a person with Type 2 diabetes will require insulin injections on a temporary basis until the stress has passed.

Glycosuria. One way the body tries to lower blood sugar is to flush it out the kidneys, which results in **glycosuria** (glucose in the urine). Frequent urination and thirst are often associated with hyperglycemia. The level of blood sugar generally has to rise unacceptably high (>180 mg/dL) before glucose is detected in the urine. This is referred to as the **renal threshold.** Thus glycosuria tests are generally not recommended except as an easy screening test and for those persons who refuse, or are unable, to test blood sugars.

TEACHING P•E•A•R•L

A good assessment question to ask a patient is whether he or she has to get up in the middle of the night to use the bathroom and how often. Persons with undiagnosed diabetes are often relieved to hear they can again expect an uninterrupted night's sleep with improved blood glucose control. This can motivate patients to adhere to medical nutrition therapy and exercise prescriptions.

Ketonuria. Without insulin, carbohydrates are unavailable for energy utilization. Instead, the body calls on fat as an energy source. Under normal conditions, the liver breaks down small amounts of fatty acids to form ketones. These ketones are further metabolized for energy. In uncontrolled diabetes, ketone production exceeds utilization. The excess is excreted in the urine. This is known as **ketonuria.** If the excess ketones are not removed adequately, the condition known as ketoacidosis develops. In ketoacidosis, the blood pH changes to a more acidic level, which can cause death. Treatment should be prompt and hospitalization will be needed if blood becomes too acidic. This condition generally occurs in Type 1 diabetes but can also occur in persons with Type 2 diabetes who are producing large amounts of counter-regulatory or "stress" hormones, such as with infection or surgery.

Dehydration. The excess fluid loss associated with high levels of blood glucose causes water to be taken from body tissues. This can result in dehydration if water is not replaced and blood sugar controlled. Dehydration with concentrated amounts of glucose in the blood can cause a condition known as **hyperglycemic hyperosmolar nonketotic syndrome (HHNK).** This condition is commonly found in elderly patients, in whom diabetes is much more prevalent and in whom there is a diminished sensation of thirst owing to the aging process. Because dehydration of the brain can occur, many elderly patients with HHNK have a history of lethargy, sleepiness, and confused state lasting from several days to weeks before progressing into a coma. Dehydration and HHNK are easily treated if caught in the early stages. All older patients, but especially those with diabetes, should be taught the importance of adequate water intake even when they are not thirsty.

Polydipsia and Polyuria. Increased thirst, known as **polydipsia,** is experienced as the body senses the need to replace excess fluids lost from frequent urination **(polyuria).** This is an attempt by the body to remove excess ketones and glucose.

Polyphagia. Increased appetite, known as **polyphagia,** is the body's response to the need for energy. However, this need is not being satisfied, because carbohydrates are not available for energy. This can be another sign that a person has undiagnosed diabetes. A health care professional should inquire about a person's appetite and whether it has changed. Polyphagia may cause weight gain.

Weight Loss. Because the sugar is staying in the blood and is not used for energy, a feeling of fatigue, hunger, and weight loss can be associated with hyperglycemia. Glucose that does not enter the body cells is excreted in the urine along with excess ketones. Both represent wasted energy sources. Weight loss results because energy demand exceeds available sources. This is more likely to happen with Type 1 diabetes or in severe cases of Type 2 diabetes in which there is insufficient or no insulin production.

WHAT ARE THE CAUSES, SYMPTOMS, AND TREATMENT OF HYPOGLYCEMIA?

Either insulin or certain **oral hypoglycemic agents** (also called diabetes pills) can cause the blood sugar to drop below a point at which the body can function. Feelings of hypoglycemia when no diabetes medication is being taken is not life-threatening and generally can resolve on its own through the release of stored glycogen in the liver. In the presence of excess alcohol in the blood, the breakdown of glycogen is impaired, which may result in hypoglycemia.

The individual with hypoglycemia may begin to perspire; experience hunger and nervousness; have skin that becomes pale, cold, and clammy; and experience mental confusion, physical tremor, weakness, headache, rapid heart beat, numbness in the tongue, and double or blurred vision (see Table 9–1). When these symptoms are noted, the blood sugar level should be checked to verify hypoglycemia. However, not all diabetic individuals experience these symptoms, especially children, elderly persons, or persons who have frequent episodes of hypoglycemia. The latter can be resolved by meticulous prevention of hypoglycemia, at least in the person who has had Type 1 diabetes for a short period of time (Bolli, 1997). The health professional or close family member should suspect hypoglycemia, and treat it accordingly, when a diabetic child becomes unusually quiet or fretful or when an elderly or other diabetic patient becomes weak or faint. A physician should be consulted if the cause is not readily apparent or if hypoglycemia happens frequently.

The treatment for a person who can swallow is to give 15 grams of a rapid-acting carbohydrate source, such as 4 ounces of orange juice, 4 teaspoons of sugar mixed in water, or three to four glucose tablets (see Table 9–4). The blood sugar should be rechecked in 15 minutes and the procedure repeated until the blood sugar returns to normal. This is referred to as the **15:15 rule.** For severe hypoglycemia, the amount of carbohydrate may be increased to 30 grams of carbohydrate, as every 15 grams of carbohydrate raises the BG level 20 to 50 points only. Squeezing cake icing or honey inside the cheek is appropriate only if the person is alert enough to swallow.

Table 9–4
Portions for Dietary Treatment of Hypoglycemic Episodes in Conscious Persons

15 g Carbohydrate	30 g Carbohydrate
3 oz apple juice	6 oz apple juice
4 oz orange juice	8 oz orange juice
5 oz regular soda pop	10 oz regular soda pop
4 tsp honey	8 tsp honey
4 tsp sugar	8 tsp sugar
¼ c sherbet	½ c sherbet

The 15:15 rule: Check blood sugar; if low (less than 70 mg/dL) treat with 15 grams of carbohydrate. Recheck blood sugar in 15 minutes; if still low repeat with another 15 grams of carbohydrate. If the blood sugar is severely low (less than 50 mg/dL) treat with 30 grams of carbohydrate and recheck in 15 minutes.

If the person becomes unconscious, glucagon can be injected or an intravenous solution of glucose may be administered in the hospital or ambulance setting. Long-term treatment includes diet, activity, insulin modification (the chart on page 227 shows factors that raise or lower blood glucose levels), or education to help prevent future episodes.

WHAT IS THE NUTRITIONAL MANAGEMENT OF DIABETES?

Meal Planning

Balanced meals are essential for the management of diabetes. Pure carbohydrate meals will raise the blood sugar level faster because carbohydrates are digested in 1 hour or less. Food has to get through the stomach before it can significantly affect blood sugar levels. Including at least a small amount of protein with a meal or snack will slow down the process of digestion, thereby limiting its impact on blood sugar. Although the macronutrient carbohydrate has the greatest impact on postprandial BG levels, a diet rich in plant foods will provide a variety of trace minerals and phytochemicals. In particular, legumes, nuts, whole grains, vegetables, and fruits contain naturally occuring phytochemicals and have other natural antioxidants that have been associated with protection and/or treatment of chronic disease including diabetes, heart disease, hypertension, and cancer (Craig, 1997).

Kilocalories

The amount of kilocalories needed by a person with diabetes should be the same as the recommended dietary allowances (RDA) for a person without diabetes. Adjustments in kilocalories may be necessary to maintain or attain normal body weight and can be made as necessary. Generally, 20 to 30 kilocalories per kilogram body weight is adequate to maintain weight. A 500 kilocalorie reduction from this level should result in a weekly weight loss of 1 pound (see Chapter 20). The person with Type 2 diabetes is more likely to need to lose weight, whereas the person with Type 1 diabetes is more likely to need to gain weight, especially at the time of diagnosis.

Carbohydrates

Carbohydrates are now recognized to be the prime factor in producing meal-related hyperglycemia. Whereas a high-fat diet is generally associated with increased insulin resistance, the effect of carbohydrate is more controversial (Daly et al., 1997). The recommended allowance for carbohydrate is 50 to 60 percent of total kilocalories. For the person with Type 1 diabetes, the amount of carbohydrate is based on preferences as insulin dose can match carbohydrate intake. Of the total carbohydrate intake, high-fiber foods should be included. Sugar may be tolerated in small quantities and should be counted as part of total grams of carbohydrate in a meal. Four grams of sugar, as listed on food labels, is the same as 1 teaspoon of sugar. Individuals can determine the impact of table sugar, or sucrose, on their blood glucose level through the use of SMBG. It was found in the DCCT study that the total amount of carbohydrate, versus the type, had the biggest impact on blood glucose levels.

Fiber promotes normal blood glucose levels **post-prandially** (after meals) by slowing the time of digestion. The recommendation for fiber intake remains the same for persons with diabetes as for the general public or 25 grams of fiber for persons requiring 2000 kilocalories. A recent study found that persons with Type 2 diabetes who consumed oatmeal bread containing 3 grams of fiber had both post-prandial blood glucose levels and insulin levels that were significantly lower than another group who ate white bread. This shows that soluble fiber, as found in oats, directly enhances the action of insulin among persons with Type 2 diabetes (Pick et al., 1996). The recommendation of the Dietary Guidelines for Americans for increased fiber is beneficial not only for the general public but also for the person with diabetes in particular. A goal of 20 to 30 grams of fiber should be promoted, with particular emphasis on legumes and other sources of soluble fiber such as greens and other vegetables, fruits, and grains with a "gummy" texture.

It is now recognized that including some sugar as part of total meal carbohydrate can be safe and will allow feelings of greater normalcy for the individual with diabetes. Sugar substitutes (see Table 9–5) are not always preferable. Sugar alcohols, such as sorbitol and xylitol, are often found in dietetic foods; they contain similar kilocalories per gram, can cause the blood glucose levels to rise, and thus should not be considered "free foods." In addition, excess intake may lead to diarrhea. Saccharin, aspartame (NutraSweet), and acesulfame-K (a new sugar substitute) have no appreciable kilocalorie content in amounts commonly consumed but may be used in foods that contain other sources of kilocalories, such as fat. These foods may give a person with diabetes the false perception that if the

Table 9–5
Nutritive and Nonnutritive Sweeteners*

Name	Composition	Sources
Nutritive Sweeteners		
Glucose	Monosaccharide	Found in blood as the end product of starch digestion
		Occurs naturally in fruit
Fructose	Monosaccharide	Found in fruit and honey
Sucrose	Disaccharide composed of glucose and fructose	Commonly known as table sugar and widely used in commercial foods
Lactose	Disaccharide composed of glucose and galactose	Found in milk and unfermented milk products[†]
Maltose	Disaccharide composed of two glucose molecules	Produced during brewing and bread-making; also made commercially
Honey	Mainly fructose and glucose	Made from plants by honeybees
Maple syrup	Primarily sucrose	Made by boiling off the liquid found in sap of mature sugar maple trees
Corn syrup	Composed of glucose molecules of different chain lengths	Produced from cornstarch
High-fructose corn syrup	Contains 40–100% fructose	Produced enzymatically from cornstarch
Molasses	Contains 50–75% sucrose	Produced during the processing of table sugar
Sorbitol, mannitol, xylitol	Sugar alcohols	Found naturally in fruit and used as a sugar substitute
Aspartame	Methyl ester of two amino acids: phenylalanine and aspartic acid (aspartate)	Commonly known as NutraSweet and widely used in low-sugar food products; kilocalories are insignificant, since small amounts are used because it is intensely sweet (180–220 times as sweet as sucrose)
Nonnutritive Sweeteners		
Saccharin	Organic compound	Originally banned in 1977 after being implicated as causing bladder tumors in rats fed high doses; currently available as a sugar substitute.
Cyclamate	Available as cyclamic acid, calcium cyclamate, and sodium cyclamate	Banned since 1969 after evidence showed it as a possible cancer-causing agent in rats; FDA may reconsider its use given more studies on its safety

*Nutritive sweeteners are those that provide kilocalories; nonnutritive sweeteners are entirely free of kilocalories because they are not metabolized.
†Lactose as found in milk is not harmful to diabetic individuals.

food is sugar-free it is also kilocalorie-free. Commercial fructose offers only minimal advantage over sucrose for the person with diabetes, although both sweeteners may be tolerated in small amounts.

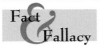

Fallacy: Although persons with diabetes need to avoid sugar, they can eat honey without a problem.

Fact: Honey is composed of glucose and fructose, two simple sugars, and as such cannot safely be used freely. Occasional moderate use, especially by a person who practices self-monitoring of blood glucose (SMBG), may be appropriate.

Protein

The percentage of kilocalories derived from protein should be 10 to 15 percent with a maximum of 20 percent. This allows the individual with diabetes from 1 to 1.5 grams of protein per kilogram of body weight and should approximate the RDA. A level of protein intake at 0.8 grams of protein per kilogram body weight or less may be desirable to control kidney disease.

Fat

Fat intake should be individualized based on weight needs, cholesterol levels, and blood glucose needs. For the person with Type 2 diabetes, a high-carbohydrate, low-fat diet can increase blood triglyceride levels whereas a diet high in monounsaturated fat but low in saturated fats may be more effective (Berry, 1997). *Note*

Calculating the Diet

Once the diet order is received from the physician, the diet can be calculated from protein, carbohydrate, and fat content. For example, if the diet order calls for 2000 kilocalories, it can be calculated as follows:

Protein:

$$2000 \times 0.15 = 300 \text{ kcal } (4 \text{ kcal/g} = 75 \text{ g protein})$$

Carbohydrate:

$$2000 \times 0.60 = 1200 \text{ kcal } (4 \text{ kcal/g} = 300 \text{ g carbohydrate})$$

Fat:

$$2000 \times 0.25 = 500 \text{ kcal } (9 \text{ kcal/g} = 55 \text{ g fat})$$

The calculations for protein, carbohydrate, and fat must now be translated into a meal pattern that will fit the person's lifestyle and insulin type. Meals are planned using food exchange lists. The foods in each list are grouped in terms of similarity of composition, and they supply approximately the same amount of protein, carbohydrate, and fat. One serving of any food may be exchanged for another serving in the same list. The full exchange list is shown in Appendix 9. Adjustments can be made until the ideal diet plan is developed—one that is appropriate for diabetes management and good nutritional intake and is suited to fit individual lifestyles. Dietitians are best qualified to develop meal pattern guides based on patient food preferences and lifestyles, although other health professionals or persons with diabetes can be trained to calculate food patterns using the exchange list system.

It is important that the diet be individually planned to facilitate patient compliance. Thus, dissemination of preplanned diet guides is not in the best interest of persons with diabetes.

Other forms of meal planning may be appropriate. As previously referred to, carbohydrate counting can be useful for someone who finds the ADA exchanges too cumbersome or whose blood glucose levels are poorly managed. The person with diabetes learns how much carbohydrate is in foods (see Table 9–3) and aims for a regular amount, such as 50 grams with each meal for the person with Type 2 diabetes or based on insulin-to-carbohydrate ratios for the person with Type 1 diabetes. SMBG is imperative to determine individual needs for carbohydrate.

Fact & Fallacy

Fallacy: Diabetic individuals must give up the foods they love.

Fact: The rule of moderation applies to both the general public and the diabetic individual in achieving the goal of good nutritional intake. Moderate amounts of all foods are acceptable. All food consists of carbohydrate, protein, fat, or a combination, and therefore can be worked into the exchange list system. The potential problem with this approach is individual definitions of moderation. Assessment of weight control and SMBG are two methods that can indicate whether moderation is truly moderate. A referral to a registered dietitian is strongly advised in order to educate persons with diabetes about how to make appropriate changes in their diets and to help manage their diabetes.

Carbohydrate Distribution

Carbohydrate should be distributed among the meals and snacks according to the type of insulin prescribed. For the person receiving oral hypoglycemic agents, meals and snacks should be guided by SMBG. Generally, an afternoon and an evening snack are desirable to prevent hypoglycemia for a person on diabetes medication. Individual blood glucose patterns can determine whether snacks are really necessary. A bedtime snack containing carbohydrate for the person with

Type 1 diabetes whose blood glucose level is less than 100 mg/dL is generally advised. Distributing carbohydrate throughout the day will help prevent both hypoglycemic and hyperglycemic reactions.

Can a Person with Diabetes Drink Alcoholic Beverages?

Alcohol contributes about 7 kilocalories per gram (carbohydrate and protein yield 4 kilocalories per gram and fat yields 9 kilocalories per gram) and thus needs to be calculated into a diabetic diet. Mixed drinks, liqueurs, and sweet wines should be avoided entirely because of the high content of simple sugars. Beer, hard liquor mixed with water or diet soda, and dry wine may be tolerated in limited quantities but should be consumed only after consultation with the patient's physician and dietitian.

It is important that the patient eat food containing carbohydrate when having a drink, because alcohol can induce hypoglycemia. Alcohol, in moderation, enhances the action of insulin and if consumed along with increased physical activity, the person needs to be alert to symptoms of hypoglycemia. The person with diabetes should tell a companion that he or she has diabetes in case hypoglycemia develops while drinking alcohol. Hypoglycemia has been mistaken for intoxication. A drink of orange juice would be recommended if a person with diabetes appears inebriated.

How Can a Person with Diabetes Eat at Restaurants?

Restaurant eating poses no problem if there is adequate selection. Simple foods without gravy or other sauces may be desirable, and sweets should be avoided or included as part of the meal carbohydrate. Dessert might be shared with a friend and portions controlled by asking for a "doggy bag." Portions might also be controlled by ordering several appetizers rather than the entree, which generally is inappropriately large for persons trying to control their weight and blood sugar.

Eating "on the road" can be a particular challenge. Low-carbohydrate snack foods might be packed for dealing with the "munchies," whereas other snacks containing carbohydrate are essential for the person taking insulin or other diabetes medication when regular mealtimes may be difficult or impossible to achieve. Persons with Type 1 need to be instructed on how to make alternative choices of food based on carbohydrate, protein, and fat content. The use of carbohydrate counting can facilitate an easy method to compare the predicted impact of various foods on blood glucose. Many fast food restaurants now make available the nutritional content of their food selections (see Appendix 4).

WHAT IS THE GLYCEMIC INDEX OF FOOD?

Not all carbohydrate foods cause blood glucose levels to rise equally. This is primarily related to the time of digestion and liquid carbohydrate foods (such as juice) raise the blood glucose quickly (which is desirable when treating hypoglycemia). Foods that contain soluble fiber generally leave the stomach slowly due to the gummy texture of these foods. This is referred to as the **glycemic index** of food. Research is still evolving as to the predictable glycemic responses with various foods and combinations of foods. Until more knowledge is acquired, specific indexes cannot be used appropriately for dietary guidance. However, it is generally known that legumes and greens have a lower glycemic index than do root vegetables and grains. High-fiber foods have a lower glycemic index than do low-fiber foods. Foods that are highly processed and easier to digest leave the stomach more quickly and can be described as having a high glycemic index. For example, cold processed cereal will often raise the blood glucose more rapidly than does oatmeal. Bagels, which are boiled before they are baked, tend to have a high glycemic index. By using SMBG, persons with diabetes can determine their own glycemic index to foods.

Protein foods that are low in carbohydrate have a lower glycemic index. Fats have the lowest glycemic index. Thus cheese would not be expected to significantly raise the blood sugar but is discouraged because of its high saturated fat content and its contribution to heart disease. Low-fat cheeses are appropriate if the sodium is taken into account.

TEACHING P•E•A•R•L

You might say to a person that the old adage that "oatmeal sticks to the ribs" is absolutely true. This food can be helpful when a person is trying to prevent his or her after-meal blood glucose level from rising too high. Legumes are also very high in soluble fiber. The adage "beans and greens" further helps a person remember which foods are high in soluble fiber.

WHAT IS THE ROLE OF EXERCISE IN DIABETES MANAGEMENT?

Exercise is an integral component of treatment in Type 2 diabetes. It is a factor in weight control and has been found to lower blood glucose levels to the point of reducing or eliminating the need for oral hypoglycemic agents or insulin. Children and adults who are on insulin may need to lower their insulin dose while also increasing their carbohydrate intake if their physical activity level is greatly increased over usual amounts.

Exercise can be beneficial in Type 1 diabetes, but greater caution is needed. For the ketotic or hyperglycemic patient (those whose blood glucose level is greater than 240 to 300 mg/dL), exercise will actually increase glucose levels further, primarily because insulin is a prerequisite for glucose usage in exercising muscles. Hyperglycemia is generally indicative of insufficient insulin availability. Exercise should be avoided unless blood glucose levels are under control. Even the patient with well-controlled Type 1 diabetes, however, needs to achieve a balance between the extra energy demands of exercise and diet and insulin. The general rule of thumb is to eat at least 15 grams of carbohydrate for every 1 hour of exercise as based on weight and intensity of exercise (see Table 9–6), to decrease the amount of insulin, or both, and to avoid exercising at the times that insulin is acting at peak levels. These guidelines help prevent the

Table 9–6

Grams of Carbohydrate (CHO) Used per Hour Based on Weight and Exercise

Activity	Grams of CHO Used per Hour (based on an individual's weight)		
	100 lb	150 lb	200 lb
Walking (3 mi/hr)	14	21	28
Jogging (5 mi/hr)	30	45	60
Running (7 mi/hr)	52	77	103
Running (9 mi/hr)	69	103	138
Bicycling (5 mi/hr)	13	20	27
Bicycling (10 mi/hr)	30	45	60
Bicycling (15 mi/hr)	52	77	103
Swimming (20 yd/min)	24	36	48
Swimming (50 yd/min)	58	87	117
Gardening (light)	8	12	16
Golf (with golf cart)	9	14	19
Mopping floors	12	18	24
Lawn mowing (power, pushing)	13	19	25
Bowling	13	19	25
Golf (pulling cart)	13	20	27
Scrubbing floors	17	25	33
Softball	17	25	33
Badminton	19	28	37
Horseback riding (trot)	19	28	37
Square dancing	19	28	37
Roller skating	19	28	37
Tennis (doubles)	19	28	37
Volleyball	19	28	37
Raking leaves or hoeing	20	30	40
Ice skating or roller skating	23	34	45
Mini trampoline	23	35	47
Digging a garden	23	35	47
Ice skating (10 mi/hr)	23	35	47
Chopping wood	23	35	47
Dancing (disco)	24	36	48
Mowing (hand mower)	25	38	51
Tennis (singles)	25	38	51
Dancing (square)	29	44	59
Waterskiing	29	44	59
Snow shoveling	30	45	60
Digging ditches	31	46	62
Rock climbing	31	46	62
Dancing (fast step)	31	46	62
Downhill skiing	33	50	67
Basketball (pickup)	39	58	77
Squash	40	60	80
Soccer	40	60	80
Basketball (vigorous)	44	65	87
Racquetball (singles)	60	90	120
Cross-country skiing (6 mph)	70	105	140

From MiniMed Inc., Sylmar, CA.

development of severe hypoglycemia, which is caused by excess insulin in relation to the amount of blood glucose available. It is important for anyone with diabetes to have a complete physical examination by a physician before embarking on an exercise program, but it is crucial for all persons with Type 1 diabetes or those with coronary heart disease or neuropathy with Type 2 diabetes. SMBG is a valuable tool for determining the best way to adjust diet and insulin before, during, and after exercise. Increased carbohydrate may need to be consumed for up to 24 hours as the body repletes its glycogen stores and allows for stable blood glucose.

WHAT ARE COMPLICATIONS OF DIABETES?

Insulin Reaction and Diabetic Coma

Insulin reaction (or insulin shock) occurs when more insulin is injected than is needed. Table 9–4 describes nutritional management of a conscious person. Insulin shock can result from omitting foods from the diet, increasing activity and exercise (which burns more kilocalories than normal), or making an error in insulin injection in relation to exercise. The result is hypoglycemia, a lowering of the blood glucose level. The onset is usually sudden. If the hypoglycemia is not treated promptly, the diabetic patient becomes mentally confused and disoriented. If this situation is prolonged, seizures, unconsciousness, and death can result. All family members should have on hand and know how to inject glucagon in order to raise blood sugar for an unconscious person. (**Glucagon,** as discussed earlier, is a counter-regulatory hormone that acts to release stored glycogen from the liver, thereby providing a blood sugar source; it is available with a physician's prescription.) Medical services should be sought in the case of insulin shock to help prevent another occurrence.

Diabetic coma is a potential result of ketoacidosis, discussed earlier in this chapter. In this condition, the blood glucose level becomes elevated, and glycosuria and ketonuria occur. The person experiences drowsiness, lethargy, and sometimes nausea with vomiting. The skin becomes hot and dry. There is a fruity odor to the breath (acetone). Breathing is deep and labored. Death can result if the patient is not treated promptly with insulin and fluids. Hospitalization is required.

Heart Disease

Deaths among persons with diabetes are highly related to cardiovascular disease. The American Diabetes Association recommends that physicians measure blood lipids and treat associated problems as a primary intervention to reduce the risk of cardiovascular disease among persons with diabetes. See Chapter 8 for management of lipid disorders.

Kidney Disease

Persons with Type 1 diabetes are at particular risk for kidney disease owing to small blood vessel damage. Kidney disease also occurs in Type 2 diabetes and is the type of diabetes found most commonly with kidney disease due to there being so many more persons with Type 2 diabetes. The Diabetes Control and Complications Trial (DCCT) study found that maintaining good blood sugar control will greatly lessen the risk of kidney disease.

Eating protein in more moderate portions is appropriate—almost no one needs more than 6 oz of meat per day—but it only becomes necessary when there is severe kidney damage as with macroalbuminuria. Aside from the protein found in meat, the type of fat is important. Omega-3 fatty acids as found in cold-water fish and fish oil has been shown to lower blood pressure and triglyceride levels in humans (Berry, 1997). Controlling blood pressure is critical to preserving kidney functioning. Regular blood pressure screening is necessary, and antihypertensive therapy, particularly the use of ACE inhibitors, helps preserve the functioning of the kidneys when there is mild hypertension with glycated albumin as found with hyperglycemia (Mangrum, 1997). Borderline hypertension needs to be treated aggressively in persons with diabetes in order to preserve kidney function.

Eye Disease

Diabetic retinopathy (a disease of the back of the eye where visual images are conveyed to the brain) occurs in about half of all persons who have had diabetes for more than 10 years and in about 80 percent of all persons who have had diabetes for more than 25 years. Controlling blood sugar levels significantly lowers the risk of retinopathy, according to the DCCT study. Hypertension should also be controlled. Regular eye exams, at least annually, with special tests to monitor for retinopathy are necessary to save vision. Treatment is available today that can preserve the sight of most persons with diabetes.

Nerve Disease

Nerve disease can occur at any location of the body but typically affects peripheral nerves (those at the periphery of the body such as the feet and legs) and the autonomic nervous system (comprising the nerves that send unconscious messages to the body, such as in the stomach, heart, or intestines). Problems with peripheral nerves (**peripheral neuropathy**) in the feet can cause burning, pain, and if severe, no feeling at all. It is paramount for persons with peripheral nerve problems of the feet to follow meticulous foot care. This can help prevent foot infections, which could lead to amputation. Any sign of a problem should immediately be taken care of by a physician or **podiatrist** (foot doctor).

Problems with the autonomic nervous system are referred to as **autonomic neuropathy. Gastroparesis** is partial paralysis of the stomach, resulting in diminished digestion and movement of food through the stomach. This can be a cause of unexplained hypoglycemia, as blood sugar levels can be raised only when food leaves the stomach. When this condition is suspected, a dye test is administered to determine the amount of time it takes for the food to leave the stomach. There is medication for this condition. Exercise may be discouraged for a person with autonomic neuropathy, as the heart may not be able to speed up to increase the oxygen intake. Another form of autonomic neuropathy affects the ability of the body to produce glucagon and epinephrine in response to low blood glucose. This is referred to as **hypoglycemic unawareness** because symptoms of hypoglycemia—shakiness, rapid heartbeat, and so on—will not be felt. It is now known that frequent hypoglycemia leads to hypoglycemic unawareness.

Times of Illness

The need for insulin increases when a person is acutely ill, even if there is a diminished intake of food. To prevent excess production of ketones, the person with Type 1 diabetes must maintain adequate insulin injections and carbohydrate intake (a minimum of 15 grams of carbohydrate per hour or 30–50 grams of carbohydrate every 3–4 hours) and contact a physician immediately when illness occurs.

The quality of the diet is less important than the quantity of carbohydrate consumed during severe illness; thus the intake of simple sugars such as those found in regular ginger ale may be recommended. Sipping juice or soft drinks throughout the day may be helpful when the intake of food is greatly diminished, as during an illness. To prevent loss of needed electrolytes that can result from vomiting and diarrhea, orange juice should be consumed for potassium and soup for sodium. Sports drinks or other commercial drinks containing electrolytes may also be consumed to provide sodium and potassium. Adequate intake of fluid sources, without carbohydrate to manage hyperglycemia, is imperative because dehydration compounds the undesirable effect of hyperglycemia and ketonuria.

WHAT COUNSELING STRATEGIES CAN NURSES AND OTHER HEALTH PROFESSIONALS USE IN DIABETES MANAGEMENT?

The nurse or other health professional needs to determine real versus perceived needs of persons who have already learned to live with diabetes. People sometimes feel their diabetes is controlled because they feel well physically. Or they may be in denial, feeling unable to cope with the demands of having diabetes. Positive verbal reinforcement for any attempt at control is always useful. Beyond that, the nurse can help patients to identify their perceived needs in relation to diabetes management, can make referrals as appropriate—for example, to the physician, dietitian, or diabetes support group—and can advocate gradual changes (small steps) in the control of diabetes. Simply being empathetic about the frustrations and challenges that are likely to be encountered by the individual with diabetes is an important role of the health care professional.

Another area to assess is the patient's knowledge of the physiology of diabetes mellitus, which is a prerequisite for effective decision making in diabetes management. Does the individual have a basic understanding of what makes blood glucose levels increase or decrease (see the following chart)? Does the individual have the skills to determine what course of action is most appropriate for the various situations likely to be encountered—such as for differing food intake or physical activity levels—and does he or she have the ability to follow through by making adjustments in diet, insulin administration, or activity? Is the person able to accept the reality of having diabetes mellitus and to take responsibility for its control? How does the person's environment (social, economic, and so on) reinforce or inhibit diabetes management? By identifying areas of strength for positive reinforcement and areas of need for referral or personal assistance, the nurse or other health care professional can have an integral and valuable role in facilitating the potential for full and productive lives in individuals with diabetes mellitus.

Factors Lowering Blood Sugar Levels	Factors Raising Blood Sugar Levels
Weight loss or reduced intake of food	Weight gain or increased food intake
Exercise*	Excess carbohydrate intake
Diabetes medication	Excess saturated and total fat intake
	Mental or physical stress
	Infections and illness
	Steroids, beta-blockers, diuretics
	Dawn phenomenon

Critical Thinking

Case Study

Chen led the way to the family table as Joey followed. Chen was glad he could bring his roommate from UCLA home for the weekend. Both of their fathers had diabetes and it seemed odd to Chen that Joey's dad had never tried ginseng as a remedy. He also thought it odd that Joey's dad included sugar as part of the carbohydrate in his diet. Chen's dad believed sugar had caused his diabetes and refused to eat any. As they sat down, Chen explained the family-style dishes in front of them, "This is oxtail soup—don't worry you'll like it, stir-fried pork with tofu (soybean curd—bland like mozzarella cheese), and bok choy (a form of greens like Swiss chard), and rice, and tea."

*If there is insufficient insulin in the body, exercise will raise blood sugar levels. If blood glucose levels are consistently elevated above 240 mg/dL or in cases of ketonuria, exercise should be postponed until diabetes is better controlled.

Applications

1. What might you ask Chen's father about the use of ginseng as a treatment for diabetes? If his father feels strongly about the importance of ginseng in maintaining health, how might this be explained?
2. How might you advise Chen's father if he chose to include a sweet food in his diet?
3. Describe which foods at this meal contain carbohydrate. Which ones are relatively high in carbohydrate (>15 grams per ½ cup) and which ones are low (<5 grams of carbohydrate) or have no carbohydrate (refer to Table 9–3)? Which foods contain soluble fiber?

Study Questions and Classroom Activities

1. Bring some convenience food labels into class. How can they be calculated into a diabetic person's diet?
2. Self-monitor your blood glucose levels using Chemstrips (strips which are visually read rather than using a blood glucose meter) for at least 1 day, prior to meals and 2 hours post-prandially. Maintain a record of your eating habits, including amounts eaten and times, and time and duration of activities. Based on this experience, discuss in class how you feel about advocating SMBG for all individuals with diabetes.
3. Determine what changes, if any, you would have to make if you were diagnosed as having diabetes. Could you consistently follow a low-fat, low-sugar meal plan? How would you feel if you had to reduce the amount of sweets and greasy foods in your diet?
4. Describe why a person with hyperglycemia is at increased risk of heart disease and kidney disease.
5. Become a member of the American Diabetes Association (for about $28 per year) and receive its monthly publication, "Diabetes Forecast." Each publication contains a feature story about a person with diabetes along with other informative articles.
6. If a person with Type 1 diabetes takes NPH insulin at 7:00 A.M., what time will the insulin peak? If this person begins to feel shaky at 3:00 P.M., what should he or she do?
7. Knowing that milk contains about 15 grams of carbohydrate per cup and that the form of carbohydrate in milk is lactose, calculate how many teaspoons of sugar equivalent it contains.
8. Determine if the following individual is likely to experience hypoglycemia:

Insulin-to-carbohydrate ratio (1 unit of insulin to 15 grams of carbohydrate)	1:15
Total units of insulin daily (*Hint:* 1500 rule)	45 units
Pre-meal blood glucose	175 mg/dL
Meal insulin dose	10 units regular insulin
Meal carbohydrate consumed (*Hint:* Insulin:carbohydrate ratio)	60 grams

9. Role-play in class a person who refuses to take control of diabetes, who has a HbA$_{1C}$ of 10 percent (average BG of 240 mg/dL). One student to role-play the nurse or other health care professional; the second student can role-play the person with diabetes. Discuss as a class the nurse's communication style and approach; was it effective or how else might the situation be handled?

References

Berry EM: Dietary fatty acids in the management of diabetes mellitus. Am J Clin Nutr. October 1997; 66(4 Suppl):991S-997S.

Bjorntorp P: Obesity. Lancet. 1997; 350:423–426.

Bolli GB: Hypoglycaemia unawareness. Diabetes Metab. September 23, 1997; (23 Suppl)3: 29–35.

Craig WJ: Phytochemicals: Guardians of our health. J Am Diet Assoc. October 1997; (10 Suppl 2):S199–S204.

Daly ME, Vale C, Walker M, Alberti KG, Mathers JC: Dietary carbohydrates and insulin sensitivity: A review of the evidence and clinical implications. Am J Clin Nutr. November 1997; 66(5):1072–1085.

Fineberg SE: Insulin analogs and human insulin lispro (humalog). Practical Diabetology. June 1997; 16(2):16–23.

Florez H: Steps toward the primary prevention of type II diabetes mellitus. Various epidemiological considerations. Invest Clin. March 1997; 38(1):39–52. [Article in Spanish]

Kimura K: Role of essential trace elements in the disturbance of carbohydrate metabolism. Nippon Rinsho. January 1996; 54(1):79–84.

Leibel RL, Rosenbaum M, Hirsch, J: Changes in energy expenditure resulting from altered body weight. N Engl J Med. 1995; 332:621–628.

Mangrum A, Bakris GL: Predictors of renal and cardiovascular mortality in patients with non-insulin-dependent diabetes: A brief overview of microalbuminuria and insulin resistance. J Diabetes Complications. November 1997; 11(6):352–357.

Mazzella M, Cotellessa M, Bonassi S, Mulas R, Caratozzolo A, Gaber S, Romano C: Incidence of type I diabetes in the Liguria Region, Italy. Results of a prospective study in a 0- to 14-year age group. Diabetes Care. October 1994; 17(10):1193–1196.

Morici ML, Di Marco A, Sestito D, Candore R, Cangemi C, Accardo F, Donatelli M, Cataldo MG, Lombardo A: The impact of coexistent diabetes on the prevalence of coronary heart disease. J Diabetes Complications. September 1997; 11(5):268–273.

Pan XR, Yang WY, Li GW, Liu J:Prevalence of diabetes and its risk factors in China, 1994. Diabetes Care. November 1997; 20(11):1664–1669.

Pick ME, Hawrysh ZJ, Gee MI, Toth E, Garg ML, Hardin RT: Oat bran concentrate bread products improve long-term control of diabetes: A pilot study. J Am Diet Assoc. December 1996; 96(12):1254–1261.

Quatromoni PA, Milbauer M, Posner BM, Carballeira NP, Brunt M, Chipkin SR: Use of focus groups to explore nutrition practices and health beliefs of urban Caribbean Latinos with diabetes. Diabetes Care. August 1994; 17(8):869–873.

Snehalatha C, Ramachandran A, Satyavani K, Vallabi MY, Viswanathan V: Computed axial tomographic scan measurement of abdominal fat distribution and its correlation with anthropometry and insulin secretion in healthy Asian Indians. Metabolism. October 1997; 46(10):1220–1224.

The DCCT Research Group: The effect of intensive treatment of diabetes on the development and progression of long-term complications in insulin-dependent diabetes mellitus. N Engl J Med. 1993; 329:977–986.

The Expert Committee on the Diagnosis and Classification of Diabetes Mellitus. Report of the Expert Committee on the Diagnosis and Classification of Diabetes Mellitus. Diabetes Care. 1997; 20:1183–1197.

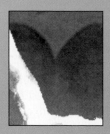

10
Renal Disease

Objectives

After completing this chapter, you should be able to:

- Describe the basic functions of the kidneys.
- Identify the clinical symptoms and serum parameters of renal disease.
- Describe the principles of nutritional management, including the control of disease and promotion of good nutritional status.
- Describe the role of the nurse and other health care professionals in the management of renal disease.

Terms to Identify

Albumin	Creatinine	Hypotension
Albuminuria	Edema	Nephrons
Anuria	End-stage renal disease	Oliguria
Azotemia	(ESRD)	Osteomalacia
Blood urea nitrogen	Erythropoietin	Osteoporosis
(BUN)	Glomerular filtration rate	Positive nitrogen balance
Carnitine	(GFR)	Proteinuria
Chronic renal failure	Hematuria	Renal insufficiency
Continuous ambulatory	Hemodialysis	Renal osteodystrophy
peritoneal dialysis	Hypercalciuria	Uremia
(CAPD)	Hypoalbuminemia	

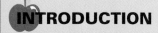 **INTRODUCTION**

Managing renal (kidney) disease is like a juggling act. Usually not just one but several nutritional components need to be controlled. Because of clearance problems, protein, phosphorus, sodium, and potassium need to be limited. If the renal disease results from complications of diabetes, carbohydrate needs to be considered for management of blood glucose levels. The remaining source of kilocalories—fat—needs to be maintained at a level that allows for slow weight loss or weight stabilization without promoting hypercholesterolemia. However, once a person with renal disease begins dialysis, the restrictions are often reversed in order to compensate for the excess losses incurred. Managing renal disease is complex and difficult for the patient and the entire health care team. But renal failure and the need for dialysis may be lessened or even prevented if the patient is willing and able to control the interrelated but diverse dietary factors that allow for normal lab values.

WHAT ARE THE FUNCTIONS OF KIDNEYS?

Kidneys have three basic functions: (1) excretion of waste material, (2) reabsorption of important body constituents, and (3) a metabolic and hormonal role. Their most widely known function is to filter body wastes, including drugs and toxins. This filtering process occurs in the **nephrons,** of which there are more than 1 million (Fig. 10–1). For renal disease patients, medications need to be adjusted to reflect diminished clearance through the kidneys. Persons on insulin therapy may need a lower dose of insulin when the kidneys fail.

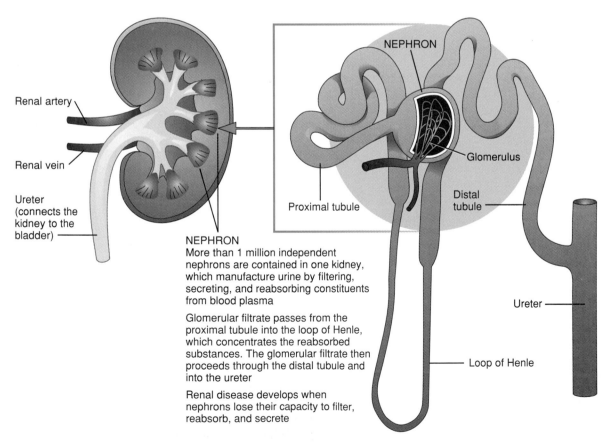

NEPHRON

Renal artery

Renal vein

Ureter (connects the kidney to the bladder)

Glomerulus

Proximal tubule

Distal tubule

Ureter

Loop of Henle

NEPHRON
More than 1 million independent nephrons are contained in one kidney, which manufacture urine by filtering, secreting, and reabsorbing constituents from blood plasma

Glomerular filtrate passes from the proximal tubule into the loop of Henle, which concentrates the reabsorbed substances. The glomerular filtrate then proceeds through the distal tubule and into the ureter

Renal disease develops when nephrons lose their capacity to filter, reabsorb, and secrete

Figure 10–1
Anatomy of a kidney.

Selectively reabsorbing nutrients as necessary is another basic function of the kidneys. This function serves an important role in maintaining the acid-base balance (pH level) and the balance of various body constituents. Thus, kidneys help maintain appropriate levels of water, electrolytes, nitrogen, fixed acids, bicarbonates, and other body constituents through the two functions of excretion of wastes and reabsorption of important nutrients.

The third and least well-known function of kidneys is the metabolic and hormonal one. Kidneys convert the inactive form of vitamin D from foods and sun exposure into the active form. Kidneys also produce the enzyme renin, which affects systemic blood pressure, and the hormone **erythropoietin,** which stimulates red blood cell production by the bone marrow. Figure 10–1 portrays the composition of the kidneys.

HOW IS RENAL DISEASE DIAGNOSED?

The general criteria for diagnosing renal disease center around the functions of the normal kidney. Given that kidneys excrete excess nitrogen, protein, electrolytes, water, and other substances, tests for abnormal levels of these constituents provide an indication of whether renal disease is present and, if so, how severe it is. Renal disease progresses along a continuum (Table 10–1). Lack of urinary excretion **(anuria)** or decreased urinary output **(oliguria)** suggests renal obstruction, which may lead to irreversible renal damage. Other clinical manifestations of renal disease include **hematuria** (blood in the urine), **albuminuria** (**albumin,** a form of protein, found in the urine), **azotemia** (nitrogen in the blood), hypertension, edema, **hypoalbuminemia** (low levels of albumin in the blood), hyperlipidemia, and **proteinuria** (protein in the urine).

Specific serum indicators routinely used for assessing the degree of renal failure and response to dietary control are the **blood urea nitrogen (BUN)** level and **creatinine** (a nitrogenous compound formed in muscle), albumin, potassium,

Table 10–1
Stages of Chronic Renal Disease

Stage	Therapeutic Dietary Measures
Glomerulonephritis	Protein restricted until kidney function improves; sodium restricted if hypertension or edema present; may be self-limiting or proceed to more severe renal disease
Nephrotic syndrome	May need to compensate for protein losses due to albuminuria; mild sodium restricted if edema present (3 g/day)
Diminished reserve	May need to control for hypertension with sodium restriction
Renal insufficiency	Restriction of protein, fluid, and electrolytes with adequate kilocalories required; level of dietary control based on renal functioning
Renal failure	Dialysis begun; diet needs to compensate for losses from dialysis; phosphorus restriction still needed
Uremia	Kidney transplant required unless uremia can be controlled through more frequent dialysis or stricter dietary control

phosphorus, sodium, and calcium determinations. The **glomerular filtration rate (GFR)** also gives an indication of how fast the kidneys are functioning in excreting wastes. A normal GFR is 125 mL per minute; less than 25 to 30 mL per minute is equated with **renal insufficiency;** and less than 15 mL per minute is associated with uremia. **Uremia** is associated with high creatinine levels of over 5 mg/dL; normal creatinine is less than 1.5 mg/dL; and levels over 10 mg/dL will require dialysis to preserve life.

WHAT ARE SOME TYPES OF RENAL DISORDERS AND THEIR NUTRITIONAL TREATMENT?

Nephrotic Syndrome

Nephrotic syndrome involves loss of the glomerular barrier to protein in the nephron (see Fig. 10–1). Protein is thus lost in the urine. This in turn causes a decreased serum albumin level. A decreased serum albumin level leads to **edema** (fluid retention). Nutritional care is aimed at improving protein status. A **positive nitrogen balance** (the amount of protein needed in the diet to allow for tissue growth or intake of protein that exceeds output) will promote an increased serum albumin level and correction of the edema.

How Much Protein Is Needed to Achieve a Positive Nitrogen Balance?

The amount of protein recommended to achieve positive nitrogen balance is based on individual needs. In the past, patients were routinely given double the recommended protein intake (1.5 g/kg body weight as compared with the normal recommendation of 0.8 g/kg). Now it appears that the quality of protein is more important than the total amount, although the goal is to still avoid excess protein (or no more than 0.8 g/kg); 60 grams of protein are often appropriate. An intake of 60 to 75 percent of the protein from high biological sources (meat, eggs, and milk products) is recommended along with adequate kilocalories to prevent weight loss. Weight measurements and estimates of kilocaloric needs can be assessed but must be verified for individual patients. For example, if weight loss is occurring on a 2000-kilocalorie level, the kilocalorie intake can be increased by 200 kilocalories for the goal of weight stablization. Kilocalorie needs can range from about 25 to 50 kilocalories per kilogram of ideal body weight for adults and up to 100 kilocalories per kilogram for children.

How Is Edema Treated in the Nephrotic Syndrome?

Because the cause of edema in the nephrotic syndrome is secondary to hypoalbuminemia, typical treatment of edema (low-sodium diet and diuretic medications) does not apply. The underlying hypoalbuminemia and subsequent edema will be corrected by achieving a positive nitrogen balance through increased protein utilization. Sodium should be restricted only mildly (to the 3 g/day range) because further reductions can cause **hypotension** (abnormally low blood pressure). Hypoalbuminemia causes a low blood volume, which would be exacerbated with very low sodium intakes (less than 2 g/day).

Nephritic Syndrome

This syndrome includes a group of inflammatory diseases of the kidney, specifically of the glomerulus (see Fig. 10–1). A term used to describe this condition is *glomerulonephritis*, or *nephritis*. Hematuria, hypertension, and mild loss of renal function are common. Recent studies have documented that excessive protein intake is toxic to the kidneys and promotes an inflammatory reaction in most forms of glomerulonephritis, which precede renal scarring. Nephritis with proteinuria is found in the presence of tubular inflammation (Remuzzi et al., 1997).

What Dietary Changes Are Made with the Nephritic Syndrome?

No routine dietary changes are made for nephritic syndrome except to maintain health during the inflammation stage. Alterations in protein intake should be based on serum lab values. Mild restrictions of protein and potassium may be indicated. Sodium restriction of 2 to 3 grams per day would be appropriate to control hypertension.

Diabetic Nephropathy

Diabetic nephropathy accounts for almost a third of cases of end-stage renal disease (ESRD) (Lapuz, 1997). Treatment becomes complicated as hypertension and dyslipidemia (elevated triglycerides and low HDL-cholesterol) are usually found in association with diabetes. Managing diabetic nephropathy is a very complex medical condition. Medical nutrition therapy as provided by a dietitian is critical when trying to balance the nutritional demands of diabetes, hypertension, hypercholesterolemia, and renal disesase.

The ideal course of action is to prevent the development of ESRD among persons with diabetes. The stages of damage leading to ESRD begin with the identification of microalbuminuria, and if diabetes and blood pressure are treated early and aggressively, the development of renal disease can be delayed if not halted. In the Modification of Diet in Renal Disease (MDRD) study it was found that patients with proteinuria should have a target blood pressure of 125/75 (Klahr, 1997). Microalbuminuria is defined as urinary albumin excretion of between 20 and 200 micrograms per minute; levels above this are referred to as macroalbuminuria. The GFR will not decrease until the macroalbuminuria stage has developed. Maintaining normal HbA_{1c} at about 7 percent (near normal blood glucose levels) is vital from allowing renal disease to progress with diabetes (Mogensen, 1997).

Acute Renal Failure

Acute renal failure (ARF) occurs when there is a sudden decrease in the GFR. In the MDRD study six factors predicted a fast decline in GFR: proteinuria, diagnosis of polycystic kidney disease (PKD), lower serum transferrin, higher arterial blood pressure, African American racial background, and low HDL-cholesterol (Hunsicker et al., 1997). Oliguria (reduced production of urine to less than 500 mL in 24 hours) may occur with ARF. Depending on the cause, ARF may be short-lived with no nutritional intervention necessary. About 25 percent of patients with heatstroke from excess physical exertion in a hot and humid environment develop ARF (Yu et al., 1997). If the patient goes on to develop **uremia** (a toxic buildup of protein by-products in the blood causing such problems as nausea and vomiting) and other problems such as fluid and electrolyte imbalances, nutritional care becomes a primary treatment. **Chronic renal failure** is a term used to describe the long-term condition of renal insufficiency.

How Is the Diet Modified in Chronic Renal Failure (CRF)?

Protein intake is based on individual lab values. Protein recommendations are usually set at 0.8 g/kg, which allows for adequate but not excessive intake (see Table 10–2). See the sample menu for a 60-gram protein diet, which is commonly prescribed; high-sugar, high-fat foods and beverages are included to show how increased kilocalories might be achieved. A vegan diet (no animal protein) was found to have comparable outcomes to a standard low-protein diet when there

Sample Menu for a 60-Gram Protein Diet

Breakfast

½ c cranberry juice
½ c cream of wheat cereal
2 slices toast
2 tsp butter

2 tsp honey
1 c whole milk
2 tsp sugar
¾ c coffee

Lunch

2 oz tuna salad
2 slices toast
½ c carrot sticks
6 slices cucumber with leaf lettuce

Italian salad dressing
½ c pineapple rings
1 tsp sugar
1 c Kool-Aid

Supper

Pear and peach halves on lettuce served with ¼ c cottage cheese
1 c pasta in olive oil and garlic sauce
½ c green beans

2 tsp butter
1 dinner roll
1 high-sugar, low-protein popsicle
1 tsp sugar
1 c whole milk

Table 10–2
Dietary Parameters in Renal Failure[a]

Energy and Nutrients	Renal Insufficiency	Hemodialysis	Peritoneal dialysis	Transplantation
Protein	0.6–0.8 g/kg/day, >50%–60% HBV[b]; 0.8–1.0 g/kg in nephrotic syndrome	1.2–1.4 g/kg/day, >50%–60% HBV	1.2–1.5 g/kg/day, >50%–60% HBV	1.3–1.5 g/kg/day after surgery; 1.0 g/kg/day chronic, stable renal function
Energy	30–35 kcal/kg/day	30–35 kcal/kg/day	23–35 kcal/kg/day, including dialysate energy; 20–25 kcal/kg for weight loss	25–35 kcal/kg/day to maintain desired body weight; limit fat to 30% total energy; <300 mg/day cholesterol
Sodium	2.0–4.0 g/day; variable with disease etiology and urine output	2.0 g/day	2.0–4.0 g/day	2.0–4.0 g/day after surgery; 3.0–4.0 g/day chronic, stable renal function
Potassium	Not usually restricted until GFR[c] <10 mL/min	2.0–3.0 g/day	3.0–4.0 g/day	Unrestricted; monitor drug effects
Phosphorus	10–12 mg/g dietary protein	12–15 mg/g dietary protein	12–15 mg/g dietary protein	Unrestricted; monitor
Calcium	1.0–1.5 g/day	1.0–1.5 g/day	1.0–1.5 g/day	1.0–1.5 g/day
Fluid	Unrestricted until urine output decreases	Urine output plus 1,000 c^3/day	Monitored; most tolerate 2,000 c^3/day	Unrestricted unless urine output decreases or fluid overload occurs
Vitamins and minerals	Daily RDA[d] of vitamins B, C, and D, iron, zinc; do not supplement vitamin A or magnesium	Daily RDA except: vitamin C = 60–100 mg/day; vitamin B-6 = 5–10 mg/day; folic acid = 0.8–1.0 µg/day; do not supplement vitamin A or magnesium	Daily RDA except: vitamin C = 60–100 mg/day; vitamin B-6 = 5–10 mg/day; folic acid = 0.8–1.0 µg/day; do not supplement vitamin A or magnesium	Daily RDA

[a]Data from references 4, 6, 19, 21, 24, 36–40.
[b]HBV = protein of high biological value.
[c]GFR = glomerular filtration rate.
[d]RDA = Recommended Dietary Allowance (19).
From Beto JA: Which diet for which renal failure: Making sense of the options, JADA. August 1995; 95(8):900.

was a good balance of amino acids from whole grains and legumes (Barsotti et al., 1996). Other factors such as diabetes, hypertension, or hypercholesterolemia need to be considered, but these chronic health conditions may have a lower priority to the goal of maintaining adequate body weight.

Usually a 1500-mg to 2000-mg level of potassium is appropriate. A normal diet may contain as much as 3000 to 8000 mg because potassium is widely distributed in foods (meats, fruits, whole-grain breads and cereals, and dark green leafy vegetables). Cooking water and the juices from canned fruits and vegetables must be discarded because potassium is water soluble. Table 10–3 lists foods low in sodium, potassium, and phosphorus.

Restricting phosphorus to 600 to 1200 mg (the RDA for adults is 800 mg) should maintain desirable serum phosphorus levels. Phosphate binders can be used as well but are now generally avoided because of possible aluminum toxicity. The use of calcium carbonate can decrease serum phosphorus while increasing serum calcium.

Fluids are restricted for patients with kidney failure; a balance between intake and output must be achieved. The general guideline is 500 to 1000 mL (about 2 to 4 cups) plus the amount lost in daily urine production and other body fluids such as with vomiting. For example, if the patient has a daily urine and fluid output of 1000 mL, the recommended fluid intake would range from 1500 to 2000

Table 10–3
Foods for Management of Renal Disease*

≤50 mg Sodium, Potassium and Phosphorus	≤100 mg Sodium, Potassium, and Phosphorus
Fruits	**Fruits and Vegetables**
Cranberry juice cocktail, ≤2 c	Blueberries, ≤½ c
Lemonade, ≤1 c	Grapes, ≤½ c
	Lettuce, ≤½ c
Sugars	Watermelon, ≤½ c
Granulated, ≤8 c	
Hard candy, ≤1½ lb	**Sugars**
Jelly beans, ≤5 c	Honey, ≤½ c
Marshmallows, ≤3½ oz	
Jam, ≤2 tbsp	**Alcohol**
Jelly, ≤3 tbsp	Beer, ≤12 oz
	Table wine, ≤4 oz
Fats	
Cooking oil (vegetable), unlimited	
Lard, unlimited	
Salt-free margarine, ≤1 c	
Salt-free butter, ≤1 c	

*Refer to food composition table (Appendix 5). Specific dietary advice should be given in conjunction with a registered dietitian and a physician. Foods contributing ≥2 g protein in common portions are not included.

mL per day; if there is anuria (no urine output), the fluid restriction would be 500 to 1000 mL per day. Thus the amount of fluid lost through urinary output needs to be estimated individually before recommended daily amounts can be determined.

Enteral liquid supplements have been developed to assist in providing amino acids (protein) and kilocalories while contributing low levels of the electrolytes sodium and potassium (see Appendix 8). If kidney function continues to deteriorate to end-stage renal disease, dialysis or kidney transplantation may be required (see later section).

Nephrolithiasis (Kidney Stones)

There are several forms of kidney stones, each with its own medical or nutritional intervention. The best prevention of kidney stones is adequate intake of fluids (1½ to 2 quarts or liters or more per day). Adequate fluid intake helps keep the urine dilute, which helps prevent crystals that lead to stone formation. Nutritional factors associated with stone formations include excessive intake of meat protein, oxalate, and sodium with inadequate intake of vegetables and fibers, calcium, and fluid (Jaeger, 1994). Once a stone has formed, treatment may best be decided after a chemical analysis of the stone. The most common form of stone is calcium oxalate.

Calcium Oxalate Stones

Calcium oxalate or phosphate stones account for almost 70 percent of all renal stones observed in economically developed countries and seem to have a genetic predisposition (Trinchieri, 1996). Calcium oxalate stones come in many forms. Medical input is necessary to determine nutritional intervention, and some calcium stones require medical or surgical intervention. Another form benefits from a low-oxalate diet. A dietitian should be consulted for such a diet, as foods high in oxalate (legumes and nuts, dark green leafy vegetables, berries, and citrus fruits) are very nutritious. The diet to control stone formation from oxalates needs to be evaluated for adequacy. If **hypercalciuria** (high levels of calcium in the urine) is noted to be the cause of stone formation, treatment with a low-calcium diet may not be appropriate. Intestinal calcium absorption can be stimulated with a low-calcium diet, which can promote stone formation (Messa et al., 1997). Only one type of hypercalciuria will improve on a low-calcium diet. The calcium restriction is now more moderate—in the range of 800 to 1200 mg of calcium per day. Patients with this form of hypercalciuria also need to follow a low-oxalate diet, which may require them to avoid such foods as legumes and dark green leafy vegetables. A magnesium supplement is also advised. A mild sodium restriction (4 to 5 g/day) can decrease urinary calcium levels in another form of hypercalciuria.

Uric Acid Stones

Limiting protein to the level of the RDA (45 to 55 g/day) is useful for treating uric acid stones. Emphasis on milk instead of meat, eggs, and legumes for protein will help prevent acidic urine. Increased intakes of fruit (except cranberries, plums, and prunes) and decreased intake of bread products may also help prevent acidic urine.

Cystine Stones

Cystine stones require a high fluid intake (greater than 4 quarts or liters per day). Following the diet to avoid acidic urine may also help prevent future formation of cystine stones.

Struvite Stones

Struvite stones are not managed nutritionally. They are usually seen in women and require long-term antibiotic therapy with surgical or ultrasonic stone removal.

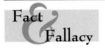

Fallacy: A person with kidney stones should follow a low-calcium diet.

Fact: Only recently it has been found that calcium restriction may be counterproductive for a person with kidney stones. Kidney stone formation now appears to be more related to oxalate intake with calcium binding to it. Oxalate is found in beets, chocolate, nuts, rhubarb, spinach, strawberries, tea, and wheat bran. Megadoses of vitamin C also contribute oxalate. The best course appears to be to avoid excess oxalate and protein while including the recommended amount of milk and increasing intake of potassium foods and water.

HOW DO THE DIETARY GUIDELINES RELATE TO MANAGEMENT OF RENAL DISEASE?

Although healthy persons are typically advised to avoid sugar and fat, their consumption may become mandatory for the renal patient to maintain adequate kilocalorie intake without contributing protein and electrolytes. The recommendation to increase sugar and fat may be met with resistance because of long-standing attempts to control health. A reduced sodium and moderate protein intake is recommended especially for the person with renal disease. Alcohol may contribute a significant source of kilocalories but ideally should be avoided. Maintenance of ideal body weight applies to the renal patient as well as to the general population.

Protein Restriction

Low-protein (and phosphorus) diets can help resolve uremic symptoms, secondary hyperparathyroidism, and metabolic acidosis in patients with CRF. It is controversial whether protein restriction slows the rate of progression of renal failure and the time until ESRD develops (Maroni & Mitch, 1997). A moderate intake of 60 grams of protein may be beneficial to stave off the development of ESRD and to meet the nutritional needs of most individuals, with or without renal disease. Once the GFR is less than 24 mL/min there is evidence that a protein-restricted diet will slow the progression of renal disease (Klahr, 1997).

WHAT ARE SOME NUTRITIONAL COMPLICATIONS ASSOCIATED WITH RENAL DISEASE OR ITS TREATMENT?

Nutrient Deficiencies

Careful planning must be undertaken to help ensure that the renal patient's nutritional status is not jeopardized while trying to prevent further kidney damage through the use of the low-protein diet. Finding foods that are low in potassium is generally the most limiting restriction in terms of food choices for the person with renal disease, as potassium is found in meats, fruits, whole-grain breads and cereals, and dark green leafy vegetables. There are other foods low in only sodium and phosphorus. Other special low-protein products may also have low electrolyte content. These food restrictions can be compounded by food dislikes or intolerances and can predispose the person with renal disease to ingest inadequate nutrients. However, even with caution, the risk of vitamin and mineral deficiency is inherent in the restrictive diet. It is prudent for renal patients to have a water-soluble vitamin supplement that does not exceed the RDA. This is especially true for the person who is restricting potassium intake, as such foods are high in other vitamin and minerals (whole grains, most fruits and vegetables, milk, and meat). Vitamin D supplementation is generally required to treat ESRD. However, the recommendation for vitamin and mineral supplementation should take place in conjunction with a physician consultation.

Protein calorie malnutrition in patients with end-stage renal disease can occur after two to three years of following a low-protein diet (0.58 g/kg/day) or a very-low-protein diet (0.28 g/kg/day supplemented with an amino acid mixture). Patients' intake of protein and kilocalories, as well as their nutritional status, must be monitored (Kopple et al., 1997).

Carnitine deficiency becomes an issue for long-term hemodialysis patients because of the combined effect of two complications: decreased availability of lysine and methionine (amino acids) and of vitamin C, niacin, vitamin B_6, and iron (micronutrients) to synthesize carnitine; and decreased metabolic activity of the kidney combined with removal of carnitine by the dialysis procedure. Carnitine, a substance produced in the kidneys, has the role of fatty acid oxidation, primarily of the heart and skeletal muscle. Oral and intravenous supplementations of L-carnitine may improve muscle cramps and weakness in patients receiving dialysis (Feinfeld et al., 1996). Carnitine may help in the use of erythropoietin in correcting renal anemia (Matsumura et al., 1996).

Lipid Abnormalities

Another situation calling for a low-sugar diet is Type IV hyperlipidemia, in which the triglyceride (very-low-density lipoproteins) level is elevated, whereas cholesterol levels are normal. This is a common occurrence in chronic renal failure and is treated with a low-sugar, high-fiber diet with moderate amounts of unsaturated fat. Small amounts of sugar may be tolerated as part of a moderate carbohydrate intake.

Renal Osteodystrophy

Renal osteodystrophy consists of a group of bone diseases resulting from the effects of chronic renal failure, such as poor bone development in children, **osteomalacia** (soft bones), and **osteoporosis** (brittle bones). Specifically, renal osteodystrophy is caused by a combination of high serum phosphorus levels, low serum calcium levels, and altered parathyroid function. Close monitoring and adherence to a controlled diet can help prevent or delay these complications.

Anemia

Problems with erythropoietin production may lead to diminished production of red blood cells and anemia. This condition is not responsive to iron supplementation; however, causes of iron deficiency should be ruled out before deciding not to treat with increased iron intake. Reversal of anemia with erythropoietin therapy slows the progression of chronic renal failure, especially in nondiabetic patients, provided blood pressure and dietary protein restriction are appropriate (Kuriyama et al., 1997).

WHAT ARE THE SPECIAL NUTRITIONAL CONSIDERATIONS FOR TREATING CHILDREN WITH RENAL DISEASE?

Children with renal disease have been noted to have stunted growth. One study found children with CRF to have inadequate intakes of calcium, zinc, vitamin B_6, and folate (Foreman et al., 1996). Children with CRF may also have a disturbance in the calcium-phosphorus balance, resulting in insufficient availability of calcium for bone growth. Once phosphorus levels are under control, the calcium and vitamin D intake can be increased to help promote bone growth.

Making mealtime fun in children is important for good nutritional intake. Liquid supplements that are designed for renal management can be given popular names such as "Barney Milkshake" for young children. Health care professionals interacting with the child should try to make foods sound appealing, provide small portions frequently, and arrange for favorite foods.

WHAT ARE THE DIFFERENT FORMS AND PROCEDURES OF DIALYSIS?

Dialysis is generally begun when a patient's creatinine level exceeds 10 to 12 and the BUN is above 100. This is indicative of **end-stage renal disease (ESRD).** A number of studies have now established plasma homocysteine to be a risk factor for vascular disease that is found in patients with ESRD. Homocysteine levels can be reduced by folic acid or vitamins B_{12} and B_6 but more research is needed to assess reduction in health risk (Gupta & Robinson, 1997).

There are two forms of dialysis, both of which have the goal of maintaining and balancing protein, electrolytes (potassium and sodium), and fluid levels. The traditional form is **hemodialysis,** which generally requires a renal patient to travel to a dialysis unit several times a week. For several hours the patient's blood is extracted and filtered through a dialysis solution. The dialyzed blood is then returned through the patient's venous system.

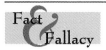

Fallacy: With dialysis, the patient with renal disease need not restrict food intake.

Fact: It is true that in order to compensate for incurred losses, some of the dietary restrictions are reversed during hemodialysis (e.g., protein, potassium, and sodium for the normotensive patient), but in general there are still restrictions. In fact, the frequency and duration of hemodialysis can be reduced when strict dietary controls are adhered to. For patients using dialysis, a more liberal dietary intake may be possible.

Continuous ambulatory peritoneal dialysis (CAPD) is a form of dialysis that was developed to improve the quality of life of the dialysis patient, as it does not require attachment to a machine. It entails filling the abdominal cavity with dialysis fluid, which has a high glucose content, which then absorbs toxins from the blood. After several hours, the dialysis fluid is drained, and fresh dialysis fluid is reinserted. This form of dialysis can also be performed intermittently, usually during sleep. This form of dialysis may not be appropriate for a person with diabetes because of the high sugar content of the dialysis fluid.

Dialysis has become commonplace since the U.S. Congress passed legislation allowing federal funds to be used for the procedure. Kidney transplants were also covered in this legislation, which was passed in 1972.

WHAT ARE SOME NUTRITIONAL RENAL TRANSPLANT ISSUES?

Steroid-induced weight gain can occur in conjunction with kidney transplants. Steroids are required to prevent rejection by the body of the new kidneys. Fat and carbohydrate restrictions help promote normal lipids and are further modified to meet weight goals. Protein intake should be high enough to prevent muscle wasting (Steiger et al., 1995). One study looked at post–renal transplant patients whose lipids were not adequately treated with the American Heart Association Step Two diet. A low dose of simvistatin (10 mg) and 6 grams of fish oil were both effective and safe, but further research was recommended (Castro et al., 1997). Restriction of sodium to 2 to 4 grams is recommended, with potassium and phosphorus restrictions based on patient serum values. Transplant goals should include control of obesity and hyperlipidemia to reduce cardiovascular mortality (Beto, 1995). Dietary selenium (0.2 mg/day) was found to be a potent antioxidant and to help prevent the atherogenic process (Hussein et al., 1997).

WHAT IS THE ROLE OF THE NURSE AND OTHER HEALTH CARE PROFESSIONALS IN THE MANAGEMENT OF RENAL DISEASE?

The nurse should be aware that nutritional treatment of kidney stones should not be undertaken lightly. Dietary changes may not be necessary, and restrictions can cause nutritional inadequacy and hardship for the patient. Nutritional advice should be made only in consultation with the patient's physician.

The patient with chronic renal disease has difficult decisions to make. Life expectancy with CRF or ESRD can be extended, but only at the expense of an impaired quality of life. Stress on other family members will likely occur. As a consequence, a patient with newly diagnosed chronic renal failure can be expected to experience typical grief reactions: denial and anger first, with the need for information and acceptance of responsibility for management of the disease appearing only later.

Through a sensitive approach and strong communication and listening skills, the health care professional can begin to determine what stage the patient with renal disease is in and thereby develop an appropriate plan of action, with referrals being a cornerstone of therapy. A referral to a social worker might be indicated when the patient is exhibiting anger or denial. A referral to a dietitian is imperative when the patient is ready to accept responsibility for dietary control. A referral to a nurse at a dialysis center is beneficial in regard to dialysis issues, such as the control of dry mouth. The nurse can further help the renal patient identify the available options and the advantages and disadvantages of each. Finally, the health care professional can help motivate the patient to recognize that life is inherently valuable irrespective of the diminished quality.

For the patient who has begun to take responsibility for the control of chronic renal disease, the health care professional can help serve as a reality tester. The person with renal disease cannot make drastic long-term dietary changes easily and thus should be verbally rewarded for the attempts made and reassured that mistakes and overindulgences will happen, and encouraged not to give up the fight.

Critical Thinking

Case Study

Little Dove and her daughter went to see the kidney doctor. They knew what was coming. Little Dove had become greatly fatigued and ill and she suspected her kidneys were failing. But she was not old. She had been a teenager when her daughter was born and had a full life, but age 60 was still too young to die. Little Dove felt that there must be a way to keep healthy awhile longer. She knew she had to be strong for her family's sake, as her son-in law was still in the hospital and her grandson was soon to be married. She hoped to live long enough to become a great-grandmother.

The doctor called them into his office. Her blood urea nitrogen (BUN) was up to 75 and her creatinine was up to 8. It was time to plan to start dialysis. Either she could come in three times weekly to have her blood filtered via a machine or she could try the newest treatment, which meant putting a solution via a catheter into her lower abdomen to dwell and then drain four times daily. Little Dove looked over at her daughter, who was holding her head in her hands. How could they all cope with this?

Before they left the hospital, they decided to go to the hospital cafeteria to have a bite to eat. They knew they could find something low in potassium and protein, such as applesauce, which Little Dove was well used to. Little Dove would taste the applesauce to see if it was sweetened. If so, she wouldn't have any other source of carbohydrate because she knew her meal limit on a stressful day like today was 30 grams of carbohydrate. She also knew if she ate more carbohydrate than that, her blood sugar level would go too high. She and her daughter looked around for a lettuce wedge and a deviled egg—only 1 ounce of meat and she could still go home and have a small amount of meat later. As they sat down at their table, they were surprised to see a man they recognized as a patient on the dialysis unit. He was eating a huge banana split sundae, and Little Dove wondered why or if he should be eating this.

Applications

1. Why might this man be eating a banana split sundae if he is diagnosed with renal disease?
2. Why did Little Dove complain of being "greatly fatigued"?
3. What might be factors in the development of Little Dove's chronic renal failure?
4. Discuss how family member's influence the management of health problems.
5. Why would applesauce be a good food choice for Little Dove? What else might she eat if the applesauce was found to be unsweetened?
6. What are some traditional Navajo foods low in potassium (see Appendix 7)?
7. Describe how you would feel if you had to insert and remove abdominal dialysis fluid four times a day. What might you say to a person undergoing this procedure?

Study Questions and Classroom Activities

1. What foods can the patient with renal disease generally consume freely, in moderate amounts, and in restrictive amounts?
2. Why does the patient with chronic renal failure need to restrict protein, electrolytes, and fluid?
3. What causes uremic symptoms to develop?
4. Record a 24-hour diet recall on yourself. Calculate the amount of protein, phosphorus, sodium, and potassium in your diet.
5. As a class, visit a dialysis unit. Arrange to have a nurse, a dietitian, and, if possible, a patient with renal disease consult with the class on the dietary control of renal disease as it pertains to dialysis.

References

Barsotti G, Morelli E, Cupisti A, Meola M, Dani L, Giovannetti S: A low-nitrogen low-phosphorus vegan diet for patients with chronic renal failure. Nephron. 1996; 74(2): 390–394.

Beto JA: Which diet for which renal failure: Making sense of the options. J Am Diet Assoc. August 1995; 95(8):898–903.

Castro R, Queiros J, Fonseca I, Pimentel JP, Henriques AC, Sarmento AM, Guimaraes S, Pereira MC: Therapy of post-renal transplantation hyperlipidaemia: Comparative study with simvastatin and fish oil. Nephrol Dial Transplant. October 1997; 12(10): 2140–2143.

Feinfeld DA, Kurian P, Cheng JT, Dilimetin G, Arriola MR, Ward L, Manis T, Carvounis CP: Effect of oral L-carnitine on serum myoglobin in hemodialysis patients. Ren Fail. January 1996; 18(1):91–96.

Foreman JW, Abitbol CL, Trachtman H, Garin EH, Feld LG, Strife CF, Massie MD, Boyle RM, Chan JC: Nutritional intake in children with renal insufficiency: A report of the growth failure in children with renal diseases study. J Am Coll Nutr. December 1996; 15(6):579–585.

Gupta A, Robinson K: Hyperhomocysteinaemia and end stage renal disease. J Nephrol. March 1997; 10(2):77–84.

Hunsicker LG, Adler S, Caggiula A, England BK, Greene T, Kusek JW, Rogers NL, Teschan PE: Predictors of the progression of renal disease in the Modification of Diet in Renal Disease Study. Kidney Int. June 1997; 51(6):1908–1919.

Hussein O, Rosenblat M, Refael G, Aviram M: Dietary selenium increases cellular glutathione peroxidase activity and reduces the enhanced susceptibility to lipid peroxidation of plasma and low-density lipoprotein in kidney transplant recipients. Transplantation. March 15, 1997; 63(5):679–685.

Jaeger P: Prevention of recurrent calcium stones: Diet versus drugs. Miner Electrolyte Metab. 1994; 20(6):410–413.

Klahr S: Prevention of progression of nephropathy. Nephrol Dial Transplant. 1997; 12 (Suppl 2):63–66.

Kopple JD, Levey AS, Greene T, Chumlea WC, Gassman JJ, Hollinger DL, Maroni BJ, Merrill D, Scherch LK, Schulman G, Wang SR, Zimmer GS: Effect of dietary protein restriction on nutritional status in the Modification of Diet in Renal Disease Study. Kidney Int. September 1997; 52(3):778–791.

Kuriyama S, Tomonari H, Yoshida H, Hashimoto T, Kawaguchi Y, Sakai O: Reversal of anemia by erythropoietin therapy retards the progression of chronic renal failure, especially in nondiabetic patients. Nephron. 1997; 77(2):176–185.

Lapuz MH: Diabetic nephropathy. Med Clin North Am. May 1997; 81(3):679–688.

Maroni BJ, Mitch WE: Role of nutrition in prevention of the progression of renal disease. Annu Rev Nutr. 1997; 17:435–455.

Matsumura M, Hatakeyama S, Koni I, Mabuchi H, Muramoto H: Correlation between serum carnitine levels and erythrocyte osmotic fragility in hemodialysis patients. Nephron 1996; 72(4):574–578.

Messa P, Marangella M, Paganin L, Codardini M, Cruciatti A, Turrin D, Filiberto Z, Mioni G: Different dietary calcium intake and relative supersaturation of calcium oxalate in the urine of patients forming renal stones. Clin Sci (Colch). September 1997; 93(3): 257–263.

Mogensen CE: How to protect the kidney in diabetic patients: With special reference to IDDM. Diabetes. September 1997; 46 (Suppl 2):S104–S111.

Remuzzi G, Ruggenenti P, Benigni A: Understanding the nature of renal disease progression. Kidney Int. January 1997; 51(1):2–15.

Steiger U, Lippuner K, Jensen EX, Montandon A, Jaeger P, Horber FF: Body composition and fuel metabolism after kidney grafting. Eur J Clin Invest. November 1995; 25(11): 809–816.

Trinchieri A: Epidemiology of urolithiasis. Arch Ital Urol Androl. September 1996;68(4): 203–249.

Yu FC, Lu KC, Lin SH, Chen GS, Chu P, Gao GW, Lin YF: Energy metabolism in exertional heat stroke with acute renal failure. Nephrol Dial Transplant. October 1997; 12(10): 2087–2092.

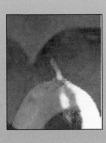

11
Gastrointestinal Diseases and Disorders

Objectives

After completing this chapter, you should be able to:

- Explain the role of diet in the treatment of diseases of the gastrointestinal tract.
- Explain how the normal diet is modified for these diseases.
- Describe the role of the nurse or other health care professional in managing conditions or diseases of the gastrointestinal tract.

Terms to Identify

Achalasia
Ascites
Celiac sprue
Cholecystitis
Cholelithiasis
Cirrhosis
Cleft palate
Constipation
Crohn's disease
Cystic fibrosis
Diarrhea
Diverticulitis
Diverticulosis
Dyspepsia

Dysphagia
Encopresis
Esophageal reflux
Esophageal varices
Gastritis
Gliadin
Gluten
Hepatic coma
Hepatitis
Hiatal hernia
Hyperchlorhydria
Hypochlorhydria
Irritable bowel syndrome

Jaundice
Lactobacillus culture
Lactose intolerance
Medium-chain
   triglycerides (MCTs)
Nontropical sprue
Obstipation
Residue
Sickle cell disease
Steatorrhea
Thalassemia
Ulcerative colitis
Videofluoroscopy

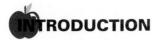TRODUCTION

Think of the gastrointestinal (GI) tract as one long tube with a couple of attachments (liver, gallbladder, and pancreas). The GI tract is far more than a tube that allows food to pass through, however. It is one of the major endocrine glands, producing a wide variety of hormones and digestive enzymes that control how food is digested, absorbed, and metabolized. An individual's nutritional status is at risk of being affected whenever the gastrointestinal tract is functionally impaired. An adequate dietary intake is important but is sometimes difficult to maintain when the normal digestion and absorption process is interrupted. (See Chapter 4 for a full description of the digestive process.)

Physical disorders can begin where digestion begins—in the mouth, or oral cavity. Problems with the oral cavity such as **cleft palate** (an opening or hole in the roof of the mouth sometimes extending to the lip; see later discussion) or lack of teeth can prevent adequate ingestion of food. The esophagus transfers food from the oral cavity to the stomach. This process is complicated and can go awry with neurological or neuromuscular disorders. Swallowing problems, referred to as **dysphagia,** are often related to stroke, head injury, cerebral palsy, and other conditions (see Fig. 4–6 regarding the swallowing process).

Organic disorders of the stomach result from a change in structural tissue. Examples include pathological lesions, peptic ulcer, hiatal hernia, carcinoma, and **gastritis** (inflammation of the gastric mucosa).

Functional disorders of the stomach (reflex disorders) involve a change in body functions without detectable changes in structural tissue. Examples include **dyspepsia** (indigestion), **hyperchlorhydria** (an excess of hydrochloric acid in the gastric juice), and **hypochlorhydria** (too little hydrochloric acid).

The small intestine, large intestine, liver, gallbladder, and pancreas all contribute to the digestive process and are susceptible to numerous diseases and disorders.

WHAT ARE PROBLEMS OF THE ORAL CAVITY?

Cleft Palate

Babies born with an opening in the roof of the mouth have difficulty creating a suction seal around their mother's nipple or a bottle nipple, which leads to inadequate ingestion of breast milk or formula. Severe cases may require surgical correction. Babies with less severe forms of cleft palate may benefit from special bottle nipples that do not require suction or from a slightly larger hole in the bottle nipple. Mothers who are motivated to continue nursing until the problem is resolved should be encouraged to do so with supplemental bottle feedings as needed (see Chapter 16).

Dental Problems

Missing teeth or severe dental caries can adversely affect food choices. Persons with dental problems may have a low fiber intake because of difficulty in chewing. Without adequate nutritional knowledge, omitting food groups may not seem important to a person with dental problems. Alternatives should be discussed, such as eating applesauce in place of fresh apples, or eating cooked or soft vegetables in place of raw or hard-to-chew vegetables. Prevention of dental caries is addressed in Chapter 19.

Dysphagia

Dysphagia is an uncomfortable and potentially life-threatening condition that affects approximately 15 million people in the United States. Dysphagia is generally a neuromuscular problem and can benefit from swallowing therapy as provided by a speech pathologist (Paterson, 1996). The assessment of dysphagia was found to be strongly predicted when patients coughed after drinking 3 oz of water (Mari et al., 1997). Patients who have had a cardiovascular accident (also called CVA or stroke; see Chapter 8) may not be able to swallow correctly, and this may result in aspiration of food into the lungs. Aspiration pneumonia is a frequent complication of cerebral vascular accidents, but with changes in the consistency of the diet according to swallowing evaluation, a significant reduction in aspiration pneumonia can occur (Gottlieb et al., 1996). Individuals who have developmental delays (see Chapter 18) with neurological impairment are at particular risk for dehydration and undernutrition, and for some the provision of gastrostomy tube feeding may be life saving (Kennedy et al., 1997).

Dysphagia requires a review of the swallowing process in order to determine the best means of feeding. A speech pathologist is trained to help assess swallowing problems. An X-ray examination called **videofluoroscopy** is used to objectively diagnose dysphagia. Liquids are usually the most difficult food to swallow for persons with dysphagia. Table 11–1 shows categories of foods rated according to swallowing difficulty. Liquids thickened with a commercial product such as THICK-IT or with baby rice cereal or other thickener may be easier for a patient with dysphagia to swallow. Feeding positions can also help (see Chapter 18). Table 11–2 lists food consistency considerations.

WHAT ARE DISEASES OF THE ESOPHAGUS?

Achalasia

In **achalasia,** the lower part of the esophagus fails to relax, and swallowing difficulty occurs. The individual senses fullness in the sternal region and may vomit; then there is danger that the contents of the esophagus may be aspirated into the respiratory passages. Weight loss may become a problem that requires nutri-

Table 11–1
Main Features of Dysphagia Diet Categories

Solid Foods*

Stage 1	All pureed foods, smooth hot cereals, strained soups thickened to pureed consistency, creamed cottage cheese, smooth yogurt, and puddings
Stage 2	All foods in previous stages plus soft moist whole foods such as pancakes; finely chopped tender meats, fish, and eggs bound with thick dressing; soft cheeses (e.g., American); noodles and pasta; tender cooked leafy greens; sliced ripe banana; soft breads; soft moist cakes
Stage 3	All foods in previous stages plus eggs any style, tender ground meats bound with thick sauce, soft fish, whole soft vegetables, drained canned fruits
Stage 4	All foods in previous stages plus foods with solids and liquids together (e.g., vegetable soup), all whole foods except hard and particulate foods such as dry breads, tough meat, corn, rice, apples
Stage 5	Regular diet

Liquids*

Thin[†]	Water, all juices thinner than pineapple, Italian ice, other clear liquids except gelatin desserts
Thick[†]	All other liquids including milk, any juice not classified as a thin liquid, sherbet, ice cream
Thickened	Liquids thickened with starch to pureed consistency for those who cannot tolerate any other liquids

*Progressing in swallowing difficulty from easiest to most difficult.
[†]Categories are unrelated in swallowing difficulty.
From Pardoe EM: Development of a multistage diet for dysphagia. © The American Dietetic Association. Reprinted by permission from J Am Diet Assoc. 1993; 93(5):568–571.

tional intervention. Dilation of the esophagus or surgical intervention can improve the condition (Anselmino et al., 1997).

Dietary Modifications. A soft diet with low bulk is advised for mild cases of achalasia. Small meals should be eaten slowly along with frequent sips of fluids to facilitate swallowing. Smooth-textured foods (for example, pudding and pureed foods) are easier to swallow. When normal swallowing resumes, a regular diet following the guidelines given in Chapter 6 should be followed.

A high-protein, high-calorie liquid diet may be prescribed. This may include milkshakes, cream soups, or commercial nutrition supplements.

Esophageal Reflux

The condition of **esophageal reflux** is the opposite of achalasia: The lower esophageal sphincter is incompetent and allows stomach matter to regurgitate into the esophagus. Symptomatic stricturing of the esophagus complicates the course of about 10 to 15 percent of patients with gastroesophageal reflux disease, particularly if they are elderly (Barkun & Mayrand, 1997). Gastroesophageal reflux disease (GERD) is considered common in the elderly and may present with various symptoms, such as heartburn, regurgitation, dysphagia, or chest pain (Triadafilopoulos & Sharma, 1997). The sphincter pressure may become low from

Table 11–2
Food Consistency Considerations

Type of Diet	Example	Potential Impact on Oral Function
Thin foods and liquids	Soup broth, juice	More difficult to control within mouth, especially with limited tongue control, i.e., quickly runs to all areas of mouth. Often promotes excessive food loss
Thick foods	Pudding, yogurt, applesauce	Improved control within oral cavity due to reduced flow and increased sensory input (i.e., weight and texture)
Pastelike or sticky foods	Peanut butter, thick cheese sauce	May be more difficult to move in oral cavity with limited tongue movement May stick to the roof of the mouth, especially with a high, narrow palate
Slippery foods	Pasta, Jell-o	Often difficult to control and either triggers reflexive swallow too quickly or runs out of oral cavity before the swallow
Smooth textures	Pudding, pureed foods	Relatively easy to swallow; promotes minimal tongue and jaw movement, especially over periods of time
Coarse textures	Creamed corn, ground foods, Sloppy Joe filling	Increases sensory input to stimulate more jaw and tongue movements Coarseness of food should be carefully graded
Varied textures	Soups with noodles or chunks of vegetables	Difficult to manage in oral cavity, especially with limited tongue movement or decreased oral sensitivity (i.e., liquid is swallowed and solid pieces remain in the mouth)
Scattering textures	Grated carrots, rice, coleslaw, corn bread	Very difficult to manage with limited tongue movement and decreased oral sensitivity
Crisp solids	Carrot sticks, celery sticks	Requires sophisticated biting and chewing in order to grind pieces into consistency that is safe to swallow
Milk-based substances	Milk, ice cream	Appear to coat mucous membranes in oral-pharyngeal cavities to interfere with swallowing
Broth	Meat broth, chicken broth	Appears to cut mucus in oral-pharyngeal cavity and facilitate swallowing
Dry foods	Bread, cake, cookie	May be difficult to chew or swallow with insufficient saliva
Whole soft foods	Slice of bread	Requires the ability to bite off appropriately sized pieces

Courtesy of the Occupational Therapy Department of the J.N. Adams Developmental Center, Perrysburg, NY.

a variety of causes including a high-fat diet and central obesity with resulting regurgitation. Medications and hormonal variations can also play a role. An increased level of progesterone during pregnancy has been found to change the motility level throughout the entire GI tract. These changes include decreased esophageal sphincter pressure leading to an increased risk of reflux and aspiration (Baron et al., 1993).

Dietary Modifications. Treatment may include weight loss (except during pregnancy) to decrease abdominal pressure on the stomach, small frequent meals to avoid stomach distention, and avoidance of chocolate and fats, which reduce sphincter competence. Avoidance of caffeine and alcohol may help reduce stomach acidity. Drinking liquids between meals and remaining upright after eating also help.

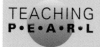

Patients with esophageal reflux are likely to follow dietary advice if the health professional gives them the rationale for doing so. This is due to the negative reinforcement of physical discomfort. Thus, you should explain that the goal of dietary treatment is to lessen physical discomfort. To achieve this, the patient should consume small frequent meals to help prevent an overly full stomach. Many individuals eat without thinking about how full they are getting. The patient with esophageal reflux may need to be taught to chew thoroughly and slowly in order to better recognize feelings of fullness. Reinforce to the patient that gravity helps keep the food in the stomach. Thus, sitting up after meals is important.

Hiatal Hernia

A **hiatal hernia** is a protrusion of a part of the stomach through the esophageal hiatus (opening) of the diaphragm (Fig. 11–1). Persons with this disorder sometimes complain of heartburn because of the reflux of gastric contents into the esophagus. Medical treatment includes ingestion of antacids to neutralize or inhibit gastric secretions and possibly surgery.

Dietary Modifications. Small, frequent meals that follow a normal balanced diet are recommended to reduce symptoms, although dietary modifications cannot eliminate the cause. Foods that are poorly tolerated should be avoided, especially those that may irritate the mucous membranes (e.g., orange juice and tomato juice). Extremes in food temperature should be avoided. No food is allowed for approximately 3 hours before bedtime, and the person should remain in the upright position after eating. For the obese person, weight loss is indicated to help relieve pressure on the diaphragm. Any source of pressure on the abdomen, such as bandages or clothes that fit too tightly, should be eliminated.

WHAT ARE DISEASES OF THE STOMACH?

Gastritis

Gastritis (acute or chronic) is an inflammation of the lining of the stomach that results in abdominal pain, nausea, and vomiting. It may be caused by food poisoning, overeating, excessive intake of alcohol, or bacterial and viral infections. A chronic condition may be related to other disease states. It often precedes the development of ulcers or cancer.

Dietary Modifications. Acute gastritis, which usually heals within a few days, is often treated first with antibiotics and neutralization of the stomach contents. The stomach is allowed to rest for a while, and then the patient drinks clear fluids for the first day or two. The patient may then progress to small amounts of soft, low-fiber foods. It may be necessary for the patient to avoid highly seasoned foods, alcohol, caffeinated beverages, decaffeinated coffee, and red (cayenne) pepper.

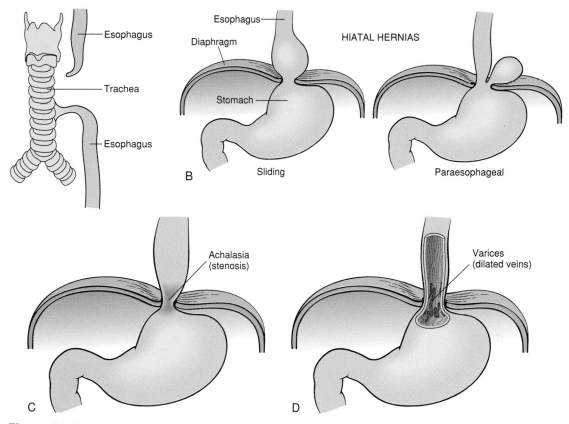

Figure 11–1
Sketch of hiatal hernia. (From Damjanov I: Pathology for the Health-Related Professions. Philadelphia, WB Saunders, 1996, p. 261.)

Peptic Ulcer

A peptic ulcer is an eroded lesion in the lining (mucosa) of the stomach (gastric ulcer) or duodenum (duodenal ulcer). Theories as to the cause of peptic ulcers have changed over the years from a focus on acid production and stomach irritants using a variety of medications from tranquilizers and antacids to histamine receptor antagonists to an increasing recognition in recent years that the *Helicobacter pylori* infection is involved (Pohle et al., 1997). In 1995, however, only 5 percent of those with peptic ulcer were found to be treated with antibiotics, whereas 75 percent were treated with antisecretory medications (Munnangi & Sonnenberg, 1997).

Symptoms include burning or gnawing pain in the pit of the stomach. Peptic ulcers are diagnosed by gastric analysis, X-ray or fluoroscopic studies, or gastroscopy.

Dietary Modifications. While an ulcer is bleeding, no food is allowed; instead, the patient may be given intravenous feedings of dextrose and amino acids. As the condition improves, the patient usually progresses from a full liquid diet to a regular diet with the omission of irritants based on individual tolerances (see Fig. 11–2; individualization of this diet is suggested). Cigarette smoke is a nondietary irritant of the gastric mucosa. The patient should be referred to a smoking-cessation program.

A liberal approach to dietary intervention is currently being used by most clinicians, as it is now known that a bland diet has little effect on the healing of ulcers. Nutritional advice should be individualized. If a patient feels that certain foods cause gastric pain, those foods should be omitted until the person feels comfortable eating them again. Coffee, whether caffeinated or not, may cause gastric distress. Food omissions should be made carefully to prevent nutritional inadequacy. Table 11–3 lists some guidelines for dietary treatment of peptic ulcers which may be appropriate.

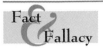

Fallacy: People with stomach ulcers need to avoid citrus juice.

Fact: Actually, the stomach produces hydrochloric acid, which is more acidic than any food. Therefore, orange juice cannot be considered harmful to the gastric mucosa, because it cannot increase the acidity of the stomach contents. However, caution should be used. The patient should be advised to try a small amount of orange juice (2 ounces) with a meal to ensure that it is tolerated. Increased amounts can be consumed based on individual tolerance.

Breakfast
Poached egg   Orange juice
Whole-wheat toast   Milk

Midmorning Snack
Fresh apple slices

Lunch
Celery and carrot sticks   Fresh peach
Macaroni and cheese casserole   Milk
Green beans

Midafternoon Snack
Graham crackers   Milk

Supper
Tossed salad with blue cheese   Sliced carrots
   dressing   Bread and butter
Baked chicken   Milk

Evening Snack
Cheese and wheat crackers

Figure 11–2
Sample menu for a peptic ulcer diet.

Table 11–3
Dietary Treatment of Peptic Ulcers

Guideline	Rationale
Eat three regular meals or six small meals	Inhibits stomach distention
Avoid caffeine-containing beverages, decaffeinated coffee	Decreases gastric secretions
Avoid alcohol	Reduces damage to stomach lining
Avoid black pepper, chili powder, cloves, nutmeg, curry powder, mustard seed	Reduces irritation to stomach lining
Avoid aspirin	Reduces irritation of stomach lining
Avoid cigarette smoking	Promotes healing of ulcer
Eat in a relaxed atmosphere	Reduces stress

WHAT ARE DISEASES OF THE INTESTINES?

Lactose Intolerance

Congenital, or primary, **lactose intolerance** refers to the inability to digest milk sugar (lactose). It is caused by a low amount of the enzyme lactase, which is necessary for converting lactose into glucose and galactose in the gastrointestinal tract. Symptoms include bloating, flatulence, cramping, and diarrhea. Different populations show variations in degrees of lactase deficiency, usually occurring after 5 years of age. Lactase deficiency is more common among persons of African, Asian, Mediterranean, Hispanic, and Native American heritage than among persons of Northern European heritage.

Acquired lactase deficiency, also referred to as secondary lactose intolerance, is associated with chronic gastrointestinal disease and disorders such as gluten-sensitive enteropathy, Crohn's disease, and other conditions leading to atrophy of the villi of the intestines (see Fig. 4–2). An estimated 50 to 90 percent of persons with celiac disease also have lactase deficiency (Ferguson, 1995). It was recently noted that persons with the diagnosis of irritable bowel syndrome frequently have lactose intolerance, which can be treated with a lactose-restricted diet (Bohmer & Tuynman, 1996).

Dietary Modifications. Many persons with lactose intolerance do not have to eliminate lactose-containing foods entirely from their diets because they can produce small amounts of lactase (Table 11–4). Varying amounts of lactose are found in milk products; hard cheeses and yogurt have the least amount of lactose. When foods containing lactose are omitted, it is important to include other sources of calcium in the diet (see Fig. 11–3 and Table 1–3). If an individual whose genetic background predisposes him or her to lactase deficiency reports these symptoms when milk is ingested, he or she should not be forced to drink it.

Table 11–4
Guidelines for Food Selection for Lactose-Controlled Diet

Food Category	Recommended	May Cause Distress
Beverages	All beverages with allowed ingredients, soybean milks, other lactose-free supplements, lactose-hydrolyzed milk	Milk, milk products, or acidophilus milk as tolerance dictates
Breads and cereals	Whole-grain or enriched breads and cereals	Depending on tolerance, some breads and cereals prepared with milk or milk products may need to be avoided
Desserts	Cakes, cookies, pies; flavored gelatin desserts; water ices made with allowed foods	Any prepared with milk or milk products (e.g., sherbet, ice cream, ice milk, custard, pudding, commercial desserts, and mixes)
Fats	Butter or margarine; salad dressings; nondairy creamer; all oils	Any prepared with lactose-containing ingredients
Fruits	All fruits and juices	None
Meats and meat substitutes	All meats, poultry; fish; eggs; peanut butter; dried peas and beans; hard, aged, and processed cheese, if tolerated; yogurt as tolerated	Cold cuts and frankfurters that contain lactose filler; cottage cheese
Potatoes and potato substitutes	Potatoes; enriched rice; barley; noodles, spaghetti, macaroni, and other pastas	Potatoes or substitutes prepared with milk or milk products; mixes prepared with lactose-containing ingredients
Soups	Broth, bouillon; soups made with allowed ingredients	Soups made with milk or milk products
Sweets	Sugar; corn syrup; pure maple syrup; honey; jellies, jams; pure sugar candies; marshmallows	Chocolate; caramels; any candies made with lactose-containing ingredients
Vegetables	All	Vegetables prepared with milk or milk products
Miscellaneous	All spices, seasonings, flavorings	Any prepared with milk or milk products

From Manual of Clinical Dietetics, 5th ed. The American Dietetic Association, 1996; pp. 421–422.

Adding commercial lactase enzymes, in tablet or liquid form, to milk reduces the lactose content of milk by 70 to 90 percent. The milk will taste sweeter than regular milk because the lactose is broken down into simple sugars. Many grocery stores now carry a new 100 percent lactose-free milk. Ensure and Sustacal are lactose-free nutritional supplements.

For some persons it is important to read all labels carefully to avoid foods containing even traces of lactose. They should look for the terms "whey milk," "dry milk solids," and "nonfat dry milk" when inspecting food labels. Lactalbumin, lactate, and certain calcium compounds do not contain lactose. There will be no long-term health problem if lactose is accidentally ingested, however, because the condition is an intolerance, not an allergy.

The patient with lactose intolerance should be encouraged to try small amounts of milk products such as low-fat cheese or yogurt. These are often tolerated in mild forms of lactose intolerance. It has been noted that up to the equiva-

Breakfast

½ cup orange juice	2 tsp milk-free margarine
½ cup farina	1 tbsp jelly
1 egg, soft cooked	2 tsp sugar
2 slices Vienna bread toasted	Coffee or tea

Lunch

2 oz sliced chicken	2 tsp milk-free margarine
½ cup rice	½ cup canned peaches
½ cup green beans	1 slice angel food cake
½ sliced tomato on lettuce	1 tsp sugar
2 tsp mayonnaise	Coffee or tea
1 slice Vienna bread	

Midafternoon Snack
1 cup apple juice

Supper

3 oz roast beef	1 slice Vienna bread
½ cup cubed white potatoes	2 tsp milk-free margarine
¼ cup beef broth gravy	Small banana
½ cup peas and carrots	1 tsp sugar
¾ cup tossed lettuce salad	Coffee or tea
1 tbsp oil and vinegar	

Evening Snack
Popcorn

Figure 11–3
Sample menu for a lactose-free diet.

lent of 4 oz of milk are tolerated by individuals with lactose-intolerance (Vesa et al., 1996). Lactose-reduced milk products should be promoted as needed. The rationale for including milk in the diet—namely, that milk provides not only calcium but also protein, vitamin B_2 (riboflavin), potassium, and magnesium—can be stressed. Health benefits attributed to milk include prevention of osteoporosis and possibly control of hypertension. There is also some evidence that lactase enzyme activity can increase with regular intake of small amounts of milk products.

Diarrhea

Diarrhea is the passage of frequent stools of liquid consistency. It may be either acute, lasting 24 to 48 hours, or chronic, lasting 2 weeks or longer. When the condition is acute, the nutritional losses are easily replaced as food and fluid intake returns to normal. Chronic diarrhea results in more serious nutritional losses. The absorption of fluids, electrolytes, and nutrients may be impaired because of their rapid transit through the gastrointestinal tract.

Dietary Modifications. Persons experiencing severe diarrhea are told to abstain from consuming any food for up to 48 hours. This will give the intestinal tract a chance to rest. Low-residue diets prescribed for acute diarrhea often restrict milk intake. Milk does not contain fiber and is a medium-residue food (that is, it leaves a moderate amount of **residue,** or undigested food matter, in the GI tract) and may not need to be restricted on a low-residue diet as long as the person can tolerate milk and is not lactase deficient. Intravenous solutions of dextrose, amino acids, electrolytes, and vitamins will help replace fluids and electrolytes and provide some nutrients. Clear liquid or an elemental diet may be given after this time. Once diarrhea has diminished, the patient can progress to a diet that is restricted in residue and high in protein, calories, nutrients, and fluids. Table 11–5 shows how residue can be restricted using the food groups of the Food Guide Pyramid. These restrictions are gradually replaced by a regular normal diet as soon as the patient is able to tolerate it.

Antibiotic treatment can cause diarrhea because it kills helpful as well as harmful bacteria. The intestinal tract normally contains certain types of bacteria that help digest food matter. A person in this situation will benefit from consuming yogurt with live bacterial culture **(lactobacillus culture).** Carbohydrate foods low in roughage such as plain white rice, white bread, pasta, or peeled potatoes are generally well tolerated.

Constipation

Constipation is a condition in which the waste matter in the bowels is difficult to pass or the emptying time of the feces is so delayed that discomfort or uncomfortable symptoms result. Prolonged constipation is called **obstipation.** Symptoms include nausea, heartburn, headache, general malaise, or distress in the rectum or intestine as a result of the nerves reacting when the rectum is distended by the contained matter.

Table 11–5
Low-Residue Diet as Modified with Food Groups from the Food Guide Pyramid

Grains	Emphasize refined grain products such as white bread, white rice, pasta, and cereals that are not whole grain
Vegetables/fruits	Emphasize those without skins or seeds such as canned fruits and fruit juice
Milk	Two cups or more as tolerated per day
Meat	Emphasize tender meats; avoid fried meats or those with gristle
	Avoid legumes and nuts

Atonic Constipation

Atonic constipation is characterized by the loss of rectal sensibility and weak peristaltic waves. It commonly occurs in elderly or obese persons, pregnant women, persons who abuse or overuse laxatives, and postoperative patients. Factors contributing to its occurrence include a low-fiber diet, irregular meals, inadequate fluid intake, lack of exercise, lack of time allowed for evacuation of stool, and prolonged use of chemical laxatives.

Spastic Constipation

This condition (also known as **irritable bowel syndrome,** spastic colitis, and mucous colitis) is characterized by irregular contractions of the bowel, resulting in either diarrhea or constipation. Factors contributing to its occurrence include excessive use of laxatives or cathartics, irregular eating habits, antibiotic therapy, and nervous tension. Its treatment requires prolonged intervention.

Encopresis

Encopresis is a condition of chronic constipation that afflicts children. Encopresis is characterized by a fecal impaction consisting of a semi-fitting "plug" of feces that allows more liquid fecal material to seep around and soil the child's pants. Parents may not understand this physiology and may wonder if their child is misbehaving. In one study 75 percent of children with encopresis remained free of soiling after following a high-fiber diet with use of laxatives after a complete bowel cleanout (McClung et al., 1993). Mineral oil, if used, should be infrequent because of associated malabsorption of food nutrients.

Dietary Modifications. A high-fiber diet (see Fig. 11–4) is used in the treatment of constipation, because it allows the feces to be easily and more quickly expelled. A variety of high-fiber foods from a variety of sources is recommended, with 20 to 35 grams of fiber recommended for adults and "age plus five" grams of fiber advised for children (American Dietetic Association, 1996).

For the management of irritable bowel syndrome the emphasis is on soluble fiber. Soluble fiber absorbs water and has a gummy texture, which allows for more stable GI transit time. Other forms of constipation will benefit with either type of fiber (soluble or insoluble). Figure 11–5 shows how this is accomplished.

Wheat bran, an insoluble fiber, increases bulk and facilitates the movement of feces along the intestinal tract. Large particles of coarsely ground bran are more effective than are finely ground fibers. Soluble fiber helps prevent constipation by absorbing water, thereby preventing dry stools that may be difficult to pass. There are many sources of soluble fiber, such as oats, barley, brown rice, legumes, and psyllium seed. A commercial laxative product that contains psyllium fiber is Metamucil. When diarrhea occurs during spastic constipation, a minimal-residue diet may be beneficial (see Table 11–5).

Breakfast

Raisins
½ cup bran cereal
1 slice toast, 100% whole wheat
1 tsp butter or margarine

1 tbsp jam
1 cup 1% milk
1 tsp sugar
Coffee or tea

Lunch

Tuna sandwich on 2 slices toast,
   100% whole wheat
½ cup green beans
Tomato slices

¾ cup lettuce salad
½ cup canned peaches
Oatmeal cookie

Midafternoon Snack

Fresh orange

Supper

½ cup split pea soup
2 oz roast beef
1 baked potato with skin
½ cup cooked carrots
1 cup tossed salad
1 tbsp French dressing

1 slice bread, 100% whole wheat
1 tsp butter or margarine
Fig bar
1 cup 1% milk
Coffee or tea

Evening Snack

½ cup bran cereal
½ cup 1% milk

1 tsp sugar

Figure 11–4
Sample menu for a high-fiber diet.

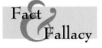

Fact & Fallacy

Fallacy: Cheese causes constipation.

Fact: There is no evidence that supports the belief that cheese causes or aggravates constipation. A lack of dietary fiber and fluids is more likely to be the problem. Occasionally, a person may be allergic to dairy products and may experience constipation as a result. Cheese, however, may take longer to digest if it has a high fat content. Whole-grain breads and cereals, fresh fruits and vegetables, and at least 64 ounces of fluids daily should counteract any tendency toward constipation in most healthy individuals. Cheese and other dairy products are the best sources of calcium and riboflavin (vitamin B$_2$) and should be included in the daily diet. Cheese is a versatile food that can be eaten cooked or uncooked and can be used in recipes from many cultures. Cheese is provided by the Women, Infants, and Children (WIC) Supplemental Nutrition Program (see Chapter 22).

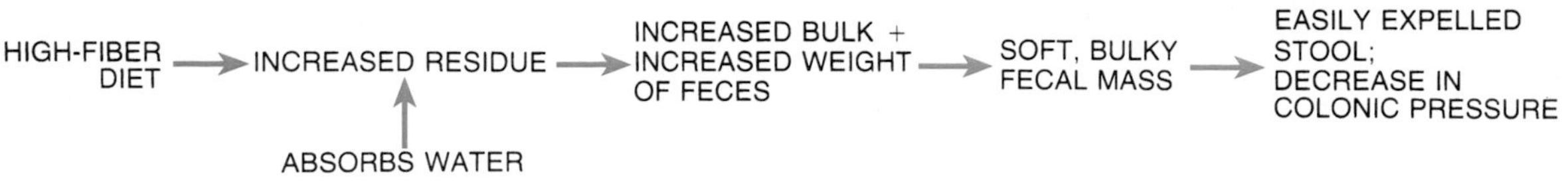

HIGH-FIBER DIET → INCREASED RESIDUE → INCREASED BULK + INCREASED WEIGHT OF FECES → SOFT, BULKY FECAL MASS → EASILY EXPELLED STOOL; DECREASE IN COLONIC PRESSURE

↑ ABSORBS WATER

Figure 11–5
How a high-fiber diet helps correct and prevent constipation.

Steatorrhea

Steatorrhea is diarrhea characterized by excess fat in stools and results from a malabsorption syndrome caused by disease of the intestinal mucosa or pancreatic enzyme deficiency. Steatorrhea usually indicates a more serious underlying organic disease. It may be seen in pancreatitis or following gastric or intestinal resection. It is often associated with diseases of the liver or gallbladder or with malabsorptive diseases such a nontropical sprue (celiac disease—see the following section) or regional enteritis. It sometimes occurs after gastrointestinal radiation. All of these disorders may involve problems with fat digestion or absorption. It is generally diagnosed from a fecal fat test, which may require 3 to 4 days of fecal material collection.

Dietary Modifications. The treatment of steatorrhea may involve the use of **medium-chain triglycerides (MCTs),** which are fats that contain 8 to 10 carbon atoms (as opposed to the 12 to 18 carbon atoms found in long-chain triglycerides [LCTs]). MCTs are used in the treatment of steatorrhea because they are more easily digested, absorbed, and transported than are LCTs. They also help reduce fecal losses of water, electrolytes, and nutrients.

In diet planning, the emphasis is on low-fat foods to decrease the amount of LCTs in the diet. More than half of the allowed fat calories are in the form of MCTs. This can be accomplished with the use of commercially available products. The two principal forms of MCT are Portagen, which is a powdered formula that can be mixed and served as a supplement to meals, and MCT oil, which can replace vegetable oil in recipes.

Celiac Disease

This malabsorptive disorder is also known as gluten-induced enteropathy and **nontropical sprue** or **celiac sprue.** The detection rate of celiac disease greatly underestimates its prevalence. This is the result of lack of awareness of the many manifestations of the condition and the requirement for at least one small intestinal biopsy for diagnosis (Murray, 1997). Celiac disease is characterized by an allergy to a protein known as **gliadin** found in foods containing gluten. **Gluten** is the protein portion of wheat, oats, rye, and barley. The exact cause of this disease is unknown but it occurs more frequently among persons of British heritage than among other groups. One interesting case suggests transmission of celiac disease by bone marrow transplantation and supports the T cell concept in celiac disease

(Bargetzi et al., 1997). An incidence rate of 1:2800 live births was noted among Arab children living in Jordan, where there is a high intake of wheat (Rawashdeh et al., 1996). Evidence suggests a linear trend toward a lower celiac disease prevalence as age increases (Corazza et al., 1997). There is some evidence that stressful events precede the onset of celiac disease. Symptoms include diarrhea, steatorrhea, and weight loss. Measurement of antigliadin antibody was found to be useful in selecting children for final testing with intestinal biopsy, which is the gold standard for diagnosis (Chartrand et al., 1997). If celiac sprue is untreated with diarrhea, vitamin and mineral deficiencies become apparent.

Dietary Modifications. The patient is prescribed a gluten-free diet, in which all products containing gluten or gliadin are eliminated (see Fig. 11–6 and Table 11–6). Lactose intolerance often accompanies celiac sprue. Because some patients are extremely sensitive to trace amounts of gluten, all potential sources (including gluten-free wheat starch and white vinegar) should be avoided. The patient's condition improves dramatically on a gluten-free diet. Dietary counseling must include a discussion of foods allowed, reading labels for even small amounts of gluten in various foods, and using alternative flours (e.g., rice, corn, and potato) in recipes. Other substitutes include tapioca and soybean and arrowroot flours. The gluten-free diet is very tedious, and referral to celiac organizations is highly recommended.

Breakfast
½ cup grapefruit juice
½ cup cream of rice cereal
1 egg, soft cooked
Cornmeal muffin
1 tsp butter or margarine

1 tbsp grape jelly
1 cup 1% milk (or lactose-reduced milk as needed)
2 tsp sugar
Coffee or tea

Lunch
2 oz sliced turkey
1 cup rice
½ cup green beans
½ sliced tomato on lettuce
Rice muffin
1 tsp butter or margarine

Fresh apple
Puffed rice bar
1 cup 1% milk (or lactose-reduced milk as needed)
Coffee or tea

Supper
3 oz roast beef
1 cup cubed white potato
½ cup cooked broccoli
¾ cup tossed lettuce salad
1 tbsp oil and lemon juice

Rice muffin
2 tsp butter or margarine
1 cup 1% milk (or lactose-reduced milk as needed)
Coffee or tea

Figure 11–6
Sample menu for a gluten-restricted diet.

Table 11–6
Guidelines for Food Selection for Gluten-Restricted, Gliadin-Free Diet

Food Groups	Recommended	Excluded
Beverages	All milk and milk products except those on excluded list; lactose-free, nondairy drinks, soy milk; pure instant or ground coffee, decaffeinated coffee, tea; carbonated drinks, fruit drinks; wines, rums; sake, vermouth, cognac, tequila, akvavit, and vodka derived from grapes or potatoes	Commercial chocolate milk, malted milk, instant milk drinks; hot cocoa mixes; nondairy cream substitutes; flavored instant coffee; some herbal teas with barley or barley malt; alcoholic beverages distilled from cereal grains such as gin, whiskey, vodka, beer, ale, malt liquor; some root beers
Breads	Breads and rolls made from tapioca, arrowroot, corn, or potato starch; corn, potato, rice, or soy flour; gluten-free bread mix; pure corn tortillas; rice cakes and wafers; breads specially prepared using only allowed flours; some crackers and chips*	Any made with wheat, rye, oats, kasha, barley, buckwheat, durum, graham, or wheat starch; commercial mixes for biscuits, cornbread, muffins, pancakes, or waffles; wheat germ, bran, bulgur; millet, triticale; breads made with low-gluten flour; quinoa; crackers; pretzels
Cereals	Corn or rice cereals containing malt flavoring derived from corn; puffed rice, cream of rice; cornmeal; hominy; grits; popcorn	Cereals containing malt flavoring or malt derived from barley; cereals containing wheat, rye, oats, barley, bran, wheat germ, buckwheat bulgur; millet, kasha, quinoa, spelt, teff; cereals made with low-gluten flours
Desserts	Ice cream, sherbet, cakes, cookies, pies, pudding, gelatin desserts, and fruit ice made with allowed ingredients; custard; tapioca and rice puddings; junket	Commercially prepared mixes of all kinds (unless gluten-free); commercial cakes, cookies, pies, doughnuts, and pastries prepared with wheat, rye, oat, or barley flour; ice cream cones; ice creams with gluten stabilizers*; commercial pie fillings*; bread pudding; pudding thickened with flour; products made with brown rice syrup prepared with barley malt enzyme
Fats	Butter or margarine; homemade salad dressings; pure mayonnaise prepared with allowed vinegar; vegetable oils	Commercial salad dressings containing gluten stabilizers
Fruits	All fruits and fruit juices	Any thickened or prepared with fruits; some fruit pie fillings*
Meats and meat substitutes	All meats, poultry, fish, and shellfish; eggs; dried peas and beans; nuts; peanut butter; aged cheese; soybean and other meat substitutes; yogurt; tofu; cold cuts, frankfurters, or sausage without fillers*	Any prepared with wheat, rye, oats, barley, gluten stabilizers, or fillers including some frankfurters, cold cuts, sandwich spreads, sausages, and canned meats*; any cheese or cheese spread containing oat gum; canned pork and beans*; turkey basted or injected with hydrolyzed or texturized vegetable protein (HVP, TVP); tuna canned with hydrolyzed protein*; breaded fish or meats

Table continued on following page

Table 11–6
Guidelines for Food Selection for Gluten-Restricted, Gliadin-Free Diet (*continued*)

Food Groups	Recommended	Excluded
Potatoes and potato substitutes	White or sweet potatoes; yams; hominy; plain potato chips; enriched or wild rice; rice noodles; pastas made with allowed flours; some Oriental rice or noodles*	Barley; regular noodles, spaghetti, macaroni, and other pastas prepared with rye, wheat, oats, or barley flour; creamed or scalloped potatoes; commercial rice or pasta mixes
Soups	Homemade broth; vegetable or cream soups made with allowed ingredients	Commercially prepared soups made with wheat, rye, oats, or barley products; most canned soups and soup mixes; bouillon and bouillon cubes with HVP*
Sweets	Sugar; most syrups*; honey; jelly, jam; hard candies; plain chocolate; pure cocoa; coconut; molasses; marshmallows*; meringues	All other sweets*
Vegetables	All plain, fresh, frozen, or canned vegetables except those listed as excluded	Any creamed or breaded vegetables (unless allowed ingredients are used); canned baked beans*; commercially prepared vegetables with cream or cheese sauce*
Miscellaneous	Iodized salt; herbs, spices, seasonings,* and flavorings*; food coloring; food flavoring extracts*; gravies and sauces made with allowed flours and starches; baking soda; baking powder; cream of tartar; dry mustard; cider, rice, and wine vinegar; monosodium glutamate and tamari made without wheat, olives, or pickles	Any condiment prepared with wheat, rye, oats, or barley, such as some ketchup,* chili sauce,* soy sauce,* mustard,* bottled meat sauces,* horseradish,* some dry seasoning mixes,* distilled white vinegar,* steak sauce,* some curry powders*; seasonings containing fillers, stabilizers, or HVP; sauces and gravies with gluten sources; some chewing gum*; chip dips*

*Check product label and contact the manufacturer to clarify questionable ingredients, especially the source of "flavoring" used in meat and poultry products.
© 1996, The American Dietetic Association. Manual of Clinical Dietetics, 5th ed. Used by permission.

Hydrolyzed vegetable protein, hydrolyzed plant protein, vegetable protein, starch, modified food starch, cereal, and millet are other ingredients that may contain gluten and are listed on food labels. The manufacturer of the product should be contacted to verify the presence of gluten or gliadin or use of the foods containing these substances (such as flour) on food conveyor belts. Celiac organizations are the best resources for current listings of acceptable foods.

Diverticulosis

Diverticulosis is the formation of outpockets of small sacs (diverticula) protruding through the wall of the intestines. They are found mainly in the sigmoid colon. Low-fiber diets favor the development of diverticulosis because intraluminal pressure is exerted against the colon wall instead of longitudinally, resulting in pouches (Fig. 11–7). These outpockets do not disappear. Thus a person with diverticulosis will always have diverticulosis but can experience diverticulitis (the inflammation stage; see next section) in cycles. Diverticulosis is common among older persons.

Dietary Modifications. The high-fiber diet is used for diverticulosis. Insoluble fiber such as wheat bran tends to increase fecal bulk and soften the stool. The weight of insoluble fiber residue in the colon helps gravity propel fecal matter through the intestinal tract. Soluble fiber sources such as legumes and oatmeal provide moisture in the stool. The effect of fiber and liquids is expected to reduce the incidence and symptoms of diverticular disease by reducing pressure inside the intestinal tract. Until recently, the diet restricted intake of seeds, skins, and nuts. If these foods are consumed, thorough chewing should be advised.

Diverticulitis

Diverticulitis is an inflammation of diverticula, which may result when food particles or materials are trapped in the outpockets (described in the previous section) and attract bacteria. Symptoms include abdominal pain, usually in the lower left quadrant, and occasionally fever. Other diseases with similar symptoms, including colon cancer, need to be ruled out. There may be many tests be-

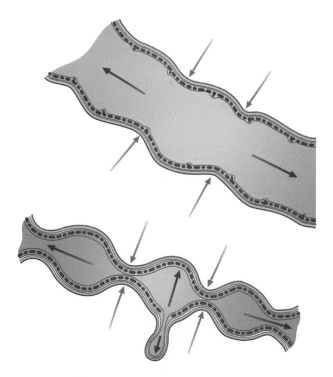

Figure 11–7
Mechanism by which low-fiber, low-bulk diets might generate diverticula. Where colon contents are bulky (top), muscular contractions exert pressure longitudinally. If lumen is smaller (bottom), contractions can produce occlusion and exert pressure against colon wall, which may produce a diverticular "blowout."

fore the diagnosis is made with assurance. Diverticulitis is a temporary condition of inflammation.

Dietary Modifications. During the acute phase, patients are put on a clear liquid diet, which is gradually changed to a restricted-residue diet (see Table 11–5). Once the symptoms have disappeared, the patient gradually switches to a high-fiber diet.

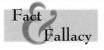

Fallacy: A person with diverticulosis should avoid seeds, nuts, and skins.

Fact: These foods have a high fiber content and help keep the pressure down inside the intestinal tract, thus preventing further outpockets. The increased weight of fecal material in the colon from high-fiber foods helps prevent constipation, which further diminishes intestinal pressure. A high-fiber diet is recommended for individuals with diverticulosis. Thorough chewing is advocated to help the digestive process. Only during diverticulitis would these foods be restricted.

Crohn's Disease

Crohn's disease (regional enteritis) is another inflammatory bowel disease, the cause of which is unknown. However, it is becoming more common, especially in young adults, and is felt to be an autoimmune disease in which the body attacks itself. Crohn's disease can affect any part of the intestinal tract, but inflammation usually occurs in the terminal ileum. Diarrhea, abdominal cramps, fever, and weakness are common symptoms. Malnutrition is likely caused by inadequate dietary intake, decreased absorption of nutrients, and excessive losses from the gastrointestinal tract.

Dietary Modifications. The goal of dietary treatment is to maintain good nutritional status, promote healing, and reduce inflammation. A well balanced high-calorie, high-protein diet is indicated. However, an elemental diet may be used in the treatment of Crohn's disease. The theory behind elemental diets is that inflammation of Crohn's disease may arise from an immunologic response to dietary protein antigens. The use of an elemental diet, which provides nitrogen in the form of amino acids instead of whole protein, may lessen or avoid this response (Sullivan, 1993). A vitamin and mineral supplement that meets the RDA is beneficial because of the malabsorption that occurs with Crohn's disease. The prescribed diet is low in residue, especially during the acute stages. When a regular diet is resumed, foods that are not tolerated should be avoided. The patient should be taught the importance of documenting foods eaten in relation to symptoms. Particular attention should be paid to medications that may adversely affect the absorption of nutrients or increase nutrient needs. See Chapter 7 regarding food and drug interactions.

Ulcerative Colitis

Ulcerative colitis is a chronic disease characterized by inflammation and ulceration of the mucosa of the large intestine. The cause of this disease is unknown. In the 1970s, however, researchers found that patients with ulcerative colitis had high levels of prostaglandins (naturally occurring chemicals that regulate acid secretion in the stomach) in the stomach mucosa. Recent studies suggest that marine fish-oil supplements, which are high in omega-3 fatty acids, may reduce the inflammation associated with ulcerative colitis (Ross, 1993). Fish-oil supplements should be used only under a physician's guidance, as they may cause undesirable side effects such as reducing the clotting time of blood, although ½ teaspoon of cod liver oil daily is likely to be safe. Symptoms of ulcerative colitis include rectal bleeding, diarrhea, fever, anorexia, dehydration, and weight loss.

Dietary Modifications. When symptoms are evident, a tube feeding of an elemental diet (a liquid supplement that does not require digestion because the food material is already broken down), peripheral parenteral nutrition (PPN), or total parenteral nutrition (TPN) may be necessary (see Chapter 14). These forms of nutritional support will provide necessary nutrients without aggravating the condition. Once solid foods are tolerated, the patient progresses to a restricted-residue diet (see Table 11–5) that is high in calories, protein, vitamins, and minerals to replace nutritional losses and provide for tissue repair. Individualizing the diet to a patient's specific food tolerances is necessary to give optimal nutritional care. Vitamin and mineral supplements may be indicated to provide additional nutritional support.

WHAT ARE DISEASES OF THE LIVER?

Enzymes produced by the liver aid in the metabolism of protein, carbohydrate, and fat (see Chapter 4). The liver stores vitamins A and D and glycogen, detoxifies harmful substances, and synthesizes many needed substances. Liver diseases have major nutritional implications.

Hepatitis

Hepatitis is inflammation and injury to liver cells caused by infections, drugs, or toxins. Symptoms include anorexia, fatigue, nausea, vomiting, fever, diarrhea, and weight loss.

Dietary Modifications. The symptoms during the early stage of hepatitis make it difficult for the patient to consume adequate nutrients. Tube feedings (see Chapter 14) may be indicated until the patient can tolerate the oral intake of food. Once oral intake is resumed, a diet high in calories, protein, vitamins, and minerals with moderate fat is planned for the patient. Several small meals are usually better tolerated than are three large ones.

Cirrhosis

Cirrhosis is a chronic liver disease in which normal liver tissue is replaced by inactive fibrous tissue. Because liver tissue is not able to function normally, there may be **jaundice** (a buildup of bile in the body causing yellowing of the skin and eyes), a prolonged bleeding time, fatty infiltration of liver tissue, lower serum albumin levels, and other complications, depending on the severity of tissue function impairment. Symptoms sometimes include nausea, vomiting, anorexia, **ascites** (accumulation of fluid in the abdomen), and **esophageal varices** (enlargement of the veins in the esophagus because of poor portal vein blood circulation).

An individual with cirrhosis may have a low energy level, which is related to inadequate metabolism of carbohydrate. Electrolyte imbalance is also common because of poor storage of minerals. A common cause of cirrhosis is chronic alcoholism. A nutritious diet does not prevent the development of cirrhosis but is still beneficial to promote health.

Dietary Modifications. Because carbohydrate metabolism is often affected by this condition, the diet for cirrhosis should be adequate in energy and nutrients to prevent further deterioration of the liver. As much as 300 to 400 grams of carbohydrate may be necessary, as well as 45 to 50 kilocalories per kilogram of body weight to spare protein. The fat intake may need to be modified because of malabsorption of fats. Protein may be restricted to 35 to 50 grams per day (see Fig. 11–8) to prevent **hepatic coma** (a toxic effect on the brain due to diminished clearance of blood toxins; see the following section). Vitamin and mineral supplementation is often necessary. Sodium and fluids are restricted if edema and ascites develop. It is not unusual for the sodium to be limited to 500 to 1500 mg per day. Fluids are restricted to 100 to 1500 mL per day, depending on the severity of the condition. Foods high in roughage (whole grains and vegetables and fruits with skin and seeds) may need to be restricted with esophageal varices to prevent rupture of these tiny blood vessels.

Hepatic Coma

When liver function becomes severely impaired, ammonia levels become abnormally high and toxic to brain tissue. The unconsciousness that may result is known as hepatic coma. Contributing factors include gastrointestinal bleeding, excessive dietary protein, severe infection, and surgical procedures. Symptoms include confusion, irritability, delirium, and flapping tremors of the hands and feet.

Dietary Modifications. The aim of this diet is to decrease the amount of ammonia that enters the general circulation. Antibiotics are administered to decrease the ammonia production from intestinal bacteria. Protein in the diet is restricted to 0 to 20 grams, depending on the severity of the condition. The amount of protein is gradually increased in increments of 10 to 15 grams as liver function improves. Supplements of branched-chain amino acids may be used (Hepatic-Aid). Kilocalorie intake must be kept high to prevent tissue breakdown. Kilocalories from carbohydrate and fat are emphasized. Sodium is restricted if ascites or edema is present. Additional vitamin and mineral supplements should be given.

Breakfast
½ cup fruit or juice
½ cup cereal with ½ cup milk, sugar

1 slice toast with margarine and jelly
Coffee or tea

Lunch
1 small potato with margarine
½ cup vegetable
Tossed salad with Italian dressing

1 slice bread with margarine
½ cup fruit
½ cup milk

Supper
1 oz meat or 1 egg
1 small potato
½ cup vegetable
Fruit salad

1 slice bread with margarine
½ cup fruit
½ cup milk
Coffee or tea

*On a 20-g protein meal pattern, 1 oz of meat and 1 cup of milk would be omitted. Extra margarine, concentrated sweets, low-protein bread and pasta, and possibly carbohydrate supplements help to provide adequate kilocalories in the diet.

Figure 11–8
Sample menu for a 35-gram protein meal.

WHAT ARE DISEASES OF THE GALLBLADDER?

Gallbladder diseases are related to stones and inflammation. The release of bile for fat digestion can cause severe pain.

Cholecystitis

Cholecystitis is an inflammation of the gallbladder. It can be caused by a bacterial infection or stones in the gallbladder. Symptoms include acute pain in the upper-right quadrant, nausea, belching, vomiting, fever, and jaundice if the bile duct is blocked.

Cholelithiasis

Cholelithiasis is the formation of gallstones. Sometimes the gallstones block the bile duct and interfere with the flow of bile. Symptoms include pain in the right upper quadrant as the gallbladder contracts and jaundice if the bile duct is obstructed.

Obesity, diabetes, familial hypercholesterolemia, cardiovascular disease, multiple pregnancies, use of oral contraceptives, fasting (such as with very-low-kilocalorie diets), and total parenteral nutrition (TPN, see Chapter 14) are all asso-

Table 11–7
Daily Food Allowances for 50-Gram Fat Diet

Food	Amount	Approximate Fat Content (gm)
Skim milk	2 cups or more	0
Lean meat, fish, poultry	6 oz or 6 equivalents	18
Whole egg or egg yolks	3 per week	3
Vegetables	3 servings or more, at least 1 or more dark leafy green or orange	0
Fruits	3 or more servings, at least 1 citrus	0
Breads, cereals	As desired	0
Fat exchanges*	5–6 exchanges daily	25–30
Desserts and sweets	As desired from permitted list	0
	Total fat	46–51

ciated with the increased incidence of gallstones. A high-fiber diet has been linked to decreased incidence of gallstones (Davis & Sherer, 1994).

Dietary Modifications. During an acute attack of cholecystitis or cholelithiasis, food may be withheld for up to 24 hours. Food is introduced gradually, starting with a clear liquid diet. As food tolerance improves, patients progress to a minimum-fat diet that contains 50 grams of fat or less (see Table 11–7). Excess fat intake will cause the gallbladder to contract, which can be very painful if gallstones are present. Foods high in fat, therefore, may not be tolerated, including foods such as sausages, bacon, and peanut butter. Other food intolerances, such as with onions, may exist in certain individuals. If stone removal by surgery or ultrasonic or chemical dissolution is necessary, the patient should follow a low-fat diet until the procedure is performed.

After stone removal, the patient should follow a low-fat diet for several weeks until fat digestion is normalized. Thereafter, a normal diet is usually well tolerated and should be encouraged, although a 50-gram fat diet is appropriate for long-term use.

WHAT ARE DISEASES OF THE PANCREAS?

The pancreas produces digestive enzymes for metabolism of protein, carbohydrate, and fat; bicarbonate ions to neutralize chyme; and hormones such as insulin (see Chapters 4 and 9).

Cystic Fibrosis

Cystic fibrosis (also called cystic fibrosis of the pancreas) consists of an insufficiency or abnormality of some essential hormone or enzyme. Excessive thick mucus is produced by the exocrine glands and interferes with breathing and digestion. Fats are poorly digested and absorbed, and a common symptom is frequent fatty, bulky, and odorous feces. Recurrent respiratory infections and excessive loss of sodium and chloride from the sweat glands are common. Pancreatic insufficiency may develop. MCTs are more easily absorbed and therefore are the best source of fat in the diet for cystic fibrosis. Pancreatic enzyme tablets given at mealtimes, however, allow for more normal intake of dietary fats and can therefore promote growth of children with cystic fibrosis. The fat-soluble vitamins (A, D, E, and K) and a high-protein, high-kilocalorie diet are the cornerstones of diet therapy for this condition. Children who have cystic fibrosis often have a good appetite, which allows for adequate intake of kilocalories and protein.

Pancreatitis

Pancreatitis is inflammation of the pancreas. It is caused by digestion of pancreatic tissue by its own pancreatic digestive enzymes. The reason for this is not fully understood. Chronic alcoholism and triglyceride levels over 1000 mg/dL are often associated with pancreatitis. Symptoms include fever, malaise, nausea, and vomiting. Treatment is aimed at resting the pancreas. A low-fat diet is often implemented during acute pancreatitis. Pancreatic insufficiency may develop and is treated by the administration of pancreatic enzyme at each meal.

Diabetes Mellitus

This disease is related to inadequate amounts of insulin produced by the islets of Langerhans found in the pancreas (see Chapter 9). Because this is a complex disease, Chapter 9 has been devoted to a full discussion of its management.

WHAT ARE DISEASES OF THE BLOOD?

Sickle Cell Disease

Sickle cell disease is a serious hereditary, chronic condition that is found mainly in African Americans but sometimes in persons of Mediterranean, Middle Eastern, and Asian Indian ancestry. In persons with this disease the red blood cells (erythrocytes) are rigid and crescent or sickle shaped and have difficulty passing through the small arterioles and capillaries. The cells clump together and obstruct blood vessels, causing pain. The major symptoms are anemia, periodic joint and extremity pain (sometimes with edema), and severe bouts of abdominal pain with vomiting and distention. The patient is prone to infection.

Children with sickle cell disease have decreased height and weight levels, which may be related to inadequate intake of food per the Food Guide Pyramid (Williams et al., 1997). Another study found that sickle cell disease was associated with malnutrition, iron deficiency, high copper levels, and low plasma zinc levels related to low stature (Pellegrini et al., 1995). Good nutritional intake should be promoted and referral might be made to community nutrition programs such as the Expanded Food & Nutrition Education Program (EFNEP) of the Cooperative Extension Association.

Thalassemia

Thalassemia is a condition in which red blood cells are small and contain less hemoglobin than is normal. It is a hereditary disease. The relationship of vitamin E to β-thalassemia is being studied, especially because this vitamin has an antioxidant effect on cells and may improve red blood cell survival.

WHAT IS THE ROLE OF THE NURSE OR OTHER HEALTH CARE PROFESSIONAL IN MANAGING DISEASES OF THE GASTROINTESTINAL TRACT?

An important responsibility of all health care professionals is to be alert to problems of the GI tract. Problems of the GI tract should be identified through noting missing teeth, absence of or failure to use dentures, weight loss indicating either inadequate nutritional intake or problems with digestion or absorption of nutrients, and constipation or diarrhea. The health care professional should carefully assess and evaluate the person's need for nutritional intervention, which may include nutritional support measures (see Chapter 14). High-risk persons should be referred to their family physician and a registered dietitian for further assessment and intervention. The planning and implementation of nutritional care must always be individualized. The health care professional must be aware of the specific portion of the gastrointestinal tract involved and understand the digestive process in relation to the need for a modified diet. Remember that many of the modified diets recommended in this chapter are for short-term use only and that the return to a normal diet should be encouraged as soon as the individual's condition allows it. The various guides for good nutrition presented in Chapter 6 should be applied whenever possible.

For long-term dietary adherence, the health belief model should be used. If the patient understands the rationale for the dietary change and recognizes that the result of those changes is feeling better and experiencing less discomfort, the likelihood of dietary compliance increases.

Critical Thinking

Case Study

Elizabeth was glad to be teaching her kindergarten class again, back with energy. She had been getting too skinny and was surprised when her doctor asked her if she had British heritage. When she replied "yes" a gleam of recognition had come into his eyes. He then told her all about celiac disease and how she would likely get better on a gluten-free diet. He had ordered an intestinal biopsy to verify the diagnosis prior to the start of the diet. Her diet was difficult to follow but easier with gluten-free products the health food store carried. She couldn't eat any wheat, oats, rye, or barley, and because so many food additives and preservatives are wheat based, she had to read food labels and ask questions at restaurants. But it was worth it. She was only in her thirties and it had become impossible for her to teach because of chronic diarrhea and feelings of fatigue.

Applications

1. Discuss the impact of gastrointestinal disease on society and personal relationships.
2. How would you feel if you were told you could never eat foods that include wheat; list some of your favorite foods that contain wheat.
2. What foods might this school teacher eat from the school lunch menu. What are some foods that could be packed from home that would be tolerated by someone with celiac disease and lactose intolerance?

Study Questions and Classroom Activities

1. Why would a low-fiber and then a high-fiber diet be helpful for someone with diverticulitis?
2. Why is a 35- to 50-gram protein diet used to treat cirrhosis and a 0- to 20-gram protein diet used to treat hepatic coma?
3. Why is a low-fat diet used to treat gallbladder disease?
4. Plan a gluten-restricted menu for 1 day that meets the minimum recommended servings of foods in the Food Guide Pyramid.
5. Go to the grocery store and identify five nutrition labels that indicate the products contain gluten. Report your findings to the class.
6. How can a person with lactose intolerance consume adequate amounts of calcium?

References

American Dietetic Association, Age Plus Five Campaign for Children's Fiber Intake, 1996.

Anselmino M, Perdikis G, Hinder RA, Polishuk PV, Wilson P, Terry JD, Lanspa SJ: Heller myotomy is superior to dilatation for the treatment of early achalasia. Arch Surg. March 1997; 132(3):233–240.

Bargetzi MJ, Schonenberger A, Tichelli A, Fried R, Cathomas G, Signer E, Speck B, Gratwohl A: Celiac disease transmitted by allogeneic non-T cell-depleted bone marrow transplantation. Bone Marrow Transplant. October 1997; 20(7):607–609.

Barkun AN, Mayrand S: The treatment of peptic esophageal strictures. Can J Gastroenterol. September 1997; 11 (Suppl B):94B-97B.

Baron TH, Ramirez B, Richter JE: Gastrointestinal motility disorders during pregnancy. Ann Intern Med. March 1993; 118(5):366–375.

Bohmer CJ, Tuynman HA: The clinical relevance of lactose malabsorption in irritable bowel syndrome. Eur J Gastroenterol Hepatol. October 1996; 8(10):1013–1016.

Chartrand LJ, Agulnik J, Vanounou T, Russo PA, Baehler P, Seidman EG: Effectiveness of antigliadin antibodies as a screening test for celiac disease in children. CMAJ. September 1, 1997; 157(5):527–533.

Corazza GR, Andreani ML, Biagi F, Corrao G, Pretolani S, Giulianelli G, Ghironzi G, Gasbarrini G: The smaller size of the "coeliac iceberg" in adults. Scand J Gastroenterol. September 1997; 32(9):917–919.

Davis JR, Sherer K: Applied Nutrition and Diet Therapy for Nurses, 2nd ed. Philadelphia, WB Saunders, 1994; pp. 870–871.

Ferguson A: Mechanisms in adverse reactions to food: The gastrointestinal tract. Allergy. 1995; 50(20 Suppl):32–38.

Gottlieb D, Kipnis M, Sister E, Vardi Y, Brill S: Validation of the 50 ml3 drinking test for evaluation of post-stroke dysphagia. Disabil Rehabil. October 1996; 18(10):529–532.

Kennedy M, McCombie L, Dawes P, McConnell KN, Dunnigan MG: Nutritional support for patients with intellectual disability and nutrition/dysphagia disorders in community care. J Intellect Disabil Res. October 1997; 41(Pt5):430–436.

Mari F, Matei M, Ceravolo MG, Pisani A, Montesi A, Provinciali L: Predictive value of clinical indices in detecting aspiration in patients with neurological disorders. J Neurol Neurosurg Psychiatry. October 1997; 63(4):456–460.

McClung HJ, Boyne LJ, Linsheid T, Heitlinger LA, Murray RD, Fyda J, Li BU: Is combination therapy for encopresis nutritionally safe? Pediatrics. March 1993; 91(3):591–594.

Munnangi S, Sonnenberg A: Time trends of physician visits and treatment patterns of peptic ulcer disease in the United States. Arch Intern Med. July 14, 1997; 157(13):1489–1494.

Murray JA: Serodiagnosis of celiac disease. Clin Lab Med. September 1997; 17(3):445–464.

Paterson WG: Dysphagia in the elderly. Can Fam Physician. May 1996; 42:925–932.

Pellegrini Braga JA, Kerbauy J, Fisberg M: Zinc, copper and iron and their interrelations in the growth of sickle cell patients. Arch Latinoam Nutr . September 1995; 45(3):198–203.

Pohle T, Hilker E, Domschke W: Development of duodenal ulcer concomitant with successful Helicobacter pylori eradication. Z Gastroenterol. July 1997; 35(7):563–565.

Rawashdeh MO, Khalil B, Raweily E: Celiac disease in Arabs. J Pediatr Gastroenterol Nutr. November 1996; 23(4):415–418.

Ross E: The role of marine fish oils in the treatment of ulcerative colitis. Nutr Rev. 1993; 51(2):47.

Sullivan, M.: Spotlight, 1993; 14(3):2–3, 16.

Triadafilopoulos G, Sharma R: Features of symptomatic gastroesophageal reflux disease in elderly patients. Am J Gastroenterol. November 1997; 92(11):2007–2011.

Vesa TH, Korpela RA, Sahi T: Tolerance to small amounts of lactose in lactose maldigesters. Am J Clin Nutr. August 1996; 64(2):197–201.

Williams R, George EO, Wang W: Nutrition assessment in children with sickle cell disease. J Assoc Acad Minor Phys. 1997; 8(3):44–48.

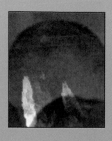

12
Cancer: Nutrition Prevention and Treatment

Objectives

After completing this chapter, you should be able to:

- Describe cancer prevention strategies.
- Explain how cancer and cancer treatments affect nutritional status.
- Describe the eating problems associated with cancer and possible solutions.
- Explain why nutritional needs must be met during cancer treatment.
- Describe the role of the nurse in counseling the patient for the prevention or management of cancer.

Terms to Identify

Anorexia	Dysgeusia	Oncology
Cancer	Esophagitis	Radiation therapy
Cancer cachexia	Gluconeogenesis	Systemic
Chemotherapy	Hyperandrogenic	

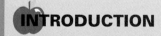

INTRODUCTION

In most western populations, cancer causes about a fifth of all deaths. One-third of all cases of cancer are considered to be caused by diet (Walker, 1996). Cancer occurs most commonly in persons aged 65 years and older (Yancik, 1997). As the U.S. population ages, the incidence of cancer will increase. Greater attention to diet can play a key role in the prevention and management of cancer. Although many questions still need to be answered, the best advice one can give the public regarding preventive nutritional practices is to follow the dietary guidelines that emphasize moderation, balance, and variety with emphasis on plant foods (whole grains, legumes, vegetables, and fruits), monounsaturated fats, and lean meats such as fish and chicken.

This chapter (1) explores current knowledge regarding the prevention of cancer; (2) discusses goals for the cancer patient; (3) explains how cancer treatment affects nutritional needs, and (4) reviews ways to cope with the nutritional problems that develop in people with cancer. Two changes that commonly occur in the course of the disease regard the way the body uses nutrients and the patient's eating habits. These changes may be caused by the tumor itself, by the cancer treatment, or by the psychological impact of having cancer.

WHAT IS CANCER?

Cancer is characterized by the uncontrolled growth and spread of abnormal cells, which continue to reproduce until they form a mass of tissue known as a tumor. A malignant tumor interrupts body functions and takes away the food and blood supply from normal cells. Cancers develop in various sites and require different methods of management. **Oncology** is the study and the sum of knowledge of tumors.

WHAT ARE THE CAUSES OF CANCER AND THE LIFESTYLE RECOMMENDATIONS TO REDUCE CANCER RISK?

The role of diet in the development of cancer is continuously being studied by the scientific community. There is strong evidence that total fat intake greater than 30 percent of total kilocalories increases the incidence of cancer. This is particularly true when the total fat intake includes mostly saturated fat. Polyunsaturated fats are now also felt to increase cancer risk (see Table 3–4). This may be due to increased oxidative damage with polyunsaturated fats. One way to decrease the intake of saturated and polyunsaturated fats is to limit the total fat intake. A fat intake of 10 to 20 percent of total kilocalories, as found in traditional Japanese diets, is associated with reduced cancer risk (Weisburger, 1997). The Mediterranean diet, which is relatively high in total fat but low in saturated fat, is also associated with low cancer risk. Olive oil, a monounsaturated fat, has a neutral effect on cancer risk. The traditional Canadian and Alaskan Native American diet includes a high intake of omega-3 fatty acids from cold-water fish. Fish and fish oil (omega-3 fats) have a strong role in preventing cancer risk and improved outcome in treatment due to improved immune functioning (Imoberdorf, 1997).

In assessing family health history, one often finds a history of cancer in association with a history of heart disease or diabetes. Recent studies have shown that hyperinsulinemia and abdominal obesity, which are recognized as markers of insulin resistance (see Chapters 8 and 9), are also risk markers for postmenopausal breast cancer. Excess weight gain linked to a high dietary intake of saturated fat is thought to be a major cause of insulin resistance (Stoll, 1996). The combination of insulin resistance and a high intake of simple carbohydrates can produce particularly high insulin levels. Hyperinsulinemia may explain why obesity, physical inactivity, and a diet low in fruits and vegetables and high in red meat and extensively processed foods, all common in the West, increase colon cancer risk (Giovannucci, 1995).

Breast cancer risk is increased in **hyperandrogenic** (excess androgen hormones) postmenopausal women and also in premenopausal women with mild hyperandrogenism. There may be a positive association between risk of breast cancer before menopause and subclinical forms of the polycystic ovary syndrome, a known risk factor of the insulin resistance syndrome (Kaaks, 1996). Up to a 50-pound weight gain is common after the diagnosis of breast cancer. It is not yet known, however, if the cause of this weight gain is due to changes in food intake, physical activity, or a change in metabolic rate. An increased weight gain is noted among premenopausal versus menopausal women with breast cancer (Demark-Wahnefried et al., 1997).

Dietary factors appear to be among the most important determinants of colorectal cancer risk. It is estimated that up to 75 percent of colon and rectal cancers could be avoided through dietary choices (American Institute for Cancer Research, 1998). Reducing red meat and fat consumption; increasing fruits, vegetables, and grains; avoiding obesity; and adopting a regular program of physical activity reduce the risk of colorectal cancer (Sandler, 1996). Consumption of green leafy and orange vegetables, broccoli, corn, carrots, bananas, garlic, and legumes (including soy products) was inversely associated with risk of colorectal cancer in a study in Hawaii, which included persons of Japanese, Caucasian, Filipino, Hawaiin, and Chinese heritage who had this form of cancer (Le Marchand et al., 1997). A high consumption of soy products and other legumes is also associated with a decreased risk of endometrial cancer (Goodman et al., 1997). Increased soluble fiber intake from fruit may be particularly helpful in reducing cancerous polyps of the colon (Platz et al., 1997). Insoluble fiber is also believed to lower cancer risk because this form of fiber moves food through the gastrointestinal tract faster. This rapid transit of food through the intestinal system decreases the amount of time carcinogens are in contact with the gastrointestinal mucosa.

Maintaining or returning to more traditional ethnic eating is important for a number of populations, one group being persons of Latino heritage who upon acculturation develop more westernized food habits and lifestyles. Educational messages should encourage Latinos to continue or return to eating traditional foods such as fruits, rice, and beans while reducing fried food and whole milk consumption (Otero-Sabogal et al., 1995). Among foreign born Asian Americans, prostate cancer risk increased with years of residence in North America and with saturated fat intake (Whittemore et al., 1995). As another example the Navajo population historically had a low prevalence of obesity and overweight but recent studies show an increased prevalence. Today an estimated two-thirds of Navajo women have been found to be overweight (White et al., 1997).

Antioxidants such as beta-carotene (found in dark green leafy vegetables and deep orange vegetables and fruits), vitamin E (found in seeds, nuts, and wheat germ), and vitamin C (found in citrus fruits and dark green leafy vegetables) appear to protect against cancer. There is no known positive impact from vitamin supplements containing antioxidants on cancer risk, whereas beta-carotene supplements actually increased risk for lung cancer (Blot, 1997).

Environmental factors such as alcohol intake and cigarette smoking are also linked to the development of cancer, especially that of the gastrointestinal tract and lungs. Individuals with a family history of cancer should be particularly careful to follow guidelines for cancer prevention.

Reduce Your Cancer Risk

The 1998 recommendations of the American Institute for Cancer Research can be summarized in seven steps:

1. Choose a diet rich in a variety of plant-based foods.
2. Eat plenty of vegetables and fruits.
3. Maintain a healthy weight and be physically active.
4. Drink alcohol in moderation, if at all.
5. Select foods low in fat and salt.
6. Prepare and store food safely.
7. Do not use tobacco in any form.

HOW DO CANCER AND CANCER TREATMENT AFFECT THE NUTRITIONAL STATUS OF THE HOST?

As the disease progresses in the cancer patient, the appetite and food intake are likely to decrease, which results in a form of malnutrition and emaciation commonly referred to as **cancer cachexia.** Figure 12–1 shows the pathways that contribute to cancer cachexia. The characteristics of cachexia include weakness, loss of appetite **(anorexia),** metabolic and hormonal abnormalities, a reduction in lean body mass, and a progressive loss of vital functions.

Cachexia may develop for several reasons. An altered sense of taste **(dysgeusia),** a lack of energy, a feeling of fullness, nausea and vomiting, food aversions, altered metabolism, and malabsorption of nutrients are commonly noted in cancer patients, even before therapy begins. Side effects of treatment often add to the patient's discomfort. Chewing and swallowing problems, a sore mouth,

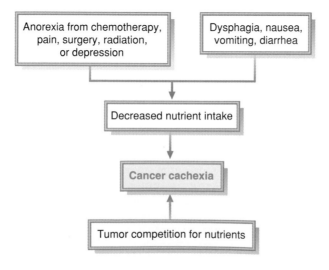

Figure 12–1
Cancer cachexia.

esophagitis (inflammation of the esophagus), and decreased saliva production may occur, but most of these conditions will cease when treatment is finished. Metabolites, which are chemical substances produced by the tumor, may have an anorexic effect on the hypothalamus, that portion of the brain believed to regulate hunger and satiety.

Among the most common taste changes are a lowered threshold for bitter flavors and an elevated threshold for sweetness. This may account for the common aversion to meat and the difficulty in tasting sweet foods. Extra sugar on fruits and cereals is a frequent request of cancer patients. Thresholds for tasting sour and salty foods tend to increase. According to a study of 169 cancer patients, the most frequently reported symptoms affecting eating were alterations in taste and smell. Anorexia or food aversions or both often accompany subjective taste changes in cancer patients. The taste for salty, sweet, sour, and bitter foods may be affected. Deficiency of vitamin B_{12}, thiamine, folacin, iron, and riboflavin have been associated with increased taste thresholds in cancer patients (Ames et al., 1993).

What Are the Nutritional Problems Resulting from Cancer Treatment?

Cancer is usually treated by surgery, radiation and chemotherapy, used alone or in combination. Each form of therapy imposes nutritional risks on the patient (see Tables 12–1 through 12–3).

Table 12–1
Cancer Surgery and Nutrition

Area of Cancer	Surgical Procedures	Possible Nutrition Problems
Head, neck, tongue	Removal of all or part of the tongue (glossectomy)	Makes chewing and swallowing difficult
Jaw	Removal of lower jawbone	Requires tube feeding
Esophagus	Removal (esophagectomy) with reconstruction using muscle from the intestine	Food may leak into the lungs or the new esophagus may narrow
Stomach	Removal (gastrectomy)	Food may travel to the intestines too quickly or low blood sugar may develop
Small intestine	Opening created outside the body (jejunostomy or ileostomy)	Poor absorption of nutrients, vitamin B_{12} deficiency, salt and water imbalance, scars, blocked bowels
Digestive organs	Removal of pancreas	Poor absorption of nutrients, diabetes
Large intestine	Removal (colectomy) with or without an opening created outside the body (colostomy)	Poor absorption of nutrients and water

From *Nutrition of the Cancer Patient.* Reprinted with permission from the American Institute for Cancer Research, 1994.

Table 12–2
Radiation and Nutrition

Area of Treatment	Short-Term Effects	Long-Term Effects
Head and neck	Irritation of mouth, tongue, esophagus	Dry mouth, tooth decay, stricture of esophagus, inability to taste
Abdomen	Irritation of stomach, diarrhea, milk intolerance, nausea and vomiting	Some of these symptoms may continue in some patients
Upper spine	Irritation of the stomach and esophagus	Some of these symptoms may continue in some patients
Lower spine	Diarrhea	
Pelvis	Diarrhea, malabsorption	Some of these symptoms may continue in some patients

From Nutrition of the Cancer Patient. Reprinted with permission from the American Institute for Cancer Research, 1994.

Surgery

Surgery is used in the treatment of cancer in an attempt to remove tumors or alleviate symptoms (e.g., obstruction). The nutritional problems that may develop depend on the type of procedure performed. Providing optimal nutrition may require dietary modifications based on the patient's ability or inability to consume, digest, and absorb nutrients. Table 12–4 lists common dietary modifications that are needed after certain surgical procedures.

Table 12–3
Chemotherapy and Nutrition

Chemotherapy-Induced Side Effects
Irritation and inflammation of the mouth
Irritation and inflammation of the tongue
Irritation and inflammation of the throat
Diarrhea
Constipation
Nausea
Vomiting
Taste changes
Appetite changes (increased, decreased)
Weight changes (increased, decreased)
Milk intolerance
Food aversions

From Nutrition of the Cancer Patient. Reprinted with permission from the American Institute for Cancer Research, 1994.

Table 12–4
Surgical Procedures Requiring Postoperative Dietary Modifications

Procedure	Nutritional Problems	Dietary Modifications
Radical neck resection	Inability to chew or swallow	Nasogastric tube feeding
Gastrectomy	"Dumping syndrome"	Small frequent meals, liquids between meals, restrict concentrated carbohydrate
Small bowel resection	Diarrhea, malabsorption	Elemental diet
Ileostomy; colostomy	Fluid and electrolyte imbalances	Replacement of fluids and electrolytes

Radiation

Radiation therapy (application of radioactive material) to the head, neck, thorax, esophagus, and abdomen can cause acute eating problems. For example, a dry mouth, sore throat, severe dental and gum destruction, and altered taste and smell sensations may develop after radiation to the head and neck. Swallowing difficulty (dysphagia) often results from radiation to the thorax, and when the abdomen is irradiated, malabsorption of many nutrients occurs if the damage to the gastrointestinal tract is severe. If damage is less severe, gastritis, nausea, vomiting, and diarrhea may result.

Chemotherapy

Chemotherapy is the use of drugs to cure or control cancer. It is **systemic,** meaning that it can affect the entire body rather than just a part of it. The drugs interfere with cells as they divide and reproduce themselves. Normal cells as well as cancer cells are affected, and when cells in the gastrointestinal tract are affected, diarrhea, constipation, or poor absorption of nutrients may occur. However, these side effects are only temporary, because the gastrointestinal tract cells replace themselves every 3 days. Chemotherapy drugs cause nausea and vomiting. Steroids are sometimes used that cause water retention and bloating. After treatment, these conditions disappear and the patient's nutritional status improves. Steroids used in chemotherapy may require the use of dietary sodium and carbohydrate restrictions because of fluid retention and high serum glucose levels. The side effects experienced during chemotherapy treatments may make it difficult for the patient to consume the optimal amounts of nutrients.

What Are the Reasons for Preventing Weight Loss in the Cancer Patient?

In several tumor categories, patients who have not lost weight survive almost twice as long as those who have lost weight. Also, the response to chemotherapy in patients with breast cancer, lung cancer, colon cancer, and acute leukemia is more favorable if pretreatment weight loss has not occurred. Weight loss appears to negatively affect the response to therapy and the likelihood of survival (Rombeau & Rolandelli, 1997). Postoperative gastric cancer mortality was found to be strongly correlated with impaired immunity, hypoalbuminemia, weight loss, and malnutrition (Rey-Ferro et al., 1997).

Why Does Weight Loss Occur in the Cancer Patient?

Decreased kilocalorie intake or increased kilocalorie expenditure (from energy demands of the tumor), or a combination, as well as decreased glucose tolerance and altered protein metabolism, all play a role in weight loss. Reduced gastrointestinal function with diminished movement of food from the stomach causes the individual to feel full too soon and further diminishes the appetite.

In conditions of stress (see Chapter 14), increased amounts of counter-regulatory hormones are produced that inhibit the action of insulin (see Chapter 9). This results in **gluconeogenesis** (production of blood glucose from protein). There is increased breakdown of proteins in the muscle of the cancer patient, which causes a loss of amino acids, resulting in muscle weakness and wasting. The ability to preserve muscle mass during periods of reduced food intake is diminished in a person with cancer. Thus, loss of muscle and protein stores is common during cancer. Significant hypoalbuminemia is frequently found (Rombeau & Rolandelli, 1997).

WHAT ARE THE NUTRIENT NEEDS AND GOALS DURING CANCER TREATMENT?

The diet of the cancer patient must supply enough protein, fat, carbohydrate, vitamins, minerals, and fluids to meet the increased energy demands of a high metabolic rate to prevent weight loss, to rebuild body tissues, and to promote a sense of well-being during treatment. Hypermetabolism may occur frequently but rarely exceeds an increase of 10 to 15 percent (Imoberdorf, 1997). Individual assessment of kilocalorie intake and weight stabilization will give insight into a particular patient's needs. Nutritionally complete liquid supplements in addition to meals are often needed to ensure adequate nutritional intake. As much as 3000 kilocalories and 100 grams of protein or more may be necessary to prevent tissue breakdown and weight loss (see Chapter 14 for more information on nutritional support). It should be noted, however, that there is debate about which cancer patients will benefit from total parenteral nutrition (TPN).

The intake of all vitamins and minerals should at least meet the recommended dietary allowance (RDA). Individual needs must be assessed carefully, because radiation, chemotherapy, and surgery impose nutritional risks. Fluids are especially important to replace losses from fever, diarrhea, and vomiting and to aid the kidneys in the removal of waste products that result from cancer treatment. The following are nutritional goals during cancer treatment:

1. Preventing weight loss (a short-term goal)
2. Achieving and maintaining normal weight (a long-term goal)
3. Replacing nutritional losses from side effects of treatment (i.e., fluid and electrolyte losses from vomiting, diarrhea, malabsorption)
4. Providing adequate kilocalories, protein, carbohydrates, fat, vitamins, and minerals

These goals cannot be achieved without knowledge of individual food tolerances and preferences.

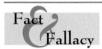

Fallacy: The high-fiber, low-fat macrobiotic diet will cure cancer.

Fact: The macrobiotic diet is low in kilocalories and cannot support the high-energy and nutrient needs of the cancer patient. Weight loss leading to cachexia would likely result; therefore, this diet is not recommended.

WHAT IS THE ROLE OF THE NURSE IN NUTRITIONAL COUNSELING FOR CANCER PREVENTION AND TREATMENT?

The nurse plays an important role in helping the cancer patient cope with eating difficulties that may arise. The nurse should establish a good relationship with the individual before explaining why it is important to eat well. Advice should then be given with sensitivity as to how to promote optimum nutrition at a time when the individual may be feeling poor physically, emotionally, and psychologically. Table 12–5 suggests possible solutions to problems such as lack of appetite, altered taste sensation, feeling full too soon, nausea, chewing and swallowing difficulties, and tiredness.

The cancer patient in the home needs encouragement to take advantage of the good days when favorite and well-tolerated nutritious foods can be prepared in advance, frozen or refrigerated, and heated and served later at mealtime. An effort should then be made to provide a pleasant dining atmosphere.

The nurse has the primary responsibility in caring for the patient in the home setting. He or she must learn what the nutritional needs really are and know when to consult a dietitian or to personally counsel the patient wisely in order to promote comfort as long as possible. Good nutritional status in the cancer patient is of utmost importance, as it greatly influences the effectiveness of therapy and the individual's overall comfort. Visiting nurses, doctors, dietitians, and volunteers are often active in hospice care (a program for the terminally ill, including cancer patients) and assist in dealing with the last stages of life in the home setting, as discussed in Chapter 22.

Table 12–5
Suggested Solutions to Dietary Problems

Anorexia	Ice cream mixed with a carbonated beverage, milkshake, frozen yogurt, eggnog (pasteurized), blended sherbet and fruit juice
	Small frequent meals
	Snacks available during the day
	Bedtime snack
	Favorite foods; novel or ethnic foods
	Foods served attractively with garnishes, variety of color and texture
Dysgeusia	Substitute chicken, turkey, or fish for red meat if necessary; avoid strong-smelling fish
	Add bacon bits, sliced almonds, ham strips, or pieces of onion to vegetable for added flavor
	Tart foods may enhance flavors (lemonade, vinegar, or lemon juice)
	Wines, beer, or mayonnaise added to soups and sauces enhance flavor
	Marinate meat, chicken, or fish in sweet fruit juices, sweet wines, sweet and sour sauce, Italian dressing
	Many foods taste better if cold or at room temperature
Feeling full too soon	Small, frequent meals
	Chew foods slowly
	Limit greasy foods, butter, and rich sauces
	Liquids consumed should be nutrient dense
	Limit the amount of liquids at meals
Nausea and vomiting	Antinausea medicine may be prescribed and taken ½ to 1 hour before eating
	Smaller portions of foods low in fat
	Salty foods recommended; very sweet foods avoided
	Clear, cool beverages recommended; liquids sipped slowly using a straw
	Liquids at mealtime not recommended—take ½ to 1 hour before meals instead
	Sit down rather than lie down after meals
	Fresh air and loose clothing may relieve nausea
Nausea and vomiting from the smell of food	Someone else may be requested to do the cooking
	Avoid greasy and fried foods
	Rather than cooking, warm already prepared foods from the freezer
Difficulty chewing and swallowing because of a sore or dry mouth	Physician may prescribe artificial saliva
	Eat soft foods—avoid rough, coarse, or dry foods
	Blend foods after cooking
	Add gravy to cut-up meats
	Use butter, gravies, or cream sauces on meats and vegetables
	Avoid very salty and acidic foods
	Add extra liquids to stews and casseroles
	Low-acid fruits and nectars may be easier to swallow
	Use a straw for liquids
	Rinse mouth as needed
	Avoid hot spices, hot food
	Use nutritional formulas to provide adequate calories if necessary
Too tired to eat	Cook easy-to-prepare foods (canned creamed soup, fruit and dairy foods, or a creamed sauce over fish or chicken)
	Small portions
	Make meals before tiredness is expected and freeze the food for future use
	Accept offers of food from friends
	Use Meals on Wheels

Modified from U.S. Department of Health and Human Services: Eating Hints. Public Health Service, National Institutes of Health, November 1994.

Critical Thinking

Case Study

Maria thought back to last week when she went for a lumpectomy with removal of breast tissue. The lump had been found to be cancerous, and she would now receive radiation therapy and probably chemotherapy too. How could this have happended to her? She thought only women with few or no pregnancies developed breast cancer. She had three children one of whom was only in kindergarten. She had breastfed her last child, which she thought would protect her against breast cancer. Maria wondered what she might have done to promote cancer. She knew that her family was eating well now but thought back to all the high-fat foods she had eaten up until a few years ago. She decided to pray that her condition would improve.

Applications

1. Discuss how positive thinking and prayer may help the recovery process.
2. What nutrition advice would be appropriate for Maria?
3. What foods might be suggested to reduce Maria's risk of recurrent cancer?
4. What advice would be appropriate if Maria develops anorexia from chemotherapy?
5. Can it be assumed if Maria gains weight with breast cancer that she is eating more food than usual? Why or why not?

Study Questions and Classroom Activities

1. Discuss some of the reasons that cancer patients experience anorexia.
2. Name some of the factors contributing to cancer cachexia.
3. What are some of the nutritional problems imposed by cancer therapies? What dietary modifications are necessary?
4. Why is it important to individualize the diet of the cancer patient?

References

American Institute for Cancer Research: Diet and Cancer Prevention. AICR Newsletter, Winter 1998, Issue 58.

Ames HG, Gee MI, Hawrysh ZJ: Taste perception and breast cancer: Evidence of a role for diet. J Am Diet Assoc. 1993; 93(5):541.

Blot WJ: Vitamin/mineral supplementation and cancer risk: International chemoprevention trials. Proc Soc Exp Biol Med. November 1997; 216(2):291–296.

Demark-Wahnefried W, Rimer BK, Winer EP: Weight gain in women diagnosed with breast cancer. J Am Diet Assoc. May 1997; 97(5):519–526.

Giovannucci E: Insulin and colon cancer. Cancer causes control. March 1995; 6(2):164–179.

Goodman MT, Wilkens LR, Hankin JH, Lyu LC, Wu AH, Kolonel LN: Association of soy and fiber consumption with the risk of endometrial cancer. Am J Epidemiol. August 15, 1997; 146(4):294–306.

Imoberdorf R: Immuno-nutrition: Designer diets in cancer. Support care cancer. September 1997; 5(5):381–386.

Kaaks R: Nutrition, hormones, and breast cancer: Is insulin the missing link? Cancer causes control. November 1996; 7(6):605–625.

Le Marchand L, Hankin JH, Wilkens LR, Kolonel LN, Englyst HN, Lyu LC: Dietary fiber and colorectal cancer risk. Epidemiology. November 1997; 8(6):658–665.

Otero-Sabogal R, Sabogal F, Perez-Stable EJ, Hiatt RA: Dietary practices, alcohol consumption, and smoking behavior: Ethnic, sex, and acculturation differences. J Natl Cancer Inst Monogr. 1995; 18:73–82.

Platz EA, Giovannucci E, Rimm EB, Rockett HR, Stampfer MJ, Colditz GA, Willett WC: Dietary fiber and distal colorectal adenoma in men. Cancer Epidemiol Biomarkers Prev. September 1997; 6(9):661–670.

Rey-Ferro M, Castano R, Orozco O, Serna A, Moreno A: Nutritional and immunologic evaluation of patients with gastric cancer before and after surgery. Nutrition. October 1997; 13(10):878–881.

Rombeau JL, Rolandelli, RH: Clinical Nutrition, Parenteral Nutrition, 3rd ed., Philadelphia, WB Saunders, 1997.

Sandler RS: Epidemiology and risk factors for colorectal cancer. Gastroenterol Clin North Am. December 1996; 25(4):717–735.

Stoll BA: Nutrition and breast cancer risk: Can an effect via insulin resistance be demonstrated? Breast Cancer Res Treat. 1996; 38(3):239–246.

Walker AR: Diet in the prevention of cancer: What are the chances of avoidance? J R Soc Health. December 1996; 116(6):360–366.

Weisburger JH: Dietary fat and risk of chronic disease: Mechanistic insights from experimental studies. J Am Diet Assoc. July 1997; 97(Suppl 7):S16–S23.

White LL, Ballew C, Gilbert TJ, Mendlein JM, Mokdad AH, Strauss KF: Weight, body image, and weight control practices of Navajo Indians: Findings from the Navajo Health and Nutrition Survey. J Nutr. October 1997; 127(Suppl 10):2094S–2098S.

Whittemore AS, Kolonel LN, Wu AH, John EM, Gallagher RP, Howe GR, Burch JD, Hankin J, Dreon DM, West DW, et al: Prostate cancer in relation to diet, physical activity, and body size in blacks, whites, and Asians in the United States and Canada. J Natl Cancer Inst. May 3, 1995; 87(9):652–661.

Yancik R: Cancer burden in the aged: An epidemiologic and demographic overview. Cancer. October 1, 1997; 80(7):1273–1283.

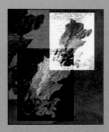

13

HIV and AIDS

Objectives

After completing this chapter, you should be able to:

- Define HIV, ARC, and AIDS.
- Describe nutritional concerns and interventions to delay the onset of AIDS.
- Describe nutritional interventions for persons with AIDS.
- Describe the nutritional needs of children with AIDS.
- Describe the role of the nurse or other health care professional in the nutritional delay and management of AIDS.

Terms to Identify

Acquired immuno-
    deficiency syndrome
    (AIDS)
AIDS-related complex
    (ARC)

AIDS enteropathy
Dementia
HIV positive
Human immuno-
    deficiency virus (HIV)

Kaposi's sarcoma
Persons with AIDS
    (PWAs)
Thrush

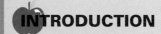 **INTRODUCTION**

As health care professionals we will all deal with **persons with AIDS (PWAs)** at some point in our career. You may already know someone who is **HIV positive** (infected with the human immunodeficiency virus), who has **AIDS-related complex (ARC),** or who has a full-blown case of AIDS. More than a half million cases of AIDS had been reported to the Centers for Disease Control (CDC) as of 1996 (CDC, 1996). HIV infection has become the fourth leading cause of premature mortality, measured in terms of years of potential life lost (years of life lost before 65 years of age), in the United States and the leading cause in a sizable number of U.S. cities (Selik & Chu, 1997). However, for the first time since human immuno-deficiency virus infection was created as a special cause-of-death category in 1987, death rates for human immunodeficiency virus infection declined from 1995 to 1996 (Guyer et al., 1997). In 1995 women accounted for 19 percent of AIDS cases in adults; the greatest increases in AIDS incidence rates were observed in heterosexually infected women born between 1970 and 1974 (Wortley & Fleming, 1997).

The AIDS virus is transmitted only through intimate personal contact in which body fluids are exchanged. HIV is spread through semen, vaginal fluids, and blood. You cannot catch HIV or AIDS from a drinking fountain or through casual contact such as handshaking. This is vital to remember when working with someone with AIDS, because a simple touch on the hand can have a very positive effect on the psyche of such a person.

Probably more than any other condition, AIDS is associated with major biopsychosocial symptoms. Physiologically it is associated with severe weight loss resulting from elevated metabolism, reduced food intake, and increased gastrointestinal losses from diarrhea. Reduced social contact, because of social stigma, can have a profound negative psychological effect on a person with AIDS. AIDS can also cause a type of **dementia** (deranged mental functioning) that prevents the person with AIDS from making appropriate health care decisions. Care of the AIDS patient requires an understanding of the physiology as well as the psychological and social needs. All members of the health care team play a major role in the multifaceted needs of the AIDS patient.

WHAT IS AIDS?

Acquired immunodeficiency syndrome (AIDS) is a condition in which the body has lost its immune system. The **human immunodeficiency virus (HIV)** is felt to be the cause of the destruction of the immune system. A person with AIDS thus has no protective defense against infection.

A person who has been infected with HIV is said to be HIV positive. AIDS-related complex (ARC) precedes AIDS. The time interval between HIV infection and full-blown AIDS varies among individuals, and it is not fully understood why there is so much variation. Older adults generally progress more quickly from HIV infection to full-blown AIDS than younger adults (Adler et al., 1997). One common complication of AIDS is **Kaposi's sarcoma,** a malignancy that may be found on the skin, mucous membranes, lymph nodes, or gastrointestinal tract and can interfere with nutritional intake (Fig. 13–1). Good nutrition and weight maintenance are believed to delay the onset of full-blown AIDS by helping to preserve immune function. It may take as many as 10 years or more for HIV infection to develop into AIDS.

WHAT IS THE ROLE OF NUTRITION IN AIDS MANAGEMENT?

As soon as a person is diagnosed as HIV positive, he or she should pay extra attention to nutritional needs. Ideally, a baseline nutrition and diet assessment by a registered dietitian should be undertaken. Because an adequate diet is a prerequisite to a healthy immune system, it is currently believed that good nutrition will at least delay and possibly prevent the onset of AIDS. Malnutrition is a common complication of HIV infection and plays a significant and independent role in morbidity and mortality (Babameto & Kotler, 1997). Malnutrition may be pre-

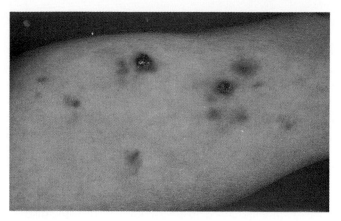

Figure 13–1
Nodular lesions of Kaposi's sarcoma. (From Friedman-Kien, Cockerell: Color Atlas of AIDS, 2nd ed. Philadelphia, WB Saunders, 1996, p. 52.)

vented and reversed by using current therapies, such as medical nutrition therapy that includes nutrition assessment, the development of an individualized nutrition therapy plan, and implementation of the therapy (Young, 1997).

Adequate protein status is imperative for a fully functioning immune system. Assessment of protein status can be determined through the following:

- Anthropometric measurements such as body mass index (see Chapter 20) or percent weight loss from usual or last recorded weight
- Tricep skin-fold measures and midarm circumference
- Lab values such as serum albumin level
- A diet history to determine whether adequate amounts of protein and kilocalories are consumed

Other nutritional concerns of newly diagnosed persons with HIV include adequate vitamins and minerals for a healthy immune system. Foods with vitamins A and C are especially important. Other nutrients that contribute to a healthy immune system include vitamin B_{12}, copper, and zinc. Many other nutrients help maintain health and thereby reduce the stress on the immune system. Minimally processed foods remain the preferred medium for nutrients (whole grains, vegetables, fruits, milk and other protein foods). This is because foods provide kilocalories as well as phytochemicals, which are not found in vitamin supplements.

The same principles that are used to establish an adequate diet for a healthy person also apply to the person with AIDS or ARC. But the amount of kilocalories and protein will need to be increased when the metabolic rate increases from infections and other stressors. Generally, the person with HIV will not have additional requirements beyond the recommendations for all healthy persons until the advanced stage of ARC begins.

What Are Some Specific Nutrition Concerns Once HIV Has Progressed to ARC or AIDS?

Increased energy needs are a result of the stress and infections associated with ARC and AIDS. Other concerns have to do with either reduced food intake or malabsorption of nutrients with resulting diarrhea. Table 13–1 lists dietary considerations of nutrition-related complications. Food safety is vital (see Chapter 22). It may be preferable to emphasize cooked foods once AIDS has developed to help ensure avoidance of food-borne pathogens. Eggs, in particular, need to be thoroughly cooked to avoid risk of salmonella.

Loss of appetite can have biopsychosocial causes. Sores of the mouth and esophagus can make eating painful and difficult. **Thrush** (an infection of the mouth) causes an increased need for kilocalories because of the accompanying fever as well as a diminished desire to eat. Medications for treatment of AIDS may also cause nausea. Abdominal discomfort and diarrhea associated with malabsorption of food nutrients compound the lack of desire to eat while increasing the need for additional nutrients. Psychologically, dementia can cause such disorientation that the person with AIDS forgets to eat. Depression is common and can reduce a desire to eat. Social isolation is a known aspect of decreased eating and desire to eat.

What Is the Role of Nutrition Support?

For an HIV-positive person to maintain a very high intake of kilocalories, liquid supplements are often required. Kilocalorie needs may be as high as 3500 kilocalories or more per day (Table 20–4 presents a sample menu for 3000-kilocalorie diet; the addition of two cans of a commercial liquid supplement will supply the additional 500 kilocalories). Regular milkshakes or more expensive commercial supplements that are designed to provide high levels of kilocalories, protein, vitamins, and minerals may be appropriate. If oral intake is inadequate, even with liquid supplements, tube feeding may be required. The tube feeding may be in addition to oral feeding. When severe gastrointestinal problems such as digestive problems and malabsorption are present, oral feeding may be withheld and total parenteral nutrition (TPN) started (see Chapter 14). However, TPN should be used as a last resort because of the increased chance of infection at the site of infusion. Elemental formulas with tube feeding are generally well absorbed and should be tried before TPN. The higher osmolarity of elemental formulas may require a cautious increase in strength and rate of delivery.

How Are Kilocalorie Needs for PWAs Determined?

Resting metabolic rates in persons with AIDS can vary due to factors such as active infections, (i.e., pneumonia or other opportunistic infections). Infection and fever will elevate the metabolic rate, resulting in an increased need for

Table 13–1
Summary of Dietary Considerations* for Nutrition-Related Complications†

Diarrhea

Follow low-lactose, low-fat diet
Offer clear liquids with dilute juice (at most 12 to 24 hours duration)
Try Lactaid milk, low-lactose milk products
Avoid caffeine-containing beverages
Include soluble fiber (pectins, gums) and avoid bran-type fiber
Offer small, frequent meals
Between meals try liquids, diluted juices, and sports drinks at room temperature
Replace potassium and fluid losses with high potassium foods, liquids
Consider flavored oral elemental diet
Avoid simple sugars, candy, honey, and jelly
Try oral rehydration solutions that use rice powder as a carbohydrate source (Ceralyte, Infalyte)
Avoid sorbitol

Nausea and Vomiting

Emphasize low-fat foods
Offer small, frequent meals
Try dry, salty foods (pretzels, crackers)
Offer foods when nausea is absent
Avoid concentration of very sweet foods
Offer high kilocalorie liquids between meals; use a straw
For drinks with strong odor, serve in cup with a lid and straw
Offer meals before taking drugs that may cause nausea
Encourage eating slowly, relaxing
Avoid gas-producing or spicy foods
Encourage rest after meals; elevate head
Try flat, carbonated beverages (add ginger to gingerale) or herbal, peppermint teas
Check with physician for antinausea medications

Mouth Pain or Dry Mouth

Apply topical medication before meals
Rinse mouth frequently with solution recommended by physician (usually hydrogen peroxide and water)
Offer semisolid foods or liquid or pureed food
Avoid acidic and spicy foods when mouth sores are present
Avoid hot foods; try cold or room temperature
Use straw to bypass painful area
Rinse mouth frequently
Provide artificial saliva (from dentist) for very dry mouth
Dip foods into beverage or soup to soften
Try popsicles or snowcones before eating to numb mouth
Maintain good oral hygiene
Keep sports bottles on hand for sipping

Swallowing Difficulties

Offer soft or semisolid foods or liquid or pureed food
Offer moist foods
Offer adequate fluids, use straws
Add commercial thickening agents to foods
Add potato flakes or mashed potatoes to soups, gravies to thicken
Avoid dry or "rough" foods (chips, popcorn) and "hard" foods (raw, crunchy fruits, vegetables)
Offer foods with even consistency versus uneven, combination foods

Table continued on following page

Table 13-1
Summary of Dietary Considerations* for Nutrition-Related Complications† (*continued*)

Dip foods into beverage or soup to soften
Avoid sticky foods
Offer acidic foods (may help thin saliva, aid in chewing)
Tilt head back or move forward to aid swallowing
See neurodiagnostics (speech pathology) for specific help with techniques and appropriate food consistency
Check with physician regarding artificial saliva

Altered Taste

Marinate meats, poultry
Use plastic utensils to help avoid "metallic taste"
Serve food cold or at room temperature
Adjust sweetness, saltiness, tartness, and sourness to increase taste

Infection and Fever

Offer high-calorie, high-protein diet
Increase high-energy fluids
Use concentrated nutritional supplements with infection/fever
Provide multiple vitamin/mineral supplements
Consider enteral feedings to supplement intake

Fatigue

Prepare and freeze meals when feeling well
Keep easy-to-prepare items on hand (sandwiches, canned foods)
Check community resources for in-home help with meal preparation, meal delivery, food banks
Encourage adequate rest
Encourage small, frequent meals
Try calorie- and nutrient-dense foods and beverages

Anorexia

Encourage small, frequent meals
Offer high-calorie, high-protein snacks
Avoid low-calorie foods and beverages (e.g., coffee, tea)
Provide pleasant, relaxing atmosphere for meals
Drink liquids between rather than with snack or meal
Keep ready-to-eat snacks at side
Try schedule for meals, snacks; "eat by clock" regardless of appetite
Check with physician regarding small amount of wine before meals
Add modular supplements, protein or glucose polymers to foods and liquids where feasible

*For oral intake only. Suggestions are not included for enteral and parenteral nutrition.
†When more than one complication is present, suggestions for one may be contraindicated by another (e.g., acidic juices may benefit those with an altered sense of taste but would likely cause pain when mouth sores are present).
Adapted from Schreiner J: Nutrition Handbook for HIV/AIDS, 3rd ed. Aurora, CO, Carrot Top Nutrition Resources, 1999.

kilocalories. Estimated kilocalorie needs can be verified through weight monitoring. For example, if the patient shows an undesirable weekly weight loss of 1 pound, an increase of 500 kilocalories per day will be required to prevent further weight loss. This can be equated to the 3500 kilocalories required per pound of weight loss (see Chapter 20 for more information on weight management and kilocalorie goals). Avoidance of diarrhea is important as kilocalorie intake is increased.

What Are the Causes of and Nutritional Intervention for Diarrhea?

Diarrhea in the PWA can result from opportunistic infections of the gastrointestinal tract, medication side effects, inadequate digestion of food and malabsorption, and malnutrition with hypoalbuminemia. An unexplainable cause, which is generally referred to as **AIDS enteropathy,** might also be responsible.

Diarrhea may be controlled by reducing intake of lactose (lactose intolerance is common with gastrointestinal upsets, see Chapter 11), reducing fat intake, or using a medium chain triglyceride oil (a commercial product available through pharmacies) if steatorrhea or fatty stool is present. Medium chain triglyceride oil does not require digestion and is well absorbed if fat maldigestion and malabsorption are present. A decrease in roughage or insoluble fiber along with an increase in soluble fiber may be of further benefit. Soluble fiber sources such as gums and pectin found in applesauce, pears, potatoes, oatmeal, barley, and banana flakes can help reduce diarrhea. Metamucil, which contains soluble fiber from psyllium seed, can also be helpful. Sometimes total bowel rest is indicated, and therefore the risks of TPN are outweighed by the positive nutritional benefits that result when the person's status is NPO (nothing by mouth). Dehydration can become an issue if the diarrhea is persistent. The person with AIDS may need to be taught to recognize the symptoms of dehydration and constipation. Constipation can result from antidiarrheal medication and insufficient water intake.

Should the Person with AIDS Take Vitamins?

A multivitamin and mineral supplement is generally recommended in amounts supplying 100 to 200 percent of the RDA, especially if there are signs of maldigestion and malabsorption, such as diarrhea. This amount is felt to be adequate without causing harm. Megadoses of some vitamins and minerals (greater than 10 times the RDA) may impair the immune system.

HOW DO CHILDREN DEVELOP AIDS?

Women are increasingly developing AIDS through heterosexual contact and are passing the HIV infection to children prenatally (during pregnancy—see Chapter 16). Perinatal transmission accounts for almost 90 percent of all pediatric HIV infections. The median age at diagnosis of AIDS in children with perinatally acquired HIV infection is 12 to 24 months (Hoernle & Reid, 1995). In the United States acquired immunodeficiency syndrome is the seventh leading cause of death in children aged 1 to 4 years and the fourth leading cause of death among women aged 25 to 44 years (Rogers, 1997). Through 1993 an estimated 15,000 HIV-infected children were born to HIV-positive women in the United States. A two-thirds reduction in the risk for perinatal transmission of HIV has been shown with the medication zidovudine (MMWR Morb Mortal Wkly Rep, 1997).

The ability to transmit HIV via breast-feeding has been established. Banked human milk is pasteurized to destroy the HIV virus but retains properties that may be helpful to infants of HIV-positive mothers. Breast-feeding by women with HIV is not recommended in developed countries as the risk for transferring HIV to the infant is outweighed by the health benefits of breast-feeding (Black, 1996). The estimated postnatal transmission rate from mothers with HIV who breast-feed is 26 percent (Van de Perre, 1995).

What Are the Nutrition Goals in Pediatric AIDS?

Malnutrition, skeletal muscle wasting, and changes in cardiac muscle mass and function have been described in children infected with HIV. In one study children infected with HIV were found to be significantly below age-adjusted standards for height, weight, triceps skinfold thickness, and arm muscle circumference (Miller et al., 1997). Infants with AIDS may require a high-calorie formula (24 to 27 kilocalories per ounce). Many of the same principles of nutrition care apply to infants and children. Kilocalorie and protein needs are more difficult to ascertain and should be based on individual needs using growth charts and nitrogen balance studies.

In an attempt to increase kilocalories, any food that the child tolerates and accepts is appropriate. General nutritional guidelines to avoid excess fat and sugar in the diet do not apply as strongly to the child with AIDS. So long as the child is consuming adequate amounts of protein, vitamins, and minerals (the child is eating at least the minimum recommended number of servings listed on the Food Guide Pyramid), added kilocalories can come from any source. Candy bars, soda pop, and potato chips provide significant amounts of kilocalories. Small amounts should be tried first to ensure tolerance to foods with a high fat content. More nutritious sources of kilocalories, such as milkshakes and puddings, are preferable; these can be made to be low in fat if needed. Important to finding sources of additional kilocalories are the child's willingness to consume the food items and a physical tolerance of them.

WHAT IS THE ROLE OF THE NURSE OR OTHER HEALTH CARE PROFESSIONAL IN THE NUTRITIONAL MANAGEMENT OF HIV-POSITIVE OR AIDS PATIENTS?

All health care professionals should encourage a person with HIV to eat well-balanced meals to preserve immune function. The health care professional may need to ensure that the patient receives meal trays in a timely fashion and may need to sit with the patient during meals to provide emotional support. Prevention of weight loss is critical. It is much more difficult for a person with AIDS to regain lost weight than it is to maintain weight.

The nurse has a unique role in caring for AIDS patients because of the complex medical conditions. The nurse should be well versed in how to care for the AIDS patient and should be alert to problems that may compromise nutritional status. The nurse may need to become actively involved in feeding the person with AIDS when weakness prevents adequate self-care. All persons with AIDS should have a baseline nutritional assessment with referral to a registered dietitian for any high-risk conditions such as being underweight or experiencing weight loss.

The health care professional can avoid acquiring HIV when caring for HIV positive or AIDS patients by avoiding the patients' bodily secretions and using special care in handling needles used by the patient. Gloves should be worn, and good hand washing is necessary after patient contact. If these precautions are taken, the health care professional does not need to worry about contracting AIDS. The disease is not spread through the air or through touch alone. When the nurse's fears about AIDS transmission are eliminated, sensitivity and compassion toward the patient are likely to increase.

Critical Thinking

Case Study

Denise thought back to her old pal "Mr. B," as she had referred to him, while she ate her whole-grain toast with peanut butter and half a grapefruit in the company's cafeteria. It had been 5 years since they worked together, but his encouragement to eat well had influenced her. When she first learned she was HIV positive, she thought her life was over and had become very depressed. Mr. B's friendship and the daily jokes he told had helped her get out of her depression. She wondered if it really was true that because she was eating well and getting adequate rest her condition had not yet progressed to full-blown AIDS. She had not lost any weight and so far was healthy. Denise was thankful she was still able to work and tried to avoid thinking about what her future held.

Applications

1. How can positive social support help in managing illness?
2. What nutrients is Denise getting in higher amounts in the meal described in the case compared to having a donut and coffee for breakfast?
3. How might Denise eat if she had diarrhea and was losing weight?

Study Questions and Classroom Activities

1. What are the different nutrition management concerns for HIV and AIDS? What nutritional monitoring technique should be done on a regular basis?
2. Why might a person with AIDS need to have a high kilocalorie intake?
3. Why is it particularly important for a person with AIDS to avoid homemade eggnog?
4. Interview nurses at the local health department to assess what measures are taken to prevent the spread of HIV and AIDS in the community.

References

Adler WH, Baskar PV, Chrest FJ, Dorsey-Cooper B, Winchurch RA, Nagel JE: HIV infection and aging: Mechanisms to explain the accelerated rate of progression in the older patient. Mech Ageing Dev. June 1997; 96(1–3):137–155.

Babameto G, Kotler DP: Malnutrition in HIV infection. Gastroenterol Clin North. June 1997; 26(2):393–415.

Black RF: Transmission of HIV-1 in the breast-feeding process. J Am Diet Assoc. March 1996; 96(3):267–274.

Centers for Disease Control and Prevention: AIDS Among Children—United States, 1996. Morbidity and Mortality Weekly Report. November 22, 1996; 45(46).

Guyer B, Martin JA, MacDorman MF, Anderson RN, Strobino DM: Annual summary of vital statistics—1996. Pediatrics. December 1997; 100(6):905–918.

Hoernle EH, Reid TE: Human immunodeficiency virus infection in children. Am J Health Syst Pharm. May 1, 1995; 52(9):961–979.

Miller TL, Orav EJ, Colan SD, Lipshultz SE: Nutritional status and cardiac mass and function in children infected with the human immunodeficiency virus. Am J Clin Nutr. September 1997; 66(3):660–664.

MMWR Morb Mortal Wkly Rep: Update: Perinatally acquired HIV/AIDS—United States, 1997. November 21, 1997; 46(46):1086–1092.

Rogers MF: Epidemiology of HIV/AIDS in women and children in the USA. Acta Paediatr Suppl. June 1997; 421:15–16.

Selik RM, Chu SY: Years of potential life lost due to HIV infection in the United States. AIDS. November 1997; 11(13):1635–1639.

Van de Perre P: Postnatal transmission of human immunodeficiency virus type 1: The breast-feeding dilemma. Am J Obstet Gynecol. August 1995; 173(2):483–487.

Wortley PM, Fleming PL: AIDS in women in the United States. Recent trends. JAMA. September 17, 1997; 278(11):911–916.

Young JS: HIV and medical nutrition therapy. J Am Diet Assoc. October 1997; 97(10 Suppl 2):S161–S166.

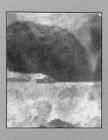

14
Nutritional Support in Physiological Stress

Objectives

After completing this chapter, you should be able to:

- Describe nutritional support.
- Describe different types, methods, and uses of nutritional support.
- Explain why the nutrition recovery syndrome might occur with nutritional support.
- Describe the role of the nurse in nutritional support.

Terms to Identify

Anabolic
Aspiration
Catabolic
D50W/D70W
Elemental
Enteral nutrition
Gastrostomy

Hyperalimentation
Jejunostomy
Nasogastric
Nutritional support
Parenteral nutrition
Peripheral parenteral nutrition (PPN)

Phlebitis
Physiological stress
Refeeding syndrome
Sepsis
Total parenteral nutrition (TPN)
Tube feeding

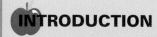 **INTRODUCTION**

Conditions of **physiological stress** (an insulin-resistant state in which increased amounts of stress-related hormones are present) are created through trauma, surgery, burns, fever, and infections (Table 14–1). Kilocalorie and protein needs can be dramatically increased under such conditions, causing weight loss and loss of muscle mass unless an adequate diet is consumed. It is often not possible to treat this condition through meals alone. Thus, medical nutritional support is generally required during times of physiological stress. Oral intake or enteral nutrition through a tube into the gastrointestinal (GI) system is the preferred route. The rule of thumb states, "When the gut works, use it."

Table 14–1
Physiological Responses to Stress

Type of Stress	Possible Physiological Response
Surgery	Blood loss, shock, hemorrhage Depletion of protein or increase in protein metabolism Negative nitrogen balance Dehydration Edema Nausea, vomiting, diarrhea Electrolyte imbalance
Fractures of long bones and other trauma	Increase in protein metabolism Loss of phosphorus, potassium, sulfur Development of osteoporosis because of immobilization and loss of calcium Electrolyte imbalance Loss of fluids Renal failure and uremia
Burns	High loss of nitrogen Increased water loss Anorexia Fluid loss Weight loss Electrolyte imbalance Mineral losses
Infection	Increased metabolism Dehydration Fever Body tissue breakdown Nausea and vomiting Anorexia Poor synthesis of B-complex vitamins related to antibiotics given Loss of sodium and potassium if fever is present
Fevers, including those of short and long duration	Increased protein metabolism Depletion of body's energy stores Lowered sodium, chloride, and potassium levels Disturbance of appetite, digestion, and absorption
Radiotherapy and chemo-therapy	Damage to gastrointestinal mucosa

WHAT IS NUTRITIONAL SUPPORT?

Nutritional support can be as simple as between-meal snacks for institutionalized patients or as complex as total parenteral nutrition (TPN). **Nutritional support** is the provision of macronutrients (carbohydrate, protein, and fat) to promote healthy weight management and nutritional status. It is used during times of physiological stress, when the oral intake from standard meals cannot keep pace with the increased metabolic needs of the stress state. TPN is used when the GI

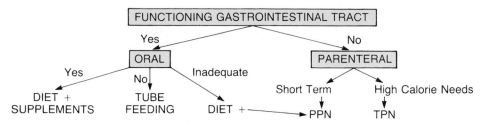

Figure 14–1
Determining the type of nutritional support for the patient.

tract is not functioning (see Fig. 14–1). After total gastrectomy (stomach removal), use of nasojejunal tube feeding (see Fig. 14–2) has been found to be well tolerated and about one-fourth as expensive as TPN (Sand et al., 1997). The use of percutaneous endoscopic gastrostomy (PEG) tubes—a permanent feeding tube surgically implanted through the stomach—has increased with children and adults who have neurological damage resulting in dysphagia (see Chapter 18). This form of nutrition support provides a major improvement for children requiring long-term tube feeding (Behrens et al., 1997). However, for children who are likely to return to oral feeding as their main source of nourishment, oral feeding needs to be encouraged whether it is by using a pacifier, drinking water, or eating small amounts of food. It has been found that infants who receive only nasogastric tube feeding for more than 9 months have significant and persistent difficulty making the transition to oral feeding. Problems encountered have included difficulties in chewing and swallowing, refusal to eat, and panic attacks from swallowing (Dello Strologo et al., 1997).

WHAT ARE INDICATIONS FOR NUTRITIONAL SUPPORT?

Nutritional support is essential for anyone who (1) has had an unplanned weight loss of 10 percent or more within 3 months; (2) shows a significant loss of muscle mass; (3) has a serum albumin level of less than 3 g/dL, a serum transferrin level of less than 150 mg/dL, or both; or (4) is scheduled for major surgery, for example, a total gastrectomy or another procedure in which there is stress as well as a potential for starvation after surgery.

Recording a patient's food intake will give a fairly accurate estimate of kilocalories and nutrients consumed in relation to weight and other lab assessments. This information can be used to assess whether the patient's nutritional needs can be met orally or if alternative methods of nutritional support should be considered. Stressful conditions resulting from cancer, surgery, burns, head injury, infections and fevers, and AIDS often require nutritional support. Patients with pressure sores and chronic obstructive pulmonary disease also can benefit from nutritional support.

Whenever possible, the patient should be encouraged to ingest a normal diet by mouth. This is the preferred and most natural method of nutritional support.

It has the psychological advantage of giving the patient control over at least one aspect of treatment. It also provides the physical benefit of promoting continued GI functioning. High-kilocalorie, high-protein foods such as milk shakes, custards, and puddings are often used in conjunction with between-meal feedings. When more complete nutritional intake is needed, commercial liquid supplements should be used. These liquid supplements include the known vitamins, minerals, and other nutrients essential for health.

Cancer. The goal of nutritional support during cancer treatment is the maintenance of lean body tissue. Because of the catabolic state induced by cancer, with rapid loss of muscle tissue and reduced intake of food, nutritional support may be critical to survival.

Enteral nutritional support is the preferred method if the GI tract is functioning. Tube feeding at rates of up to 150 mL/hr is usually tolerated (the flow rate should start at about 50 mL/hr and should be increased daily by about 25 mL/hr to ensure tolerance). Most liquid supplements provide 1 kcal/mL. Thus at 150 mL/hr for 24 hours, the intake will be 3600 kilocalories. This diet should meet the needs of the cancer patient. The dietitian, in consultation with the patient's physician, is the person who determines patient kilocalorie needs.

Patients undergoing resection of an upper GI tract malignancy are at increased risk for malnutrition, as well as postoperative morbidity and mortality. Early enteral feeding significantly improves protein metabolism in upper GI cancer patients (Hochwald et al., 1997).

During the 1980s, TPN use in cancer treatment became more common. Children with cancer often are good candidates for TPN because of their high nutrient needs to support growth. TPN is not appropriate for terminal cancer patients.

A common problem among cancer patients is glucose intolerance, which should be considered in the provision of nutritional support. Glucerna is a commercial liquid supplement designed for persons with diabetes and may be an appropriate supplement for cancer patients if glucose intolerance is a problem (the patients' lab values for glucose should be monitored at least daily; glucose levels over 200 mg/dL warrant intervention). TPN solutions can be modified to be lower in dextrose (sugar) and higher in fat content to provide adequate kilocalories. Insulin injection may be required, or insulin may be infused into the TPN solution.

Surgery. Even well-nourished individuals under stressful conditions, such as surgery, experience a **catabolic** (cell breakdown) phase before the **anabolic** (cell growth) phase of healing occurs. For the patient to benefit from nutritional support, the anabolic phase must occur. This occurrence can be confirmed with the finding of a positive nitrogen balance. When new tissue is formed to repair damage, the body reaches a positive nitrogen and potassium balance and bodily functions such as digestion, urination, and hydration return to normal. By supplying the patient with sufficient nutrients and fluids to help counteract the depletion caused by stressful situations, this anabolic phase should be reached as quickly as possible.

To prepare a patient for such a stressful situation, preoperative dietary treatment may be required for a time, depending on the patient's condition and whether the operation is major or minor. Patients at increased risk of mortality and morbidity postsurgically include those who have nutritional deficiency severe enough to cause a loss of reaction to skin antigens. One study found 36 percent mortality and 52 percent morbidity in patients with negative skin antigen test results, compared with only 2 percent to 7 percent in patients with positive skin antigen test results (Rombeau & Caldwell, 1997). Special attention is given to providing high-protein, high-carbohydrate meals, with mineral and possibly vitamin supplementation (particularly ascorbic acid and minerals such as zinc and magnesium) and fluids. Obese patients, anemic patients, and diabetic patients may need medical nutrition therapy.

Adequate kilocalorie and protein intake should be the prime consideration in helping the patient reach the anabolic phase of healing after surgery. Otherwise, the patient will lose weight and become weak. Blood loss, dehydration, edema, nausea, vomiting, and diarrhea are all postoperative conditions requiring prompt nutritional intervention.

After major surgery, small amounts of clear fluid are offered first, and the diet gradually progresses to normal as soon as the patient can tolerate it. Recommended nutritional guidelines after surgery are as follows:

- No patient is on a clear-liquid diet/nothing by mouth (NPO) without nutritional support for more than 7 days.
- No patient has weight loss greater than 10 percent of admission weight at discharge; kilocalorie and protein or volume goals for patients on enteral or parenteral nutrition are documented in the medical record.
- Patients on enteral or parenteral nutrition receive at least 1000 kilocalories per day by the fourth day after an operation, although total kilocalorie needs will be greater than this (Queen et al., 1993).

Burns. Nutritional assessment and support are essential to promote wound healing and prevent weight loss in patients with burn injury. The increase in energy expenditure that accompanies burns exceeds that of any other injury. These patients appear to become and remain hypermetabolic in response to a characteristic set of hormonal signals. The postburn elevated metabolic rate is proportional to the size of the thermal injury and lasts until the majority of the wound is closed. If the increased protein and kilocalorie requirements are not supplied externally through nutritional support, the patient's skeletal muscle is broken down for fuel. Inadequate nutritional support can result in weight loss, loss of lean body mass, negative nitrogen balance, delayed wound healing, skin graft failure, decreased immunological response, burn wound sepsis, and increased mortality.

Many methods exist for estimating the nutritional requirements of burn patients. All have some limitations. The Curreri formula is used widely to determine calorie requirements and is probably best at estimating peak energy expenditure.

Adult:

$$(25 \text{ kcal} \times \text{kg preburn weight}) + (40 \text{ kcal} \times \% \text{ of body burned})$$

Child (<12 years of age):

$$(60 \text{ kcal} \times \text{kg preburn weight}) + (35 \text{ kcal} \times \% \text{ of body burned})$$

Adequate protein is critical. A goal of 1.5 to 2.0 grams of protein per kilogram of body weight can be used as a guideline. Patients should receive a high-kilocalorie, high-protein diet. Most also receive therapeutic vitamin and mineral supplementation. Adequacy of nutrient intake should be monitored by daily weight measurements and kilocalorie counts. Oral dietary supplements, tube feedings, or parenteral nutrition is included as needed.

No benefits to overfeeding have been demonstrated. In fact, overfeeding can be detrimental. Overfeeding a malnourished patient can also result in congestive heart failure. Maintaining the patient's weight within 10 percent of preburn weight is suggested as a guideline to prevent the problems associated with over- or underfeeding (University of Iowa Hospitals and Clinics, 1996).

Head Injuries. Head injuries greatly increase the rate of metabolism. Head injury patients at risk of Wernicke-Korsakoff syndrome from alcoholism should receive thiamine in order to prevent an additional insult to the damaged brain (Ferguson et al., 1997).

Infections. The goal of nutritional therapy for patients with infections is to combat the effects of increased metabolism, dehydration, and electrolyte imbalance. Fever often accompanies infections, and the patient's kilocalorie needs are increased by about 50 percent over the basal metabolic needs. Protein needs are also increased when the body is trying to produce antibodies and lymphocytes to fight the infection. Extra fluids are necessary to match the increased kilocalorie needs associated with fever and increased metabolic rate (an increase of 13 percent with each degree centigrade above normal temperature). Fluids help the body eliminate toxins that enter the circulatory system and are carried out by the kidneys. Sodium chloride and potassium levels are lowered as a result of diarrhea and vomiting. Antibiotics used in treating the infections interfere with intestinal synthesis of B-complex vitamins. Nutritional support of patients with infection is summarized as follows:

1. An increase in kilocalorie intake (35 to 45 kcal/kg body weight)
2. An increase in protein intake (1.5 to 2 g/kg body weight)
3. An increase in B-complex vitamins as kilocalories are increased
4. Vitamin and mineral supplements
5. Frequent small feedings
6. Tube feeding as necessary

Intestinal Diseases. Malnutrition is caused by inflammation associated with Crohn's disease or inflammatory bowel disease and may be worsened with lack of appetite. In children, nutritional therapy should be considered to prevent growth problems. Protein intake should be 150 percent of the RDA. Nutritional support, using either elemental or polymeric diets, has been shown to be as effective as steroids in achieving remission of inflammatory bowel disease (Buller, 1997).

Pressure Sores. Patients with pressure sores (bed sores) need nutritional support to help with the healing process. Kilocalorie and protein needs may be doubled. Vitamin C and zinc are needed to help wounds heal. Liquid nutritional supplements or tube feeding can help meet this need. Adequate fluid is needed to help prevent and manage pressure sores.

Chronic Obstructive Pulmonary Disease. This condition often results in weight loss, and nutritional support will be needed. A higher intake of fat and moderate amounts of carbohydrate may help ease the work required of the lungs. It is primarily important to avoid overfeeding the patient when attempting to wean him or her from a ventilator.

Special supplemental formulas that are low in carbohydrate and higher in fat content, such as Pulmocare, are available. If TPN is used, the percentage of dextrose should not exceed 50 percent of kilocalories, with fat up to 40 percent as tolerated, with emphasis on avoiding excess kilocalorie intake.

AIDS. The use of nutritional support is always appropriate. Milk shakes, puddings, or commercial liquid supplements between meals can significantly increase kilocalorie and protein intake and help prevent weight loss. Tube feeding may also be desirable when oral intake is not adequate.

As with cancer, the question regarding the use of TPN has to do with the patient's prognosis. TPN should not be used for any terminally ill patients. If the person with AIDS has a reasonable life expectancy, and quality of life can be improved by correcting malnutrition but the person cannot achieve adequate nutrition with enteral support, TPN should be considered. Strict infection control guidelines should be adhered to with tube feeding and TPN.

WHAT ARE THE METHODS OF DELIVERING NUTRITIONAL SUPPORT TO THE PATIENT?

The techniques for providing the patient with optimal kilocalorie and nutrient requirements range from very simple to complex. Figure 14–1 shows how the type of nutritional support is determined. A patient receives nutritional support by oral feedings, tube feedings, peripheral parenteral nutrition, or total parenteral nutrition, all of which are discussed in the following sections. One major concern is providing adequate nutritional support without being too aggressive. One means to help determine kilocalorie needs of critically ill patients is use of the metabolic cart (see Fig. 4–3). The metabolic cart measures oxygen intake and carbon dioxide output to best estimate needed kilocalories.

Liquid Supplements. Supplemental foods must also adhere to the diet order prescribed for the patient. When selecting these foods or liquid commercial supplements, it is important that the patient sample various supplements and choose those preferred for between meals. This has three advantages: (1) it gives the patient control over an aspect of treatment; (2) it increases the likelihood of the supplement's being consumed; and (3) it avoids intolerance of foods caused by changes in taste perception.

Commercial formulas as well as pasteurized eggnog and milk shakes are among the most popular supplements. Commercial eggnogs should be used because they are pasteurized. Homemade eggnog made with raw eggs has a high risk of carrying salmonella (see Chapter 22). High-kilocalorie and high-protein puddings, gelatins, and soups have also been developed. The nutritional contents of some commercial products and specialized formulas are listed in Appendix 8.

Tube Feeding. Enteral nutritional support is also known as **tube feeding.** Tube feeding requires a functioning gastrointestinal tract. A tube feeding consists of blenderized foods or a commercial formula administered by a tube into the patient's stomach or small intestine. The enteral method of administering nutrients most closely resembles the body's own metabolic routes. The role of the liver in tube feeding is especially important because this organ extracts, processes, alters, and metabolizes the nutrients as they pass through it. Liver disease can inhibit the impact of nutritional support.

For temporary nutritional support, a small, flexible tube is inserted through the nose and placed either into the stomach **(nasogastric tube)** or beyond the stomach into the duodenum. The latter approach is used when there are concerns about vomiting and **aspiration** (food or liquid entering the lungs). The duodenal or jejunal positioning of the tube is also appropriate at times when stomach emptying may be impaired, such as after surgery. The tube may be left in place for several days and changed on an occasional basis as needed. Or the tube may be removed daily and repositioned each night, for example, in the case of home enteral nutritional support.

Long-term enteral nutrition may be required, such as with throat cancer or with neurological damage that causes swallowing difficulties. Long-term nutritional support is best done with the feeding tube implanted directly into the stomach (a **gastrostomy**) or the jejunum (a **jejunostomy**). The liquid supplement may be provided through gravity, by simply pouring the supplement at a slow rate directly into the tube (this is not recommended for jejunal feedings), or through the use of a pump set at the desired rate of flow. The supplement should not be excessively cold when administered. Possible complications of enteral feeding are listed in Table 14–2, with suggested solutions if problems arise.

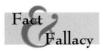

Fallacy: If diarrhea develops with tube feeding, the feeding must stop immediately.

Fact: The cause of diarrhea may be unrelated to formula use, especially if the formula is isotonic and lactose-free. Other problems should be ruled out such as the presence of hyperosmolar electrolyte solutions or sorbitol in some medications (Table 14–2).

What Are Common Sites for Tube Feeding?

The following are common routes for tube feedings (Fig. 14–2):

1. *Nasogastric:* The tube is passed through the nose to the stomach.
2. *Nasojejunal:* The tube is passed through the nose to the small intestine (also called nasoenteric).

Table 14–2
Enteral Feeding Complications and Problem Solving

Problem	Cause	Prevention/Treatment
Mechanical		
Aspiration pneumonia	Delayed gastric emptying, gastroparesis	Feed beyond the pylorus or ligament of Treitz Reduce administration rate Select isotonic or lower-fat formula Regularly check gastric residuals, tube placement, and abdominal girth Keep head of bed elevated 30° to 45° during and after feeding
	Gastroesophageal reflux Diminished gag reflex	Use small-bore feeding tubes to minimize compromise of lower esophageal sphincter Keep head of bed elevated 30° to 45° during and after feeding Initially and regularly check tube placement
Pharyngeal irritation, otitis	Prolonged intubation with large-bore NG tubes	Use small-bore feeding tubes whenever possible Consider gastrostomy or jejunostomy sites for long-term feeding
Nasolabial, esophageal, and mucosal irritation and erosion	Prolonged intubation with large-bore NG tubes Use of rubber or plastic	Use small-caliber feeding tubes made of bicompatible materials Tape feeding tube properly to avoid placing pressure on the nostril Consider gastrostomy or jejunostomy sites for long-term feeding
Irritation and leakage at ostomy site	Drainage of digestive juices from stoma site	Attention to skin and stoma care Use gastrostomy tubes with retention devices to maintain proper tube placement
Tube lumen obstruction	Thickened formula residue Formation of insoluble formula-medication complexes	Irrigate feeding tube frequently with clear water or use an enteral pump that provides a water flush Avoid instilling medications into feeding tubes, when possible Use liquid forms Irrigate tubes with clear water before and after delivering medications and formula, and after aspirating gastric contents
Gastrointestinal		
Diarrhea	Low-residue formulas	Rule out non-formula-related causes Select fiber-supplemented formula
	Rapid formula administration	Initiate feedings at low rate Temporarily decrease rate
	Hyperosmolar formula	Reduce rate of administration Select isotonic formula or dilute formula concentration and gradually increase strength
	Bolus feeding using syringe force	Reduce rate of administration Select alternate method of administration
	Hypoalbuminemia	Use hydrolyzed, peptide-based formulas or parenteral nutrition until absorptive capacity of small intestine is restored

Table continued on following page

Table 14–2
Enteral Feeding Complications and Problem Solving (*continued*)

Problem	Cause	Prevention/Treatment
Diarrhea (*continued*)	Nutrient malabsorption	Select a hydrolyzed, peptide-based formula that restricts offending nutrients
	Microbial contamination	Avoid prolonged hangtimes Use sanitary handling and administration techniques
	Disuse atrophy of the GI tract	Use enteral nutrition support whenever possible
	Rapid GI transit time	Select fiber-supplemented formula
	Prolonged antibiotic treatment or other drug therapy	Review medication profile and eliminate causative agent if possible
Cramping, gas, abdominal distention	Nutrient malabsorption	Select a hydrolyzed formula or one that restricts offending nutrients
	Rapid, intermittent administration of refrigerated formula	Administer formula by continuous method Administer formula at room temperature Advance administration rate according to patient tolerance
	Intermittent feeding using syringe force	Reduce rate of administration Select alternate method of administration
Nausea and vomiting	Rapid formula administration	Initiate feedings at low rate and gradually advance to desired rate Temporarily decrease rate
	Gastric retention	Select isotonic or dilute formula Reduce rate of administration Select low-fat formula Consider need for postpyloric feeding
Constipation	Inadequate fluid intake	Supplement fluid intake
	Insufficient bulk	Select fiber-supplemented formula
	Inactivity	Encourage ambulation, if possible
Metabolic		
Dehydration	Elevated fluid needs or losses of GI fluid and electrolytes	Supplement intake with appropriate fluids Monitor and intervene to maintain hydration status
Overhydration	Rapid refeeding	Use a calorically dense formula
	Excessive fluid intake	Reduce rate of administration, especially in patients with severe malnutrition or major organ failure
Hyperglycemia	Inadequate insulin production for the amount of formula being given	Select low-carbohydrate formula Initiate feedings at low rate Monitor blood glucose
	Metabolic stress Diabetes mellitus	Use insulin if necessary
Hypernatremia	Inadequate fluid intake or excessive losses	Assess fluid and electrolyte status Increase water intake

Table 14–2
Enteral Feeding Complications and Problem Solving (*continued*)

Problem	Cause	Prevention/Treatment
Hyponatremia	Fluid overload Syndrome of inappropriate antidiuretic hormone secretion (SIADH) Excessive GI fluid losses from diarrhea, vomiting Chronic feeding with relatively low-sodium enteral formulas as the sole source of dietary sodium	Assess fluid and electrolyte status Restrict fluids, if necessary Use diuretics, if necessary Use a rehydration solution such as EquaLYTE Enteral Rehydration Solution to replace water and electrolytes Supplement sodium intake, if necessary
Hypophosphatemia	Aggressive refeeding of malnourished patients Insulin therapy	Monitor serum levels Replenish phosphorus levels before refeeding
Hypercapnia	Excessive carbohydrate loads given patients with respiratory dysfunction and CO_2 retention	Select low-carbohydrate, high-fat formula
Hypokalemia	Aggressive refeeding of malnourished patient	Monitor serum levels Provide adequate potassium
Hyperkalemia	Excessive potassium intake Decreased excretion	Reduce potassium intake Monitor serum levels

Used with permission of Ross Products Division, Abbott Laboratories, Columbus, OH 43216. © From Enteral Nutrition Handbook © 1996. Roos Products Division, Abbott Laboratories.

3. *Gastrostomy:* The tube is surgically inserted into the stomach.
4. *Jejunostomy:* The tube is surgically inserted into the small intestine.

How Is the Type of Liquid Supplement Determined?

Digestive and absorption processes and nutrient needs should be ascertained to determine the type of liquid supplement required. If the person has the ability to digest all nutrients and can absorb all nutrients, any liquid preparation that meets the RDA for the person's kilocalorie needs is appropriate. Some supplements are designed for high-kilocalorie needs and other supplements are designed for low-kilocalorie needs. Thus, the kilocalorie needs might dictate the appropriate type of supplement. Formulas that provide 2 kcal/mL are useful for the fluid-restricted patient.

Often during times of stress the body is unable to break down lactose, which results in abdominal distention, bloating, and diarrhea. For this reason, many commercial supplements are lactose-free. Fat malabsorption is also common in many disease states. Medium-chain triglyceride (MCT) oil is another common in-

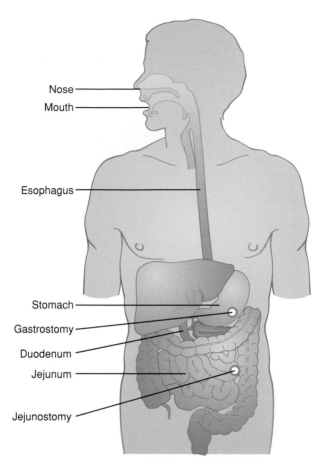

Nose
Mouth
Esophagus
Stomach
Gastrostomy
Duodenum
Jejunum
Jejunostomy

Figure 14–2
Tube feeding routes.

gredient in commercial supplements. MCT oil does not require bile salts so the fat is better absorbed.

A person's condition may require other diet restrictions such as low sodium, low sugar, low protein, or low potassium. There are specially developed formulas for these restrictions or related conditions, such as for kidney disease or diabetes. There are also formula modules that allow the patient to follow a "recipe" to meet individual needs.

If the patient's gastrointestinal tract is not fully functioning, a formula containing digested nutrients can be administered. These formulas are referred to as **elemental** or defined formula diets (e.g., Vivonex, Vital). They are commonly used for short bowel syndrome, intestinal malabsorption, and pancreatitis, depending on the severity of the condition. These formulas are absorbed in the upper part of the small intestine. Elemental formulas generally are given via tube feeding, as most patients do not like their taste.

All formulas should be refrigerated once they are mixed or opened to prevent bacterial contamination. Any unused portion of the formula should be discarded after 24 hours.

How Is the Amount or Rate of Flow Determined?

The amount of liquid supplement is determined by assessing the person's need for kilocalories, protein, fluid, vitamins, and minerals. The rate of flow when a pump is used can be calculated by a mathematical equation to meet the needs. For example, if the person can easily have the pump run for 12 hours and the supplement desired contains 1 kilocalorie per milliliter, 125 mL per hour for 12 hours would be required to meet 1500 kilocalories (divide 1500 mL by 12 hours to equal 125 mL per hour). However, this is too high an amount to start. Thus, a steady progression in flow rate is recommended, starting at about 50 mL per hour and increasing by about 25 mL every 12 to 24 hours until the desired rate is achieved. Or the length of time of tube feeding could be increased to allow for a slower rate of delivery while meeting the kilocalorie needs sooner.

If a pump (Fig. 14–3) is not used, the flow rate is more difficult to manage; however, management can be achieved using a clamp and timing the flow rate. Manual delivery through a gastrostomy should take at least 15 minutes. To help with tolerance, the solution should not be excessively cold.

How Are Fluid Needs Determined?

A good rule of thumb is that 1 mL of water is needed for each kilocalorie provided. The actual water content of commercial liquid supplements can be obtained from the manufacturer (see Appendix 2 for phone numbers of the major suppliers) but usually is about 75 to 80 percent of the total formula volume. Thus

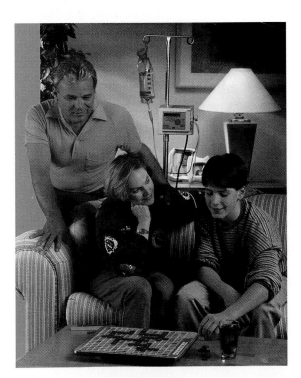

Figure 14–3
Tube feeding systems have been developed so that patients are not confined to a hospital bed. Some may even be used in the home. (Used with permission of Ross Products Division, Abbott Laboratories, Columbus, OH 43216. From Tube Feeding at Home, 1995 Ross Products Division, Abbott Laboratories.)

the volume of a 2000-kilocalorie solution is generally 2000 mL, but only about 1600 mL of that is actual water content. Water flushes to keep the tube clean are recommended each time a bag of formula is used. The amount of water for this purpose needs to be calculated into the patient's nutritional support regimen. All sources of fluid taken by the patient, including those taken for medication delivery, may need to be considered to avoid fluid overload.

Peripheral Parenteral Nutrition. The simplest form of **peripheral parenteral nutrition (PPN)** is intravenous dextrose (a 5 percent sugar solution—D5W— delivered into a vein of the arm). PPN is used in addition to oral intake and is often used in conjunction with delivery of a saline solution to treat dehydration. PPN can provide only minimal amounts of nutrition, as the route of access is a small vein. Therefore, although a patient may receive only PPN, he or she must receive it for a limited time period, and the catheter site should be rotated every 2 to 3 days.

Carbohydrate is the primary substrate used in PPN. Amino acid solutions that provide protein may also be used. Fat is generally not provided in PPN, but if it is, it should be in solutions of soybean or safflower oil (10 to 20 percent solutions).

Parenteral Nutrition. Parenteral nutrition is the most aggressive form of nutritional support and is often referred to as **total parenteral nutrition (TPN)** or **hyperalimentation.** TPN is best used when the GI tract is not functioning or in cases of severe vomiting when potential aspiration is a concern, such as in hyperemesis of pregnancy (see Chapter 16 for more concerns of pregnancy). TPN solutions are delivered directly into a large vein, which is necessary because of the amount of nutrients provided and the high osmolarity of the solutions.

TPN consists of a dextrose solution, such as **D50W** or **D70W.** D50W stands for 50 percent dextrose in water, which provides 1.7 kilocalories per milliliter of water. A protein solution—as well as vitamins, minerals, and trace elements in liquid form—is also provided with the dextrose on a daily basis. The protein source is amino acids. Fat emulsions are generally given about twice a week or daily to provide essential fatty acids and supplement the kilocalories provided by carbohydrate (dextrose) and protein (amino acids). A person with TPN sometimes is still able to eat or may do so in the transition to an oral diet.

Two important goals of TPN are to maintain a positive nitrogen balance and to prevent electrolyte imbalance. Weight gain should be no more than ½ pound per day. For patients in some stressed states, such as those with cancer, achieving a positive nitrogen balance can be very difficult. One problem may be a too aggressive use of glucose administration. A slow increase in glucose/dextrose delivery is important to increase the rates of insulin production without causing hyperglycemia.

HOW IS NUTRITIONAL SUPPORT MONITORED?

Serum glucose levels need to be monitored at least daily. In any physiological stress condition, glucose intolerance is common. Because many nutritional support preparations are high in sugar, a patient can easily reach unacceptably high levels of serum glucose. No patient should have a blood glucose (BG) level exceeding 200 mg/dL, and pregnant women should maintain a BG less than 120 g/dL at all times. Excess intake of carbohydrate can also elevate serum triglycerides, which should be monitored. Another indicator of excess carbohydrate intake is increased carbon dioxide production. Respiratory therapists can play a role in identifying tolerance to nutrition support. Modifications of supplement use, decreased rate of delivery, or implementation of insulin may be required to avoid hyperglycemia.

The serum albumin level should be monitored for all patients receiving tube feeding or TPN. A low level (less than 3.5 mg/dL) may hinder the patient's ability to absorb the formula. Albumin may then be administered parenterally (intravenously), and the formula should be diluted to one-quarter strength until the desired albumin level is reached (if the formula is isotonic, dilution is not necessary). Blood urea nitrogen (BUN) is a lab value that can indicate how the body is accepting the increased protein intake. A very high level can indicate too much protein in the feeding regimen but can also be a sign of dehydration or excessive protein breakdown due to inadequate kilocalorie intake. A low BUN level may indicate excess fluid intake, severe malnutrition, or impaired liver function.

Patients receiving tube feedings should be weighed daily to ensure that the patient is receiving adequate kilocalories to promote weight gain. Adequate fluid intake is especially important with formulas containing high amounts of protein so that the kidneys can efficiently excrete nitrogenous waste products. Encouraging the patient to drink fluids as well as rinsing the tube with water between feedings will help increase fluid intake. Electrolytes and appropriate nutritional assessment tests should be monitored weekly.

Patients receiving TPN need to have essential trace minerals such as chromium, copper, manganese, molybdenum, selenium, and zinc added to parenteral fluids to prevent the development of deficiency syndromes. Trace-metal monitoring is critical in infants and those on long-term TPN to prevent deficiency or toxicity (Leung, 1995).

Phlebitis (inflammation of a vein) is a potential complication of PPN, so the infusion site should be closely observed. The nursing staff is called on to pay strict attention to the care of the TPN catheter to avoid **sepsis** (infection) at the site of the catheter, which is one of the more common problems associated with TPN.

WHAT IS THE NUTRITION RECOVERY SYNDROME?

Also referred to as the **refeeding syndrome,** the nutrition recovery syndrome can occur when nutritional support is provided too aggressively, particularly in the malnourished person. As the cells begin to be renourished, they take nutrients from the plasma first. Thus low serum phosphorus levels are common when nutritional support is undertaken, and death can result if they become too low. Monitoring lab values is imperative to the safe use of nutritional support.

Overestimation of kilocalorie needs can cause the refeeding syndrome. An increase in the heart rate, temperature, and respiration rate may occur.

WHEN IS NUTRITIONAL SUPPORT DISCONTINUED?

Nutritional support should be gradually discontinued whenever the individual starts consuming enough food orally to maintain adequate nutritional intake. Small, frequent feedings are recommended. A low-residue and lactose-free diet may be necessary if diarrhea occurs, as is sometimes the case with patients who have been receiving TPN. If parenteral feedings are withdrawn too rapidly, hypoglycemia may result. Intravenous dextrose can help, or tube feedings may be needed to supplement the oral diet until the patient makes the final adjustment to oral feeding. Kilocalorie intake studies and daily weight records will indicate whether nutritional support can be withdrawn.

WHAT IS THE ROLE OF THE NURSE OR OTHER HEALTH CARE PROFESSIONAL IN NUTRITIONAL SUPPORT?

All health care professionals share the responsibility for identifying patients at risk for malnutrition. Routine weight assessments are critical. Unintentional weight loss should be a red flag, and a significant weight loss of 5 to 10 percent of the usual body weight should be brought to the attention of the primary care physician and a registered dietitian.

Once nutritional support is implemented, the health care professional should be aware of any potential complications. Diarrhea, constipation, abnormal lab values, continued weight loss or excessive weight gain, or deviation from the prescribed regimen should be brought to the attention of all health care professionals working with the patient.

It is also of vital importance that all health care professionals provide positive patient support. Expressing negative comments related to the taste of liquid supplements or squeamishness toward a catheter site is unprofessional and counterproductive to patient health.

Critical Thinking

Case Study

It had been one week since Nellie's husband was found unconscious in his mangled car after being hit by a drunk driver. The nurse was explaining to the family that he had been on total parenteral nutrition (TPN), initally due to the head injury which caused a fast rate of metabolism. However, the concern now was that he needed to use his "gut" to help make the transition to a regular diet. The doctor would place a tube through the patient's nose and go past his stomach to be sure he didn't accidently aspirate this feeding into his lungs. The nutrition department would provide a standard low-lactose formula to help prevent diarrhea.

Applications

1. Why might lactose be an issue with tube feeding?
2. Why might the health professionals have elected to use TPN before enteral feeding in treating this patient's head injury?
3. List clinical indicators that would suggest that this man had an intolerance to an enteral feeding regimen.

Study Questions and Classroom Activities

1. Why is the diet for patients with fractures, burns, and infections high in protein?
2. Taste-test a variety of liquid nutrition supplements such as Carnation Instant Breakfast, Ensure, and Sustacal. Compete with other classmates in a contest to develop the milk shake highest in kilocalories and protein that also tastes good.

References

Behrens R, Lang T, Muschweck H, Richter T, Hofbeck M: Percutaneous endoscopic gastrostomy in children and adolescents. J Pediatr Gastroenterol Nutr. November 1997; 25(5):487–491.

Buller HA: Problems in diagnosis of IBD in children. Neth J Med. February 1997; 50(2): S8–S11.

Dello Strologo L, Principato F, Sinibaldi D, Appiani AC, Terzi F, Dartois AM, Rizzoni G: Feeding dysfunction in infants with severe chronic renal failure after long-term nasogastric tube feeding. Pediatr Nephrol. February 1997; 11(1):84–86.

Ferguson RK, Soryal IN, Pentland B: Thiamine deficiency in head injury: A missed insult? Alcohol Alcohol. July 1997; 32(4):493–500.

Hochwald SN, Harrison LE, Heslin MJ, Burt ME, Brennan MF: Early postoperative enteral feeding improves whole body protein kinetics in upper gastrointestinal cancer patients. Am J Surg. September 1997; 174(3):325–330.

Leung FY: Trace elements in parenteral micronutrition. Clin Biochem. December 1995; 28(6):561–566.

Queen PM, Caldwell M, Balogun L: Clinical indicators for oncology, cardiovascular, and surgical patients: Report of the ADA Council on Practice Quality Assurance Committee. J Am Diet Assoc. 1993; 93(3):338.

Rombeau JL, Caldwell MD, eds: Clinical Nutrition: Parenteral Nutrition, 3rd ed. Philadelphia, WB Saunders, 1997.

Sand J, Luostarinen M, Matikainen M: Enteral or parenteral feeding after total gastrectomy: Prospective randomised pilot study. Eur J Surg. October 1997; 163(10):761–766.

University of Iowa Hospitals and Clinics: Recent Advances in Therapeutic Diets, 5th ed. Ames, IA, Iowa State University Press, 1996.

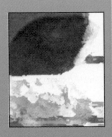

15

Physiological and Psychological Food Allergies and Food Intolerances

Objectives

After completing this chapter, you should be able to:

- Explain how food allergy and intolerance are diagnosed and treated.
- Explain the difference between food allergy and food intolerance.
- Identify common food allergens.
- Describe assessment and intervention strategies for psychological eating disorders.

Terms to Identify

Anaphylactic shock	Bulimarexia	Food intolerances
Anorexia nervosa	Bulimia	Immunoglobulin E (IgE)
Attention deficit hyper-activity disorder (ADHD)	Elimination diets	antibody
	Fight or flight response	Purging
Bipolar disorder	Food allergens/antigens	Schizophrenia
	Food allergy	

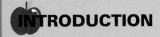

INTRODUCTION

Inadequate or inappropriate food intake can result from physiological or psychological problems, whether real or imagined. Food allergies are physiological conditions involving the immune system. Food intolerances may be either physiological or psychological. For example, lactose intolerance is a physiological problem related to the inability to digest milk sugar. Anorexia nervosa is a psychological problem in which the person may have a strong fear of eating. Persons with mental health problems may have altered thinking about food needs, tolerances, and intolerances.

The fields of medicine and psychology should be utilized in diagnosing and treating food allergies and intolerances. Problems need to be correctly diagnosed in order for health care professionals to plan the most effective intervention. Negative family functioning may be part of the cause of a patients eating disorder or may result from attempts to deal with food allergies and intolerances. Involving families in the assessment and planning stage promotes their support of the intervention plan. The school setting and the peer group also have an important impact on food choices. For example, how does the child with a wheat allergy deal with classroom birthday parties? This chapter explores physiological and psychological food intolerances.

WHAT IS A FOOD ALLERGY?

A **food allergy** is a condition that develops when a person is hypersensitive to certain proteins found in food. It is an immune response that can be mildly annoying or severe enough to induce death through **anaphylactic shock** (a life-threatening condition in which the breathing passages can be blocked). Peanuts, tree nuts, seafood and seeds, as well as milk and eggs can cause anaphylaxis in highly allergic children, and reexposure to such foods presents the risk of life-threatening reactions. All children at risk for food anaphylaxis should be identified, and their parents or caretakers should be prepared to administer epinephrine (adrenalin) before taking the child to the emergency room (Anderson, 1997).

The immune system is designed to destroy harmful foreign substances in the body. With food allergies, the body reacts to certain food proteins as if they were harmful substances. For this immune response to be avoided, the offending foods need to be reduced or entirely eliminated from the diet.

More young children than adults experience food allergies. Infants who are exposed to highly allergenic foods, such as egg whites, may have an increased risk of food hypersensitivity. Fortunately many children outgrow their food sensitivities and intolerances. However, millions of Americans suffer from food allergies.

Food allergens/antigens are the proteins or other large molecules from food that induce an immune response. The **immunoglobulin E (IgE) antibody** is produced in response to these "foreign" substances in an attempt to rid the body of them. IgE causes the typical allergy symptoms. Symptoms affect the skin, nasal passages, and respiratory or gastrointestinal tract. Hives, diarrhea, nausea, vomiting, cramps, headache, and asthma are common symptoms of food allergy. If the entire circulatory system is affected, shock occurs.

There are two major types of allergic reaction to foods: immediate and late. Immediate reactions are characterized by the rapid appearance of symptoms, often within minutes after the offending food is eaten or upon contact. The immediate allergic response is generally the more severe, and life-threatening, form of allergy. Late reactions are more subtle. Up to 48 hours may elapse between eating the allergenic food and the appearance of symptoms such as nasal congestion.

The foods that most often cause allergic reactions are milk, fish, shellfish, nuts, berries, egg whites, chocolate, corn, wheat, pork, and legumes (green peas, lima beans, and peanuts) and some fresh fruits, such as those in the peach family. As much as 31 percent of children and 80 percent of adults with food allergies are allergic to eggs. One form of egg protein, lysosyme, is used in cheese production but is not declared on food labels (Fremont et al., 1997). Peanut allergy is characterized by more severe symptoms than other food allergies and by high rates of symptoms on minimal contact (Hourihane et al., 1997).

Atopic dermatitis is one allergic condition that has a genetic basis but needs to be provoked by environmental influences. There is some hope that by identifying infants with a high risk for this condition, early avoidance of allergens may prevent its development. This approach should only be taken in consultation with a physician and registered dietitian to avoid possible adverse growth and development if food intake is being restricted (Hide, 1997). Breast-feeding or use of a partial whey hydrolysate formula was shown to reduce the incidence of eczema, food allergies, and asthma in children up to age 5 (Chandra, 1997).

HOW IS FOOD ALLERGY DIAGNOSED?

Medical Diagnostic Tests

Skin testing involves scratching or puncturing the skin with extracts of food. A skin reaction such as raised bumps around this area may be indicative of an immune response to the causative food extracts. The radioallergosorbent test (RAST) uses a blood sample. Both the skin test and the RAST can be incorrectly interpreted and thus are not considered infallible. The skin test should be performed under medical supervision to avoid or safely treat anaphylactic shock that can ensue.

Nutritional Diagnostic Tests

A detailed allergic history is important in diagnosing and managing food allergy. Specific details of foods, beverages, and medications ingested are recorded along with any noted symptoms for a period of 2 to 4 weeks. This close observation may help pinpoint problematic substances in the diet.

Elimination diets are used to determine the causative food allergen. These diets contain a few carefully chosen foods, with common allergens omitted. The elimination diet should be followed for 1 to 2 weeks. An improvement in physical symptoms may indicate that an allergenic food has been eliminated. Foods are slowly and cautiously put back into the diet, one food at a time for a few days. If no symptoms are noted, another food is added for another couple of days. This procedure is continued to ensure tolerance and to identify those foods that are linked to the redevelopment of allergic symptoms.

HOW ARE FOOD ALLERGIES TREATED?

Once food allergens are identified, a nutritionally adequate diet that eliminates the offending foods needs to be developed. Education is critical. A person may know he or she has a milk allergy but may not think of all foods made with milk, such as cream soups, margarine with milk solids, cheese, and milk chocolate. Alternative terms for milk protein on the food label—such as lactalbumin, lactoglobulin, casein, nonfat milk solids, or whey—may not be familiar to the patient. The services of a registered dietitian are helpful in patient education and may be required when the patient has multiple food allergies in order to avoid nutritional inadequacies. Tables 11–6, 15–1, and 15–2 list common foods to be

Table 15–1
Egg-Free Diet*

Food Group	Foods Allowed	Foods Excluded
Beverages	All plain milks, creams, and buttermilks Cocoa, tea, coffee Carbonated beverages	Eggnogs, malted beverages Beverages "cleared" with egg or shells
Soups	Creamed meat, fish, and vegetable soups prepared without egg (such as egg noodles)	Any soups "cleared" with egg or shells, egg powder, dried egg, and albumin
Protein sources	All plain meats, fish, and poultry (some severely allergic individuals cannot eat the meat of egg-laying chickens) Cheese	All breaded or batter-dipped foods if egg was used in the mix Sausages, croquettes, or loaves using egg as a binding agent
Vegetables	Fresh, frozen, canned, raw, or cooked	None unless combined with egg
Fruit	All fresh, frozen, canned, or dried All juices	None
Breads and cereals	Rye-Krisp, corn pone, beaten biscuits, and plain crackers Any homemade breads without egg Any breakfast cereal Rice Pasta made without egg	Gingerbreads, griddle cakes, muffins, waffles, fancy breads, pretzels, saltines Commercial breads and rolls containing eggs or that have been brushed with egg
Fats	All butters, creams, homemade salad dressings without eggs	All others unless label shows made without egg, albumin, or egg powder
Combination	Any made without egg or egg products	Any made with egg or egg products; avoid biscuit toppings, thickened sauces
Sweets and snacks	Plain fruit-flavored gelatins Fruit pies Ices Cookies, frostings, cakes and puddings made without eggs Popcorn, nuts, olives, pickles Sugars, hard candy	Prepared mixes for pancakes, cakes, cookies (may contain egg powder), cream-filled pies, meringues, ice cream, sherbet Some commercial candies that contain egg or albumin

*Adequacy: Since a perfectly well-balanced diet can be planned without eggs, if an individual eats the food provided, this diet can meet the recommended dietary allowances (1989 and 1997) for all nutrients.

Courtesy of the Bureau of Nutrition Services, Office of Mental Retardation and Developmental Disabilities, Albany, NY.

Table 15–2
Milk-Free Diet

Food Group	Foods Allowed	Foods Excluded
Beverages	Soft drinks Soya milk products Coffee, tea Decaffeinated coffee	All milk and milk-containing beverages
Soups	Any broth-based soup with no milk products	All creamed soups
Protein sources	All fresh meats Kosher luncheon meats, hot dogs, bologna, and salami labeled "Parve" (may be very spicy) All-beef hot dogs All poultry without stuffing All fish Eggs Dried beans, peas Peanut butter	Non-Kosher luncheon meats: bologna, salami, wieners, sausage, meat loaf, cold cuts Poultry with stuffing Meat balls, meat loaves Cheese Yogurt Breaded items that contain milk in batter or bread crumbs made with milk
Vegetables	Any fresh, canned, or frozen vegetables Pasta Rice	All creamed vegetables Any creamed sauces, including au gratin Mashed potatoes (unless made without milk)
Fruit	Any fresh, frozen, or canned fruit or juice	None
Breads and cereals	Rye-Krisp, homemade brands made without milk, rye breads Italian breads	Other baked goods
Fats	Poultry, meat, and pure vegetable fats and oils Dressings made without milk or milk products Margarine (without milk solids)	Butter Any salad dressings containing milk or cheese Gravy made with milk or cream
Combination	Any made without milk or milk products	Any dishes containing milk or milk products
Sweets and snacks	Plain fruit-flavored gelatin Angel and sponge cakes Fruit ices Jellies and jams Sugars, hard candy	Prepared mixes: waffle, cake, muffin, pancake Puddings, creams Ice cream, sherbet Milk chocolate candy

Courtesy of the Bureau of Nutrition Services, Office of Mental Retardation and Developmental Disabilities, Albany, NY.

omitted on the wheat-, rye-, and oat-free diets, the egg-free diet, and the milk-free diet.

Individuals who are sensitive only to wheat products can follow a gluten-restricted diet (see Table 11–6) in which wheat, rye, oats, and barley are omitted. However, the person with a wheat allergy may need to restrict only wheat. Persons with celiac disease and dermatitis herpetiformis (an allergic skin disorder) need to avoid all sources of gluten. There is new evidence that oats may be consumed in moderation for both persons with celiac disease and dermatitis herpetiformis (Hardman et al., 1997). Food products with cornmeal or rice flour are acceptable for persons with wheat allergy or gluten intolerance. Cornstarch can be used as a thickening agent. The American Dietetic Association can provide sources for allergy recipes (see Appendix 1). Many commercial products for allergy diets are available. Careful reading of the labels on such products is necessary to detect any specific allergen to be omitted in the diet. Writing to food manufacturers to inquire about possible cross-contamination (such as dusting the food conveyor belt with flour) can be helpful.

Often a person who is allergic to one food will be allergic to others in the same food family. For example, someone allergic to peanuts usually cannot eat peas or beans either, simply because they are members of the pea family.

HOW DO FOOD INTOLERANCES DIFFER FROM FOOD ALLERGIES?

Food intolerances do not involve the immune response; food allergies do. Food intolerances are not life threatening because the immune response is not evoked. Food allergies usually begin in childhood, whereas food intolerances can begin at any age. Food intolerances may have a biological basis, such as a lack of a digestive enzyme, or a psychological basis.

The general public often confuses intolerances and allergies, but it is important to know the difference. A person with milk allergy may become seriously ill from any trace of milk. But a person with lactose intolerance may be able to tolerate small quantities of milk or low-lactose forms of milk such as yogurt and cheese.

Psychosomatic illness, even though psychological in origin, can have physical consequences. This is because of the **"fight or flight" response** of the sympathetic system (the hormonal response to stress that induces increased heart rate and blood pressure). The overstimulation of the sympathetic nervous system can produce psychosomatic symptoms such as diarrhea. It is important to accurately diagnose physical intolerances as opposed to psychological ones so that effective intervention can be more appropriately planned.

WHAT ARE SOME COMMON FOOD INTOLERANCES?

Some food intolerances are well documented, whereas others are not understood or recognized. A common food intolerance that is well known throughout the world is lactose intolerance. See Chapter 11 for further discussion.

Fat Intolerance

Fat intolerance is often related to pancreatitis and gallstones. Alcoholism is commonly associated with pancreatitis and problems digesting fat. Vegetarians or others who normally follow a low-fat diet often report nausea and indigestion as a result of increased meat or fat intake. These are both physiological intolerances to fat. A person with psychological intolerance may think any fat listed on a food label is harmful. A low-fat meal containing 15 grams of fat should be physiologically tolerated. Although the person with psychological intolerance might find this amount of fat unacceptable for a meal, he or she should be told that this amount is safe, especially if the fat consumed is primarily monounsaturated fat.

Intolerance to Vegetables and Fruits

Intolerance to vegetables and fruit is highly individual. The problem may not be the food as much as the style of eating. Thorough chewing and eating slowly will lessen symptoms of intolerance. Many people avoid legumes (dried beans) because of excessive flatulence. Such people may benefit by slowly increasing amounts eaten. Chewing thoroughly and including adequate fluid in the diet are important. Some people find a commercial enzyme preparation such as Beano to be helpful (although persons with an allergy to mold should avoid this product as it is derived from mold). Older persons often find that lettuce causes indigestion or abdominal pain. Again, small amounts of lettuce that are thoroughly masticated may help. Jerusalem artichokes contain a type of carbohydrate that humans cannot digest. Undigested carbohydrate allows bacteria to multiply in the gastrointestinal (GI) tract, which leads to flatulence. Apple skin may be a problem for some people. The cause of intolerance may be a sudden increase in the fiber content of these foods. Gradually increasing the amounts of fruits and vegetables eaten may be beneficial.

Intolerance to Hot, Spicy Foods

An intolerance to hot, spicy foods is often associated with peptic ulcers, pancreatitis, and gallbladder disease. The intolerance may be physical or psychological in the case of persons who believe they cannot tolerate spicy foods. Intolerance to spicy foods is not diagnostic of peptic ulcers, although the amount of spicy food eaten may be related. Small amounts may be tolerated.

WHAT ARE SOME PSYCHOLOGICAL EATING DISORDERS?

Psychological eating disorders are increasingly recognized. Anorexia nervosa and bulimia not only are problems of weight control but also involve biological, psychological, and social factors. Obsessive dieting, refusal to eat, binge eating, gorging, purging, fasting, and laxative and diuretic abuse can lead to malnutrition, electrolyte imbalance, and cardiac arrhythmia, which can result in death. There are a variety of forms of eating disorders. The most common include anorexia nervosa (food restricter), bulimia (purging behavior), bulimia nervosa (food restricter with purging behavior), and binge eating disorder. Any nonphysiological reason to restrict or alter food intake might be termed an eating disorder when health is adversely affected.

Family relationships seem to contribute to the development of psychological and behavioral traits for risk of some eating disorders. One study found that bulimia nervosa is the result of exposure to general risk factors for psychiatric disorder and risk factors for dieting. Negative self-evaluation and certain parental problems were noted among those with bulimia nervosa (Fairburn et al., 1997). Disordered eating behavior is common and persistent in young women with diabetes and is associated with poor blood glucose control and a higher risk of diabetic retinopathy (Rydall et al., 1997). There is new evidence that eating disorders are not limited to younger persons. Eating disorders may occur whenever self-starvation or binge-purge behaviors become entrenched as sustaining behaviors in relation to bereavement, mood disorders, or interpersonal distress (Beck et al., 1996). "The emerging picture is that psychosocial factors seem to provide the most compelling factors in the etiology and onset of anorexia, while biological factors—in most cases induced by severe malnutrition and strenuous overexercising—predominate in the maintenance of the disorder" (Davis, 1997).

Other psychiatric problems, such as bipolar disorder (see later discussion) and schizophrenia, are associated with behavioral eating problems. Monitoring weight and diet is important in the management of psychiatric illness.

Anorexia Nervosa

Anorexia nervosa is characterized by a refusal to eat. Initially there is no real loss of appetite. However, once severe weight loss has occurred, hormonal changes are believed to take place that alter perception. The syndrome occurs mainly in girls after puberty, but about 10 percent of all cases of anorexia occur in boys and young men (Davis & Sherer, 1994). There is an increased risk of anorexia nervosa among high achievers and upper socioeconomic populations. Some common correlates of anorexia are as follows:

- An intense fear of becoming obese that does not lessen as weight loss progresses
- A disturbance of body image, such as claiming to feel fat even when emaciated
- Weight loss of at least 25 percent of original body weight
- Refusal to maintain body weight over a minimal healthy weight for age and height
- No known physical illness that would account for the weight loss
- Amenorrhea due to altered hormonal states
- Bizarre eating habits such as cutting food into tiny pieces or limiting intake to only a few foods
- Underlying low self-esteem
- Compulsive exercise habits

Dietary Treatment. The goal of treatment should be to restore good nutritional status and resolve the underlying psychological problems. Outpatient treatment is the preferred method. The person with anorexia nervosa who is 30 percent below normal weight and fails to gain weight, is in complete denial, or is suicidal should be hospitalized. Mortality rates of anorexia nervosa have been estimated between 5 and 20 percent (Neumarker, 1997). All members of the health care team must be aware of the need to individualize the care plan. The nurse's role includes closely supervising and encouraging the patient to eat all of the food provided. A trusting relationship between patient and health care professional is absolutely essential. It should be recognized that treatment will require a long-term, family-based approach, and a considerable amount of time is needed. Treatment is not always successful.

Bulimia

Bulimia is characterized by binge eating followed by purging through self-induced vomiting, abusive use of laxatives, or both. The person is afraid of becoming overweight and is aware that the eating pattern is abnormal. However, the bulimic patient loses control over eating and often eats large amounts of food rapidly. High-kilocalorie, easily ingested foods are chosen during binge episodes. Fasting then follows, often resulting in a weight fluctuation of as much as 10 pounds. **Bulimarexia** or bulimia nervosa is the term used to describe cycles of binge eating and **purging** (vomiting or laxative abuse) with undereating.

Dietary Treatment. In the hospital, food intake should be normalized to appropriate mealtimes, with close supervision after eating to control vomiting. Psychological assessment should take priority, and plans should be made for long-term, outpatient, family-based counseling with a health care professional trained in eating disorders. A total health care team effort is essential to ensure effective treatment. Short-term mortality, as compared to anorexia nervosa, is significantly lower but bulimia nervosa was found to become an entrenched pattern of eating in 20 percent of women studied (Keel & Mitchell, 1997). Outpatient dietary treatment of bulimia emphasizes regular mealtimes with appropriate food portions to satisfy hunger needs. Food is discouraged as a means of reward or comfort.

Attention Deficit Hyperactivy Disorder

Attention deficit hyperactivity disorder (ADHD) is the official term sanctioned by the American Psychiatric Association. The term attention deficit disorder (ADD) is an older but still used term. This disorder relates to a child's inability to pay attention and to sustain effort.

Many dietary theories have evolved over the years. One study demonstrated a beneficial effect of eliminating reactive foods and artificial colors from the diets of children with ADHD. Children with atopic dermatitis and ADHD had a significantly higher response rate than the nonatopic group (Boris & Mandel, 1994). Sugar has not been found to induce ADHD. Megavitamin therapy has also been advocated by some, however, megavitamins have not been proven to be effective in reducing the symptoms of ADHD in children, whereas they may increase blood levels of vitamins to toxic levels. Families and caregivers of ADHD children may need to be reminded of the adage "cause no harm" when it comes to restricting foods from the child's diet. This is especially true with ADHD because there is no proven dietary treatment at this time.

Bipolar Disorder

Bipolar disorder is characterized by alternating periods of mania and depression. During the manic stage, such persons are hyperactive and may have grandiose ideas that they do not require food as most people do. In the depressive stage, appetite for nutritious foods may be diminished while appetite for sweets and other non-nutritious foods may be increased. Lithium, a commonly used medication for treatment of bipolar disorder, is associated with increased blood glucose levels via increased glucagon production (Hermida et al., 1994).

Schizophrenia

Schizophrenia is a chronic mental disorder that causes bizarre perceptual disturbances such as visual hallucinations and delusions of hearing voices. A person with schizophrenia may feel that food has been poisoned. A health care team approach is strongly advised. Any attempts to encourage eating may cause the person to become even more suspicious that the food has been poisoned. A great deal of patience and a matter-of-fact approach are advisable when working with a person with schizophrenia.

WHAT IS THE ROLE OF THE HEALTH CARE PROFESSIONAL IN MANAGING FOOD ALLERGIES, INTOLERANCES, AND AVOIDANCES?

The nurse or other health care professional needs to be aware of the medical biases and unknowns when it comes to problems with food. The nurse should be supportive in listening to patients and their families describe food intolerances. Judgments should be avoided, such as the idea that psychosomatic illness is "all in the patient's head." The nurse should determine what valid testing has been undertaken to diagnose food allergies and intolerances. Assessment should include asking patients what foods they cannot tolerate. If major food groups, such as milk, are being omitted from the diet, the nurse or other health care professional should refer as needed to the patient's primary physician or a registered dietitian or both. The diagnosis should be confirmed when needed, and patient education should be provided to ensure good nutritional intake.

Critical Thinking

Case Study

Elizabeth was slowly increasing the amount of milk she drank. She had had lactose intolerance since she was diagnosed with celiac disease, but her dietitian had said that once her intestines healed she may again be able to tolerate regular milk. She had been able to use a lactose-reduced milk product but wanted to use regular low-fat milk because it was easier to find. Since she was a woman of Northern

European heritage, was thin, and had used steroids, Elizabeth was told she was at particular risk for osteoporosis (see Chapters 16 and 21).

Applications

1. Why might Elizabeth be able to safely resume drinking regular milk?
2. What symptoms might occur if Elizabeth drank too much regular milk?
3. How would you describe the difference between a milk allergy and lactose intolerance?
4. Do a nutrient analysis on milk (see Appendix 5). What nutrients are found in high amounts in milk (greater than one-third the RDA)? List food alternatives that might be consumed by someone with a milk allergy. By someone with lactose intolerance.

Study Questions and Classroom Activities

1. What are some symptoms of food allergy?
2. What is the difference between food allergy and food intolerance?
3. What are the characteristics of anorexia nervosa and bulimia?
4. Plan a day's menu for someone who is allergic to wheat and milk.

References

Anderson JA: Milk, eggs and peanuts: Food allergies in children. Am Fam Physician. October 1, 1997; 56(5):1365–1374.

Beck D, Casper R, Andersen A: Truly late onset of eating disorders: A study of 11 cases averaging 60 years of age at presentation. Int J Eat Disord. December 1996; 20(4):389–395.

Boris M, Mandel FS: Foods and additives are common causes of the attention deficit hyperactive disorder in children. Ann Allergy. May 1994; 72(5):462–468.

Chandra RK: Five-year follow-up of high-risk infants with family history of allergy who were exclusively breast-fed or fed partial whey hydrolysate, soy, and conventional cow's milk formulas. J Pediatr Gastroenterol Nutr. April 1997; 24(4):380–388.

Davis C: Eating disorders and hyperactivity: A psychobiological perspective. Can J Psychiatry. March 1997; 42(2):168–175.

Davis JR, Sherer K: Applied Nutrition and Diet Therapy for Nurses. Philadelphia, WB Saunders, 1994.

Fairburn CG, Welch SL, Doll HA, Davies BA, O'Connor ME: Risk factors for bulimia nervosa. A community-based case-control study. Arch Gen Psychiatry. June 1997; 54(6): 509–517.

Fremont S, Kanny G, Nicolas JP, Moneret-Vautrin DA: Prevalence of lysozyme sensitization in an egg-allergic population. Allergy. February 1997; 52(2):224–228.

Hardman CM, Garioch JJ, Leonard JN, Thomas HJW, Walker MM, Lortan JE, Lister A, Fry L: Absence of toxicity of oats in patients with dermatitis herpetiformis. N Engl J Med. December 25, 1997; 337(26):1884–1887.

Hermida OG, Fontela T, Ghiglione M, Uttenthal LO: Effect of lithium on plasma glucose, insulin and glucagon in normal and streptozotocin-diabetic rats: Role of glucagon in the hyperglycaemic response. Br J Pharmacol. March 1994; 111(3):861–865.

Hide DW: Early intervention for the prevention of atopic dermatitis. Pediatr Allergy Immunol. February 1997; 8(1):7–10.

Hourihane JO, Kilburn SA, Dean P, Warner JO: Clinical characteristics of peanut allergy. Clin Exp Allergy. June 1997; 27(6):634–639.

Keel PK, Mitchell JE: Outcome in bulimia nervosa. Am J Psychiatry. March 1997; 154(3):313–321.

Neumarker KJ: Mortality and sudden death in anorexia nervosa. Int J Eat Disord. April 1997; 21(3):205–212.

Rydall AC, Rodin GM, Olmsted MP, Devenyi RG, Daneman D: Disordered eating behavior and microvascular complications in young women with insulin-dependent diabetes mellitus. N Engl J Med. June 26, 1997; 336(26):1849–1854.

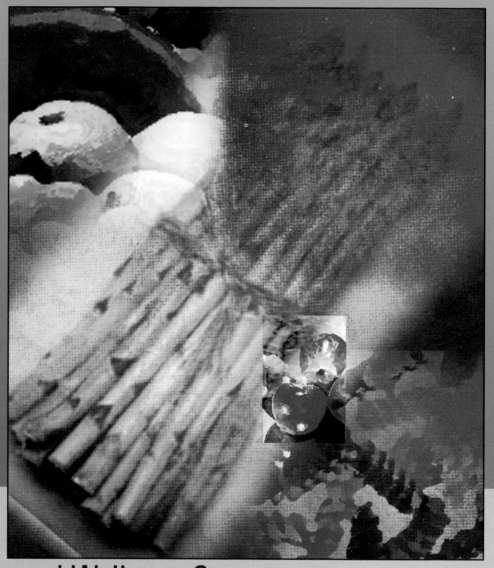

Lifespan and Wellness Concerns in Promoting Health and Managing Illness

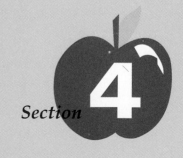

Section **4**

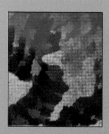

16
Maternal and Infant Nutrition

Objectives

After completing this chapter, you should be able to:

- Describe nutritional needs during pregnancy, lactation, and infancy.
- Describe lactation management techniques.
- Describe infant feeding strategies.
- Describe women's health concerns.

Terms to Identify

Antidiuretic hormone
Colostrum
Denver Developmental
    Screening Test
Diuresis
Embryo
Esophageal sphincter
Failure to thrive (FTT)
Fetal alcohol syndrome
Fetus
Fore milk
Gavage feeding
Gestational
Hind milk

Immunoglobulin A (IgA)
Lactation
La Leche League
Let-down reflex
Milk anemia
Nursing-bottle mouth
Obstetrician
Otitis media
Oxytocin
Pediatrician
Physiological anemia
Pica
Pincer grasp
Placenta

Postpartum blues
Preconception
Preeclampsia
Pregnancy-induced
    hypertension (PIH)
Premenstrual syndrome
    (PMS)
Prenatally
Preterm milk
Products of conception
Unsaturated fat
Spina bifida
Toxemia
Weaning

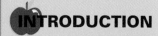 **INTRODUCTION**

The human species is very resilient, having survived over the centuries with wide differences in nutritional intake. Many adults are healthy today even though as infants they were fed under less than ideal circumstances. Only in this century have nutritional health, reproduction, and ways to promote the healthiest babies

Table 16–1
Fetal Development

First Trimester (Embryo; Critical Stage)	Second Trimester (Fetus)	Third Trimester to Birth
Organs develop (4–12 weeks) Central nervous system develops (4–12 weeks) Skeletal structure hardens from cartilage to bone (4 weeks)	Growth and development continue (13–40 weeks) Teeth calcify (20 weeks) Fetus can survive outside womb (24 weeks)	Growth and development continue Storage of iron and other nutrients (36–40 weeks; premature babies often deficient in iron) Development of necessary fat tissue (36–40 weeks)

been fully understood. It is now widely accepted that nutrition plays a vital role in a healthy pregnancy and baby.

Growth of the **fetus** (the unborn baby; Table 16–1) may be affected by various maternal factors, for example, the ingestion, digestion, and absorption of food materials (nutrients) from the mother's intestinal tract. The fetus is dependent on these processes as well as on maternal metabolism of the absorbed nutrients and transfer of nutrients through the **placenta** (an organ that allows the transfer of maternal nutrients to the fetus via the umbilical cord). An intact placenta of good size is critical for the ideal growth of the fetus.

The impact of maternal nutrition does not stop at birth. Breast-feeding, preparation for a future successful pregnancy, and even the infant's meal environment are all influenced by the mother's nutrition. A well-nourished mother is better able to cope with the demands of infant care, and a well-nourished infant displays a pleasant disposition, facilitating the return of the mother's strength and vitality. Maternal and infant nutrition is very much a reciprocal relationship.

HOW DOES NUTRITION INFLUENCE THE OUTCOME OF PREGNANCY?

The development of the **embryo** (the fetus during the first trimester) is the critical period of pregnancy (see Table 16–1), although pregnancy is often not recognized until a significant amount of time in the first trimester has passed. It is for this reason that the **preconception** (prior to conception) nutritional status is now considered so important. This is especially true for a woman with diabetes (see later discussion). Maternal nutritional counseling should cover the preconceptual and postpartum periods as well as the more traditional **gestational** (time of pregnancy) period.

Adequate nutrition without excess mineral or vitamin intake can help prevent some birth defects. For example, **spina bifida** (a neural tube birth defect in which the spine does not close) is associated with inadequate intake of folate. Neural tube defects are among the most common and serious birth defects (Tinkle & Sterling, 1997). Certain foods are now fortified with folate as a means to reduce the nation's incidence of neural tube defects. Adequate nutrient availability during the first trimester can help the embryo form well-developed organs such as heart, lungs, liver, kidneys, and intestines. It is important that the preconception nutritional status be good because pregnancy is often not confirmed, or even suspected, until the end of the first trimester. Appropriate weight gain and avoidance of excess nutrients such as vitamin A **prenatally** (during pregnancy) are further associated with reduced morbidity and mortality. Much more information needs to be learned about the prevention of birth defects. It is known that not all defects are amenable to nutritional intervention. Nutrition has no affect, for example, on genetic disorders.

WHAT NUTRITIONAL ADVICE IS RECOMMENDED DURING PREGNANCY?

Weight Gain. A major determinant of fetal outcome during pregnancy is maternal weight gain. Prior to 1960, pregnant women were encouraged to restrict their weight gain to less than 15 pounds. Current research shows that more liberal weight gain improves fetal growth. A woman who is underweight prenatally needs to gain more weight than is typically recommended in order to best promote growth of the **products of conception** (Fig. 16–1). It is imperative that the placenta grow adequately, because it transfers maternal nutrients to the fetus.

Ideal weight gain is now considered to be about 25 to 35 pounds for normal-weight women, (that is, those who have a body mass index [BMI] of 20 to 26; body mass index equals body weight in kilograms divided by the square of the height in centimeters—see Chapter 20 and Appendix 12 for a nomogram to easily determine BMI), 28 to 40 pounds for an underweight woman (BMI < 20), and 15 to 25 pounds for an overweight woman (BMI > 26) with an average weight gain of about 1 pound per week in the second and third trimesters of pregnancy. A general weight gain grid can be used to plot weight gain throughout the pregnancy (Fig. 16-2). Excess weight gain during pregnancy should be discouraged, but not if doing so would cause nutrient deficiencies.

Women who are malnourished, such as those raised in third-world countries, with consequent small hip growth may be at higher risk for cesarean sections if their diet greatly improves during pregnancy. This is due to the prenatally well-nourished fetus's head or shoulders growing larger than the mother's pelvis will allow (Abitbol et al., 1997).

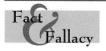

Fallacy: Because a pregnant woman is "eating for two," she should eat twice as much.

Fact: It should be remembered that the second person is very small—about 7 pounds at birth. Although some nutrient requirements increase dramatically during pregnancy, the overall kilocalorie needs increase only about 15 percent, amounting to about 150 extra kilocalories a day during the first trimester and 350 additional daily kilocalories for the remainder of the pregnancy. Thus, it is important that a pregnant woman consume mainly nutrient-dense foods (foods that have a lot of nutrients for the amount of kilocalories).

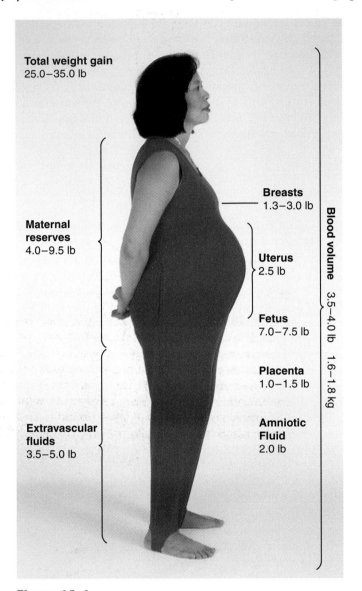

Figure 16–1

Components of weight gain during pregnancy. (From Gorrie TM, McKinney ES, Murray SS: Foundations of Maternal-Newborn Nursing, 2nd ed., Philadelphia, WB Saunders, 1998, p. 192, Fig. 9–1.)

Nutrient Needs. To promote maternal and infant health, a pregnant woman should be encouraged to consume at least the minimum number of servings from the Food Guide Pyramid (Table 16–2), with a focus on the use of whole grains and unprocessed or minimally processed foods. Protein intake needs to be adequate. One study found that a diet containing 20 percent protein versus 9 percent

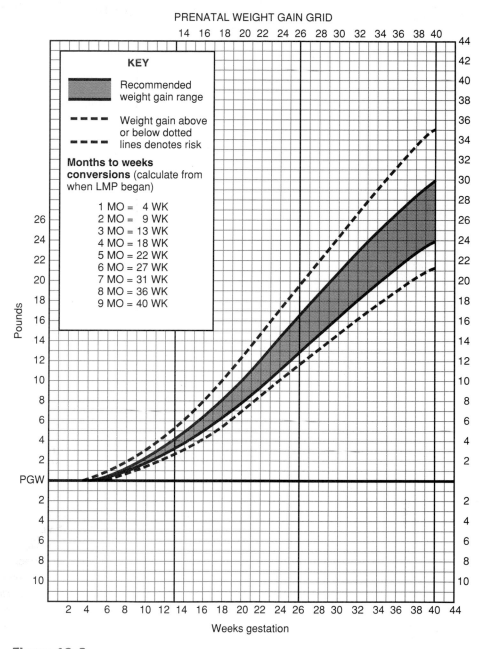

Figure 16–2

Recommended prenatal weight gain. Chart to monitor weight gain throughout pregnancy. KEY: PGW = pregestational weight (weight prior to conception). (From the New York State Health Department, WIC Program.)

Table 16–2

Changes in Foods from the Food Guide Pyramid Groups during Pregnancy and Lactation

Food Guide Pyramid Groups*	Nonpregnant Women	Pregnant Women (second half of pregnancy)	Lactating Women
Milk			
Adult	2 cups or more	3 cups or more	4 cups or more
Adolescent	4 cups or more	5 cups or more	5 cups or more
Vegetable and fruit			
Citrus and substitute	1 serving	2 servings	2–3 servings
Dark green leafy or deep orange vegetable	1 serving at least every other day	1 serving daily	1–2 servings daily
Other fruits or vegetables, including potatoes	3–4 servings	2 servings	2 servings
Meat or alternate	2 servings or more	3 servings or more (6 oz cooked or more)	
Cereal and bread whole grains	6 servings or more	6 servings or more	6 servings or more
		If fortified milk is not used, obtain physician's instructions for vitamin D supplementation Use iodized salt Use water or other beverages—at least 6 to 8 cups daily	

*Additional servings of these or any other food may be added as needed to provide the necessary calories and palatability.

led to different outcomes that may have life-long implications. The low-protein diet had a long-term adverse impact on glucose transport and insulin use (Ozanne et al., 1997).

Minerals such as zinc, copper, and magnesium are found in whole grains and legumes. Adequate consumption of dark green leafy vegetables and deep orange vegetables and fruits should be encouraged for a source of beta-carotene (vitamin A). Vitamin C foods, such as citrus fruits and dark green leafy vegetables, should be increased during pregnancy and lactation. A well-balanced diet will help the fetus grow well and allow the mother to stay healthy for future pregnancies. Table 16–3 shows a sample menu.

Intake of nonessentials such as fats and sugars can be safely restricted in pregnancy as needed to achieve appropriate weight gain. A minimum intake of 20 to 30 grams of fat is needed to prevent essential fat deficiency but 0 grams of added sugar is still healthy. Salt intake can be moderated but should not be rigidly restricted. The food label guidelines of 2400 mg of sodium is appropriate for the pregnant woman. Vitamin supplements should be used only as added insurance, not as a replacement for nutrients found in foods. Supplements should not exceed 100 percent of the recommended daily allowance (RDA; Table 16–4). Iron is the only nutrient routinely supplemented during pregnancy. One study found that infant length and Apgar scores were significantly higher in infants whose mothers received iron during pregnancy (Preziosi et al., 1997). Pregnant women following a

Table 16–3
Sample Meal Plans for Pregnancy

	Pregnant Woman	Pregnant Adolescent*
Breakfast	Orange juice, 1 cup[†] Shredded wheat Scrambled egg Toast, 1 slice Milk, 1 cup Decaffeinated coffee	Orange juice, 1 cup[†] Shredded wheat Scrambled egg Toast, 2 slices Butter or margarine Marmalade[†] Milk, 1 cup
Lunch	Tuna sandwich Carrot and green pepper sticks Oatmeal cookies[†] Milk, 1 cup	Tuna sandwich on whole-wheat bread Carrot and green pepper sticks Cheese cubes Oatmeal cookies[†] Fresh fruit Milk, 1 cup
Midafternoon	Milk, 1 cup	Chicken sandwich Milk, 1 cup
Dinner	Broiled steak Steamed broccoli Baked potato Tomato salad with French dressing Apple slices	Broiled steak Steamed broccoli with melted cheese Baked potato with sour cream Vegetable salad with French dressing Apple with peanut butter Milk, 1 cup
Bedtime	Hot milk or cocoa,[†] 1 cup	Milk or cocoa,[†] 1 cup

*Needs more kilocalories, protein, and calcium.
[†]For women with gestational diabetes, juice may be contraindicated for control of blood glucose; oranges or other vitamin C-containing fruit may be advised later in the day rather than at breakfast, and desserts should be restricted based on values obtained from the woman's self-monitoring of blood glucose levels (SMBG).

vegan diet need to ensure adequate intake of vitamin B_{12} through fortified foods or as a supplement. Vitamin D is also difficult to obtain in a vegan diet and the pregnant woman's diet should be supplemented unless she receives adequate sun exposure of at least 15 minutes daily. Good nutritional intake should be maintained after delivery for healthy lactation and in preparation for a future pregnancy.

Women who have difficulty adhering to these guidelines or who have high-risk pregnancies are encouraged to consult a registered dietitian or qualified nutritionist.

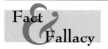
Fact & Fallacy

Fallacy: A few cups of coffee per day poses no risk during pregnancy.

Fact: There is conflicting evidence about how much caffeine is safe during pregnancy. Caffeine is known to cause blood vessels to constrict, thus potentially limiting blood flow through the placenta to the growing fetus. Until more is known, the prudent approach is to cut back on coffee and other caffeine sources gradually to no more than one cup or 200 mg daily.

Table 16–4
RDAs during Pregnancy and Lactation

	Nonpregnant Women				Lactation	
	14–18 Years	19–30 Years	31–50 Years	Pregnancy	First 6 Months	Second 6 Months
Kilocalories	2200	2200	2200	2500	2700	2700
Protein (g)	44	46	50	60	65	62
Vitamin A (RE)	800	800	800	800	1300	1200
Vitamin D (μg)*	10	10	5	10	10	10
Vitamin E (mg TE)	8	8	8	10	12	11
Vitamin C (mg)	60	60	60	70	95	90
Folate (μg)†	180	180	180	400	280	260
Niacin (mg)	15	15	15	17	20	20
Riboflavin (mg)	1.3	1.3	1.3	1.6	1.8	1.7
Thiamine (mg)	1.1	1.1	1.1	1.5	1.6	1.6
Vitamin B_{12}	2	2	2	2.2	2.6	2.6
Calcium (mg)*	1200	1200	800	1200	1200	1200
Phosphorus (mg)	1250	700	700	700	700	700
Iodine (μg)	150	150	150	175	200	200
Iron (mg)	15	15	15	30	15	15
Magnesium (mg)	360	310	320	350	310	310
Zinc (mg)	12	12	12	15	19	16
Iodine (μg)	150	150	150	175	200	200
Selenium (μg)	50	55	55	65	75	75

*Adequate intake (AI) level differs from the RDA (see inside front cover).
†It is now recommended that all women of child-bearing years include 400 μg of folate either from foods or from supplements in order to reduce the incidence of neural-tube defects.
From National Academy of Sciences National Research Council: Recommended Dietary Allowances, 10th and 11th eds. Washington, DC, National Academy of Sciences, 1989 and 1997.

WHAT ARE SOME COMMON AND CLINICAL PROBLEMS DURING PREGNANCY?

Nausea

Nausea sometimes occurs in the first trimester and on occasion throughout the entire pregnancy. The cause of the nausea is not fully understood but is probably related to hormonal changes during pregnancy. In line with this, an increased level of progesterone in pregnancy has been found to change the motility throughout the gastrointestinal (GI) tract. Changes in the gastric and small bowel motility can lead to nausea and vomiting with abdominal bloating and constipation (Baron et al., 1993). Fried foods and other high-fat foods further reduce GI motility and should be avoided unless tolerated and allowable within weight gain goals.

Another theory on the cause of nausea is related to low blood sugar levels, since nausea seems to increase when a woman has not eaten for a period of time.

Eating high-carbohydrate foods, such as dry toast or crackers, before arising may alleviate the problem. A gradual increase of food intake during the late afternoon and evening can replace nutrients that were not consumed in the morning (a common time for nausea).

Hyperemesis

Hyperemesis is characterized by excessive and prolonged vomiting. It probably is more common than statistics show, since treatment may be in a physician's office rather than in a hospital setting. One study found a 1.5 percent rate of hyperemesis among pregnant women and noted a low incidence of psychiatric disorder, which has been a theory in the past (Tsang et al., 1996). One cause of hyperemesis has been found to be hyperthyroidism (Nader & Mastrobattista, 1996). Hyperemesis can cause serious dehydration, and weight loss of over 5 percent is considered indicative of hyperemesis. The effects of prolonged vomiting can be serious. Charlotte Brönte, the famous writer, died of hyperemesis in 1855.

Hospitalization with administration of intravenous fluids may be necessary, as may more aggressive medical management. When total parenteral nutrition (TPN) is indicated, it can be lifesaving for both the mother and the fetus (Badgett & Feingold, 1997). Caution still needs to be exercised, as there are at least two published cases of maternal and fetal demise in connection with TPN. Enteral nutrition has been effective and can be considered as an alternative to total parenteral nutrition in the management of hyperemesis gravidarum (Hsu et al., 1996).

One study of women with hyperemesis found that more than 60 percent had suboptimal biochemical status of thiamine, riboflavin, vitamin B_6, vitamin A, and retinol-binding protein with evidence of dehydration. Thus repletion of fluid status and the correction of malnutrition are important in managing hyperemesis (van Stuijvenberg et al., 1995).

When severe nausea and vomiting are adversely affecting weight gain, all foods that are tolerated are considered acceptable. Nutrient density becomes a minor issue when kilocalories are paramount in promoting weight gain. Chocolate, potato chips, donuts, and other foods generally not considered the healthiest choices are appropriate if tolerated when increased total kilocalorie intake becomes necessary to prevent weight loss.

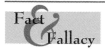

Fallacy: Hyperemesis is psychological in origin.

Fact: There is little evidence that hyperemesis is caused by psychological problems. It is more likely that hyperemesis is the cause of psychological distress. Hyperemesis is known around the world. The evidence is much stronger that hormonal or other physical causes are the basis of the development of hyperemesis. Smells, odors, and motion often precipitate the nausea and vomiting.

Anemia

Anemia from iron deficiency may occur during pregnancy when iron intake and stores do not meet the demand. This is preventable and treatable by daily supplements of 30 to 60 mg of ferrous salts.

Anemia from folate deficiency may occur if the intake of food and nutrients is poor. A daily supplement of 400 µg of folacin and improvement in eating habits will correct the anemia. Anemia from folate deficiency is likely to decrease in incidence with recent food fortification of this vitamin.

Physiological anemia also results from the expanded volume of blood (plasma increases without a concomitant increase in red blood cells). There is controversy in the medical field over whether this form of anemia needs to be treated. However, until further research indicates otherwise, increased intake of iron is advised.

Constipation

Constipation can be related to iron supplementation as well as to decreased intestinal motility, which is believed to be a normal physiological process that assists in nutrient absorption during pregnancy. Adequate fiber, fluid, and appropriate exercise can help control constipation. Laxatives should only be used on the advice of an **obstetrician** (a physician specializing in pregnancy).

Heartburn

Heartburn in pregnancy is believed to be caused by the pressure of the growing fetus on the stomach, resulting in the stomach's hydrochloric acid content being forced into the esophageal area. For this reason, pregnant women may find it helpful to eat more frequent, smaller meals and to avoid a reclining position after meals. Excess fat intake can contribute to heartburn by allowing stomach contents to remain in the stomach for longer periods. Excess fat is also associated with relaxed muscle tone of the **esophageal sphincter** (the muscle connecting the stomach and esophagus), which further promotes hydrochloric acid being forced back up into the esophagus. The woman should not take over-the-counter medication for heartburn without consulting her obstetrician.

Pica

The practice of **pica** (eating nonfood items, especially clay or laundry starch) during pregnancy is a carryover from a tradition in Africa, where it is still practiced in some areas. The consumption of clay can provide a source of calcium, iron, and other minerals. However, it can also provide toxic contaminants. When clay is not available in this country, laundry starch is sometimes substituted. Intake of these substances can interfere with consumption of adequate nutrients and their absorption and their use should be discouraged.

The practice of pica is not often revealed, especially if the health care professional appears to have a judgmental attitude. Great sensitivity needs to be used by the health care professional in order to elicit an accurate assessment of the practice of pica. Because pica is generally related to cultural heritage and beliefs, changing the practice may be difficult. Using objective measures, such as informing the woman about the danger of anemia or lead poisoning, may help her understand the negative consequences of pica.

Closely Spaced Pregnancies

Although many parents plan to space their children close together so that the children can be playmates, it is healthier for the mother and the fetus for pregnancies to be at least 12 to 18 months apart. Longer spacing helps the mother reestablish good nutritional stores.

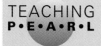

TEACHING P•E•A•R•L   Two effective assessment questions concerning nutritional preparation for subsequent pregnancies could be, "Are you planning to have another pregnancy in the future?" and if so, "What have you heard is the ideal spacing between pregnancies?"

Weight Reduction

A weight reduction regimen should not be initiated at any time during pregnancy. Overweight women should observe the same principles of prenatal nutrition as do women of normal weight. The total weight gain, however, should be smaller, averaging about 15 to 20 pounds, thus limiting sugar and fat intake becomes important.

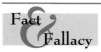

Fallacy: You can safely avoid gaining too much weight during pregnancy by taking calcium supplements instead of drinking milk.

Fact: Milk provides more nutrients than just calcium. A calcium supplement will not give you the extra 30 grams of protein found in the recommended four cups of milk. Riboflavin and other nutrients, such as potassium, magnesium, phosphorus, vitamins A and D, and other trace elements, are found in milk as well. Low-fat or skim milk can be used by weight-conscious women.

Pregnancy-Induced Hypertension

Pregnancy-induced hypertension (PIH), formerly known as **toxemia,** is a condition that may occur during the third trimester of pregnancy. Its cause is not known, but it is no longer felt to be a toxic condition; therefore, the term toxemia is no longer used. PIH is characterized by proteinuria, elevated blood pressure, and rapid weight gain caused by edema.

Preeclampsia is associated with symptoms of PIH. Eclampsia (the most severe form of preeclampsia) is associated with convulsions and coma. Some symptoms that can indicate its development include a sudden rise in blood pressure, severe headache, blurred vision, and proteinuria (protein in the urine). One study found significant risk factors for the development of preeclampsia were body mass index, blood pressure, ethnic heritage, and smoking (Sibai et al., 1997).

The former practices of restricting kilocalories and sodium to reduce the risk of PIH complications are now considered obsolete. To the contrary, there is a greater incidence of PIH among underweight women who fail to gain weight normally during pregnancy. The evidence indicates that the total amount of weight gain per se is not the significant factor. Sodium restriction is no longer recommended and may actually be harmful as sodium needs increase during pregnancy. However, avoiding excessive salt intake is recommended for pregnant women, as well as for the general population.

Diabetes

Type 1 diabetes, also called insulin-dependent diabetes mellitus (IDDM), was once considered an automatic cause for alarm if pregnancy developed. We now know that if a pregnant woman with this type of diabetes achieves near normal blood glucose control prior to conception and throughout the pregnancy, she is as likely to bear a healthy, normal infant as is for a woman without diabetes. It is paramount, however, that tight control over blood sugar levels be obtained prior to conception to help prevent birth defects from developing during the critical first trimester of organ development. For women with preexisting Type 2 diabetes (formerly called non-insulin dependent or NIDDM), the same precautions need to be taken.

Gestational diabetes mellitus (GDM, a form of diabetes that occurs only during pregnancy) is not associated with birth defects, because the elevated blood sugar does not develop until after the critical first trimester is over. The consequences of uncontrolled GDM are more problematic at the time of birth. A woman with GDM has an increased likelihood of delivering a large baby who is very susceptible to hypoglycemia in the first few hours after birth. Strict control of blood glucose during pregnancy will increase the chances of normal labor and delivery of a healthy baby without complications. Routine screening for GDM now is done between the 24th and 28th weeks of pregnancy. Women who have a family history of Type 2 diabetes, are of older age, or are overweight are all at increased risk of GDM (Solomon et al., 1997). Childhood obesity and developmental disturbances are found associated with diabetic pregnancies (Rizzo et al., 1997).

Control of pregnancy with diabetes is best handled with a medical team approach so that the most appropriate plan and means of control are developed, including aspects such as insulin, diet, and home glucose monitoring. Maternal blood sugar levels should range from 60 to 90 mg/dL (fasting) to a maximum of 120 mg/dL (1 to 2 hours after meals). High post-prandial blood sugar levels may indicate a need for further carbohydrate restriction (breakfast often needs to be very limited in carbohydrate), a need for insulin, or both. Morning urine ketones also need to be monitored. Too little intake of carbohydrate, too little insulin production, or weight loss of any amount can cause the mother's body fat to be broken down excessively. The resulting ketone buildup is potentially detrimental to the growing fetus and needs to be corrected with increased carbohydrate, at night especially, insulin, or both.

Alcohol Use

Fetal alcohol syndrome is caused by excessive alcohol intake by the mother during pregnancy. It is characterized by wide-set eyes, along with mental retardation and other physical characteristics. Because the safe limit of alcohol intake is not known, the best advice for the pregnant woman is to drink no alcohol. Professional counseling may be necessary.

Drug Addiction

The use of illegal drugs, as well as legal drugs, such as tobacco and alcohol, impairs fetal growth. Women who are addicted before conception often deny the problem and present a challenge to the health care professional. Good nutrition is vital so that complications associated with drug use are not exacerbated.

Adolescent Pregnancy

Depending on the age of the teenager as well as other risk factors, an adolescent pregnancy may be perfectly normal or extremely high risk. Younger teenagers and those who become pregnant near the time of menarche are most at risk. The proportion of teenagers who have ever had sexual intercourse decreased slightly in the 1990s and use of condoms increased, which appears related to the decreased teen birth rate observed during this time (Abma et al., 1997). Pregnant teenagers may have dietary habits that include foods low in essential nutrients, resulting in lower than recommended intake of nutrients that are especially important during pregnancy. A concern over body image may result in inadequate weight gain.

Programs for pregnant teenagers, common in most communities, offer social support, encouragement to seek good medical care, and assistance in completion of school. The Women, Infants, and Children Supplemental Nutrition Program (WIC) (see Chapters 2 and 22) is generally available to all lower-income pregnant teenagers, and referral should be made by the health care professional. This is a nutrition program that provides food vouchers for the pregnant teenager to use for purchasing specified foods that meet needs for calcium, vitamin C, and iron. Nutrition assessment and education is also provided.

Breast-feeding is possible for the motivated teenager, although other life concerns may take precedence. However, breast-feeding should be promoted for all women and teens unless specifically contraindicated by a doctor. Even a few days or weeks of breast-feeding can be beneficial to the newborn infant.

HOW DOES DIET INFLUENCE THE NURSING COUPLE?

The impact of maternal diet on infant growth does not end at delivery. This is true even for non-nursing mothers, who need to maintain their nutritional status in order to best cope with the demands of a new baby. During **lactation** (production of milk for breast-feeding; also referred to as "nursing"), adequate diet becomes more critical. Kilocalorie intake can affect the quantity of milk produced, and thus it is important for a breast-feeding woman to lose any excess weight slowly (an initial rapid loss will result from fluid loss after delivery, which is unrelated to kilocalories). Other nutrients vary in their impact on the quality of breast milk. In general, problems are limited to the excessive intake of fat-soluble vitamins through the indiscriminate use of supplements in megadoses and insufficient intake of water-soluble vitamins. Minerals do not generally affect the quality of breast milk, since development of maternal deficiency and toxicity states is uncommon. Drinking milk is not a prerequisite for successful lactation, contrary to what is often believed. However, to help prevent maternal bone loss, other calcium-rich foods—for example, cheese, yogurt, pudding, or soybean products such as tofu (see Table 16–2 for recommended intakes of food during lactation)—should be encouraged for the breast-feeding woman who cannot or will not drink milk. Women who avoid drinking milk and who live in cloudy regions may have inadequate vitamin D, which is reflected in breast milk. A vitamin D supplement may be indicated in such situations.

So long as the mother's nutritional intake is adequate, breast milk provides all the necessary vitamins for the infant, with the possible exception of fluoride. During both pregnancy and lactation, vegans may need vitamin D and vitamin B_{12} supplements, and supplements for their infants may be necessary.

The primary known health benefit to the infant from breast milk is increased immune responses (Golding et al., 1997). Breast-feeding is related to reduced incidence of childhood diarrhea, respiratory virus, and **otitis media** (ear infections) (Riordan, 1997). Recent research has identified breast-feeding as a key factor in the prevention of sudden infant death syndrome and increased cognitive functioning (Moxley et al., 1997). The improved learning ability of infants who are breast-fed may be due to the high level of essential fatty acids naturally found in breast milk but not in cow's milk. These fats are likely involved in improved neurological development of the growing infant. In **colostrum** (the substance that precedes breast milk) and breast milk, a substance called **immunoglobulin A (IgA)** helps guard against the penetration of intestinal organisms and antigens, the latter of which are a cause of allergy development.

WHAT ARE LACTATION MANAGEMENT ISSUES?

Although many people believe that breast-feeding is both beneficial and natural, several important pieces of "how-to" information are not widely known. Nurses who see lactating mothers during the first weeks following delivery can play a vital role in the success (or failure) of breast-feeding. Positive verbal encouragement and support are of crucial importance.

Frequency of Feeding

A primary rule of thumb is that the more frequently a woman nurses, the more breast milk she will produce (Fig. 16–3). This is referred to as supply and demand. Because the quantity of breast milk production is difficult to ascertain, other guidelines are used to determine adequacy. These guidelines are (1) adequate weight gain by the infant of 1 to 2 pounds per month, (2) 8 to 12 nursings per 24-hour period, and (3) six or more wet diapers per 24-hour period (assuming that the infant is not given any bottles of water).

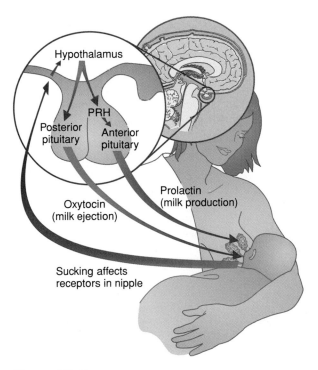

Figure 16–3
Milk release during breast-feeding.

Infant Weight Gain

Some breast-fed infants gain more than the recommended 2 pounds per month, but generally this is not a cause for concern because it is not possible to force-feed an infant who is fed only breast milk.

If the infant gains less than the recommended 1 to 2 pounds per month, great care must be taken not to discourage the lactating mother but to assess possible causes and provide appropriate counseling in a highly sensitive way. On average breast-fed infants gain weight more slowly than formula-fed infants after the first 2 to 3 months. However, this slower weight gain should not necessarily be viewed as a problem so long as there are indicators of good intake of breast milk and the infant is healthy.

Inverted Nipples

A simple exercise can determine whether a woman has inverted nipples (Fig. 16–4). Either the Hoffman technique or a milk cup (not a soft rubber shield) can be used to alleviate the problem (Fig. 16–5).

Poor Let-Down Reflex

Particularly for a first-time nursing mother, anxiety can be high and can inhibit the let-down reflex. **Oxytocin** (a hormone) promotes the let-down reflex. The **let-down reflex** occurs when the milk from the upper parts of the breast **(hind milk)** comes down to the areola (the darker skin around the nipple). A lactating woman can usually identify when the let-down reflex is occurring, as there is a momentary "pins-and-needles" feeling in the breast area.

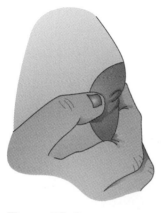

INVERTED NIPPLE

An inverted nipple looks like a slit or a fold. A partly inverted nipple folds in on one side only.

A woman can tell if she has an inverted nipple by gently pinching the nipple at the base using the thumb and forefinger. If the nipple shrinks back, it is an "inverted" nipple.

Many woman with inverted nipples have successfully breast fed, but special preparation is very helpful. Using the Hoffman Technique and wearing a hard plastic cup such as the Confi-Dry will encourage the nipples to stick out.

Figure 16–4
Inverted nipple. (From Health Education Associates, Sandwich, MA.)

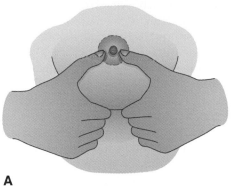

HOFFMAN TECHNIQUE
For women with flat or inverted nipples

Place your thumbs opposite each other on either side of the nipple. Gently draw your thumbs away from the nipple. Then place your thumbs above and below the nipple and repeat.

Do this twice a day for a few minutes.

A

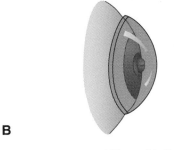

MILK CUP
For women with flat or inverted nipples

Begin by wearing the Cup under the bra for short periods of time and gradually work up to 8 to 10 hours a day.

You can allow your skin to breath by removing the Cup for short periods of time, or by wearing only the base part.

Wearing the Cup is painless. It is not noticeable when worn in the bra unless the woman is wearing a tight-fitting jersey.

B

Milkcups/shells can be purchased from La Leche League International, 1400 N. Meacham Road, P.O. Box 4079, Schaumburg, IL 60168–4079 or call 1-800-LALECHE.

Figure 16–5
(*A*) Hoffman technique. (*B*) Milk cup. (From Health Education Associates, Sandwich, MA.)

The hind milk is richer and higher in fat content than milk from other parts of the breasts. Because of the high kilocalorie content of fat found in the hind milk, the let-down reflex is crucial for the infant's adequate weight gain. Relaxation techniques are thus important to successful lactation. Humor is useful in helping the nursing mother relax; it should be encouraged by the nurse or other health care professional.

Insufficient Feedings

If the let-down reflex does not seem to be an issue (you can ask the mother if she feels a tingling sensation during nursing, which is a sign of let-down), the nurse should ask how often breast-feeding occurs. Often women try to maintain a feeding schedule and ignore the hunger cues of their baby, thinking "the baby can't be hungry yet," or the infant may be a "sleepy baby" who does not indicate his or her own hunger. Generally about every 2 to 3 hours is a good feeding schedule, but for infants who gain weight slowly, more frequent feedings may be in order until the milk supply and weight gain are increased.

During periods of growth spurts the baby may want to nurse more often than usual. Growth spurts often occur during the third week after delivery (just when the mother is likely to be going through **"postpartum blues"**—a feeling of depression) and again at 6 weeks and 3 months. This is not a sign of needing to add formula; rather, it is nature's way of increasing milk production to meet additional needs. Good advice is to encourage bed rest with continuous nursing (although strong family support is a prerequisite for this approach). After a couple of days of very frequent nursing, the milk production will have increased and the baby will go for longer periods between feedings.

Another helpful point concerning frequency of feeding is that the total number of feedings is more important than their spacing. For example, an infant who sleeps through the night but feeds more frequently during the day and has the recommended 8 to 12 feedings will most likely gain weight as well as the infant who wakes up regularly all night and day but nurses the same number of times.

Breast Engorgement

Breast engorgement is a common occurrence in the first few days after delivery. Temporary measures to release excess milk include taking a warm shower or leaning over a sink full of warm water with exposed breasts. When engorgement is diminished, the infant will be better able to grasp the nipple, thereby allowing emptying of the breasts. Short, frequent nursings can help keep engorgement under control. Eventually the amount of milk produced by the new lactating mother will even out to meet the infant's needs.

Sore or Cracked Nipples

Comfort measures for sore or cracked nipples include the following:

1. Relaxation techniques, such as deep-breathing, at the beginning of each feeding and warm washcloths with gentle breast (not nipple) massage to encourage milk flow prior to the infant's suckling
2. Nursing on the less sore side first
3. Changing feeding positions, using the football hold (baby's feet pointing outward from mother rather than inward toward mother), the regular position, or even lying down with the baby's feet pointing up toward the mother's head (awkward but effective in getting the baby's tongue off the sore spot on the woman's nipple)
4. Giving short, frequent nursings (the major portion of breast milk is removed within about 5 to 10 minutes; frequent nursings will prevent the baby from becoming overly hungry, thereby lessening excessive suckling)
5. Making sure the baby's mouth is well back on the areola, with the baby's tongue underneath the nipple

6. Making sure that the baby is removed properly from the breast, breaking suction with the mother's finger inserted into the corner of the baby's mouth
7. Air drying the nipples after each feeding
8. Using cold compresses or washcloths between nursings

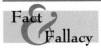

Fallacy: A lactating woman who is experiencing sore nipples should be advised to wear a soft rubber nipple shield while breast-feeding.

Fact: Although this solution may provide relief in the short term, in the long term it can cause severe problems. Because tactile stimulation is necessary to continue producing milk, the physical barrier of the shield between the mother's nipple and the baby's jaw and tongue will inhibit milk production.

Twins

Many people believe that twins preclude the option of breast-feeding. However, because milk supply is most strongly influenced by frequency of feeding (supply and demand: the more one nurses, the more milk is produced), it is feasible to nurse twins. Babies can be positioned at each breast simultaneously with the infants' feet both facing the same direction or with each twin's feet facing outward from the mother.

Inappropriate Fluid Intake

Milk production necessitates increased fluid intake; however, the mother need drink only that amount of fluid necessary to satisfy her thirst. A sudden excess in fluid intake may actually decrease milk yield, as release of **antidiuretic hormone** (a hormone that regulates water loss through the kidneys) is inhibited when fluid intake is in excess of need, resulting in **diuresis** (excess water loss through the kidneys).

The Premature Infant

Premature infants or infants with cleft palate may be fed breast milk or commercial formula using bottles with special nipples. **Gavage feeding** (a form of force-feeding through a flexible tube or pump) may be required for those premature infants who do not have adequate suckling ability for survival. Premature infants have special nutritional needs, primarily because of immature gastrointestinal functioning. These infants now use either special formula or fortified breast milk. This breast milk ideally comes from the infant's own mother, and thus it is referred to as **preterm milk.** In addition, commercial fortifiers are added to the breast milk to increase the kilocalories and other nutrients.

The mother who is collecting milk for her premature infant probably will need extra support in order to maintain breast-feeding. She particularly needs extra support in order to relax in this high-tension situation. A picture of the baby that she can look at during the collection process can help elicit that good feeling of, "Oh, don't I have a beautiful baby!"—a feeling that is difficult to experience while the baby lies in the intensive care unit hooked up to tubes and other paraphernalia. A relaxed nursing staff is of particular importance; again, the use of humor is a positive approach to help encourage the let-down reflex. It is difficult to achieve the same high level of tactile stimulation to the nipple by artificial means, because no pumping machine fully mimics the action of the baby's tongue and jaw movements.

Weaning

The **La Leche League** (a breast-feeding support group) generally advocates baby-led **weaning** (accustoming the baby to nourishment other than breast milk). However, if the mother needs or wants to wean before the baby does, a variety of strategies may be used. The early morning and late night feedings are often the most difficult for the baby to give up. This can be the ideal situation for the working woman who wants to continue partial breast-feeding, as she can continue to breast-feed her baby in the mornings before work. Then when the mother is ready to stop the morning feeding, often the baby is old enough to sit in a high-chair. When babies are fed cereal before the morning nursing, they often begin to wean themselves. The mother may need to try a variety of bottle nipples before the baby accepts one. Older infants (after 9 to 12 months of age) may be weaned directly to a cup.

WHAT ARE BOTTLE-FEEDING CONCERNS?

Although it is preferable for infants to be breast-fed because of the nutritional benefits, fortunately commercial formulas that closely resemble breast milk have been developed for those women who cannot breast-feed because they are taking medications that contraindicate it or for women with medical problems. The perfect food for human babies is clearly breast milk, but many successful adults were bottle-fed as infants.

Recently it has been shown that infants fed formulas devoid of the essential long-chain polyunsaturated fatty acids, arachadonic acid and DHA (see Chapter 3) have poorer retinal and neurologic development than babies who have been breast-fed. The exact cause of this problem is not known (Carnielli et al., 1996). Preterm infants are at the greatest risk for deficiency of these essential fats. Preterm infants who are receiving formula devoid of these essential fats may be at increased risk of impaired blood vessel development, leading to conditions such as hemorrhage and retinopathy (Crawford et al., 1997). One study found that very low birthweight infants fed formula supplemented with arachadonic acid and DHA in amounts typical for breast-milk had outcomes similar to those fed breast milk (Boehm et al., 1996). Formula-fed infants do reach similar levels of plasma lipids as breast-fed babies but not until at least 2 months after birth (Decsi et al., 1995).

Although bottle-feeding may be the more practical method of feeding for the working mother, many working mothers find that a combination of bottle- and breast-feeding works well, particularly if their work is part time. Expression of breast milk for use in a bottle can be an alternative, as shown in Figure 16–6.

It is helpful for a woman to be told that if she expresses only 1 or 2 ounces of breast milk initially, she is doing very well. Expressed milk cooled in the refrigerator can be added to previously frozen expressed milk in order to obtain full bottles (4-ounce bottles are the handiest for collecting and storing expressed milk). Such bottles are visually very interesting with blue layers (**fore milk,** the milk from the front of the breast) and thick white layers (fat-rich hind milk) being formed. Women expressing milk should be relaxed, and may find expressing milk easier after a warm shower. After a woman is comfortable with the technique and her ability, she can easily express milk any time, such as during her lunch break at work. The milk can then be stored in a portable ice chest or refrigerator (if available). Expressed milk can be kept for 1 to 2 days in sterile bottles at refrigerator temperature, for 1 to 2 weeks in a freezer, or for up to 6 months if the freezer maintains a constant temperature of $0°$ F (about $17.8°$ C) or lower.

Nursing-Bottle Mouth

Nursing-bottle mouth (also known as baby-bottle tooth decay; see Fig. 19–2) is a condition in which the two front top teeth are severely decayed or completely eroded away in the older infant or child. This condition is caused by the infant's continuously suckling on a bottle that contains a source of carbohydrate. Sleeping

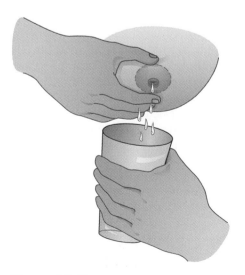

1. Do breast massage.

2. Place the thumb and index finger on the areola or darker skin around the nipple—about an inch back from the nipple. Press inward toward the chest wall and squeeze the thumb and finger together gently: push back and squeeze. Don't slide the thumb and finger. Don't pull the nipple out.

3. Keep the thumb and finger in that position and express until no more drops come out. Then move to another location around the nipple and repeat.

4. Lean over the sterile container and catch the milk. Switch to the other breast and again massage before beginning to express.

Figure 16–6
Instructions for hand expression of milk. (From Health Education Associates, Sandwich, MA.)

with a bottle is particularly harmful because of decreased production of saliva that helps cleanse the teeth. As a general rule, juice should be given in a cup and only water bottles should be allowed at bedtime, if needed. It is also possible for a breast-fed infant who continually nurses throughout the night (the infant who sleeps with the mother) to develop similar tooth decay.

Milk Anemia

Milk anemia is caused when so much milk (not iron-fortified formula) is consumed that it replaces the intake of foods high in iron. Older children who use bottles may drink excess milk. A reduction in milk intake to that recommended in the Food Guide Pyramid may be in order, with water bottles substituted as necessary. When the young child begins to drink from a cup, milk intake will likely decrease to the recommended amount. Juice intake, when excessive, can also contribute to anemia by replacing foods high in iron.

Microwave Heating

The excess steam that results when bottles are heated in a microwave oven can cause bottles to explode in the infant's face. Also, since "hot spots" in the liquid can develop, a seemingly safe temperature can actually cause the infant's mouth to be severely burned if there is contact with the hot spot. The safest way to heat a bottle is to allow very warm water from a faucet to flow over it until the chill is gone.

Use of Inappropriate Liquids

The only appropriate liquids for regular use in a bottle are expressed breast milk, formula, and water. Although occasional use of juice is acceptable (such as in a car, when drinking from a cup is prohibited), the regular use of juice in a bottle can cause nursing-bottle mouth (see earlier discussion). Other sweet liquids such as Kool-Aid or soft drinks should be avoided entirely. Formula replacements, such as nondairy creamer or other milk products that are not specifically designed for infant use, should never be used. Formula should be mixed according to directions, not under- or overdiluted unless specifically recommended by a **pediatrician** (physician specializing in the care of infants, children, and adolescents) or a registered dietitian.

Types of Infant Formulas

Commercial Cow's Milk–Based Formulas

Made from cow's milk, these formulas closely approximate human milk. They are available in powder, liquid concentrated, and ready-to-feed form. Powdered forms are more economical but require mixing and careful measuring. Liquid concentrated formulas require proper dilution with water (a 1:1 ratio) before they are used. Commercial formulas are fortified to meet all the known vitamin and mineral requirements of the infant. Formulas containing iron are available and are recommended by the American Academy of Pediatrics. Examples of infant commercial formulas are Enfamil, Similac, and SMA.

TEACHING P•E•A•R•L

A good question to ask is, "Are you aware of what formula is made from?" followed by an explanation that it is cow's milk with the excess protein removed and vitamins and minerals added to make it more nutritious like breast milk. A further explanation can be provided by saying that so much protein is needed in cow's milk to help the baby cow grow that it causes gastrointestinal irritation (stomach bleeding) in the human baby (using your hands to depict the size difference between a calf and a human baby can be very effective). This can support the continued use of formula versus changing to whole milk before the infant is physiologically ready to do so.

Soybean-Based Formulas

If the infant shows signs of allergy to cow's milk or if the parents are strict vegetarians (vegans), soybean-based formulas are generally used. Soybean-based formula is often the formula of choice as a supplement to breast-feeding because of the reduced likelihood of allergies. Commercially prepared formulas are fortified with vitamins and minerals. Bottle-fed infants who have an intolerance to lactose can use soy formulas. Examples of soybean-based formulas are ProSobee, Neo-Mull-Soy, and Isomil. Soy formulas have vitamin B_{12} added.

Special Formulas

Special formulas may be necessary for infants with digestive disturbances, allergies, or inborn errors of metabolism. Examples are Portagen, Pregestimil, Lonalac, and Lofenalac. For infants with strong family history of allergies, the elemental formulas may be the best choice if the mother cannot breast-feed.

WHAT ARE THE FEEDING GUIDELINES DURING THE FIRST YEAR?

Although many parents today feel that waiting until the infant is 4 months of age to start introducing cereal and other solid foods is too long, this was once a common practice. Before 1920 solid foods were seldom offered to infants younger than 1 year of age. As time progressed, our knowledge of infant nutrition, expanded and women relied more on bottle-feeding. By the 1960s the age at which solid foods were commonly introduced had become a couple of months or even weeks. This trend, however, was a rational response to the nutritionally inadequate formulas used at that time (often evaporated milk mixed with water and corn syrup). A vitamin C source, such as orange juice, and iron-fortified cereal were necessary then at an early age.

With the current return of breast-feeding and the development of highly nutritious commercial infant formulas, the risks associated with early introduction of solids (such as development of an allergy caused by the use of orange juice and cereal at an early age) outweigh any benefits. Other reasons to delay the introduction of solid foods until 4 to 6 months are the following:

1. Inability of the young infant to digest complex carbohydrates such as those found in cereal, vegetables, and fruits (thus infants can fill up their stomachs without getting the nutrients they need to grow; breast milk is considered the ideal food and source of nutrients for young infants)
2. Immature intestinal tract of the young infant that allows large, undigested food molecules to pass through the intestinal wall (which can activate an allergic reaction and may become a permanent condition)
3. Inadequate physiological readiness of the infant to use tongue-thrust (it is felt that biologically the human species may have developed this characteristic to prevent inappropriate ingestion of food)
4. Inability of the infant to indicate a desire for food by opening his or her mouth when a spoonful of food is presented or to indicate satiety by leaning back and turning away; it is felt that until an infant can respond in this manner (at about 5 months of age), feeding solid food may represent a type of force-feeding

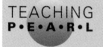

TEACHING
P•E•A•R•L   With regard to the introduction of solid foods, a good assessment question is, "Have you thought about when you are going to start solid foods such as cereal?" followed by, "What have you heard from other people about when to start?" This will help you tailor the message to the beliefs the parents may hold.

Neither breast milk nor a milk formula will furnish adequate amounts of all nutrients required by the infant in later months. One important reason for introducing some solid foods into the infant's diet is to replenish the depleting stores of iron between 4 and 6 months of age (Table 16–5 shows the RDAs for infants up to 1 year old). The general guidelines for the introduction of foods are as follows:

1. Introduce iron-fortified baby rice cereal at about 4 to 6 months of age.
2. Add pureed vegetables and fruits, one at a time, at about 6 to 8 months (starting with vegetables may help to increase acceptance by the infant not yet exposed to the sweet taste of fruits).
3. Add pureed meats at about 6 to 8 months.
4. Add juice when the infant is old enough to drink from a cup at about 9 months of age.
5. Add foods with more texture and finger foods at about 9 months of age (chopped meats, crackers, and so on).
6. Add allergenic foods, such as egg whites (or whole eggs), whole milk, and orange juice, after 1 year of age (especially important for the infant with a family history of allergies or asthma).

Table 16–5
RDAs for Infants: Birth to 1 Year

	0–6 Months	6–12 Months
Energy	108 kcal/kg	98 kcal/kg
Protein	13 g	14 g
Vitamin C	30 mg	35 mg
Folate	25 µg	35 µg
Niacin	5 mg	6 mg
Riboflavin	0.4 mg	0.5 mg
Thiamine	0.3 mg	0.4 mg
Vitamin B_6	0.3 mg	0.6 mg
Vitamin B_{12}	0.3 µg	0.5 µg
Vitamin A	375 µg of RE	375 µg of RE
Vitamin D*	5–7.5 µg	5–10 µg
Vitamin E	3 mg of TE	4 mg of TE
Calcium	210–400 mg	270–600 mg
Phosphorus	300 mg	500 mg
Iodine	40 µg	50 µg
Iron	6 mg	10 mg
Magnesium	40 mg	60 mg
Zinc	5 mg	5 mg
Selenium	10 µg	15 µg

Abbreviations: RE = retinol equivalent; TE = tocopherol equivalent.
*The lower value is the 1997 adequate intake (AI) level; the higher value is the 1989 RDA level.
Modified from National Academy of Sciences National Research Council: Recommended Dietary Allowances, 10th and 11th eds. Washington, DC, National Academy of Sciences, 1989 and 1997.

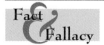

Fact & Fallacy

Fallacy: Cereal helps babies sleep through the night.

Fact: There is no scientific evidence to support this belief. Many experienced parents admit that their babies wake up regardless of how much food they have eaten. Parents should be strongly discouraged from giving an infant cereal before the baby is 4 to 6 months old, particularly when there is a family history of allergies.

At about the time the growing infant develops the **pincer grasp** (the ability to put the thumb and index finger together—at about 8 months of age), a sense of independence also begins to grow. This can be exasperating to a parent, particularly as the baby begins to spill food on the floor or decides to empty a full bowl of food on his or her own head. Because this is believed to be a normal part of development, parents are advised to cope with this behavior through positive strategies. An old shower curtain can be placed under the high-chair to catch spills, a large bib can help prevent damage to the baby's clothes, small quantities of food can be given at one time to lessen waste and bath time can be scheduled after meal time. Because the infant is being allowed additional servings, adequate intake can occur simultaneously with a lowered frustration level of the parents. Bribing and coaxing the infant to eat and not spill food can cause repetition of the negative behaviors as the infant learns he or she can control the parents' actions ("Let's see if I can get Mom and Dad to jump up and down if I drop this glass of juice"). Finger foods are preferred by the older infant.

Food Contraindications. Aside from the special requirements for allergy-sensitive infants or for those who have metabolic disorders (a referral to a registered dietitian or a qualified nutritionist is in order in these cases), it should be stressed that parents should not give honey to babies because of the potential for botulism, as honey contains botulism spores (in a quantity too low to cause adverse effects in older children and adults).

The high sodium content of some processed foods (such as canned vegetables or cured meats) can be detrimental to the immature renal functioning of infants. Steamed fresh vegetables, fruits, and other low-sodium foods may be safely used in preparing homemade baby foods. Special baby food grinders can be purchased for a reasonable price and allow the baby to eat the same foods as the family. It is important to avoid excess salt and sugar in baby foods, whether store-bought or prepared at home.

To prevent choking, foods that have a hard texture (such as a raw apple or carrot) or food in large pieces should be avoided until the infant is old enough to chew adequately. Hot dogs should never be given to an infant and can also be problematic for older children unless the hot dogs are sliced into thin strips so they cannot cause choking if chewed inadequately.

HOW DOES AN INFANT GROW AND DEVELOP?

A well-nourished infant shows a steady gain in weight and height (with some fluctuations from week to week), is happy and vigorous, sleeps well, has firm muscles, has some tooth eruption at about 5 to 6 months (about six to twelve teeth will have erupted by 12 months), and has good elimination characteristic of the type of feeding—breast or formula. The nutrients found in milk, especially the protein, are essential in the development of the new tissues that accompany this growth.

Each infant has an individual rate of growth, but all grow faster in weight than in height. A steady weight gain is more important than a large amount gained. In interpreting growth with the National Center for Health Statistics growth charts (see Appendix 10), percentiles are used. A child at the 50th percentile for age is considered average. There is no concern with growth if the length and weight for age are above the 10th percentile and are consistent (not dropping in percentile). Weight for height should be between the 25th and 90th percentile without showing a significant decrease or increase in percentiles.

WHAT ARE SOME CLINICAL PROBLEMS IN INFANCY?

Babies born before they have had a chance to grow adequately are at nutritional risk. Babies less than 5 pounds at birth generally stay in the hospital after delivery until they have reached at least this weight. Lung function may be compromised. The ability to suckle may be impaired because of immature muscle development. Special feeding devices, including tube-feeding, may be required until the infant is strong enough to suck. Oral stimulation, such as use of a pacifier, is important for the infant who is tube-fed. Guidance on the introduction of solid foods needs to take into account the amount of prematurity. For example, cereal is usually started at 4 months of age. If the infant was born 3 months prematurely, the introduction of cereal should be delayed until the infant is 7 months old. This is especially true if there is a strong family history of allergies.

Failure to Thrive

The **failure to thrive (FTT)** syndrome was first observed in infants raised in institutional settings in which they did not receive adequate amounts of attention (physical touch and emotional warmth). As a result of this recognition, volunteers are now used to cuddle premature infants in hospital settings in order to help their growth and survival.

Failure to thrive is associated with physical illness such as cystic fibrosis (Giglio et al., 1997), poor nutrition, and maternal deprivation, which can lead to severe retardation of physical growth and developmental delays. Failure to thrive is a medical diagnosis, but it includes a weight and height of less than the third percentile for the infant's age (see Appendix 10) and less than normal ability in the **Denver Developmental Screening Test** (an observational test based on infant developmental progress). A total health care team approach may be in order.

WHAT ARE SOME OTHER NUTRITION ISSUES FOR WOMEN?

Premenstrual Syndrome

Premenstrual syndrome (PMS) occurs the first few days before the onset of the monthly menstrual cycle and disappears after menstruation. The majority of American women experience some degree of PMS, with an estimated 10 to 15 percent experiencing severe or disabling symptoms, including symptoms of hypoglycemia such as increased appetite, nervousness, irritability, and headaches. However, eating does not always relieve these symptoms as would be predicted in treating hypoglycemia. One interesting study found that the thermic effect of food (the increased metabolism related to digestion of food) decreased significantly after ovulation, which may be a result of impaired glucose uptake into body cells or slower transit of food through the upper gastrointestinal tract (Tai et al., 1997). One study found a hormonal difference related to progesterone with women experiencing PMS, which may be associated with the mood symptoms of anxiety, tension, and depression (Rapkin et al., 1997). Nutrition has no known impact on PMS. However, eating balanced meals at regular times is a prudent approach.

Osteoporosis

This condition of brittle bones is more prevalent in women than in men. Women have less bone mass than men and often have inadequate calcium intake. Women of Northern European and Asian heritage are especially at risk of osteoporosis. Thin women are at high risk as well. Bone loss increases after menopause. Emphasizing milk or other calcium-rich foods in the diet helps maintain bone integrity. The equivalent of 3 to 4 cups of milk is recommended to help prevent bone loss. Hormonal therapy with estrogen and weight-bearing exercise further help maintain bone integrity (see Chapter 20 for the benefits of exercise). For more information on osteoporosis, see Chapter 21.

WHAT IS THE ROLE OF THE NURSE OR OTHER HEALTH PROFESSIONAL IN MATERNAL AND INFANT NUTRITION?

During Pregnancy

A nurse or other health care professional should be aware of potential barriers to adequate nourishment during pregnancy. Examples are poor attitude (denial of pregnancy or desire to maintain slimness), misinformation (belief that salt restriction and low weight gain are desirable), or physical barriers to adequate nourishment (insufficient food money, lack of adequate food preparation facilities, or hyperemesis). Once such a barrier is identified, referral to a registered dietitian or a qualified nutritionist, such as one associated with the WIC program, may be in order; immediate contact with the woman's obstetrician is also recommended.

It is especially important for health care professionals to recognize the strong need of pregnant teenagers and all adolescents to rebel against authority figures. Rather than telling a pregnant teen what she must do, the health care professional should inform her of alternative actions and their likely outcomes. Work as the teen's advocate and ask her in a positive manner how you can best assist her. Ask her what her perceived needs are and how she feels about your concerns. Encourage her involvement in other supportive programs in your community. Be a good listener and a supportive advocate for her.

After Pregnancy

After delivery, women should be encouraged to maintain good nutritional status for themselves to help promote adequate energy for infant care as well as to help restore nutritional stores for subsequent pregnancies. Counseling can be provided as needed to encourage adequate spacing between pregnancies and nutritional intake to prepare a woman's body for a future healthy pregnancy.

Women should be monitored for postpartum depression. A prepregnancy personal history of mood disorder (bipolar or major depression) or premenstrual syndrome places a woman at high risk for postpartum mood disorders, which can lead to serious psychological and social consequences and in some cases can even lead to suicide or infanticide. Psychological intervention is warranted prior to the pregnancy for women at high-risk for mood disorders (Pariser et al., 1997).

During Lactation

The obstetrical nurse plays an important role in promoting successful breast-feeding in the hospital setting. Of crucial importance is positive verbal encouragement and support. Flippant remarks can damage a woman's already sensitive emotions (related to hormonal changes associated with birth) and may impair her ability to breast-feed successfully.

The use of humor can help a tense new mother relax, which is important for a successful let-down reflex. All new breast-feeding women should be alerted to support and information services such as the following:

- A local La Leche League
- The Women, Infants, and Children's Supplemental Nutrition Program (WIC), which supports breast-feeding education
- The Cooperative Extension's Expanded Food and Nutrition Education Program (EFNEP), which may have breast-feeding support available through trained nutrition teaching assistants (see Chapter 22)
- The local hospital's obstetrics department, which will likely have nurses trained in lactation management; this can be especially helpful for problems that occur in the middle of the night

Breast-feeding "buddy systems" also exist in many communities. Volunteers experienced in breast-feeding are paired up with new breast-feeding mothers until breast-feeding is fully established. A nurse or other health professional can help set up such a system or make referrals to one already in existence.

For Bottle-Fed Infants

In the case of a bottle-fed infant, it is important for the nurse or other health care professional to be aware of the parents' philosophy and knowledge about feeding. Do they adhere to rigid feeding schedules that impair the infant's intake of formula or do they go solely by the infant's crying with the potential for either over- or underfeeding? Are the parents receiving conflicting advice (which is likely) that undermines their confidence or that makes them follow inappropriate feeding practices? Do they believe that formula is made from "a bunch of chemicals" and that therefore whole milk is better? Do they realize that formula requires refrigeration after it has been prepared? Do they know how to properly prepare formula?

Is nursing-bottle mouth a potential problem? If so, recommend water bottles at bedtime (an older child may be given a choice: water bottle or no bottle).

Regarding the Introduction to Solid Food

Explaining why a grandmother or a mother-in-law may be giving one piece of advice while you are giving another can go a long way in building a new mother's trust in her own common sense. Since many new mothers are anxious and insecure in their first encounters with their infants, your efforts are best aimed at building confidence and strengthening decision-making skills.

Critical Thinking

Case Study

Lanisha was scared but she was not going to act like it. She was sitting in a room with a lot of other, mostly older, women who were also pregnant. But what else could she do? Her dad recently had a heart attack and was out of work. Fortunately he wasn't too upset with the news of her pregnancy. She knew she needed to eat right to help her baby grow. She could manage being hungry. She'd been hungry many times in her life, especially at the end of the month when the food ran out. But she knew she couldn't do that now. This clinic was supposed to give her milk, eggs, cereal, juice, and peanut butter or beans. She wasn't sure she wanted the milk, however, since she couldn't drink it anyway. She wondered why she had to wait so long. She needed to get back to school.

Applications

1. What nutritional program provides the foods Lanisha describes?
2. What unique nutritional concerns might Lanisha have during her pregnancy?
3. How would you respond to Lanisha's belief that she cannot drink milk? What alternatives could be suggested?
4. What resources are available in the local area or your community to help others in Lanisha's situation?

Study Questions and Classroom Activities

1. What benefits may the mother-to-be expect if she is well nourished?
2. Why should the pregnant teenager be sure she receives adequate kilocalories as well as sufficient amounts of all important nutrients?
3. How and why do the foods needed in the daily diet during pregnancy and lactation differ from those needed by nonpregnant women?

4. What can a nurse do to support breast-feeding in the hospital setting? What are immediate concerns versus long-term concerns and their possible solutions?

5. What guidelines would you give to a breast-feeding mother to help her determine if breast-feeding is going well once she leaves the hospital?

6. Describe the likely impact of "growth spurts" on the nursing behavior of babies.

7. What are the advantages of breast-feeding? Why is breast milk so suitable for the infant?

8. What considerations for meal planning would be indicated for a pregnant or breast-feeding woman who has diabetes (see Chapter 9)?

9. Class members each provide at least one joke that can be compiled for later use with new lactating mothers in order to help promote the let-down reflex.

References

Abitbol MM, Taylor-Randall UB, Barton PT, Thompson E: Effect of modern obstetrics on mothers from Third-World countries. J Matern Fetal Med. September 1997; 6(5): 276–280.

Abma JC, Chandra A, Mosher WD, Peterson LS, Piccinino LJ: Fertility, family planning, and women's health: New data from the 1995 National Survey of Family Growth. Vital Health Stat 23. May 1997; 19:1–114.

Badgett T, Feingold M: Total parenteral nutrition in pregnancy: Case review and guidelines for calculating requirements. J Matern Fetal Med. July 1997; 6(4):215–217.

Baron TH, Ramirez B, Richter JE: Gastrointestinal motility disorders during pregnancy. Ann Intern Med. Mar 1, 1993; 118(5):366–375.

Boehm G, Borte M, Bohles HJ, Muller H, Kohn G, Moro G: Docosahexaenoic and arachidonic acid content of serum and red blood cell membrane phospholipids of preterm infants fed breast milk, standard formula or formula supplemented with n-3 and n-6 long-chain polyunsaturated fatty acids. Eur J Pediatr. May 1996; 155(5):410–416.

Carnielli VP, Wattimena DJ, Luijendijk IH, Boerlage A, Degenhart HJ, Sauer PJ: The very low birth weight premature infant is capable of synthesizing arachidonic and docosahexaenoic acids from linoleic and linolenic acids. Pediatr Res. July 1996; 40(1):169–174.

Crawford MA, Costeloe K, Ghebremeskel K, Phylactos A, Skirvin L, Stacey F: Are deficits of arachidonic and docosahexaenoic acids responsible for the neural and vascular complications of preterm babies? Am J Clin Nutr. October 1997; 66(4 Suppl):1032S–1041S.

Decsi T, Thiel I, Koletzko B: Essential fatty acids in full term infants fed breast milk or formula. Arch Dis Child Fetal Neonatal Ed. January 1995; 72(1):F23–F28.

Giglio L, Candusso M, D'Orazio C, Mastella G, Faraguna D: Failure to thrive: The earliest feature of cystic fibrosis in infants diagnosed by neonatal screening. Acta Paediatr. November 1997; 86(11):1162–1165.

Golding J, Emmett PM, Rogers IS: Does breast feeding have any impact on non-infectious, non-allergic disorders? Early Hum Dev. October 29, 1997; (49 Suppl):S131–S142.

Hsu JJ, Clark-Glena R, Nelson DK, Kim CH: Nasogastric enteral feeding in the management of hyperemesis gravidarum. Obstet Gynecol. September 1996; 88(3):343–346.

Moxley S, Sims-Jones N, Vargha A, Chamberlain M: Breastfeeding: A course for health professionals. Can Nurse. October 1997; 93(9):35–38.

Nader S, Mastrobattista J: Recurrent hyperthyroidism in consecutive pregnancies characterized by hyperemesis. Thyroid. October 1996; 6(5):465–466.

Ozanne SE, Nave BT, Wang CL, Shepherd PR, Prins J, Smith GD: Poor fetal nutrition causes long-term changes in expression of insulin signaling components in adipocytes. Am J Physiol. July 1997; 273(1 Pt 1):E46–E51.

Pariser SF, Nasrallah HA, Gardner DK: Postpartum mood disorders: Clinical perspectives. J Womens Health. August 1997; 6(4):421–434.

Preziosi P, Prual A, Galan P, Daouda H, Boureima H, Hercberg S: Effect of iron supplementation on the iron status of pregnant women: Consequences for newborns. Am J Clin Nutr. November 1997; 66(5):1178–1182.

Rapkin AJ, Morgan M, Goldman L, Brann DW, Simone D, Mahesh VB: Progesterone metabolite allopregnanolone in women with premenstrual syndrome. Obstet Gynecol. November 1997; 90(5):709–714.

Riordan JM: The cost of not breastfeeding: A commentary. J Hum Lact. June 1997; 13(2):93–97.

Rizzo TA, Silverman BL, Metzger BE, Cho NH: Behavioral adjustment in children of diabetic mothers. Acta Paediatr. September 1997; 86(9):969–974.

Sibai BM, Ewell M, Levine RJ, Klebanoff MA, Esterlitz J, Catalano PM, Goldenberg RL, Joffe G: Risk factors associated with preeclampsia in healthy nulliparous women. The Calcium for Preeclampsia Prevention (CPEP) Study Group. Am J Obstet Gynecol. November 1997; 177(5):1003–1010.

Solomon CG, Willett WC, Carey VJ, Rich-Edwards J, Hunter DJ, Colditz GA, Stampfer MJ, Speizer FE, Spiegelman D, Manson JE: A prospective study of pregravid determinants of gestational diabetes mellitus. JAMA. October 1, 1997; 278(13):1078–1083.

Tai MM, Castillo TP, Pi-Sunyer FX: Thermic effect of food during each phase of the menstrual cycle. Am J Clin Nutr. November 1997; 66(5):1110–1115.

Tinkle MB, Sterling BS: Neural tube defects: A primary prevention role for nurses. J Obstet Gynecol Neonatal Nurs. September 1997; 26(5):503–512.

Tsang IS, Katz VL, Wells SD: Maternal and fetal outcomes in hyperemesis gravidarum. Int J Gynaecol Obstet. December 1996; 55(3):231–235.

van Stuijvenberg ME, Schabort I, Labadarios D, Nel JT: The nutritional status and treatment of patients with hyperemesis gravidarum. Am J Obstet Gynecol. May 1995; 172(5):1585–1591.

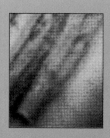

17

Growth and Development

Objectives

After completing this chapter, you should be able to:

- Describe nutritional needs during childhood and adolescence.
- Describe methods to promote good nutritional intake.
- Apply knowledge of the nutrient needs to the meal environment.

Terms to Identify

Adipose tissue	Food distribution system	Hematocrit
Bone growth	Food jags	Lean tissue
Development	Growth	

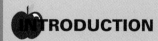

INTRODUCTION

Although the rapid growth that occurs prenatally and during infancy slows in childhood and only picks up in adolescence, developmental changes are rapid. From learning to walk to climbing trees, from uttering first words to chattering nonstop and monopolizing phone lines, from being totally dependent to growing into independence, the changes that take place from early childhood to adolescence are truly remarkable.

Nutrition plays a key role in this process. Sources of food that provide good nutrition change throughout the period of childhood. Breast-feeding may continue for the first few years. Some children need to rely on bottle use beyond the first year, although this is generally discouraged because of concerns about dental health. The texture of foods also changes as children begin to eat more solid food as they develop the full ability to chew. Peer pressure becomes more of a factor in food choices as childhood advances (Table 17–1).

Table 17–1
Age-Related Childhood Food Guidelines

Ages (years)	Suggestions
1 to 2	Provide plain, simple finger foods Place small amounts on the plate (about 1 tbsp of each food for each year of child's age) Provide cups with handles that do not tip easily, large-handled silverware, and plates with edges (for pushing food against) Trust child's hunger cues, as appetite can vary from day to day
2 to 3	Encourage the "one-taste" rule to expose children to new foods but do not force child to eat Make mealtimes pleasant and enjoyable Offer structured food choices to allow for a growing sense of independence Recognize that "food jags" (eating the same food day after day) is common at this age and beyond Continue to increase the variety of foods offered
3 to 5	Begin to include the child in food shopping (the young child can recognize numbers on food labels; give guidelines such as cereals with no more than 6 grams of sugar per serving) Include child in simple cooking techniques such as stirring and pouring Avoid using food as a bribe or as a reward Continue to increase the variety of foods offered
5 to 10	Continue to provide breakfast, which is especially important for better school performance Help child categorize foods into groups of the Food Guide Pyramid Be sensitive to the effects of food advertising; help the child understand that many foods advertised are high in fat and sugar
10 to 18	Recognize that increased body fat often precedes puberty Be sensitive to the influence of friends on food and beverage choices Provide information on healthy food choices at fast food restaurants and for snacks Help child find time to eat breakfast and to eat around sports and school events

WHAT IS MEANT BY GROWTH AND DEVELOPMENT?

Growth is the increase with age in weight and height, or size as it is popularly designated, that comes about as a result of the multiplication of cells and their differentiation for many different functions in the body. Growth is a continuous but not uniform process from conception to full maturity. During fetal life and infancy the rate of growth is very rapid. This period is followed by one of slower growth during early and middle childhood. Another period of very rapid growth occurs during adolescence, followed by a tapering off until the growth period ends.

Development refers to the increasing ability of body parts to function. For example, being able to use a knife and fork successfully is a fine-motor skill that is age dependent (see Table 17–1). Factors affecting the rate of growth and development include heredity, or inborn capacity to grow, and environment. An extremely important environmental factor is nutrition. Better diets, which accompany improved economic conditions, are credited for the taller stature of children and adults in the United States today. Adults were significantly smaller in past decades. In technologically advanced countries, the average height and weight of children of any given age have increased over the past 100 years, which is evidence that well-nourished children reach the potential set by their heredity, not only in physical growth but also in mental development.

What Is the Importance of Nutrition to Healthy Growth and Development?

Without an adequate supply of nutrients, optimal growth and development to adulthood would not be possible. Nutrients supplied by food that the child consumes provide energy and the necessary building blocks for synthesis of new tissues. Foods for growth include those in the three lower levels of the Food Guide Pyramid.

Breast milk can continue to provide good nutrition for several years. Breast milk is a source of protein as well as calcium and other nutrients needed for good growth. With the ample food supply in the United States, the nutritional component of breast-feeding the older child is secondary to the emotional needs provided by close contact with the mother. All children will eventually become weaned (stop nursing or using the bottle) without assistance (see Chapter 16 for weaning guidelines).

Brain growth stops in early childhood, but other important organs continue to grow. Although the weight of the child (specifically **adipose tissue**—body fat) is more affected by the total quantity of kilocalories consumed, **bone growth** (the growth that occurs in length and thickness of bones) and **lean tissue** (muscle) growth are affected by both the quantity and quality of the diet. Parents should strive for a high-quality diet as well as an adequate quantity of kilocalories.

Every child has different nutrient requirements based on factors such as chronological age, individual growth rate, stage of maturation, level of physical activity, and the efficiency of absorption and utilization of nutrients. Guidelines, such as recommended dietary allowances (RDAs) and the Food Guide Pyramid give general indications of needed nutrients for growth. Growth charts are another important tool (see Appendix 10). If the child's growth is appropriate, it can be generally assumed that nutritional intake is adequate. Health problems can lead to poor growth even though an adequate diet is being consumed.

Because the human is a social being, appropriate interaction is important for growth and development. Food often serves as a social link, such as at mealtimes (see Fig. 1–2). Children should eat as part of a family unit, ideally at the table. Eating with others can stimulate appetite and reinforce that eating is a pleasurable experience.

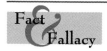

Fact &
Fallacy

Fallacy: All children should take a multivitamin and mineral supplement.

Fact: Although commercial vitamin and mineral supplements contain much of what is needed for good health, food contains even more such as protein and phytochemicals. A balanced diet consisting of a variety of foods is more likely to supply all the necessary nutrients for growth and repair than a vitamin preparation will. In addition to being unnecessary most of the time (and therefore a waste of money), excess vitamin intake can be fatal. If a parent feels safer giving vitamins, he or she should make sure that the content does not exceed 100 percent of the RDA.

WHAT ARE THE EFFECTS OF MALNUTRITION ON GROWTH AND DEVELOPMENT, LEARNING, AND BEHAVIOR?

An estimated 4 million American children—8 percent of the children under the age of 12 in this country—experience prolonged periodic food insufficiency and hunger each year (Kleinman et al., 1998). Children who do not get enough to eat and are malnourished tend to be smaller and are more likely than well-fed children to become ill because of decreased immunity. Such children may also be less able to learn. The extent to which malnutrition occurs in the United States means that many children will not be able to achieve their full potential. For developing nations worldwide, where children may constitute a large percentage of the population, malnutrition may limit the country's future social and economic development.

A prolonged lack of one or more nutrients retards physical development or causes specific clinical conditions to appear. For example, anemia, goiter, and rickets reflect a state of malnutrition. Severe malnutrition, which is characterized by clinical manifestations, is of two basic types: kwashiorkor (protein deficiency) (Fig. 17–1) and marasmus (overall deficit of food, especially kilocalories; also known as PEM—protein energy malnutrition) (Fig. 17–2). Kwashiorkor generally occurs at or after weaning, when milk high in protein is replaced by a starchy staple food providing insufficient protein. A child with this type of malnutrition usually has stunted growth and edema, skin sores, and discoloration of dark hair to red or blond. Infantile marasmus is frequently the result of early cessation of breast-feeding, overdilution of formula, or gastrointestinal infection early in life, and it is accompanied by wasting of tissues and extreme growth retardation. See Chapter 3 for a more detailed discussion of kwashiorkor and marasmus.

Undernourished children are identified most often by biochemical and clinical signs, but the value of these signs is limited to identifying an extremely inadequate diet. Chronic long-term undernutrition generally results in stunting of growth (Fig. 17–3). The degree of malnutrition is often proportional to the degree to which the child is subnormal in height or weight. Therefore, anthropometric measurements (height, weight, and amount of body fat; see Chapter 7 for more on anthropometrics) are the most commonly used indices of undernutrition.

Types of moderate malnutrition include (1) that caused by chronic food reduction (manifested by growth retardation) and (2) that resulting from vitamin or mineral deficiency and accompanied by clinical symptoms such as rickets or pellagra. Malnutrition is most often associated with poverty resulting from a **food distribution system** (how food is allocated to the world's population) that is based on purchasing power. Exact determination of the effect on the individual is difficult, because other factors influence human growth and behavioral development, including individual innate potential, health status, and environment.

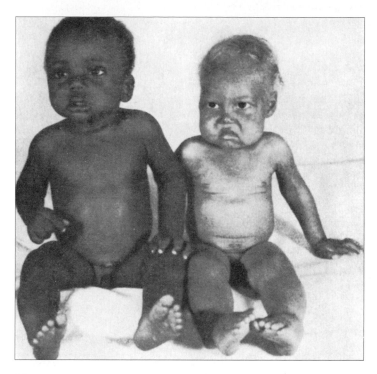

Figure 17–1

(*Right*) Infant with "sugar baby" kwashiorkor, attributed to a high-sugar, low-protein diet. The infant has stunted growth, edema of the feet and hands, fatty liver, moon face, and dyspigmentation of the skin and hair. (*Left*) Normal infant. (From Jelliffe DB: Hypochromotrichia and malnutrition in Jamaican infants. J Trop Pediatr. 1955; 1:25; by permission of Oxford University Press.)

Marasmus and kwashiorkor do occur in the United States but are quite rare. Chronic undernutrition occurs more commonly. This can lead to iron deficiency and anemia, which is relatively common, especially in growing children. A child's growth record is a more accurate measure of whether he or she is receiving sufficient nutrients than are RDAs because the gross estimates of nutritional needs are not designed to assess an individual's nutritional status.

Malnutrition impairs the body's defense against disease. Therefore infection, which is rampant in underdeveloped regions of the world because of poor sanitary conditions, occurs more frequently in malnourished children.

Very low birthweight infants generally did not survive prior to 1945, but today up to 70 percent of such infants do. Complications of very low birthweight include cerebral palsy, mental retardation, blindness, and deafness. The rates of these complications have remained steady since the 1980s, but other functional limitations may be increasing (Vohr & Msall, 1997). Very severe malnutrition in infancy, if of long duration and followed by childhood undernutrition, can pro-

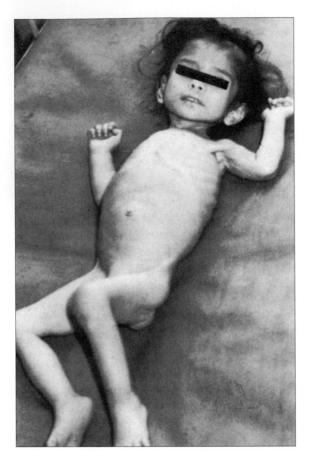

Figure 17–2
Marasmus in a child 2 years and 4 months old. (From
Cotran RS, Kumar V, Robbins SL: Robbins Pathologic Basis
of Disease, 4th ed. Philadelphia, WB Saunders, 1989.)

duce irreversible effects on neurological development, which in turn can impair a
child's ability to learn later in life.

WHY IS IRON-DEFICIENCY ANEMIA SO COMMON AMONG CHILDREN?

Young children and adolescents are particularly susceptible to iron-deficiency
anemia because of the rapid use of iron during growth and the love of foods that
are generally low in iron (see Fig. 17–4). Other reasons include blood loss caused
by parasites or menstruation. Teenaged girls are at an increased risk of anemia
because of the start of menstruation, the rapid growth of adolescence, and insufficient iron in their diets.

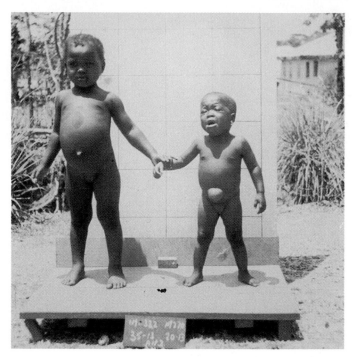

Figure 17–3
Stunting is shown with Nigerian children, born in the same month in the same village, who have genetically similar parents. (Photo courtesy of Michael Latham, Division of Nutritional Sciences, Cornell University, Ithaca, New York, and David Morley, Institute of Child Health, London, England.)

With regard to diet, children often find eating meat difficult. This may be because the meat is too tough from being overcooked (meat cooked at low temperatures using moist methods, such as the meat cooked in stews, is more tender), because they have not acquired a taste for meat (such as with liver), or because the family avoids meat for economic, religious, moral, or other reasons.

Prevention of Iron-Deficiency Anemia

Aside from increased meat intake, other foods that are high in iron should be consumed freely. As noted in Chapter 5, the iron found in meat, referred to as heme iron, is well absorbed, whereas other food sources of iron (called nonheme iron) need to be eaten with a vitamin C food in order to enhance absorption. For example, iron-fortified cereal followed by a glass of orange juice or other food high in vitamin C will greatly enhance the absorption of iron (see Chapter 5 for other iron sources and Table 17–2 for suggested vitamin C foods that can be packed for school lunches).

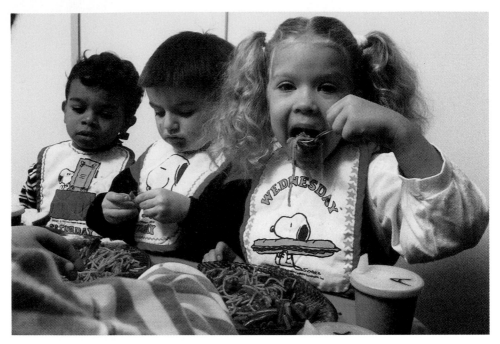

Figure 17–4
Pasta is a favorite dish of young children.

Diagnosis and Treatment of Iron-Deficiency Anemia

Because iron-deficiency anemia continues to be a major health problem in the United States, there is widespread screening among children (particularly children from low-income families, who tend to have difficulty obtaining adequate amounts of iron in their diets). Programs such as the Well Child Clinic (operated out of Public Health Departments), and the Women, Infants, and Children Supplemental Nutrition Program (WIC) commonly screen for iron-deficiency anemia using either the test for hemoglobin (the part of the blood that carries oxygen and is rich in iron) or the test for **hematocrit** (the amount of packed red blood cells) values.

Controversy exists regarding the blood levels that constitute iron-deficiency anemia. Generally, hemoglobin values greater than 12 g/dL and hematocrit values greater than 37 percent are considered normal. Hemoglobin readings of less than 11 g/dL and hematocrit readings of less than 33 percent should be evaluated further, and complete blood counts will often show low transferrin saturation levels (transferrin is an important constituent of red blood cell formation). Hemoglobin values of less than 10 g/dL (which is roughly equivalent to a hematocrit value of less than 30 percent) are signs of iron-deficiency anemia and require immediate medical attention with iron supplementation. A test dose of iron may be used to help determine whether anemia is the result of iron deficiency. Increased focus on dietary intake of iron is also imperative to help resolve the anemia and prevent future episodes.

Table 17–2
Home-Packed School Lunch Ideas

Choose one food or a combination of foods from each group to meet one-third of the RDA

Vitamin A ½ cup or equivalent	Vitamin C ½ cup or equivalent
Apricot or apricot nectar Broccoli (raw florets)* Cantaloupe* Carrot sticks or juice Peaches Spinach (raw for a salad)* Sweet potato (as in pudding) Tomato slices, juice, or soup* Watermelon (½ slice)*	Cabbage (for coleslaw) Cauliflower (raw florets) Grapefruit or juice Orange or juice Strawberries Tangelo or juice Tangerine or juice
Protein 1 oz or ¼ cup or equivalent	**Calcium** 1 cup or equivalent

Any meat, chicken, or fish
Peanut butter (2 tbsp)
Egg (hard-cooked or egg salad)
Cottage cheese
Hard cheese
(Meat and peanut butter are also high
  in iron and B vitamins)
	Milk
	Yogurt
	Hard cheese (1½ oz)
	Cream soup
	(These foods are also high in protein and
	  vitamins D and B$_2$)

Other foods are important, for example, whole-grain or enriched white flour products such as muffins, graham crackers, bread, noodles, rice, or pasta and other foods, for variety and to contribute other essential nutrients.

*Also contributes one-third of the RDA for vitamin C.

IS CHILDHOOD OBESITY RELATED TO ADULT OBESITY?

Obese children under three years of age who do not have obese parents are at low risk for obesity in adulthood, but among older children, obesity is an increasingly important predictor of adult obesity, regardless of whether the parents are obese. Parental obesity more than doubles the risk of adult obesity among both obese and nonobese children (Whitaker et al., 1997). Obesity is a common nutritional disturbance in children, ranging from 18 percent to 30 percent in children of various ages. It is even more problematic among certain ethnic populations (Keller & Stevens, 1996).

Obesity is increasing in a number of countries around the world, such as in Japan (Kotani et al., 1997). There is an increasing rate of Type 2 diabetes in children, which is believed to be due to increased obesity and decreased activity levels. Because there is a genetic predisposition to Type 2 diabetes, those children of high-risk ethnic populations with a strong family history of diabetes may benefit from diabetes screening and education to lessen the risk of diabetes development (Glaser, 1997). Some adolescents have been shown to have cardiovascular risk factors, which are also correlates of the insulin resistance syndrome, including higher blood pressure levels, dyslipidemia, and obesity, all of which continue into young adulthood (O'Neil et al., 1997).

Great care needs to be taken to ensure that an overweight child's self-esteem is not damaged in attempting to control weight gain. One study noted that lower self-esteem was found in children who believed they were responsible for their overweight condition as compared to those who attributed their overweight condition to an external cause. Lower self-esteem was also found in the children who believed that being overweight hindered their social interaction (Pierce & Wardle, 1997). Thus it is important to use a positive approach with obese children, with an emphasis on good nutritional choices in a variety of social settings. Care needs to be taken to avoid labeling foods as good or bad. The causes of weight gain should be assessed, such as inactivity (for example, excess television watching), eating for emotional reasons, drinking beverages high in sugar content, or physiological reasons that can predispose some children for obesity even though they may be eating the same amounts of food as their friends. It has been noted that fasting insulin levels are significantly higher and growth hormone significantly lower among obese children. Obese children also have lower resting metabolic rates (Laessle et al., 1997). The health care professional needs to address the underlying causes of obesity appropriately, rather than simply giving the child's parent or guardian a diet sheet for weight loss (see Chapter 20).

IS CHILDHOOD HYPERACTIVITY RELATED TO NUTRITION?

It is widely believed that sugar and food additives cause hyperactivity among children, although research has shown this to be generally false. Food additives may cause hyperactivity, but this is rare and is felt to be limited to children who are allergic to the additives. Sugar may actually slow a child down through its role in the production of serotonin in the brain. Often a very active child is falsely labeled as being hyperactive. Part of the public's confusion with the belief that sugar causes hyperactivity is that the consumption of sweets often coincides with stimulating activities such as school recess, birthday parties, or holidays (at which time the activity or excitement, and not the sugar, causes excess activity).

There does appear to be a genetic predisposition to attention deficit–hyperactivity disorder (ADHD) and major depression (Faraone & Biederman, 1997). Factors in the diet may one day be better understood in the management of depression and ADHD.

WHAT ARE IMPORTANT CONSIDERATIONS IN FEEDING THE PRESCHOOL-AGED CHILD (1 TO 5 YEARS OLD)?

As children grow, their eating habits change. These changes are reflective of their stage in development. Among toddlers, simple foods that are fun to eat are favorites (see Table 17–1 and Fig. 17–4). Mixed foods are generally unpopular with this age group. Differences in food textures interest children. Each meal might include something soft (such as macaroni and cheese), something chewy or crunchy (such as pineapple chunks and thinly cut carrot sticks), and something dry (such as peas). Small portions of a variety of foods at a meal can enhance satiety—the recognition of hunger being satisfied.

The child should be equipped with eating utensils and dishes that are easy to handle. The child should be offered only small amounts of food at a time. By eating at the table with the family, children are likely to develop an interest in food that mirrors that of their parents. By the age of 3 or 4 years, the child will be able to dish food onto a plate if smaller serving dishes and utensils are used. This further helps the child develop a sense of mastery over eating.

When compared with the infant, the preschool-aged child experiences a slowing rate of growth and development. A decrease in the consumption of food generally parallels this decrease in metabolic rate. A parent should not become alarmed if the following changes in eating behavior occur; rather, these changes are considered normal for the preschool child:

- Wanting foods plain, with no sauces and not mixed together
- Varying interest and lack of interest in food, with appetites that go up and down
- **Food jags**—eating only a few foods day after day or week after week until the next food jag starts

Keeping a record of food portions may help to allay parents' fears that their child is not eating enough. Being able to see the whole day or a whole week very often makes it apparent that the child is eating the recommended food servings of the Food Guide Pyramid. This knowledge, along with comparison of the child's growth with a growth chart, can be very helpful in calming parents' fears of nutritional inadequacy. A healthy appearance and high levels of energy in children is further evidence of good nutritional status (Fig. 17–5).

If the child's diet does appear to be lacking in a food group that is affecting growth, offering previously omitted foods at the times when the child is most hungry can help. Getting children to accept new foods may take time and patience. A child may need to be exposed to the food on several occasions before deciding that it is worth eating. Seeing the food in the grocery store or being prepared in the kitchen and a small portion served on the plate all help. The use of choice also helps.

Juice has increasingly become a staple beverage for toddlers. Because of excess kilocalories or replacement for milk, the amount of juice should be limited. A maximum of 12 oz per day of juice is recommended for children. Excess juice has been associated with reduced stature and increased obesity (Dennison et al., 1997).

Snacks should be planned to enhance the nutritional value of the diet (Table 17–3). Snacks should be served at least 1 hour before the meal to allow sufficient intake of food at mealtime. However, sometimes a compromise is needed if the child is very hungry. A premeal snack before dinner can be considered an appetizer. Good choices for snacks include a dish of peaches or yogurt, both nutritious for the young child.

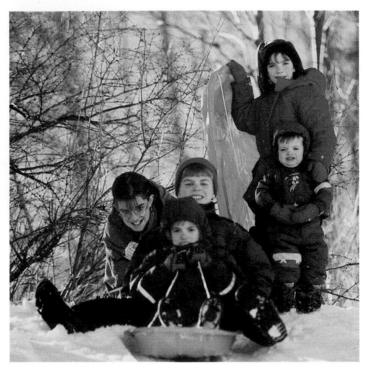

Figure 17–5
Healthy children love to play.

For a guide to the foods that should be included and amounts that should be provided for the preschool-aged child, see Table 17–4. Good food habits developed at this time will help ensure an adequate diet throughout life.

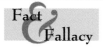

Fallacy: Once a picky eater, always a picky eater!

Fact: It takes time for food likes to develop. Children do not like many foods when they first try them, but with repeated exposure in a positive environment, even the most finicky eaters can learn to appreciate a wide variety of foods. Children should be encouraged to have one taste of all foods served but beyond that, forcing or begging a child to eat has no place in the development of long-term food preferences. It may be helpful for the anxious parent to follow the advice of Ellyn Satter, registered dietition, social worker, and author of "How to Get Your Kid to Eat . . . Not Too Much," who asserts that it is the parent's responsibility to offer nutritious foods in a positive meal setting, but that it is the child's responsibility to determine how much and what he or she eats. Children seem to eat better if they perceive they are eating because it makes them feel good and not simply to please their parents.

Table 17–3
Suggested Snacks and Finger Foods

Fruits	Vegetables
Apple wedges	Cabbage wedges
Banana slices	Carrot sticks
Berries	Cauliflower florets
Dried apples	Celery sticks*
Dried apricots	Cherry tomatoes
Dried peaches	Cucumber slices
Dried pears	Green pepper sticks
Fresh peach wedges	Tomato wedges
Fresh pear wedges	Turnip sticks
Fresh pineapple sticks	Zucchini or summer squash strips
Grapefruit sections (seeded)	
Grapes	**Meats and Meat Substitutes**
Melon cubes or balls	Cheese cube
Orange sections (seeded)	Cooked meat cubes
Pitted plums	Hard-cooked eggs
Pitted prunes	Small sandwiches (quartered)
Raisins	Toast fingers
Tangerine sections	Whole-grain crackers

*May be stuffed with cheese or peanut butter.
From U.S. Department of Agriculture: A Planning Guide for Food Service in Child Care Centers, FNS-64. Food and Nutrition Service, Washington, DC.

WHAT ARE SOME NUTRITION ISSUES IN THE PROCESS OF GROWTH AND DEVELOPMENT?

A Growing Sense of Independence among Preschoolers

A growing sense of independence occurs naturally in preschoolers. Parents will be well advised to offer the preschooler structured choices to allow for a sense of independence. This applies to food as well as to other daily activities (for example, "Are you going to put on your shoes or am I?"). Recognition of this facet of the growing child can foster positive parent-child interaction and healthy food selection. A structured food choice at the dinner table might be, "Would you like apple slices or a banana for dessert?" A structured food choice at the supermarket might be to allow the child a choice of cereals with less than 6 grams (1.5 teaspoons) of sugar.

Promoting Sound Food Values

The manner in which food is offered is fundamental to the development of interest in a variety of nutritious foods. If you reflect for a moment on the types of holiday foods promoted, such as chocolate on Valentine's Day and candy at Hal-

Table 17–4
Pattern of Feeding for Preschool-Aged Children

Meal	Children 1 to 3 Years	Children 3 to 6 Years
Breakfast		
Milk, fluid*	½ cup	¾ cup
Juice or fruit	¼ cup	½ cup
Cereal or bread, enriched or whole-grain[†] cereal or bread	¼ cup[‡]	⅓ cup[§]
	½ slice	½ slice
Midmorning or Midafternoon Supplement		
Milk, fluid* or juice or fruit or vegetable	½ cup	½ cup
Bread or cereal, enriched or whole-grain[†] bread or cereal	½ slice	½ slice
	¼ cup[‡]	⅓ cup[§]
Lunch or Supper		
Milk, fluid*	½ cup	¾ cup
Meat or meat alternate[¶]		
Meat, poultry, or fish, cooked**	1 oz	1 ½ oz
Cheese	1 oz	1 ½ oz
Egg	1	1
Cooked dry beans and peas	⅛ cup	¼ cup
Peanut butter	1 tbsp	2 tbsp
Vegetables and fruits[††]	¼ cup	½ cup
Bread, enriched or whole-grain[†]	½ slice	½ slice

*Includes whole milk, low-fat milk, skim milk, cultured buttermilk, or flavored milk made from these types of fluid milk, which meet state and local standards.
[†]Or an equivalent serving of an acceptable bread product made of enriched or whole-grain meal or flour.
[‡]¼ cup (volume) of ⅓ oz (weight), whichever is less.
[§]⅓ cup (volume) or ½ oz (weight), whichever is less.
[¶]Or an equivalent quantity of any combination of foods listed under Meat and Meat Alternates.
**Cooked lean meat without bone.
[††]Must include at least two kinds.
From U.S. Department of Agriculture: A Planning Guide for Food Service Child Care Centers, FNS-64. Food and Nutrition Service, Washington, DC, p. 5.

loween, you will quickly realize the value our society places on food. However, it is possible to promote nutritious foods. Kiwi fruit might be offered in Easter baskets and dried fruit at Halloween.

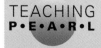

TEACHING
P•E•A•R•L

One woman captured the idea of positive values associated with vegetables. When someone commented on the wide variety of vegetables her children liked, her reply was, "Do you know how I did it? Whenever I offered a reward I would say, 'If you are good you can have a vegetable!'" Rewarding with food is not recommended, especially because candy is often the reward of choice. Rewarding with vegetables in this scenario, however, allowed the children to develop a strong appreciation for a healthy food group.

Parents and caregivers are the most effective nutrition educators of children. They teach by example and by attitude. Parents and daycare providers should be encouraged to promote positive food choices in an enjoyable manner.

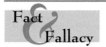

Fallacy: Once a sweet tooth, always a sweet tooth.

Fact: Children whose diets are continually high in sugar can lose their ability to appreciate the natural taste of foods. As with salt and other substances, the taste for sweetness can be both learned and unlearned. Gradual reduction in quantities used is the easiest and surest way to overcome a "sweet tooth."

Coping with Food Advertisements

Because many television or written advertisements promote foods that are not very nutritious (when was the last time you saw an ad for broccoli?), children need to be empowered to resist the negative messages. One approach is to divide food into two categories: foods that help you grow and those that do not, or foods that make you grow tall versus those that make you grow wide. This approach can help the child appreciate that the adult is being helpful by providing nutritious foods that are not advertised on television.

Working Mothers

Two parents working or single mothers working can put added stress on mealtime. Finding time to prepare meals and to offer meals in a relaxed, positive manner can be difficult. Quick meal ideas for the working family may be helpful. Examples include a meal of scrambled eggs, whole-grain toast, mini carrots, and milk, or a meal might consist of bean and cheese burritos using either commercial or home-made refried beans rolled into flour tortillas and served with fresh fruit and beverage of choice.

WHAT ARE THE IMPORTANT CONSIDERATIONS IN FEEDING SCHOOL-AGED CHILDREN (5 TO 11 YEARS OLD)?

Meeting the nutritional requirements of the 5- to 11-year-old child takes larger amounts of the same foods needed by the preschool-aged child. Growth during prepuberty is slow and steady, with gradual increases in height and weight.

With the introduction of school into the child's daily routine, the child's meal pattern is likely to change. The child may have to eat breakfast earlier to allow sufficient time to get to school. Children who skip breakfast are less well fed because it is difficult to make up missed nutrients at other meals. If the family has good breakfast habits, the child will likely continue this practice. The child may be taught to prepare a simple but nutritious breakfast. Parents should eat breakfast with their children; even setting aside 5 minutes for eating a quick bowl of non-sugar-coated cereal is helpful.

At school the child is introduced to group feeding. Peers and teachers may influence eating behavior, and the child may be more or less willing to try an unfamiliar food, depending on the eating behavior of others in the group. A child who has been exposed to a wide variety of foods at home is more likely to try new foods at school or at a friend's house.

Whether the child brings a lunch prepared at home or buys lunch from the National School Lunch Program, lunch should supply approximately one-third of the RDA for all nutrients (see the table on the inside front cover). Nutrition education may occur at school through such means as cooking and identifying foods. Ideally, this food exposure at school should positively promote sound food choices without labeling foods as good or bad.

HOW DO THE CHANGES OF ADOLESCENCE AFFECT EATING PATTERNS?

Although children may be best friends and equals in elementary school, the onset of adolescence creates vast differences. Girls especially tend to increase their amount of body fat just prior to puberty and their "growth spurt" (the time of increased long-bone growth). Their male peers, who do not reach puberty as early and retain their boyish frames, may begin to question their masculinity. Eventually boys catch up to the girls with increased muscle mass and long-bone growth. All this is happening as the adolescent's face begins to look like a war zone covered with acne—or so it is perceived, even if there is only one pimple. All of these changes are hormonally related.

Intense concern with nutritional intake develops as a consequence of these changes, but too often in a negative way. Some teenagers try weight-control diets either to lose their baby fat or to regain a sense of control over their rapidly changing bodies. This can result in conditions such as anorexia and bulimia (see Chapter 15). Others ignore sound nutritional practices (such as eating potato chips in place of fruits or drinking soft drinks in place of milk) in order to feel accepted among their peers. The need for a sense of self-worth and of identity can take priority over good nutritional practices.

Other barriers to good nutritional intake that adolescents encounter include the following:

1. *Society's emphasis on slimness.* Television advertisements now promote "the perfect size 6." Women still aspire to the 19-inch waists once common among 19th-century women, who achieved their hourglass figures by wearing tight-laced corsets. We tend to forget that we are 20th-century women who are taller and proportionally larger than our earlier counterparts. Good nutrition can suffer, particularly among female adolescents, in the attempt to achieve this unrealistic image.
2. *Access to jobs and spending money.* This allows the adolescent greater freedom in purchasing food as well as restricting the time to eat, since teenagers often

dash to part-time work directly from school. Fast food outlets are a common lure for this population. Adolescents' sense of immortality can overshadow their knowledge of the importance of good nutrition, which can result in an increased intake of fat and sugar. If this type of eating habit becomes entrenched, it can be difficult to alter eating habits as an older adult, when the need becomes more apparent.

3. *Athletic sports.* After-school sports, while a positive influence on teen's physical and mental health (see Fig. 20–1), can make it difficult for the student to eat appropriately. Dinnertime with family is often usurped by practice or game times. Limited mealtime promotes reliance on processed foods, which often are high in fat and sugar. Safe portable foods can be packed by the teen, such as a peanut butter sandwich and banana or dried apricots with bottled water or juice as a beverage. Milk intake can be promoted at other meals and as a bedtime snack in the form of yogurt or a bowl of cereal with milk.

4. *More time spent away from home.* Adolescents are increasingly in a position to determine what or if they eat. This, coupled with adolescent rebellion, can result in their consuming the opposite of what they know they should. If this is a problem for the adolescent's health needs, problem-solving with the teen should be emphasized. Just as young children better accept and practice desired behaviors when they are given choices, so do persons of all ages.

5. *Alcohol as a rite of passage.* Alcohol increasingly becomes an issue for teenagers. Television advertising can lure them into thinking that alcohol, such as beer, brings with it fun and glamour. Alcohol use can make teenagers feel more adult and independent. Many teenagers regularly drink beer and wine. Alcoholism occurs in teenagers. Alcohol can seriously impair the final stages of growth and development by replacing foods or more nutritious beverages such as milk and juice. Chronic alcohol intake can impair the body's ability to absorb and use food nutrients.

WHAT ARE THE NUTRITIONAL REQUIREMENTS OF THE ADOLESCENT (12 TO 18 YEARS OLD)?

During the rapid growth period of adolescence, kilocalorie and nutrient needs are higher to provide for increases in bone density, muscle mass, and blood volume and for the developing endocrine system. There is an increased need for kilocalories, calcium, iron, and iodine (see the table on the inside front cover). Unfortunately, this message has not been adequately "heard" by teens. Average intakes of female adolescents have been found to be below recommendations for vitamin E, calcium, iron, and zinc; for adolescent males there was inadequate intake of vitamin E, calcium, and zinc. In addition, the diet of adolescents generally has inadequate fiber and excess fat and saturated fat (Levine & Guthrie, 1997). There is increasing evidence that calcium intake up to the threshold amount, about 1500 mg, increases bone mass during growth. The National Institutes of Health recommends increasing the dietary allowance of calcium to 1500 mg per day in adolescence, which has been shown to be safe (McKenna et al., 1997). Nutrient needs can be met by increasing the serving size or number of dairy servings to four per day with the addition of other calcium foods such as legumes and certain leafy green vegetables (see Tables 1–2 and 1–3). A minimum of 3 cups of milk equivalent (or about 1000 mg of calcium) needs to be recommended to all teens (Albertson et al., 1997). A vegan or macrobiotic diet (no animal products including milk) can result in decreased bone mass in adolescents, which may increase the risk of fracture in later life (Parsons et al., 1997).

WHAT IS THE ROLE OF THE NURSE OR OTHER HEALTH CARE PROFESSIONAL IN PROMOTING GOOD NUTRITION DURING CHILDHOOD?

For Children

The terminology used with children needs to be concrete and nonscientific. Children cannot understand abstract concepts, such as the role of nutrients in foods, even though a young child can pronounce the words. Therefore, it is more appropriate to focus on promoting positive attitudes toward eating nutritious foods. Children can appreciate the concept that eating is fun, and this concept should be applied to nutritious foods. One method that strongly appeals to children (and even to the parents who may be present) is the use of puppet shows. Stick puppets are made easily with food pictures, and with the addition of paper eyes and mouths they "come alive." Children's books such as *Green Eggs and Ham,* or *Stone Soup* can also favorably influence a child's willingness to try new foods.

For Teenagers

A sensitive approach to teenagers' needs, recognizing their need for autonomy and acceptance by their peers, should be used in counseling or educational settings. The use of appropriate humor can help the teenager recognize that the health care professional is a caring human being, not merely an authority figure. Comments should be positive ones that help promote positive self-worth and do not undermine a teenager's already fragile self-image. Teenagers should be told about realistic body perceptions and eating patterns such as those represented in growth charts and the Food Guide Pyramid.

Nutrition counseling is especially important for the teenager who has failed to develop good food habits up to this point and for the teenager who has strayed from previously good habits. Information should be presented in an interesting and motivating manner. Because teenagers are very interested in their physical appearance, it should be emphasized that adequate nutrients allow for optimal growth and development of their bodies. A teenaged girl who feels that she is overweight and starts to lose weight too rapidly can use a growth chart to gain a better sense of normalcy. This tool can be particularly helpful to a teenager with anorexia or bulimia when she can visualize her growth fall from the normal curve (Fig. 17–6). Although relatively rare, boys are also known to experience anorexia and bulimia (see Chapter 15).

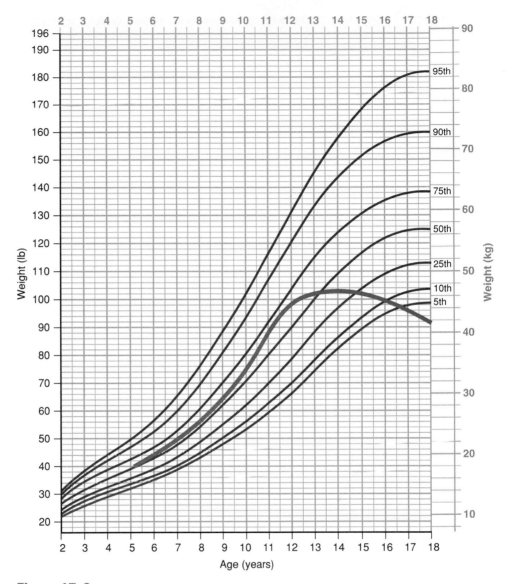

Figure 17–6

Sample growth fall from normal curve as assessed using the weight-for-age chart for girls 2 to 18 years of age.

It is important that the counselor respect the teenager's independence. Presenting the adolescent with flexible eating styles instead of a rigid eating pattern will increase the effectiveness of counseling. Special problems of teenagers, such as obesity, alcoholism, anorexia nervosa, and pregnancy, should be an important focus of nutrition counseling, as should prevention of heart disease, cancer, diabetes, osteoporosis, and other diseases that may occur later in life.

Critical Thinking

Case Study

Cindy kept losing weight and she did not know why. She was always so thirsty and tired. She decided she was tired because she was up all night in the bathroom. Her parents said if she did not stop losing weight that they were going to take her to the doctor. They seemed surprised at the amount of food she could eat and still lose weight. Cindy figured it was because she was playing the mid-field position on the soccer team. Her mother had asked her if she was vomiting every time she went to the bathroom. Cindy thought that was an odd question. She just had to urinate.

Applications

1. What is the likely cause of Cindy's weight loss based on her symptoms?
2. What might Cindy's parents think the reason for her weight loss is?
3. How might Cindy react to the diagnosis of a chronic illness?
4. What advice could you offer Cindy if she needs to purchase food from a school vending machine to treat hypoglycemia?

Study Questions and Classroom Activities

1. How would you explain the terms *growth* and *development*?
2. List all the reasons that a good breakfast is important from early childhood throughout life.
3. What effects might be expected later in life from foods inadequate in quantity and quality during the growing period?
4. Why is it particularly important for an adolescent girl to have a nutritious diet?
5. What issues would a teenager who has diabetes face (refer to Chapter 9)?

References

Albertson AM, Tobelmann RC, Marquart L: Estimated dietary calcium intake and food sources for adolescent females: 1980–92. J Adolesc Health. January 1997; 20(1):20–26.

Dennison BA, Rockwell HL, Baker SL: Excess fruit juice consumption by preschool-aged children is associated with short stature and obesity. Pediatrics. January 1997; 99(1): 15–22.

Faraone SV, Biederman J: Do attention deficit hyperactivity disorder and major depression share familial risk factors? J Nerv Ment Dis. September 1997; 185(9):533–541.

Glaser NS: Non-insulin-dependent diabetes mellitus in childhood and adolescence. Pediatr Clin North Am. April 1997; 44(2):307–337.

Keller C, Stevens KR: Childhood obesity: Measurement and risk assessment. Pediatr Nurs. November 1996; 22(6):494–499.

Kleinman RE, Murphy JM, Little M, Pagano M, Wehler CA, Regal K, Jellinek MS: Hunger in children in the United States: Potential behavioral and emotional correlates. Pediatrics. January 1, 1998; 101(1):E3.

Kotani K, Nishida M, Yamashita S, Funahashi T, Fujioka S, Tokunaga K, Ishikawa K, Tarui S, Matsuzawa Y: Two decades of annual medical examinations in Japanese obese children: Do obese children grow into obese adults? Int J Obes Relat Metab Disord. October 1997; 21(10):912–921.

Laessle RG, Wurmser H, Pirke KM: A comparison of resting metabolic rate, self-rated food intake, growth hormone, and insulin levels in obese and nonobese preadolescents. Physiol Behav. May 1997; 61(5):725–729.

Levine E, Guthrie JF: Nutrient intakes and eating patterns of teenagers. Family Economics and Nutrition Review. 1997; 10(3):20–35.

McKenna AA, Ilich JZ, Andon MB, Wang C, Matkovic V: Zinc balance in adolescent females consuming a low- or high-calcium diet. Am J Clin Nutr. May 1997; 65(5): 1460–1464.

O'Neil CE, Nicklas TA, Myers L, Johnson CC, Berenson GS: Cardiovascular risk factors and behavior lifestyles of young women: Implications from findings of the Bogalusa Heart Study. Am J Med Sci. December 1997; 314(6):385–395.

Parsons TJ, van Dusseldorp M, van der Vliet M, van de Werken K, Schaafsma G, van Staveren WA: Reduced bone mass in Dutch adolescents fed a macrobiotic diet in early life. J Bone Miner Res. September 1997; 12(9):1486–1494.

Pierce JW, Wardle J: Cause and effect beliefs and self-esteem of overweight children. J Child Psychol Psychiatry. September 1997; 38(6):645–650.

Vohr BR, Msall ME: Neuropsychological and functional outcomes of very low birth weight infants. Semin Perinatol. June 1997; 21(3):202–220.

Whitaker RC, Wright JA, Pepe MS, Seidel KD, Dietz WH: Predicting obesity in young adulthood from childhood and parental obesity. N Engl J Med. September 25, 1997; 337(13):869–873.

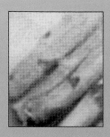

18
Nutritional Care of the Developmentally Disabled

Objectives

After completing this chapter, you should be able to:

- Define developmental disability.
- Describe specific nutritional problems and conditions of the developmentally disabled.
- Discuss the role of each health care team member in feeding and weight control programs.
- Discuss mealtime skills and feeding techniques in relation to eating problems.

Terms to Identify

Autism
Cerebral palsy
Developmental disability
Down syndrome
Epilepsy
Hyperkinesis

Inborn errors of
  metabolism
Mental retardation
Neurological
  impairment

Phenylketonuria (PKU)
Prader-Willi syndrome
  (PWS)
Spasticity
Tongue thrust

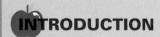 INTRODUCTION

The developmentally disabled population is at nutritional risk because of feeding problems, food and drug interactions, altered growth patterns, and metabolic disorders. The maintenance and promotion of good nutritional status ultimately spares society an economic burden by facilitating independent living versus care through institutions. They also help society realize a moral obligation to ensure that all citizens are allowed the pursuit of a high-quality life.

Caregivers of persons with developmental disabilities have to deal with issues such as difficulty in understanding and implementing diet instructions, inappropriate feeding practices, lack of nutritional information, and lack of knowledge regarding appropriate food selection and preparation. They may also have difficulty limiting food intake out of sympathy for the child or adult with a developmental disorder (Cloud, 1997).

Appropriate nutrition programs and services can have a positive impact on the health of the developmentally disabled population by helping to prevent further disabilities, improving overall health and nutritional status, and maximizing educational, vocational, and social potential.

WHAT IS MEANT BY A DEVELOPMENTAL DISABILITY?

The term **developmental disability,** according to the Developmental Disabilities Assistance and Bill of Rights Act, refers to a severe, chronic disability that

1. is attributable to a mental or physical impairment or a combination of mental and physical impairments;
2. is manifested before the person reaches the age of 22 years;
3. is likely to continue indefinitely;
4. results in substantial functional limitations in three or more of the following areas of major life activity: self-care, receptive and expressive language, learning, mobility, self-direction, capacity for independent living, and economic self-sufficiency; and
5. reflects the person's need for a combination and sequence of special interdisciplinary or generic care, treatment, or other services that are lifelong or of extended duration and individually planned and coordinated.

The subcategories of developmental disabilities are **mental retardation** (a general term for a wide range of conditions resulting from many different causes, some of which are directly related to various diseases); **autism** (characterized by extreme withdrawal and an obsessive desire to maintain the present status; temper tantrums and language disturbances are evident); **cerebral palsy** (characterized by a persistent qualitative motor disorder caused by nonprogressive damage to the brain; may involve sensory deficits and mental retardation; exhibits varying levels of **spasticity** [movements of the body]; Figure 18–1 shows individuals with cerebral palsy and Down syndrome); **epilepsy** (a group of symptoms or conditions that overstimulate nerve cells of the brain, resulting in seizures); and **neurological impairment** (involves sensory, mentation, and consciousness functions; Table 18–1).

HOW IS THE NUTRITIONAL STATUS OF THE DEVELOPMENTALLY DISABLED INDIVIDUAL ASSESSED?

The same steps in the nutrition assessment process that were discussed in Chapters 2 and 7 are followed for the developmentally disabled population, but standard criteria are not yet available, thus making it more difficult to assess nutritional status. Growth charts, except in the case of **Down syndrome** (a genetic

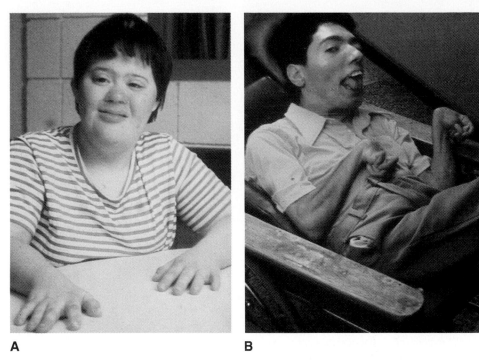

A   B

Figure 18–1
(*A*) Client with Down syndrome. (*B*) Client with cerebral palsy. (Courtesy of Ross Laboratories, Personal Touch Slides.)

defect that consists of an extra gene and results in varying levels of retardation, short stature, and characteristic facial features; Fig. 18–1), have not been developed, and ways to determine dietary needs have not been clearly established. Height is used in determining energy needs of a child with developmental disabilities (Table 18–2).

Weighing and measuring someone with bony deformities and severe contractures may be more difficult than it is for a normally developed person. Segmental measurements taken from joint to joint with a flexible metal tape are totaled, giving an approximate length, which is then plotted on a growth chart. Nonambulatory persons can be weighed in a sling-type balance such as a Hoyt lift (Fig. 18–2).

When assessing the nutritional status of the developmentally disabled individual, the dietitian addresses several areas. Figure 18–3 shows a flowchart for attaining nutritional goals. A detailed assessment is necessary if any of the following are present or suspected:

Unusual food habits
Inadequate or imbalanced dietary intake
Inadequate feeding skills
Problems with sucking, swallowing, or chewing
Marked overweight or underweight condition

Table 18–1
Description and Nutritional Implications of Some Conditions

Common Characteristics	Nutritional Implication
Down Syndrome (Caused by Chromosomal Abnormalities)	
Reduce muscle tone in varying degrees	Chewing, swallowing, sucking and tongue control may be affected
	Appetite and behavior at mealtime may be affected
Growth retardation:	Weight control
Small flattened skull	
Narrow nasal passage	
Delayed tooth development	Dental caries
Narrow palate	Eating problems
Cerebral Palsy	
Neuromuscular impairment:	Weight control
Motor disability	
Poor occlusion	Difficulties in chewing, swallowing, tongue control, and drooling
Types:	
Spastic: disharmony of muscle movements	Overweight condition possible because of limited movement
Athetoid: involuntary movements of extremities	Underweight condition possible
Ataxic: inability or awkwardness in maintaining balance	
Hypotonic: muscles fail to respond to stimulation	
Hypersensitivity	Sensitivity to taste temperatures and consistency of food
Prader-Willi Syndrome (Endocrine, Hypothalamic Disorder)	
Hyperphagia	
Obesity	Weight control
Short stature	Feeding difficulties in infancy
Small hands and feet	Dental caries
Hypogenitalism	
Mild mental retardation	
Bizarre eating behaviors (gorging, food stealing, eating inappropriate foods, e.g., pet food)	
Poor sucking ability and failure to thrive in infancy	
Rapid weight gain after 1 year of age	
Slow motor development	
Obesity-related diabetes in later childhood	
Frequent lack of emotional control	

Table 18-2
Energy Requirement Chart for Individuals with Disabilities

Diagnosis	Energy Requirement
Cerebral palsy (mild spasticity), 5–11 years old	13.9 kcal/cm
Cerebral palsy (severe spasticity), 5–11 years old	11.1 kcal/cm
Down syndrome, boys	16.1 kcal/cm
Down syndrome, girls	14.3 kcal/cm

From Rhudy NT, Kristopher L, Miller A, Murphy P: Calculating Nutritional Requirements for Individuals with Disabilities. Morgantown, WV, Nutrition and Dietary Services, University Affiliated Center for Developmental Disabilities (UACDD).

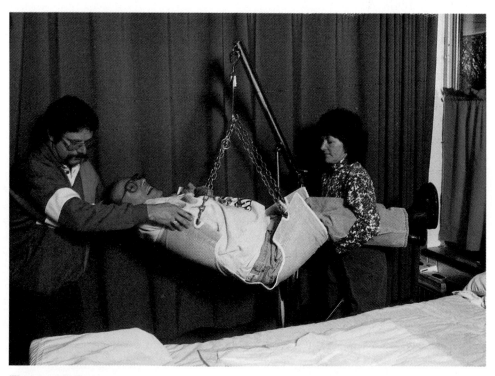

Figure 18-2
Weighing a nonambulatory person in a Hoyt lift.

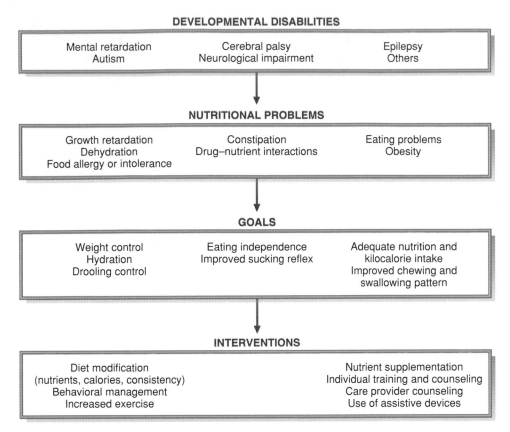

Figure 18–3
Flowchart for attaining nutritional goals for the developmentally disabled population.

WHAT ARE THE NUTRITION-RELATED PROBLEMS AND CONCERNS?

Eating problems may result from neuromuscular dysfunction such as hyperactive gag reflex, tongue thrust, poor lip closure and inability to chew or obstructive lesions, psychological factors, or a combination of factors (ADA Position Paper, 1997). *Neuromuscular dysfunction* refers to abnormal sensory input and muscle tone and is manifested in sucking, swallowing, and chewing movements that are hampered when oral muscles do not function properly. When chewing reflexes are lacking, ways must be found to stimulate them. For example, sweet and cold foods are found to be effective. Also, the act of chewing stimulates saliva production and facilitates swallowing.

Neuromuscular dysfunction is common in cerebral palsy, Down syndrome, and the Prader-Willi syndrome. One study found that more than 90 percent of children with cerebral palsy had clinically significant oral motor dysfunction. One-third of these children were severely impaired and therefore at high risk of chronic undernourishment (Reilly et al., 1996).

Anatomic defects and *malformations,* such as cleft palate, may cause food to pass into the nasal passages. Choking is a major concern in such a condition. Poor lip closure and tongue control, a strong bite reflex, tongue thrust, excessive drooling, choking, and delayed hand-to-mouth coordination are likely to cause inadequate nutrient intake. **Tongue thrust** is a term used to describe the condition in which the teeth are not brought together to initiate swallowing, the tongue pushes out saliva, and drooling occurs. It should be noted that special feeders are available for babies with anatomic defects and that surgery can largely correct cleft palate.

Just as a period of anxiety can cause gastric distress in the normally functioning population, *behavioral problems* such as tantrums, agitation, rocking, and flailing of arms (forms of self-stimulation) can result in esophagitis, aspiration of food, dehydration, and malnutrition in the developmentally disabled. Pica behavior (the ingestion of nonfood items) may cause malabsorption of certain nutrients or even intestinal blockage. Food stealing is another behavioral problem that often occurs in conditions such as the Prader-Willi syndrome.

Dental Problems

Dental caries, periodontal disease, and other oral conditions, if left untreated, are impairments that can limit a child's development (American Academy of Pediatric Dentistry, 1996). Poor oral hygiene, the inability to perform self-help skills, or both, as well as the excessive intake of sweets, will result in dental caries. Certain medications can cause gum hyperplasia (especially anticonvulsants); therefore, good dental hygiene and regular checkups, as well as intake of foods that stimulate gums, should be encouraged. Sweet, sticky snacks should be discouraged and not used as rewards. Appropriate food reinforcers are sometimes needed, however, to help modify behavior (see later discussion).

Dental caries and periodontal disease are major problems. Suppressed immune function, drug therapy, oral motor dysfunction, and modified diets put the developmentally disabled person at high risk for oral infections. Three-fourths of congenital anomalies affect the head and facial regions of the body. Cleft lip, cleft palate, misaligned jaws and teeth, and malocclusion can have a serious effect on speech, socialization, chewing ability, the enjoyment of eating, and nutritional status. The tissues of the oral cavity are sensitive to nutrient imbalances. Caregivers are often so overwhelmed with medical, physical, psychological, and feeding concerns that regular home dental care can be neglected.

To alleviate dental problems, sugar and sweets should be limited in frequency and vegetable consumption encouraged on a daily basis. Soft foods and modified texture are necessary if gums are swollen and chewing is painful.

Individuals with Down syndrome have a normal size tongue, but because of their facial structure, the oral cavity is frequently too small to accommodate the tongue, which may have deep fissures that can retain food particles. Consequently, tongue brushing should be part of daily oral hygiene.

Autistic children may pouch their food rather than swallow it and prefer soft foods that require little chewing. This puts them at greater risk for dental caries.

Growth Problems and Weight Disorders

Growth retardation, being underweight, and obesity are common problems among developmentally disabled persons and require nutritional intervention. Nutritional factors influencing growth and weight abnormalities include the following:

Inadequate dietary intake caused by feeding problems (such as oral abnormalities), reflux, or food scarcity
Chronic conditions such as congenital heart disease that increase nutrient needs
Lack of weight-bearing resulting from a disability that prevents mobility
Metabolic disorders such as phenylketonuria and maple syrup urine disease
Inability to absorb food, such as in celiac disease and galactosemia

Excessive weight compounds the health problems already present. The goals of independent care and mobility are impaired with excess weight. Health care costs will be increased for those individuals requiring braces and wheelchairs if they have to be modified as weight increases. And, as in the general population, hypertension, diabetes, hyperlipidemia, and decreased pulmonary function may develop.

Persons with Down syndrome and the **Prader-Willi syndrome** (**PWS;** a genetic condition of unknown etiology) are frequently identified as being obese. Obesity is likely to occur whenever there is limited mobility, poor muscle tone, altered growth, lack of nutritional knowledge, hyperphagia, and feeding and eating problems, unless a preventive approach is taken by caregivers and parents. Unfortunately, some well-meaning people believe that food is the only source of enjoyment for those who are physically and mentally disabled. Such an attitude will only lead to more health problems.

People with PWS need fewer kilocalories than are normally required to maintain weight. However, hyperphagia is often present. A clear preference for carbohydrate foods has been found among persons with PWS, followed by protein and then fat (Fieldstone et al., 1997). Large, soft cage balls, Sittercize records, simple dance routines, and walks are all effective in promoting weight loss (Fig. 18–4). Kilocalorie needs are increased with **hyperkinesis** (excessive movement) and seizure activity. Persons with cerebral palsy often have very rigid muscles, which can increase kilocalorie needs (hypertonia). The hypotonic form of cerebral palsy will require reduced kilocalories to allow for appropriate weight.

WHAT ARE SOME COMMON DRUG-NUTRIENT INTERACTIONS IN THE DEVELOPMENTALLY DISABLED?

Long-term drug therapy is frequently needed for controlling seizures, behavioral problems, recurrent infections, chronic constipation, and attention deficit disorders. The medications that are prescribed include anticonvulsants, central nervous system stimulants and depressants, and laxatives. These drugs may affect nutritional status in different ways (Pronsky, 1997).

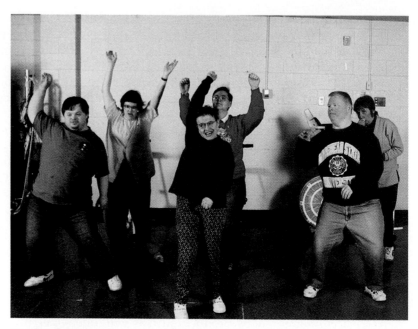

Figure 18–4
Clients exercising to promote weight loss in a simple dance routine.

Chronic use of anticonvulsants can result in abnormal nutrient and bone metabolism and gingival hyperplasia. These drugs may also result in folate deficiency and may increase serum iron levels and decrease serum ferritin. Therefore, consumption of dark green leafy vegetables, whole grains, and legumes should be encouraged.

Central nervous system stimulants can cause a loss of appetite (anorexia), insomnia, and stomach pains, which may result in weight loss. Some antidepressants and tranquilizers are known to promote weight gain because of fluid retention and an increase in appetite.

Laxatives, bulk preparations, stimulants, and stool softeners for bowel management programs require additional fluids and fiber-rich foods in the diet. The excessive use of laxatives for constipation may affect nutrient absorption. Mineral oil may decrease the absorption of fat-soluble vitamins, calcium, and phosphate.

Inactivity (physical and peristaltic), inadequate fiber and fluid intake, and certain medications contribute to the problem of constipation in the developmentally disabled population. Chewing and swallowing difficulties caused by the disability may mean that fibrous fruits and vegetables are not tolerated. However, bran and prune juice (natural laxatives) can be incorporated into the daily diet.

The individual who experiences drooling or who is prone to urinary tract infections is especially in need of extra fluids. Some developmentally disabled individuals are unable to express their thirst or are unaware of the need for fluids and must be encouraged and assisted in obtaining beverages. It must be remembered, however, that plain water satisfies thirst best and that sweetened beverages and salty liquids may increase the body's need for fluids. At least 64 oz (about 2000 mL, or 1 mL of fluid for each kilocalorie in the diet) of fluids should be offered daily, and physical activity as tolerated should be encouraged to promote bowel regularity. Thickened liquids may be necessary to ensure adequate intake if swallowing problems are present. Appropriate commercial thickeners, baby rice cereal, or yogurt may also be used to thicken liquids.

It is important, therefore, that nutrition counseling be provided. Vitamin and mineral supplements may be recommended to offset any nutritional problems that result from long-term drug therapy. Tables 7–7 and 7–8 show drug-nutrient interactions, including drugs that are commonly prescribed for conditions of the developmentally disabled individual.

WHAT ARE CONDITIONS OF INBORN ERRORS OF METABOLISM?

The term **inborn errors of metabolism** refers to a group of diseases that affect a wide variety of metabolic processes. Certain enzymes are lacking because of a genetic defect, requiring the diet to be modified to prevent toxicity from the excessive accumulation of by-products such as with phenylketonuria (PKU; discussed below). Failure to detect inborn errors of metabolism at an early age results in a variety of severe problems such as damage to the central nervous system and many body organs if an effective treatment is not started soon after birth. Many inborn errors of metabolism require specific diets for treatment. A specific diet order from the physician should be obtained, and the dietitian should provide a list of acceptable foods for various special occasions.

Galactosemia. Features that characterize galactosemia include a lack of transferase (a liver enzyme that converts galactose to glucose), toxic levels of galactose in the blood, diarrhea, drowsiness, edema, liver failure, hemorrhage, and mental retardation.

The lack of the enzyme transferase requires elimination of all milk products or other milk ingredients such as lactose, nonfat dry milk solids, casein, whey, and whey solids (see Table 15–2). Acceptable infant formulas are Isomil, Neo-Mull-Soy, ProSobee, Soylac, meat-based formulas, Nutramigen, and Pregestimil. Additional nutrients are provided according to the RDA.

It is very important that all ingredient labels for processed and packaged foods be read carefully. Any foods containing milk, lactose, nonfat dry milk solids, casein, whey, or whey solids cannot be tolerated. Lactate, lactic acid, and lactalbumin are acceptable. The complete list of ingredients may not be found on some foods, such as bread and imitation milk. Therefore, frequent monitoring of red blood cell levels of galactose and galactose-1-phosphate is recommended to assure adherence to the diet.

Phenylketonuria. Phenylketonuria (PKU) is an autosomal recessive disorder characterized by a lack of the enzyme necessary to metabolize phenylalanine, one of the essential amino acids. As phenylalanine is not metabolized, high levels accumulate and there is a characteristic excretion of phenylketones in the urine. Infants are usually blond, blue-eyed, and fair and often have eczema. The genetic heritage of PKU in Northern Ireland can be traced back to Palaeolithic people of western Europe who first colonized Ireland. Several less common forms of PKU can be traced to the Norwegian Atlantic coast and were probably introduced into Ireland by Vikings (Zschocke et al., 1997). All infants are now tested at birth for PKU. When untreated, the infants are hyperactive and irritable with an unpleasant personality and a musty or gamy odor. Severe retardation results if treatment is delayed. However, some studies have shown improvement in behavior in untreated individuals later in life even when the diet was not started at birth.

Breast-feeding is possible with children who have phenylketonuria (Duncan & Elder, 1997). Bottle-fed infants require special infant formulas that prevent buildup of toxic levels of phenylalanine. Lofenalac, Phenyl-Free, and PKU-Aid are acceptable. A 10 to 30 percent increase of protein over the RDA is necessary to assure adequate utilization of amino acids. Kilocalories need to be adjusted for the age, appetite, and growth pattern of the child. Special tables showing the phenylalanine content of various foods are available. Only one-fourth of the phenylalanine provided by the protein of the RDA should be consumed. Many products on the market contain aspartame, which is a source of phenylalanine and can be a problem for individuals with PKU.

Maternal phenylketonuria (PKU) in untreated women has resulted in offspring with microcephaly, mental retardation, congenital heart disease, and intrauterine growth retardation. Women with PKU should begin a low-phenylalanine diet to achieve phenylalanine levels less than 360 µmol/L prior to conception and should maintain this throughout pregnancy (Rouse et al., 1997).

Homocystinuria. This disease is characterized by a lack of the enzyme necessary for sulfur amino acid metabolism. The purpose of the diet for homocystinuria is to lower blood methionine and homocystine levels. Adequate L-cystine must be supplied. It is used to prevent the buildup of methionine and homocystine in the plasma and homocystine in the urine. Typically, the untreated child is retarded, with a fair complexion and detached retinas. Death usually occurs from spontaneous thrombosis.

Tyrosinosis. This disorder is a result of an error in tyrosine metabolism. The purpose of the diet for tyrosinosis is to reduce plasma tyrosine and phenylalanine levels and to prevent liver and kidney damage. It may prevent mental deterioration if started early in life.

Maple Syrup Urine Disease. In maple syrup urine disease (MSUD) there is an inability to utilize branched-chain amino acids. The purpose of the diet for this disease is to reduce leucine, isoleucine, and valine plasma levels to normal. The diet is used to prevent neurological damage and rapid death by reducing these branched-chain amino acids in the diet.

Histidinemia. This condition is caused by a lack of the enzyme for histidine metabolism. The purpose of the diet is to lower the plasma histidine level and to treat the symptoms of histidinemia, which results in speech disorders and mental retardation. Special formulas are available for homocystinuria, tyrosinosis, MSUD, and histidinemia.

WHAT OTHER CONDITIONS ARE ASSOCIATED WITH DEVELOPMENTAL DISORDERS?

Epilepsy. People with this condition have intermittent or chronic seizure activity. Grand mal seizures are those in which seizure activity is very pronounced and the person may be harmed through the extreme physical movements. Petit mal seizures may go unnoticed and last for only seconds at a time. An underweight child who has intermittent periods of "staring" may be having chronic seizure activity that increases the need for kilocalories but diminishes the ability to consume adequate amounts of food.

The ketogenic diet was originally introduced in the 1920s and is once again increasingly being used to control seizure activity. In one study, 40 percent of the children experienced at least half of their usual seizure activity and another 25 percent became seizure free while on a ketogenic diet (Batchelor et al., 1997). The effect of the ketogenic diet can exceed that of medications. The effect of the ketogenic diet appears to be a change in the brain's metabolism from glucose to ketones (Swink et al., 1997).

Autism. The serotonin system has been implicated as a factor in some cases of autism. Because serotonin acts as a neurotransmitter, low levels of serotonin may explain the problems with language and sensory integration of persons with autism (Chugani et al., 1997). Medications called serotonin reuptake inhibitors increase the length of time serotonin is available for the body to use and have been found to reduce ritualistic behavior and aggression in many persons with autism (Cook & Leventhal, 1996). Short-term depletion of tryptophan (an amino acid) in the diet was shown to result in a significant increase in behaviors such as whirling, flapping, pacing, banging and hitting self, rocking, and toe walking with increased levels of anxiousness (McDougle et al., 1996). Tryptophan is a precursor to the formation of serotonin. The genetics of autism is not well understood; however, one study found that of parents with autistic children, over 60 percent had been diagnosed with major depressive disorder prior to the birth of the child (Smalley et al., 1995).

Fetal Alcohol Syndrome. Fetal alcohol syndrome (FAS) is a leading cause of congenital mental retardation (Spohr et al., 1993). Children born to mothers who abused alcohol throughout pregnancy have been found to have severe behavioral and intellectual problems that remain at age 11 to 14 years (Aronson et al., 1997).

WHAT IS A SUCCESSFUL FEEDING PROGRAM?

The success of a feeding program is dependent on several factors:

1. Selection of an appropriate diet (see Chapter 7)
2. Proper positioning
3. Use of appropriate feeding techniques and devices
4. Relaxation of individual before feeding
5. Staff's abilities to interact and handle the disabled individual

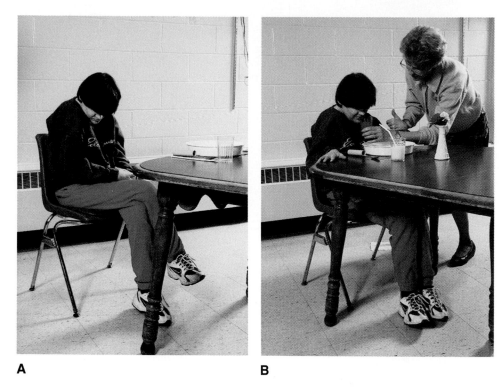

A   **B**

Figure 18–5
Improper (*A*) and proper (*B*) positioning at mealtimes.

Proper Positioning

An individual is properly positioned for eating if the following is true:

The head and upper trunk are as upright as possible
The feet are adequately supported
The hip and knees are flexed to approximate an 85-degree angle.
The head is tipped slightly forward.
The table height is appropriate.
The arms are centered close to the body.
The person is seated close to the table.

Figure 18–5 shows a person positioned properly for mealtimes. If a patient must eat in bed, wedges and pillows can be used to achieve a nearly upright position. Figure 18–6 is a sample form that may be used to screen eating skills.

EATING SKILLS SCREENING FORM (SAMPLE)

Client Name: _____ Date of Intake: _____

Date of Birth: _____ Age: _____ Sex: _____ Height (in): _____ Weight (lb): _____

General Status of Health: Excellent ☐ Good ☐ Fair ☐ Poor ☐

POSITION OF INDIVIDUAL FOR FEEDING
_____ Upright Unsupported
_____ Upright Supported
_____ Held
_____ Bed/Lying Down

METHOD OF FEEDING
_____ Independently spoon feeds
_____ Spoon feeds with assistance
_____ Finger feeds
_____ Fed by caregiver

PRESENT DIET
_____ Blended
_____ Soft
_____ Chopped
_____ Regular
_____ Dietary Restrictions

SAMPLE DAILY INTAKE
  (Explain on reverse side, including snacks and
  schedule.)

APPETITE
_____ Good
_____ Fair
_____ Shows preference for certain foods
_____ Allergies

PRIOR FOOD EXPERIENCES
  (Explain on reverse side.)

ALERTNESS
_____ Focuses attention on eating
_____ Responds to presence or absence of food
_____ Responds to environment
_____ Unresponsive or apathetic

SENSORY FUNCTIONS
Intact Impaired
_____ _____ Visual
_____ _____ Auditory
_____ _____ Tactile

EATING SKILLS
Good   Fair   Poor
____ ____ ____ Head/Trunk Control
____ ____ ____ Jaw Control
____ ____ ____ Lip Closure
____ ____ ____ Tongue Movements
____ ____ ____ Swallowing
____ ____ ____ Chewing

ORAL REFLEXES
_____ Rooting
_____ Suckling
_____ Bite Reflex
_____ Hyperactive Gag
_____ Hypoactive Gag
_____ Tongue Thrust
_____ Hypersensitivity Around Mouth

MOTOR DEFICITS AFFECTING SELF-FEEDING
  (Explain on reverse side.)

DENTAL CARE AND STATUS
  (Explain on reverse side.)

SUDDEN AND/OR LARGE WEIGHT CHANGE
_____ Loss _____ Gain

COMMENTS _____
_____
_____
_____
_____

Figure 18–6
Sample of an eating skills screening form. (Courtesy of Ross Laboratories, Columbus, Ohio.)

Feeding Techniques and Environmental Conditions

Feeding techniques and dietary considerations include the following (see also Table 18–3):

Food consistency modification (thickened liquids are easier to swallow and manage than thin liquids; Table 18–4)
Vitamin and mineral supplementation as either a milk-based beverage or tablets
Small, frequent meals
Provision of straws for beverages
Provision of plate guards, special spoons, forks, knives, and other adaptive devices (Fig. 18–7)
Encouragement and reminders to eat
Feeding techniques specialized for abnormal reflex responses and problems

Food consistency should be appropriate to the individual's ability to chew and swallow. It can be classified as grainy, lumpy, smooth, heavy, light, or mass consistency (one texture of food or a mixed consistency). Table 18–4 lists the effects that various food textures have on oral function; for example, certain foods stimulate sucking and other foods such as solids and chopped foods stimulate the lips and tongue to promote chewing and prevent choking. Foods that hold some shape also stimulate the swallowing reflex.

The temperature of the food served should also be considered. Extremely hot or cold foods should be avoided when the mouth is hypersensitive in order to avoid burning or numbing the tongue.

If acidic foods such as citrus juice increase salivation to the extent of excessive drooling, they should be offered at the end of the meal rather than at the beginning. Sweets are also known to increase saliva production.

Mealtimes should be relaxing in order to aid digestion and increase the enjoyment of food. Unless the mealtime environment is pleasant, even appealing food may be rejected. Avoidance of loud noises, bright lights, and sudden movements will help individuals with developmental disabilities eat better.

Food and Nonfood Rewards

Sometimes a specific reinforcer is needed to help someone modify his or her behavior. When the interdisciplinary team agrees that food items are the most effective means of reinforcing client behaviors, the following health issues should be addressed and considered:

Maintenance of dental health (see Chapter 19)
Avoidance of empty kilocalories, especially when the potential for becoming overweight is a problem
The negative consequence of food as a reward must be outweighed by the positive behavioral outcomes

Appropriate foods that may be used for reinforcers include popcorn or nuts for those persons without chewing or swallowing problems, fruit sections, low-

Table 18–3
Feeding Techniques for Resolving and Improving Feeding Problems

Possible Abnormal Reflex or Problem	Feeding Technique
Rooting Reflex Mouth opens and head turns in the direction of the stimulus when cheeks or lips are touched beyond 3 months of age.	Avoid stimulation to face between swallows or bites, such as wiping face with a cloth.
Suck-Swallow Rhythmical suck and simultaneous swallowing movement that continues as long as stimulus is present.	Occupational therapy program for oral normalization such as mouth and tongue stimulation, lip closure, stroking the throat, and so on. Follow OT program to progress from sucking to chewing. When using stimulation techniques, use firm, deep pressure rather than light pressure, which may tickle or irritate. Gradually increase texture and thickness of food.
Tonic Neck Reflex Develops at 4 weeks. Stimulated by receptors in the neck, it aids in eye-hand coordination. Position of the arms depends on position of the head.	
Asymmetrical Tonic Neck Reflex When the head is turned toward the right, the right arm extends outward. If to the left, the left arm extends. Prevents individual from keeping the head in position to be fed and interferes with jaw control. When self-feeding, it prevents proper hand-to-mouth coordination.	Position head and whole body in midline. (Refer to Positioning discussed previously.)
Gag Reflex Prevents passage of food into the windpipe. Present from birth on through life, although it weakens in later life.	Gagging is a "yellow light, not a red light." The feeder may think that gagging on a new food means that the individual is not ready for more complicated textures. This may not be so but just a warning to take things more slowly. To prevent behavioral problems, handle gagging in a very matter-of-fact way. Simply place hand over the child's mouth and close it until he swallows. Be careful to prevent food from entering the windpipe. Keep the head forward. Neck extension can cause aspiration.
In hypertonicity, a gag is elicited by tactile stimulation to the anterior half of the tongue. Caused by hypersensitive tongue, and difficulty in swallowing.	Tongue stimulation at other than mealtime to decrease hypersensitivity to touch. To control tongue activity, place food on the middle of the tongue with a slightly downward pressure of the spoon.
In hypotonicity, no gag response occurs regardless of what part of the tongue is prodded.	Feeder must be extremely careful in feeding this individual to prevent choking. Feed slowly. Walk the tongue with a tongue depressor or fingers in small steps to the point of gag, then withdraw depressor, close client's mouth, and wait for a swallow.
Bite Reflex Rapid rhythmical opening and closing of the jaw as long as the stimulus is present. This reflex is integrated by 4 months.	Use small Xylon spoon when feeding to prevent injury to oral structures. Wait for relaxation before removing spoon (do not try to pull spoon out).

Possible Abnormal Reflex or Problem	Feeding Technique
Chewing Rotatory movement in which food is positioned between the teeth for mastication and then repositioned for swallowing. Do not mistake tongue mashing (mashing food against the roof of the mouth) for chewing.	To encourage chewing, place dried fruit, beef jerky or cracker between the molars. Use jaw control to stimulate chewing while giving a slight tug on the food. Placement of food should be alternated from one side of the mouth to the other.
Tongue Thrust Food is pushed out of the mouth in an upward forward motion. Caused by inability to control tongue movements, improper positioning (head too far back), mouth breathing or being given too large a spoonful of food at one time.	Position client as described in positioning. Do not let client push his head back. Exercise jaw control. Use thickened pureed food. Place pressure on the tongue with the spoon. Hold the pressure briefly to stop tongue from protruding. Hold mouth closed until a swallow occurs. If mouth breather, allow time for breathing between bites.
Jaw Control Necessary to facilitate chewing. In hypertonia, jaw deviation is due to persisting asymmetrical tonic neck reflex. Will also have poor jaw control if head is tilted back too far.	Follow procedure for good positioning. When the client has poor head control, the feeder sits beside or behind the individual. The jaw is controlled with the nonfeeding hand (See Diagram A). For the client with good head control, the feeder sits in front of him (See Diagram B).

Diagram A

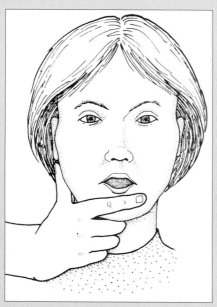

Jaw control (arm around client's head) with thumb on jaw joint, index finger between chin and lower lip.

Diagram B

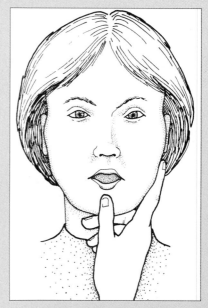

Jaw control (applied from front) with thumb between chin and lower lip, index finger on jaw joint, middle finger applied firmly just behind the chin.

Table continued on following page

Possible Abnormal Reflex or Problem	Feeding Technique
Lip Closure Necessary for removing food from the spoon and for preventing drooling.	Prefeeding stimulation of lips and jaw control in which the index finger is above the upper lip, pulling downward slightly as the spoon is removed. Never scrape food off the spoon with the client's teeth. A spoon with a flat bowl will work better than a deep-bowled spoon. Do not try to scrape any excess food from the lips with the spoon or wipe the client's mouth or chin after every bite. This may give the client the wrong signal to open his mouth, rather than keeping it closed to masticate and swallow. Allow for a little messiness while the client learns that the touch of the spoon means that he is to open his mouth and withdrawal of the spoon means he is to close his mouth.
Tongue Mobility Used in moving food to the back of the mouth for swallowing and relocating food from the sides of the mouth.	Encourage lip-licking with the tongue by placing something tasty on the lips such as peanut butter. Also place small pieces of cereal between the lips and gums.
Drooling Caused by ineffective swallowing of saliva. It is evident when there is poor jaw and tongue control and poor lip closure.	The therapist must solve the drooling problem indirectly by correcting the other feeding problems first.
Refusal to Eat Solid Food Hypersensitivity to touch. Dislikes change. May have very tight mouth.	Eliminate canned pureed food. Introduce wide variety of regular table food that has been pureed. Gradually introduce thickened consistency. Then food with general lumpiness such as rice pudding rather than discrete lumps. When introducing vegetables, initially avoid vegetables with an outer shell such as corn, peas, and lima beans.
Refusal to Drink from a Cup Poor coordination to suck-swallow. Previous experience from choking on liquids.	Begin cup drinking by using thickened liquids that flow more slowly and give the client more time to swallow. Alternate spoonfuls of thickened liquid with spoonfuls of client's other food at the meal. Gradually increase the number of spoonfuls of liquid given in succession but give client enough time to swallow between spoonfuls. Gradually thin down liquid. For example: Add apricot nectar to pureed apricots. Then reduce strained fruit gradually until the client is drinking juice alone. Use jaw control to close lips and jaw, and reinforce "normal" swallowing pattern.

Information approved by an occupational therapist of Broome Developmental Services, Ithaca, NY.

Table 18–4
Food Consistency Considerations

Type of Diet	Example	Potential Impact on Oral Function
Thin foods and liquids	Soup broth, juice	More difficult to control within mouth, especially with limited tongue control, i.e., quickly run to all areas of mouth Often promote excessive food loss
Thick foods	Pudding, yogurt, applesauce	Improve control with oral cavity owing to reduced flow and increased sensory input (i.e., weight and texture)
Pastelike or sticky foods	Peanut butter, thick cheese sauce	May be more difficult to move in oral cavity with limited tongue movement May stick to the roof of the mouth, especially with a high, narrow palate
Slippery foods	Pasta, Jell-o	Often difficult to control and either trigger reflexive swallow too quickly or run out of oral cavity before the swallow
Smooth textures	Pudding, pureed foods	Relatively easy to swallow; promote minimal tongue and jaw movement, especially over periods of time
Coarse textures	Creamed corn, ground foods, Sloppy Joe filling	Increase sensory input to stimulate more jaw and tongue movements Coarseness of food should be carefully graded
Varied textures	Soups with noodles or chunks of vegetables	Difficult to manage in oral cavity, especially with limited tongue movement or decreased oral sensitivity (i.e., liquid is swallowed and solid pieces remain in the mouth)
Scattering textures	Grated carrots, rice, coleslaw, corn bread	Very difficult to manage with limited tongue movement and decreased oral sensitivity
Crisp solids	Carrot sticks, celery sticks	Require sophisticated biting and chewing in order to grind pieces into consistency that is safe to swallow
Milk-based substances	Milk, ice cream	Appear to coat mucus in oral-pharyngeal cavities to interfere with swallowing or appear to increase congestion*
Broth	Meat broth, chicken broth	Appears to cut mucus in oral-pharyngeal cavity and facilitate swallow
Dry foods	Bread, cake, cookie	May be difficult to chew or swallow with insufficient saliva
Whole soft foods	Slice of bread	Require the ability to bite of appropriate-sized pieces

*However, there is no scientific evidence to support this belief by some people.
Courtesy of the Occupational Therapy Department of the J.N. Adams Development Center, Perrysburg, NY 14129.

fat cheese cubes, unsweetened cereal pieces such as Cheerios, pretzels, fruit juice popsicles, or diet soda. The dietitian should approve specific individual food reinforcers if they are deemed necessary. Nonfood reinforcers are preferred in order to avoid the development of adverse eating habits. Such rewards include stickers and stars, grooming supplies, and other small items. Verbal praise and outings are often excellent rewards that can be used instead of food. The staff's positive attitude about nonfood reinforcers increases the value of such rewards.

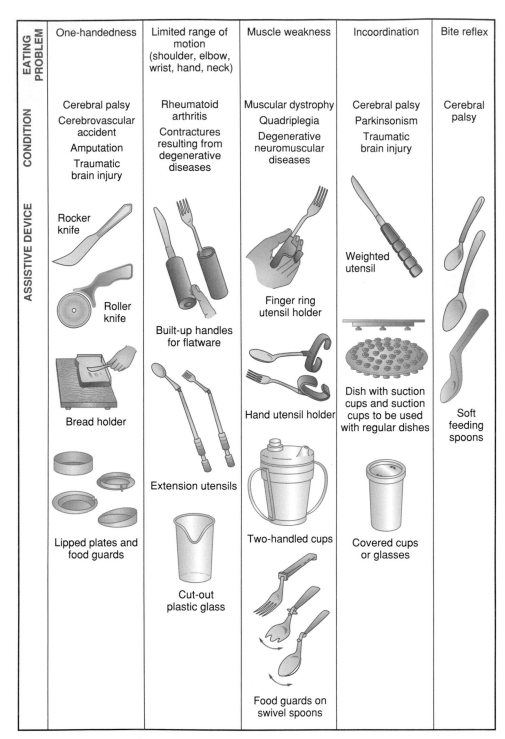

EATING PROBLEM	One-handedness	Limited range of motion (shoulder, elbow, wrist, hand, neck)	Muscle weakness	Incoordination	Bite reflex
CONDITION	Cerebral palsy Cerebrovascular accident Amputation Traumatic brain injury	Rheumatoid arthritis Contractures resulting from degenerative diseases	Muscular dystrophy Quadriplegia Degenerative neuromuscular diseases	Cerebral palsy Parkinsonism Traumatic brain injury	Cerebral palsy
ASSISTIVE DEVICE	Rocker knife Roller knife Bread holder Lipped plates and food guards	Built-up handles for flatware Extension utensils Cut-out plastic glass	Finger ring utensil holder Hand utensil holder Two-handled cups Food guards on swivel spoons	Weighted utensil Dish with suction cups and suction cups to be used with regular dishes Covered cups or glasses	Soft feeding spoons

Figure 18–7

Assistive devices for eating problems. (From Consultant Dietitians in Health Care Facilities: Feeding Is Everybody's Business: A Manual for Health Care Professionals Involved in Feeding Programs. Mead Johnson Nutritional Division.)

HOW DO HEALTH CARE PROFESSIONALS WORK AS A TEAM IN DEVELOPING FEEDING PROGRAMS FOR THE DEVELOPMENTALLY DISABLED?

Table 18–5 shows the varied responsibilities of the health care team in working with the developmentally disabled population. Various health care professionals need to be involved with weight control interventions, for example, increased ex-

Table 18–5
The Team Approach to Health Care in Feeding

Health Care Professional	Responsibility
Dietitian	Meal planning Supervision of food and modified diet preparation Delivery of meals Execution of diet orders Diet modification Nutrition counseling Nutrition assessment
Nurse	Mealtime supervision Proper positioning Charting of food and fluid intake Communication with dietitian and physician regarding acceptance of food served Implementation and integration of total care plan
Occupational therapist	Assessment of oral motor function Instruction of staff on appropriate alignment for feeding Assessment of need for assistive devices Working with client on chewing, swallowing, and other functional skill necessary to achieve feeding independence
Physical therapist	Evaluates mobility deficits Prescribes appropriate feeding activities May assist in evaluating oral motor problems
Speech pathologist	Provides assessment of oral motor functions and recommends appropriate treatment May provide help in solving problems and work with problems of bite reflex and tongue thrust
Psychologist	Evaluates specific behaviors that affect nutrition (such as food stealing, pica behavior, obsessive eating, and bizarre eating habits) and plans ways to manage them
Social worker	Collects social history and demographic data regarding patient and family Summarizes client's financial status and reaction to proposed therapy Provides financial information if needed by client in acquiring funds
Dentist	Provides assessment of patient's dental health (condition of gums, oral structure, and sensitivity related to teeth)
Physician	Identifies feeding problems Requires consultation in writing to appropriate health care professional
Recreational therapist	Provides premeal activities (music for dining, socialization)

Data from Consultant Dietitians in Health Care Facilities: Feeding Is Everybody's Business—A Manual for Health Care Professionals Involved in Feeding Programs. Mead Johnson Nutritional Division, Evansville, IN 47721.

ercise, dietary modification, and behavioral management. However, it is a challenge to develop good eating habits and appropriate levels of exercise in the developmentally disabled person.

Critical Thinking

Case Study

Juanita was at her brother's house along with the rest of the family waiting for the public health nurse to arrive. The nurse was going to do some testing to see if Juanita's baby nephew, Joshua, was behind in his development. Juanita suspected he was. At birth his eyes were set wide apart, a common sign of fetal alcohol syndrome, which Joshua was suspected of having. Now, at 2 months of age, he still had difficulty sucking on a bottle and made little eye contact. She prayed he was going to be okay, but she was afraid it was too late to help baby Joshua. She knew her brother hoped for more children. Juanita would have to see how she could help her sister-in-law stop drinking even though she claimed that she only had two glasses of wine her entire pregnancy. What else could it be? Juanita remembered her sister-in-law had a chronic cough throughout the pregnancy and wondered how much alcohol was in the cough syrup—maybe that was the problem.

Applications

1. How does Joshua meet the definition of developmental delay?
2. How might the family's reaction to the diagnosis of a child's chronic health problem help or hinder appropriate care?
3. What nutritional advice would be appropriate to help Joshua attain the best health outcomes?
4. List some over-the-counter products that may contain alcohol.

Study Questions and Classroom Activities

1. Define developmental disability and name some specific diseases.
2. How are nutritional problems of the developmentally disabled population grouped?
3. Name the growth retardation characteristics of Down syndrome.
4. With what type of cerebral palsy is obesity likely to develop? What type may involve one becoming underweight?
5. As a class activity, try to drink water in the following positions: head tipped to one side; head facing downward; trunk leaning backward with no support; correct position as described in this chapter.
6. Describe the techniques used when feeding a person with tongue thrust.
7. How does the environment play a role in the mastery of mealtime skills?
8. Describe how the assessment process is different in the developmentally disabled population.

9. How might hypertension be controlled in an adult with a developmental disability? What dietary advice might be appropriate?
10. In what ways is a child limited because of dental handicaps?

References

American Academy of Pediatric Dentistry, Oral Health Policies, Definition of the Dentally Handicapped. Reviewed and reaffirmed May 1996.

American Dietetic Association, Position of The American Dietetic Association: Nutrition in comprehensive program planning for persons with developmental disabilities. JADA; 1997; 97(2):189–193.

Aronson M, Hagberg B, Gillberg C: Attention deficits and autistic spectrum problems in children exposed to alcohol during gestation: A follow-up study. Dev Med Child Neurol. September 1997; 39(9):583–587.

Batchelor L, Nance J, Short B: An interdisciplinary team approach to implementing the ketogenic diet for the treatment of seizures. Pediatr Nurs. September 1997; 23(5):465–471.

Chugani DC, Muzik O, Rothermel R, Behen M, Chakraborty P, Mangner T, da Silva EA, Chugani HT: Altered serotonin synthesis in the dentatothalamocortical pathway in autistic boys. Ann Neurol. October 1997; 42(4):666–669.

Cloud HH: Expanding roles for dietitians working with persons with developmental disabilities. JADA 1997; 97(2):129–130.

Cook EH, Leventhal BL: The serotonin system in autism. Curr Opin Pediatr. August 1996; 8(4):348–354.

Duncan LL, Elder SB: Breastfeeding the infant with PKU. J Hum Lact. September 1997; 13(3):231–235.

Fieldstone A, Zipf WB, Schwartz HC, Berntson GG: Food preferences in Prader-Willi syndrome, normal weight and obese controls. Int J Obes Relat Metab Disord. November 1997; 21(11):1046–1052.

McDougle CJ, Naylor ST, Cohen DJ, Aghajanian GK, Heninger GR, Price LH: Effects of tryptophan depletion in drug-free adults with autistic disorder. Arch Gen Psychiatry. November 1996; 53(11):993–1000.

Pronsky ZM: Powers and Moore's Food Medication Interactions, 10th ed. Published and distributed by Food-Medication Interactions, Pottstown, PA, 1997.

Reilly S, Skuse D, Poblete X: Prevalence of feeding problems and oral motor dysfunction in children with cerebral palsy: A community survey. J Pediatr. December 1996; 129(6): 877–882.

Rouse B, Azen C, Koch R, Matalon R, Hanley W, de la Cruz F, Trefz F, Friedman E, Shifrin H: Maternal Phenylketonuria Collaborative Study (MPKUCS) offspring: Facial anomalies, malformations, and early neurological sequelae. Am J Med Genet. March 3, 1997; 69(1):89–95.

Smalley SL, McCracken J, Tanguay P: Autism, affective disorders, and social phobia. Am J Med Genet. February 27, 1995; 60(1):19–26.

Spohr HL, Willms J, Steinhausen HC: Prenatal alcohol exposure and long-term developmental consequences. Lancet. April 10, 1993; 341(8850):907–910.

Swink TD, Vining EP, Freeman JM: The ketogenic diet: 1997. Adv Pediatr. 1997; 44:297–329.

Zschocke J, Mallory JP, Eiken HG, Nevin NC: Phenylketonuria and the peoples of Northern Ireland. Hum Genet. August 1997; 100(2):189–194.

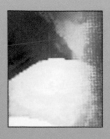

19
Oral and Dental Health

Objectives

After completing this chapter, you should be able to:

- Describe the causes of dental decay.
- Identify the factors related to dental health.
- Describe public health measures to control dental decay.
- Identify good snack foods for dental health.

Terms to Identify

Baby-bottle tooth decay	Dental enamel	Periodontal disease
Cariogenic	Dental erosion	Purging
Decalcification	Dental plaque	Salivary glands
Dental caries	Fluoride	Xerostomia

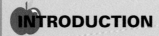

INTRODUCTION

Dental caries develops from a complex process of demineralization of the tooth (**decalcification**—removal of calcium from the tooth structure) and acid destruction. Acid is formed from the combination of carbohydrate and oral bacteria. Saliva helps neutralize this normal acid production. But when acid is continually in contact with **dental enamel** (the outer hard surface of the teeth) the structure can be quickly decalcified. Another source of acid destruction is related to erosion of the dental enamel. **Dental erosion** does not involve bacterial action but happens in cases such as bulimia, in which constant purging of meals allows the acid contents of the stomach to severely erode the dental enamel. A new role for the dental profession in diagnosing bulimia has evolved as a consequence of this nation's obsession with weight.

Dental decay is difficult to control through food choices alone. Limiting the frequency of carbohydrate snacks can help. Snacks containing sucrose in particular should be limited. Including a protein source at snack time can also help. Good dental hygiene with regular dental checkups and the use of topical fluoride are the most effective and appropriate preventive measures. The role of the dental professional should include the assessment of eating disorders (see Chapters 15 and 18) and between-meal snacking patterns.

HOW DOES DENTAL DECAY DEVELOP?

It has long been believed that sugar causes cavities. Although this is true, we know today that there is a more complex cause of dental caries. Tooth decay is caused by loss of calcium from the tooth enamel. This process is exacerbated by acidic destruction of the dental surface, the enamel. Bacteria, normally present in the oral cavity, feed on both sugar and starch. The combination of bacteria and carbohydrate results in acid production that decalcifies tooth enamel. Thus, the acidic demineralization of dental enamel normally occurs after the consumption of most carbohydrate foods and drinks. Erosion also occurs through other means of acid contact with teeth, including the repeated purging of acidic stomach contents associated with bulimia or excess intake of acidic beverages such as some soft drinks.

Bacteria, found in **dental plaque** (a buildup on dental surfaces that provides a medium for bacteria to grow) on and between the dental surfaces, use carbohydrate to grow. The chemical end product of this carbohydrate "meal" by the bacteria is acid. This process occurs whether the carbohydrate is sugar or starch. Thus, oral bacteria and carbohydrate act in concert to cause acid destruction of dental enamel.

Given an ideal situation of a plaque-free mouth, the carbohydrate in our foods would not cause dental decay, even if the diet consisted entirely of sugar. Because a bacteria-free oral cavity is not feasible, the elimination of carbohydrate from our diet would also prevent dental decay. However, because we need carbohydrate for good health, we need to make certain compromises to control and prevent dental decay.

WHAT STEPS CAN BE TAKEN TO PROMOTE GOOD DENTAL HEALTH?

The optimum approach to good dental health is thorough, frequent cleansing of the mouth, regular dental visits to remove plaque buildup, limiting the intake of carbohydrate foods and drinks to meals and snacks that include a protein source, and using fluoridated toothpaste, mouthwash, or both after each meal. If brushing the teeth cannot or does not occur immediately after eating, the mouth should be rinsed with water after eating. Chewing sugar-free gum after meals stimulates the flow of saliva. Other means to protect the enamel surface of the teeth include avoiding harsh abrasives on the teeth, not chewing ice (which can chip the teeth), not opening bottles with the teeth, and using pliable mouth guards in sports.

Proper diet, which includes adequate amounts of calcium, contributes to strong enamel formation. The formation of enamel begins in utero; thus a pregnant mother's diet should contain adequate amounts of calcium (the equivalent of 3 to 4 cups of milk daily: 1000 mg or more). A strong and thick enamel dental surface helps resist the destructive effect of acid production in the mouth.

Fluoride, a mineral that helps promote the formation of strong enamel in childhood, can be obtained through fluoridated drinking water or, for children under the age of 12, from fluoride drops or tablets. Once the adult teeth are fully formed, fluoride rinses continue to be an effective preventive treatment by promoting retention of the enamel surface. Fluoride is believed to actually promote remineralization of the dental surface.

In addition to the use of fluoride, good dental hygiene and control of carbohydrate foods help control loss of dental enamel. All carbohydrate foods, especially sugar, contribute to acid production in the presence of oral bacteria. Eating sweet foods with a meal containing protein, fat, or both will further promote dental health. Eating carbohydrate foods with a thoroughly clean mouth will also be of great benefit. Acid production begins shortly after eating is begun, so brushing the teeth and flossing before eating may be as helpful as brushing after a meal. Limiting the time of exposure to acidic beverages is also important.

The supporting structure of the teeth, the gums or gingiva, requires a good nutritional status to remain strong and healthy. Irritants, such as plaque, can increase the risk of gingivitis. Brushing the teeth regularly and flossing daily, along with at least annual dental visits for plaque removal, can help decrease the risk for **periodontal disease** (a painless gum disease that results in tooth loss in adulthood).

WHAT ARE ORTHODONTIC CONCERNS?

Orthodontists often advise their patients to eat soft foods after orthodontic treatment to avoid pressure sensitivity. One study found a decreased intake of copper and manganese after orthodontic adjustment, which may affect bone metabolism (Riordan, 1997). Thus it may be beneficial to provide nutritional guidance to patients in choosing soft-food diets.

WHAT IS THE ROLE OF GASTRIC ACID IN DENTAL DECAY?

Purging. Bulimia nervosa includes **purging** (intentional vomiting) after eating, which can ultimately cause irreversible enamel erosion by increasing the acid content of the mouth (Fig. 19–1). **Xerostomia** (diminished or absent production of saliva) and irritation of the lining of the mouth can also occur in connection with frequent purging. Dehydration and a resulting dry mouth are caused by other forms of purging such as laxative and diuretic abuse. Persons with a dry mouth might suck on sugar-based candies, which further exacerbates dental decay. Use of sugar-free candies does not promote tooth decay but adequate fluid intake is still important.

Gastroesophageal Reflux. The impact of this disorder on dental erosion is limited primarily to persistent reflux over a long period of time. There are varied

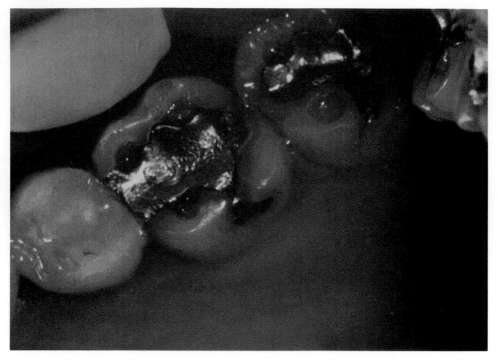

Figure 19–1
Bulimia-induced dental erosion. (Courtesy of Ruff J, Milwaukee, WI 53217. Journal of the American Dental Association.)

causes of gastroesophageal reflux, including metabolic and endocrine disorders and medication side effects (Scheutzel, 1996).

Hyperemesis of Pregnancy. Chronic vomiting during pregnancy (see Chapter 16) can also contribute to severe dental decay through the combination of vomiting and dehydration. Frequent mouth rinsing with water is important.

HOW DOES SALIVA PRODUCTION HELP PREVENT DENTAL DECAY?

Saliva surrounds the dental surfaces, acting as a lubricant. More importantly, saliva neutralizes the acidic pH level induced by the combination of oral bacteria and carbohydrate foods. Saliva also contains calcium, which helps prevent the loss of dental calcium in the enamel surface. Finally, saliva helps rinse the teeth of food debris.

Individuals at high risk of dental decay should be encouraged to use their natural saliva production to bathe each tooth with the tip of the tongue. The action of chewing or biting down can also release saliva from the salivary glands. High-risk individuals may need to chew sugar-free gum or eat other crunchy foods such as vegetable sticks or salads to promote saliva production.

What Is the Impact of Xerostomia on Dental Decay?

Xerostomia is a diminished or absent production of saliva. Severe and rapid dental decay has been observed in individuals with xerostomia, such as patients with throat cancer whose radiation therapy damaged the **salivary glands** (glands near the mouth that produce saliva). This same effect can be induced through medications that cause dryness of the mouth, such as antihistamine medications and diuretics (Pronsky, 1997). Breathing through the mouth can also cause dryness of the mouth. Patient complaints of dry mouth should be taken seriously with regard to prevention of dental decay. In the geriatric population, there is a diminished sense of thirst, which increases risk of dental caries.

What Are Some Other Contributors to Dental Decay?

Diabetes increases the risk of periodontal disease as a result of impaired immunity together with elevated levels of glucose available for bacterial growth. It is believed that gum disease can be decreased with good blood glucose control (NIH, 1994).

Acidic drinks such as some soft drinks (e.g., cola drinks, citrus fruits, or juices) can erode tooth enamel. The length of exposure to the acid is important. Drinking a glass of orange juice or cola in 10 minutes is less detrimental than sipping the drink for an hour. Chewable vitamin C tablets, also known as ascorbic acid, have also been found to be destructive to dental enamel.

ARE SOME FOODS MORE CARIOGENIC THAN OTHERS?

Most foods containing carbohydrate can be used by oral bacteria to allow acid production. Thus most carbohydrate foods are **cariogenic** (able to induce dental caries or cavities). The form of carbohydrate that does not induce dental decay is fiber. Potato chips and other sources of cooked starches may be just as harmful to dental health as candy. Harm is done in part because the public does not know that starch can cause decay. Without this knowledge a person may not be as ready to undertake preventive toothbrushing when starches are eaten. Sugar and cooked starches are the most cariogenic foods. Sticky carbohydrate foods are also more cariogenic because of their prolonged contact with the dental surface.

Foods containing protein generally are low in carbohydrate (exceptions are milk and legumes) and provide some fat (exceptions are egg whites and skim milk). The fat content of protein foods can coat the teeth and provide some protection to the dental surfaces. Thus, not only are protein foods and fats the least cariogenic food sources, they may also help prevent dental caries through their protective action. Emphasis on monounsaturated fat sources such as olives along with crackers can reduce the ability of the crackers to cause dental decay while the fat in the olives does not promote heart disease—moderate amounts of olives can fit into a low-sodium, low-fat diet.

WHAT IS BABY-BOTTLE TOOTH DECAY
AND WHAT IS ITS SIGNIFICANCE?

Baby-bottle tooth decay (also referred to as nursing-bottle mouth) occurs in babies and young children who use a bottle excessively, especially at bedtime (Fig. 19–2). Sweet liquids such as juice and other soft drinks are felt to be the primary culprits in baby-bottle tooth decay. But even formula and cow's milk contain sugar in the form of lactose. Bedtime bottles are the most harmful because there is a decreased production of saliva during sleep. Water bottles are acceptable for bedtime if no sugar is added to the water. It is best, however, if the infant does not take a bottle to bed at all. The teeth that are most at risk are the upper front teeth (see Fig. 19–2).

The physical significance of baby-bottle tooth decay is that removal of the decayed teeth can cause jaw misalignment, preventing normal spacing for adult teeth as they erupt. The pain of dental decay is not pleasant for the infant or child and can cause crying and screaming. Further, a young child with dental decay experiences a frightening and painful first dental visit. It is best to prevent dental caries in infants and young children for the sake of the child, the parent, and the dental professional. A visit to the dentist by the age of 1 or 2 years for a dental checkup and cleaning is a good idea. Baby-bottle tooth decay is entirely preventable. However, current efforts at reducing milk-bottle tooth decay are inadequate (Sonis et al., 1997).

Follow these recommendations to prevent baby-bottle tooth decay (American Academy of Pediatric Dentistry, 1996):

1. Infants should not be put to sleep with a bottle. Ad libitum nocturnal breast-feeding should be avoided after the first primary tooth begins to erupt.
2. Parents should be encouraged to have infants drink from a cup as they approach their first birthday. Infants should be weaned from the bottle at 12 to 14 months.

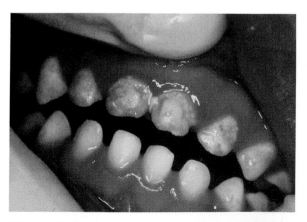
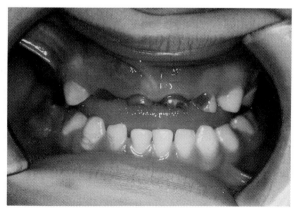

Figure 19–2
Examples of baby-bottle tooth decay. (Courtesy of Ferguson F, Department of Children's Dentistry, School of Dental Medicine, SUNY at Stony Brook, Stony Brook, NY 11733.)

3. Consumption of juices from a bottle should be avoided. When juices are offered it should be from a cup.
4. Oral hygiene measures should be implemented by the time of eruption of the first primary tooth.
5. An oral health consultation visit within 6 months of eruption of the first tooth is recommended to educate parents and provide anticipatory guidance for prevention of dental disease.

WHAT ADVICE SHOULD A NURSE OR OTHER HEALTH CARE PROFESSIONAL PROVIDE FOR DENTAL HEALTH?

Suggesting good oral hygiene with specific advice is appropriate for all health care professionals. The importance of good dental care spans all ages, from infants to the very old. Emphasizing good oral hygiene with regular dental checkups for plaque removal is in order. Infants can have their teeth cleaned with a wet washcloth. Young children can be taught to brush their teeth or have their parents do it for them. Older adults or others at risk of inadequate saliva production or other dental concerns need special care in promoting dental health (see Chapter 18 regarding the dental needs of the developmentally disabled). The use of fluoride tablets should be promoted for children under 12 years of age if it is not in the local water supply. Adults can benefit from fluoride rinses.

Assessment of dietary practices is important, especially that of between-meal snacking habits (see Fig. 19–3). Sugar is a known cariogenic food. If sweetened foods are eaten at mealtimes, they are less cariogenic. Cheese as part of a snack can help prevent dental decay, possibly because of the calcium and phosphate content but certainly because of the protein and fat content. However, in the attempt to prevent dental caries we do not want to promote heart disease. To avoid excess intake of fat, food models might be used to show what 1 ounce of cheese looks like. A referral to a registered dietitian would be in order for someone with

Carrot and celery sticks
Zucchini "matchsticks"
Radishes
Green and red pepper rings
Cucumber slices
Peanuts and other nuts (for children over 3 years, to avoid choking)
Cheese, regular in moderation or low-fat varieties
Hard-cooked egg, with or without the yolk (for cholesterol control)
Grain products (crackers, toast, bagels) with peanut butter or cheese
Apple wedges with peanut butter
Milk or yogurt

Figure 19–3
Good snack foods for dental health.

a strong family history of cardiovascular disease to make sure he or she does not eat too much fat or the wrong type of fat in an attempt to control dental decay.

Health care professionals need to be aware of the existence of bulimia and its detrimental effect on dental health. A health care team approach is advised for bulimia but also for dental care in general. Local educational programs on dental health are usually offered by the health department or the WIC program (see Chapter 22). These programs generally focus on children's dental health. The health care professional should be aware of local programs in order to make referrals.

Critical Thinking

Case Study

"With diabetes there is an increased risk of periodontal disease," explained Tony's dentist. He explained that the high blood sugar and problems with the immune system inherent with diabetes increase the risk of plaque formation and oral infections. The dentist advised Tony to have his teeth cleaned professionally at least once a year but preferably every 6 months and to floss daily along with brushing at least twice a day.

Tony's dentist suggested including a few nuts with between-meal snacks so that the fat would help prevent dental caries. Tony thought that was a good idea since nuts did not raise his blood sugar because the carbohydrate was mostly in fiber form. He had also learned from his dietitian that he could eat a small handful of nuts without adding excess fat to his diet. He also decided to pay better attention to at least rinsing his mouth with water after eating when he didn't have access to his toothbrush.

Applications

1. Why might Tony need to have professional dental cleaning every 6 months?
2. List between-meal snacks that would help Tony to control his diabetes without causing dental concerns?

Study Questions and Classroom Activities

1. Why is it important to prevent baby-bottle tooth decay?
2. What would you advise parents who insist their toddler needs a bedtime bottle?
3. Why are persons with bulimia at high risk of dental erosion? What steps should be taken by one's dental hygienist if bulimia-induced dental caries are suspected?
4. What are some strategies to make snacking less harmful to dental health?
5. Contact your local health department to determine if the water supply is fluoridated. If not, what means are available for children to receive fluoride supplementation in your area?

References

American Academy of Pediatric Dentistry, Oral Health Policies, Baby Bottle Tooth Decay/Early Childhood Caries, Revised May 1996. National Institutes of Health, National Institute of Dental Research. Diabetes & Periodontal Disease, A Guide for Patients. 1994, Publication No. 94–2946.

Pronsky ZM: Powers and Moore's Food Medication Interactions, 10th ed. Published and Distributed by Food-Medication Interactions, Pottstown, PA, 1997.

Riordan DJ: Effects of orthodontic treatment on nutrient intake. Am J Orthod Dentofacial Orthop. May 1997; 111(5):554–561.

Scheutzel P: Etiology of dental erosion—intrinsic factors. Eur J Oral Sci. April 1996; 104 2 Pt 2):178–190.

Sonis A, Castle J, Duggan C: Infant nutrition: Implication for somatic growth, adult onset diseases, and oral health. Curr Opin Pediatr. June 1997; 9(3):289–297.

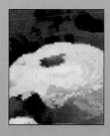

20

Weight Management and Physical Activity in Achieving Wellness

Objectives

After completing this chapter, you should be able to:

- Relate the importance of physical fitness to healthy weight management.
- Describe obesity and the condition of being underweight and discuss prevention and treatments of each condition.
- Describe the nutritional needs of the physically active and the athlete.

Terms to Identify

Aerobic exercise	Energy balance	Overweight
Amenorrhea	Fad diet	Physical fitness
Anaerobic exercise	Hyperplasty	Satiety
Body mass index (BMI)	Hypertrophy	Set point theory
Carbohydrate loading	Morbid obesity	Sports anemia
Desirable weight	Obesity	Underweight

INTRODUCTION

Physical fitness and nutrition are closely related. An adequate diet in combination with physical exercise has long been recognized as essential for building and maintaining strong, healthy bodies, and stamina. Being physically fit helps achieve good weight management.

According to a 1995 National Center for Health Statistics study, 4.7 million American children ages 6 to 17 years are severely overweight (Noonan, 1997). The proportion of overweight children and adolescents has increased by 6 percent since 1980 and that of adults by 9 percent. Over 12 percent of all children and adolescents and 35 percent of adults are overweight. Obesity has increased in all age groups (HHS News, 1997).

Millions of dollars are spent trying to control weight in the United States, with little positive impact. Many persons are easily allured by dieting gimmicks because they feel helpless to control their intake of food. They refuse to make food choices and so are able to rely on the rigidness of a **fad diet** (a diet that promises quick weight loss and an easy cure). When the desired weight loss is achieved, or the diet becomes too difficult to maintain, most overweight persons will regain the lost weight. This can be very costly psychologically. In addition, chronic dieting impairs health, especially when diets are nutritionally inadequate.

Unfortunately, in today's society, extremes of behaviors are sometimes encouraged. This is certainly true with athletic competition and weight control. Aiming for a very low body fat percentage and high lean muscle mass can be detrimental to health if not done in a sensible manner. The use of anabolic steroids by some athletes in an attempt to build muscle is a detrimental practice. And popular culture's emphasis on high-fat, high-sugar foods can create conflict in the fitness-minded person. Anorexia and bulimia have increasingly become problems of our athletic youth. Eating disorders are even found in the military men, with an estimated prevalence of anorexia of over 2 percent and bulimia nervosa almost 7 percent. Use of laxatives, diuretics, diet pills, vomiting, and fasting for standards increased during the body measurement and fitness periods (McNulty, 1997).

All persons, whether overweight or not, benefit from a diet that contains a wide variety of foods to ensure an adequate intake of nutrients. Energy needs depend on the percentage of lean body tissue present and the level and duration of activity performed. Optimum health and performance are generally promoted by a diet with 50 percent or more of the kilocalories supplied by complex carbohydrate, up to 20 percent by protein, and no more than 30 percent by fat, with ample water to prevent dehydration. Weight control and increased muscle stores can be achieved by carefully adjusting diet and exercise patterns.

WHAT STANDARDS ARE USED TO DETERMINE DESIRABLE WEIGHT?

Healthy Weight Management. Achieving a weight that is conducive to physical health as well as psychological health is part of healthy weight management. **Desirable weight,** however, may be higher than ideal body weight according to predetermined weight-for-height charts. For this reason, the term "healthy weight" is increasingly gaining acceptance. Other factors such as age, general health status, and potential for obtaining and maintaining weight loss are also considered when determining desirable weight.

Aiming for an unrealistic weight that cannot be permanently maintained is not a healthy goal. Losing weight only to gain it back can be worse than never losing any weight at all. Generally, a 10 percent weight loss for the overweight person is feasible and can have a significant impact on health. Slow weight loss of approximately ½ to 1 pound per week is more likely to be permanent and therefore falls within the boundaries of healthy weight management.

The Metropolitan Life Height and Weight Tables. This tool has been commonly used in the past for determining desirable weight. The term **overweight** refers to an excess of body weight and is usually determined by comparing a person's weight against the standard height and weight chart. If a person's weight is

10 percent greater than the standard, he or she is considered to be overweight. **Obesity** is a term used to describe an excess of body *fat*. Although weight alone does not indicate the degree of body fat, an individual is still classified by many health professionals as obese if weight is 20 percent or more than the standard weight for height; **morbid obesity** is when one weighs in excess of 30 percent of the standard. A person is **underweight** if he or she is 10 percent below recommended weight for height. However, these tables should not be used without taking into account their shortcomings. Several considerations must be kept in mind when using the Metropolitan Life tables follow:

1. Tables are not representative of the whole population, especially not of minority populations.
2. Tables are based on mortality data. Morbidity is not considered.
3. Frame size was not measured. Thus a small-framed person may appear underweight on this table while large-framed persons may appear overweight when they are not.
4. Weight tables do not provide information on the amount of weight contributed from muscle, fat, and bone. Thus a person whose weight is mostly from bone and muscle (such as a body builder) may appear overweight.

The **body mass index (BMI)** is considered one of the simpler tools that more accurately determines appropriate body weight. The formula used for the BMI was developed over a hundred years ago by a mathematician named Quetelet. As only a mathematician can, he realized that dividing a person's weight in kilograms by the square of the height in meters (kg/m^2) gives a better sense of body proportion. A healthy BMI is between 21 and 24, with an upper limit of 27—see Appendix 12 for a nomogram version of the BMI (American Dietetic Association, 1993). A BMI under 30 may be acceptable if there are no health problems. A BMI of 30 equates to being 20 percent overweight. Morbid obesity refers to a BMI greater than 40 (30 percent overweight). Someone who is underweight has a BMI of less than 19.

Other Body Fat Measurements

More precise methods of determining body fat percentage include the following:

- Skinfold measurements taken at different body sites
- The bioelectric impedance machine, which sends an imperceptible electrical current through the body
- Underwater weighing (usually done only at research centers).

WHAT ARE THE CAUSES OF AND TREATMENTS FOR OBESITY AND THE CONDITION OF BEING OVERWEIGHT?

Causes of Obesity

The causes of obesity are numerous and complex and are not thoroughly understood. Generally speaking, obesity occurs as a result of long-term positive **energy balance** for individual needs. In other words, weight gain occurs when kilocalorie intake exceeds kilocalorie expenditure (see Table 20–1) over an extended period of time. Many factors can affect energy balance in an individual. Factors such as age, gender, heredity, body composition, job type, and exercise habits all affect energy expenditure. Eating habits, cooking methods, family customs, emotional problems, peer pressure, food advertising, and food availability all have their influence on kilocalorie intake.

There are indications of genetic susceptibility to obesity (Bouchard, 1995). However, the environment seems to allow the genetic predisposition to be realized. One study found that offspring of diabetic parents were significantly heavier and more obese, with higher blood pressure, fasting insulin, glucagon, and triglycerides. Approximately half of the offspring and siblings of diabetic parents had 30-minute postprandial blood glucose levels greater than 160 mg/dL (Berenson et al., 1995). Obesity, high blood pressure, elevated insulin and triglyceride

Table 20–1
Kilocalories Expended per Hour for Various Types of Activities

Type of Activity	kcal/hr*	Type of Activity	kcal/hr*
Sedentary Activities Reading, writing, eating, watching TV or movies, listening to radio; sewing; playing cards; typing, office work, and other activities done while sitting that require little or no arm movement	80–100	**Moderate Activities** Making beds; mopping and scrubbing; sweeping; light polishing and waxing; laundering by machine; light gardening and carpentry work; walking moderately fast; other activities done while standing that require moderate arm movement; and activities done while sitting that require more vigorous arm movement	170–240
Light Activities Preparing and cooking food; doing dishes; dusting; handwashing small articles of clothing; ironing; walking slowly; personal care; miscellaneous office work and other activities done while standing that require some arm movement; and rapid typing and other activities done while sitting that are more strenuous	110–160	**Vigorous Activities** Heavy scrubbing and waxing; handwashing large articles of clothing; hanging out clothes; stripping beds; other heavy work; walking fast; bowling; golfing; gardening	250–350
		Strenuous Activities Swimming; playing tennis; running; bicycling; dancing; skiing; playing football	350 and more

*A range of caloric values is given for each type of activity to allow for differences in activities and in persons. Of the sedentary activities, for example, typing uses more kilocalories than watching TV. And some persons will use more kilocalories in carrying out either activity than others; some persons are more efficient in their body actions than others. Values closer to the upper limit of a range will give a better picture of kilocalorie expenditures for men and those near the lower limit a better picture for women.
From U.S. Department of Agriculture: Food and Your Weight. Home and Garden Bulletin No. 74. Washington, DC.

levels are part of the insulin resistance syndrome. Many populations have shown an increase of these health conditions with a change to a more westernized lifestyle. For example, the prevalence of overweight and obese Australian Aboriginal populations ranges from 0 percent in communities with a traditionally orientated lifestyle to well over 50 percent in those who developed a more westernized lifestyle (Rowley et al., 1997). The Native American population also has only recently developed high rates of obesity. It has been suggested that Native Americans have a genetic predisposition to becoming overweight that is only realized when there is abundant food and decreased energy expenditure (Broussard et al., 1995). Native Hawaiins have one of the highest rates of obesity in the world, with 66 percent being overweight or obese and 70 percent having central adiposity and other correlates of the insulin resistance syndrome including hyperinsulinemia (Mau et al., 1997). Incidence of being overweight among Native Alaskans is significantly higher than was found 25 years ago. Those who maintained a diet of indigenous carbohydrate and protein foods including seal oil were less likely to develop obesity and diabetes over this time frame (Murphy et al., 1995). This reinforces the concept that not all fats are equal in respect to obesity. Seal oil is high in the unsaturated fat, omega-3. The change in dietary fat to more saturated fats, including hydrogentated fats, and increased intake of refined carbohydrate foods are implicated in the growing obesity problem of Native Alaskans.

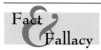

Fallacy: A person with central obesity should avoid all carbohydrate foods.

Fact: It is true that many persons with the insulin resistance syndrome have better outcomes on a low carbohydrate diet. The majority, however, do well with 40 to 50 percent of carbohydrate or less than 200 grams of carbohydrate for 1500 kilocalories. Restricting the diet to fewer than 100 grams of carbohydrate can be potentially harmful because of concommitant reduction in vitamins, minerals, and phytochemicals, which are all found in plant foods that also contain carbohydrate. These foods are important to long-term health. Milk is another natural source of carbohydrate, which should be included to help prevent osteoporosis. Emphasis on legumes, greens, and other low-carbohydrate vegetables, with moderate amounts of whole grains and fruit, low-fat or skim milk and lean meats such as fish and chicken, is the foundation of a healthy diet. These foods can be worked into a low carbohydrate meal plan that is appropriate to meet both weight loss and long-term health goals.

Thrifty Gene Theory

Some populations may have survived over the centuries because of an ability to preserve body mass during times of famine and to gain body mass easily during times of plenty. This would have been particularly important historically during the hunter-gatherer lifestyles prior to agricultural development. This is referred to as the "thrifty gene." This theory helps explain the occurrence of the insulin resistance syndrome and central obesity when there is exposure to conditions associated with westernization (Fujimoto et al., 1995).

Hyperinsulinemia

Some researchers believe that high levels of circulating insulin (or hyperinsulinemia), as found with the insulin resistance syndrome, is the cause of obesity. Others feel the increased levels of insulin is simply a marker for the degree of obesity. Much more research is needed on the cellular physiology of obesity before the causal factor of obesity is known conclusively.

A study involving Pima Indian children concluded that fasting hyperinsulinemia may be a risk factor for the development of obesity in young children (Odeleye et al., 1997). Another study found that a high sucrose intake in rats caused accumulation of abdominal adipose tissue with marked hyperinsulinemia and hyperlipidemia (Toida et al., 1996). Carbohydrate, both sugars such as sucrose and starches, is the primary cause of increased levels of blood glucose, which is the stimulus for insulin production. Researchers in Japan have shown that the combination of fat and sugar in a meal, such as with cake, cookies, and ice cream, may cause more weight gain than expected by kilocalories alone (Lepke, 1993).

The Fat Cell Theory

During childhood, excess kilocalorie intake can result in increased numbers of fat cells **(hyperplasty).** At any age, but especially after puberty, enlargement of fat cells **(hypertrophy)** can occur. Once a fat cell is created, it exists for life. Therefore, when an obese person loses weight, fat cells do not disappear, they only shrink. A person with hyperplastic obesity is believed to have more trouble losing weight and an increased likelihood of regaining any lost weight (Davis & Sherer, 1994).

The Set Point Theory

The set point theory holds that each individual has a "natural" weight, which is predetermined by a number of biological factors. Attempts to change weight below the set point are thwarted by various mechanisms in the body. In other words, the body defends its set point, even though it may be a greater weight than what is considered ideal. The set point can be a contributing factor when one is of normal weight or underweight as well; thus attempts to change one's predetermined biological weight may be thwarted by physiological mechanisms (Davis & Sherer, 1994).

Leptin

Leptin is a hormone that is believed to be involved in body weight regulation and that may serve as a **satiety** (the feeling of hunger being satisfied) factor (Schonfeld-Warden & Warden, 1997). Recent studies in ob/ob mice, which lack circulating leptin, have shown dramatic reductions in food intake and body weight after leptin treatment. However, animals that developed obesity, hyperglycemia, and hyperinsulinemia have also developed hyperleptinemia (high levels of leptin in the blood). The implication is that obese persons may have leptin resistance at the cell level. Thus more research is needed to verify the role of leptin in the prevention and management of obesity (Collier et al., 1997).

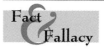

Fallacy: Obesity is caused by lack of willpower.

Fact: Many overweight persons do not consume a total amount of kilocalories in excess of what their thinner counterparts consume. There may be metabolic differences between the obese and the thin person, and the obese person may be better able to conserve kilocalories consumed. More research is needed to fully establish the metabolic differences contributing to obesity.

Obesity Treatments

Obesity is a very difficult condition to treat successfully in the long term. Up to 95 percent of overweight persons regain all or most of weight lost if the weight loss is rapid. It is imperative that all health professionals reinforce a slow, steady rate of weight loss in order to promote long-term weight management. The only exception to this is if the individual's life is at risk because of sleep apnea or need for surgery when a rapid loss of body fat is imperative. Rapid weight loss needs to be medically supervised.

The majority of all obese persons can be categorized as mildly obese, that is, less than 30 percent heavier than the ideal. For these mildly obese individuals, the comprehensive treatment plan includes some basic components: (1) a nutritionally adequate diet plan, (2) physical activity, (3) behavior modification, and (4) cognitive-behavioral therapy.

Extreme morbid obesity has been treated with various surgical techniques, such as gastric bypass, jaw wiring, gastric stapling, fat suctioning, and modified fasting. These treatments had limited success and are not currently routinely recommended.

Food intake for any individual attempting to lose weight should meet the body's needs for all nutrients but not kilocalories. It takes a deficit of about 500 kilocalories per day to lose 1 pound of fat in 1 week, because 3500 kilocalories are equal to 1 pound of body fat. For safe and permanent weight loss, an individual should lose a maximum of 1 to 2 pounds per week. This is a much slower weight loss than most people are willing to accept as the media continually advertises quick weight loss approaches. Persons with a history of diet failures or weight cycling may be more accepting of a slow weight loss approach, having learned first hand that rapid weight loss is not maintained in the long run.

Because of the way the body uses fuel from carbohydrate, fat, and protein, a rapid weight loss will compel the body to use protein (muscle) instead of fat for energy. This is highly undesirable because it decreases muscle mass, which will lower the person's needs for kilocalories. Weight cycling can change the body's composition so that muscle percentage decreases (muscle loss with each dieting attempt) and body fat percentage increases (regain of mostly body fat with each failed dieting attempt).

Experience has shown that in order to lose weight at the optimal ½ to 1 pound per week, most women need to consume about 1200 kilocalories per day; men will lose this amount with an intake of about 1500 to 1800 kilocalories per day. These kilocalorie levels may vary, however. And too much emphasis on kilocalories can be counterproductive. Reducing fat and sugar intake and learning to eat based on internal hunger cues rather than for nonhunger reasons can go a long way toward normalizing intake and weight management. Vitamin and mineral supplementation should be ordered when energy intake is less than 1200 kilocalories per day. Before embarking on any weight loss program, an individual should be examined by a physician. The dieting plan should also be individualized and flexible, and referral to a registered dietitian can allow for an individualized meal plan. See Table 20–2 for general dieting tips.

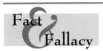

Fallacy: Skipping meals is a good way to lose weight.

Fact: Studies have shown that eating three to six meals a day is the best and most healthful approach. Skipping meals tends to suppress metabolism (the rate at which food kilocalories are burned) and can lead to overeating later in the day.

Meal Planning

Any long-term eating plan for weight management must be easy to follow if it is to be successful. Variety, flexibility, and consideration of an individual's lifestyle and food preferences must be part of the plan. Individual health needs also must

---

Table 20–2
Dieting Tips

1. Eat regularly, choosing foods low in fat and sugar.
2. Chew thoroughly and slowly.
3. Stop eating when stomach is comfortably full.
4. Make diet changes that can be maintained for life; temporary quick-fixes are counterproductive for healthy weight management.
5. Wait 15 minutes before having second helpings.
6. Include exercise for healthy weight management.
7. To deal with the "clean your plate" practice, remember that excess food goes either to waste or to the waist.
8. When faced with an indulgence, ask yourself, "How will I feel tomorrow if I don't eat this food today?" Give yourself permission to eat if feelings of deprivation may arise.
9. When ready to give up on dieting efforts, remember Ann Landers' quote, "The difference between a successful person and an unsuccessful person is that the successful person never stops trying."
10. For individualized meal-planning tips, consult a registered dietitian, the expert in nutrition.

be considered. Persons with correlates of the insulin resistance syndrome often note feelings of hypoglycemia such as physical tremors or headaches when overly hungry. Such persons can benefit from eating small, frequent meals that are moderate in carbohydrate (50 percent) and have moderate amounts of fat (30 to 35 percent) with emphasis on low saturated fat (less than 10 percent). Changes in eating habits must be viewed as a permanent change in lifestyle or "way of eating" rather than a diet, which implies a temporary and restrictive change. Most individuals who successfully lose weight and maintain their weight loss have made lifelong changes in eating patterns.

Alcohol in moderation (1 to 2 ounces or drinks) may be included in a weight loss plan so long as the minimum number of servings of the Food Guide Pyramid are included in the daily diet. A small glass of wine or one light beer provides about 100 kilocalories (roughly the equivalent of 2 teaspoons of added fat). Persons taking diabetes medications should be forewarned that their blood glucose levels generally will fall after they drink moderate amounts of alcohol. Persons who take any medications should consult their physician or pharmacist for guidance on alcohol use.

The Food Exchange System. This is a tool most often used in reducing kilocalorie intake. Originally developed by the American Diabetes Association and the American Dietetic Association, the exchange system aims to control carbohydrate intake and kilocalorie intake in the management of diabetes (see Appendix 9). This system can also be used for weight management alone. The exchanges break all foods into six separate groups. Foods in the same group have similar proportions of carbohydrate, fat, and protein and about the same number of kilocalories. The exchange list for each food group provides the portion size of each food that is nutritionally equivalent to all other foods in the group. By allowing a given number of exchanges in each group, a daily diet pattern can be developed that offers the dieter a choice of a variety of foods within the given pattern. The famous Richard Simmons' Deal A Meal card system is based on the exchanges. Weight Watchers has also used the exchange system. This system can be overly complicated for many persons unless they learn how to generalize food portions and equivalents.

The Food Guide Pyramid. Although this meal planning approach was not directly developed as a weight loss plan, it can be used as such. The minimum number of servings shows a kilocalorie range of as little as 1200 kilocalories if only lean meats and skim milk and no added fats or sugars are consumed (Table 20–3). It can be further reduced to 1000 kilocalories in a safe way if five servings of low-carbohydrate vegetables are consumed in preference to fruits since most vegetables have fewer than half the kilocalories of fruit for similar nutritional value. This needs to be based on individual acceptance of nutrient-dense vegetables such as greens, broccoli, and brussel sprouts (which all provide both vitamins A and C). The upper limit of recommended servings of the Food Guide Pyramid is about 2000 kilocalories, which may be adequately low for an overweight but active man. Table 20–4 shows how a normal 3000-kilocalorie diet, which may be needed with an active adolescent teenager, can be modified to give one family member a 1200-kilocalorie diet without preparing separate meals. Some items are omitted, some are served in smaller portions, and some are

Table 20-3
The Food Guide Pyramid as a Healthy Weight Loss Plan

Food Group	Serving Size	Comments
Bread, cereal, rice, and pasta group (6–11 servings)*	1 slice of bread 1 ounce of ready-to-eat cereal (check labels: 1 ounce = ¼ cup to 2 cups, depending on cereal) ½ cup of cooked cereal, rice, or pasta ½ hamburger roll, bagel, english muffin 3–4 plain crackers (small)	Count each serving of starch as 80 to 100 kilocalories Based on carbohydrate content and kilocalories, count dry vegetables (potatoes) and sweet vegetables (sweet corn, sweet peas, and sweet winter squash) as a starch
Vegetable group (3–5 servings)*	1 cup of raw leafy vegetables ½ cup of other vegetables, cooked or chopped raw ¾ cup of vegetable juice	One serving of vegetables is about 25 kilocalories Vegetables that are low in carbohydrate and kilocalories are high in water content and are not sweet
Fruit group (2–4 servings)*	1 medium apple, banana, orange, nectarine, peach ½ cup of chopped, cooked, or canned fruit ¾ cup of fruit juice	One serving of fruit is about 60–100 kilocalories Fruits that are dry (bananas) or are in portions greater than ½ cup contain more kilocalories
Milk, yogurt, and cheese group (2–3 servings)*	1 cup of milk or yogurt 1½ ounces of natural cheese 2 ounces of processed cheese	One cup of skim milk contains about 80 kilocalories One-percent milk has 100 kilocalories, 2-percent 125 kilocalories, and whole milk, 170 kilocalories Two ounces of full fat cheese contains 200 kilocalories
Meat, poultry, fish, dry beans, eggs, and nuts group (2–3 servings)*	2–3 ounces of cooked lean meat, poultry, or fish (1 ounce of meat = ½ cup of cooked dry beans, 1 egg, or 2 tablespoons of peanut butter)	One ounce of most meat contains 75 kilocalories Lean meat contains 50 kilocalories per ounce and high fat meat contains 100 kilocalories One tablespoon peanut butter contains 100 kilocalories and is counted as 1 ounce meat in the Exchange System One ounce equals ¼ cup; 3 ounces is the size of a deck of cards

*Recommended number of servings per day.

Table 20–4
Modified 3000-Kilocalorie Diet

1200 Kilocalories		3000 Kilocalories	
Breakfast			
Orange juice	½ cup	Orange juice	½ cup
Soft-cooked egg	1 egg	Soft-cooked egg	1 egg
Whole wheat toast	1 slice	Bacon	2 medium strips
Butter or margarine	1 tsp	Whole wheat toast	2 slices
Skim milk	1 cup	Butter or margarine	2 tsp
Coffee (black), if desired	1 cup	Whole milk	1 cup
		Coffee	1 cup
		Cream	1 tbsp
		Sugar	1 tbsp
Lunch			
Sandwich		Tomato soup with milk	1 cup
Enriched bread	2 slices	Sandwich	
Boiled ham	1½ oz	Enriched bread	3 slices
Mayonnaise	2 tsp	Boiled ham	3 oz
Mustard	free	Mayonnaise	2½ tsp
Lettuce	1 large leaf	Mustard	free
Celery	1 small stalk	Lettuce	2 large leaves
Radishes	4 radishes	Celery	1 small stalk
Dill pickle	½ large	Radishes	4 radishes
Skim milk	1 cup	Dill pickle	½ large
		Apple	1 medium
		Whole milk	1 cup
Dinner			
Roast meat	3 oz	Roast meat	4 oz
Rice, converted	½ cup	Rice, converted	⅔ cup
Spinach	¾ cup	Spinach, buttered	¾ cup
Lemon	¼ medium	Lemon	¼ medium
Salad		Salad	
Peached, canned	1 half peach	Peaches, canned	2 halves
Cottage cheese	2 tbsp	Cottage cheese	2 tbsp
Lettuce	1 large leaf	Lettuce	1 large leaf
		Rolls, enriched	2 small
		Butter or margarine	1 tsp
		Plain cake, iced	1 piece, 3 × 3 × 2 inches
Between-Meal Snack			
Apple	1 medium	Saltines	4
		Peanut butter	2 tbsp
		Whole milk	1 cup

From U.S. Department of Agriculture: Food and Your Weight. Home and Garden Bulletin No. 74. Washington, DC.

served in modified form—for example, skim milk instead of whole milk or black coffee instead of coffee with cream and sugar.

Food Labels. Reading food labels can be a good way to help plan meal goals. A low-fat meal is defined as 15–20 grams of fat or less. Snacks might be planned around 3 grams of fat or less. Daily protein intake should be at least 60 grams with a low-calorie intake. Carbohydrate content of food is also included on labels. The total carbohydrate number listed on food labels is the sum of the sugar and fiber, which are indicated, as well as the amount of starch (generally not listed separately). Usually weight loss can be achieved with 150–200 grams of carbohydrate and 30–50 grams of fat per day.

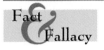

Fallacy: If the food label states 0 grams of fat, the food may be eaten freely.

Fact: The low-fat message has been very successful, almost too successful in some cases. It is possible to have too low an intake of fat, and an absolute minimum of 20–30 grams per day should be promoted. In the quest to achieve a low-fat diet, many persons have forgotten about the carbohydrate and sugar content. Pointing out the equivalents of sugar on the label with 4 grams of sugar equating to 1 teaspoon can be an eye-opener to many. A handful (½ cup) of jelly beans, or other pure-sugar candies, which contains about 100 grams of sugar (carbohydrate) at 4 kilocalories per gram equates to nearly 400 kilocalories.

High Fiber, Low Fat. Many persons have found emphasis on foods containing fiber, especially soluble fiber, helps promote satiety while losing weight. Legumes, greens, oatmeal, barley, and other plant foods with a "gummy texture" can allow for more stable blood glucose and insulin levels, which may explain the satiety value. These foods are relatively low in kilocalories and carbohydrate per volume. Emphasising foods with a high satiety and low kilocalorie level allows individuals to trust their natural hunger and satiety cues. This can be a common-sense and easy weight loss plan for many individuals.

Behavior Modification. This strategy includes principles that are used to assist the obese individual in identifying the personal eating behaviors that have been promoting weight gain and maintaining obesity. A person may know how much food he or she should eat but may have eating habits that are not conducive to change. Once these habits or factors are recognized, various techniques can be used to minimize their effects or remove them from the environment. For example, a person may have become conditioned to eat a high-fat snack upon returning home after work. The first change might be to change to a lower-calorie snack or having a smaller portion. Ultimately, the person may decide to break the habit of an afternoon snack. Or the goal might be to learn to eat more slowly. For another person the behavior might be to drink beverages that are low in sugar. For another it might be relearning alternatives to stress management other than turning to food. Many older adults who lived through the Great Depression of the 1930s find it exceedingly difficult to leave food on their plates. Strategies to prepare or order more appropriate food portions at restaurants might be helpful. By focusing on small, gradual behavioral changes, the individual learns to gain control of eating behaviors, with the goal of permanent changes in eating habits.

WHAT CAUSES A PERSON TO BE UNDERWEIGHT AND HOW IS THE CONDITION TREATED?

An individual may weigh less than is desirable for many reasons. For example, food intake that is insufficient for needs in quality and quantity (because of inadequate intake or poor absorption and utilization of food), wasting disease (e.g., cancer), increased metabolic rate (e.g., fevers, infection, hyperthyroidism, or burns), mental strain and worry, and excessive activity can all contribute to one's being underweight. If sudden or excessive weight loss occurs, serious organic illness or psychological problems should be ruled out.

An increase of 500 kilocalories a day in excess of need should result in a weight gain of 1 pound per week. An additional intake of two slices of bread, 2 tablespoons of peanut butter, or 2 ounces of cheese, and an extra two glasses of skim milk provides 500 kilocalories. If there is an adequate nutritional intake (at least the minimum number of recommended servings according to the Food Guide Pyramid), the additional kilocalories can appropriately come from added fats and sugars. Adding gravy, butter, mayonnaise, or heavy cream to foods can increase the kilocalorie density of foods. Between-meal snacks, such as milkshakes, puddings, and ice cream, can also help promote weight gain. Treatment is aimed at developing appropriate food habits so that good nutritional status and weight gain can be maintained. Persons with a family history of heart disease or diabetes would benefit from increased amounts of unsaturated fats (liquid oils and mayonnaise) versus solid fats (butter and hydrogenated fats).

WHAT IS THE ROLE OF PHYSICAL FITNESS IN HEALTHY WEIGHT MANAGEMENT?

Physical Fitness

According to the President's Council on Physical Fitness, **physical fitness** is "the ability to carry out daily tasks with vigor and alertness, without undue fatigue, and with ample energy to enjoy leisure time pursuits and to meet unforeseen emergencies." Physical fitness increases cardiovascular endurance, muscle strength, stamina, and flexibility of muscles and joints in the full range of movement. A body that is physically fit utilizes more kilocalories (muscles require more energy to be maintained than adipose tissue does). A physically fit person has a positive outlook (see Fig. 20–1) and can cope more easily with stress.

The first and most obvious reason that exercise is important for weight management is that it "burns" kilocalories. The duration of the activity, the intensity of the activity, and the weight of the individual performing the activity are all factors that affect just how many kilocalories are expended (see Table 20–1).

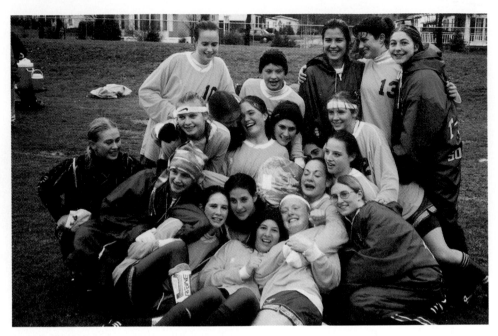

Figure 20–1
Team spirit soars after winning a regional varsity soccer game.

Activity is also important because it causes more kilocalories to be expended even *after* the exercise is finished. Research shows that physical activity can increase the metabolic rate for as long as 24 hours after the activity ceases. This is especially true of aerobic exercise.

Regular exercise, either alone or in combination with dietary modification, can have an important role in weight management. Exercise is a necessary component of daily living but one that is often forgotten. Exercise will help do the following:

- Decrease body fat while helping to preserve and tone muscle tissue
- Manage mental stress
- Increase energy levels
- Provide a sense of control over health and lifestyle
- Control appetite

The amount of exercise recommended for persons with health problems will depend on the physician's advice. Generally, walking and swimming are safe exercises for all persons. Those who are bedridden (see Fig. 21–1) or are in wheelchairs can use upper arm exercises to help maintain muscular strength and health.

Aerobic versus Anaerobic Exercise for Weight Management

Aerobic exercise is any exercise that requires more air (just like the term sounds: "air-o-bic"). It is this type of activity that tends to use the highest percentage of body fat for fuel, thus promoting the most beneficial weight loss. Aerobic exercise involves large muscle groups and builds cardiovascular endurance. Aerobic exercise includes cycling, jogging, walking briskly, soccer, basketball, cross-country skiing, rowing, and dancing. When such activity is performed continuously for at least 20 minutes three to five times per week, there is considerable benefit for weight management and cardiovascular health. But there is increasing acceptance that even "5 minutes here or there" is better than no exercise and can encourage a person to slowly increase physical activity.

Anaerobic exercise means exercise without air. Weight training is an example of anaerobic exercise. It will produce an increase in lean body mass. An increase in lean body mass will indirectly help in weight management because more energy is required to maintain muscle than adipose tissue. For the short term, muscle development can be associated with weight gain. This is a healthy gain and is often in conjunction with decreased inches related to loss of body fat. (A pound of muscle takes up less space than a pound of fat because it is denser; thus weight loss may not occur even though inches decrease.)

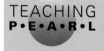 **TEACHING P•E•A•R•L** A good analogy for the impact or aerobic exercise in patient education is that of a fire in a fireplace that is going out. You can say, "When you blow on the fire, or give it more air, it burns faster. And while it is true that we do not have a fire in our stomachs, we still use air (oxygen) to burn our food kilocalories. Aerobic exercise causes us to take in more oxygen and thus we burn food kilocalories faster."

Other Benefits of Exercise

Exercise is associated with improved blood sugar control for the person with diabetes, reduced blood pressure, increased amounts of the good high-density lipoprotein cholesterol (HDL cholesterol), and improved bone density. Weight-bearing exercise can slow down bone loss after menopause. Prior to or during menopause, lifting weights actually increases bone density (Johns Hopkins Medical Letter, 1994).

Exercise-Associated Problems

It is wise to seek medical clearance before embarking on an exercise program. This is particularly true for persons with diabetes who have complications. Diabetic neuropathy can affect the ability of the heart rate to increase during times of exercise. This is a problem because the body cannot increase the flow of blood and oxygen to the working body cells.

Stress injury to the bone is a problem in female athletes with white ethnicity, low body weight, lack of weightbearing exercise, amenorrhea, and inadequate intake of calcium and kilocalories (Nattiv & Armsey, 1997). A triad consisting of osteoporosis, amenorrhea, and eating disorders often occurs in female athletes. Those with bulimia may be observed to have lesions on the skin of the hand used during self-induced vomiting (Daluiski et al., 1997). Physically active girls and women should be educated about the Female Athlete Triad and should develop plans to prevent, recognize, treat, and reduce its risks (Otis et al., 1997). For example, female crosscountry runners have shown evidence of body dissatisfaction, disordered eating patterns, and concern for weight control—traits that make health education particularly important (Parks & Read, 1997).

In some sports, such as wrestling, athletes take great pride in attaining a weight lower than their usual weight. To achieve peak performance and maintain health, the athlete must be well nourished and have a healthy minimal fat reserve. One study of teenaged wrestlers found that inadequate intake of kilocalories (less than 30 kcal/kg) and protein (0.9 g/kg) resulted in reduced muscular performance (Roemmich & Sinning, 1997). This is because of loss of muscle through rapid weight loss and depleted glycogen stores with precompetition fasting. Adequate glycogen is needed to fuel the muscles during the sports event.

Athletes, especially teenaged ones, should never be encouraged to lose weight by excessive loss of body mass or body fluids. Methods such as starvation, the use of diuretics or cathartics, the restriction of fluids, and prolonged sauna sessions are dangerous. Such methods lead to nutritional deficiencies and dehydration, with increased risk of heat stress and renal problems.

WHAT ARE THE NUTRITIONAL NEEDS OF THE PHYSICALLY ACTIVE?

Energy Requirements

Specific energy needs depend on one's age, gender, type of exercise, and degree of exertion. According to the Food and Nutrition Board of the National Academy of Sciences, the energy requirement for an adult to maintain weight with moderate activity is about one and a half times the basal energy requirement. For very active persons, such as athletes, the allowance may be two or more times the basal energy requirement (National Academy of Sciences, National Research Council, 1989 and 1997). Male athletes may require as many as 6000 kilocalories to maintain weight. With a few exceptions, an adolescent male athlete should eat no fewer than 2000 kilocalories per day, and a female athlete should eat at least 1700 to 1800 kilocalories per day.

Calculation of Kilocalorie Needs

A simple formula can also be used to calculate approximate kilocalorie needs as follows:

20 to 25 kcal/kg body weight for low to moderate activity (10 to 12 kcal/lb body
    weight)
30 kcal/kg body weight for high activity (15 kcal/lb body weight)
38 kcal/kg body weight for active adolescent females
45 kcal/kg body weight for active adolescent males

Carbohydrate Needs

Most of the energy that is used during exercise comes from carbohydrate, especially for nonathletes and for long-distance or marathon athletes and those involved in endurance sports. Carbohydrate is the nutrient that is most readily digested, stored, and metabolized. It is found in the form of glucose in the blood, and the storage form, glycogen, is found in both the liver and muscle. Glycogen is readily available during exercise, assuming the glycogen stores are not depleted. For endurance events, carbohydrate intake at regular intervals should be emphasized to maintain blood glucose levels and to help prevent the depletion of the glycogen stores. Glycogen is the limiting factor in the length of time exercise can be sustained. **Carbohydrate loading** is a means of manipulating diet and exercise in an effort to maximize glycogen stores during an endurance competition. It is most often practiced by long-distance runners, cyclists, and swimmers. Athletes practicing carbohydrate loading may eat large quantities of pasta, bagels, fruits, and other carbohydrate foods for a few days prior to an athletic event. Exhaustion is delayed simply by increasing muscle glycogen stores. Athletes should ingest carbohydrate during endurance exercise even if they have carbohydrate loaded before exercise (Dennis et al., 1997).

Carbohydrate loading is not required for short-term exercise such as a half hour of walking. Persons who are not physically fit may find their glycogen stores become depleted if they are involved in intense bouts of exercise or sports events. They should be forewarned to consume carbohydrate during or after exercise of long-duration or intense bouts of physical activity. Persons taking diabetes medication, in particular, should be warned that blood glucose can drop hours after exercise as the body attempts to replenish glycogen stores. Extra carbohydrate as a bedtime snack and a check of the 3 A.M. blood sugar level is good advice for the person with diabetes who suddenly increases the amount of his or her usual physical activity. This will decrease the risk of severe nighttime hypoglycemia (see Chapter 9). After an intense therapy session, physical therapists should alert persons with diabetes on insulin of this increased need for carbohydrate in relation to their usual insulin needs.

Role of Protein for Physical Fitness

The major role of protein is to build and repair body tissues. Recent evidence suggests that the RDA of 0.8 grams of protein per kilogram of body weight is too low for an athlete. The suggested protein requirement is now set at 1 to 1.5 g/kg/day. This protein level is easily met by a diet containing 1800 to 2000 kilocalories per day. With such a diet protein supplements are not necessary and are potentially detrimental to health and athletic performance. Dehydration and renal complications may result, for example. Also, a high-protein diet is often high in fat and kilocalories and can increase the risk for cardiovascular disease and obesity. Recreational sporting activities do not require an increased intake of protein.

Physical Fitness and Body Fat

For a well-trained athlete body fat is a major source of fuel during endurance activity. This spares glycogen stores and helps prevent exhaustion. For a person who is not physically fit, exercise is best done at a slow, steady pace until the body is better conditioned. Extremely lean athletes or anorexic athletes who have very low body fat stores may have better endurance levels if the body fat level is increased to more normal amounts. An increased intake of carbohydrate along with increased fat intake is the ideal fuel mix to promote weight gain as needed.

The Role of Vitamin and Mineral Supplementation in Sports Nutrition

Calcium. For women with **amenorrhea** (no menstrual period), a calcium intake of 120 percent of the RDA (about 1400 to 1500 mg) is recommended (American Dietetic Association, 1993). Food is still the recommended source. No supplementation is necessary for women with normal menses who have a balanced diet, including the recommended calcium intake, and who perform weight-bearing exercises that promote bone resorption of calcium. Both calcium and iron intakes are frequently deficient among adolescent female athletes. In addition to amenorrhea, such athletes may experience an increased risk of stress fractures and future osteoporosis (Timmerman, 1996). Hormonal therapy and calcium supplementation may be appropriate in women with amenorrhea and low levels of estrogen production (Kiningham et al., 1996).

Iron. Sports anemia is a condition observed in healthy athletes. The cause appears to be related to an increase in plasma volume (causing a dilution of the amount of iron in the blood) that is associated with the initiation of training. **Sports anemia** is not a clinical iron-deficiency anemia. Adequate iron intake, according to the RDA, should be ensured. Iron status should be evaluated periodically in athletes before a supplement is prescribed (American Dietetic Association, 1993).

Other Vitamins and Minerals. Athletes appear to use vitamin and mineral supplements more than the general population, and some take high doses that may lead to nutritional problems. Elite athletes have been found to use supplements more often than college or high school athletes (Sobal & Marquart, 1994). There are no conclusive studies on humans that justify supplementation of choline, antioxidant vitamins, or carnitine for athletes (Kanter & Williams, 1995). One study found that routine chromium supplementation had no beneficial effects on body composition or strength gain in men (Lukaski et al., 1996).

What Is the Role of Water and Electrolytes in Sports Activities?

Water is probably one of the most critical nutrients for athletic performance, yet it is the nutrient that so many active individuals tend to forget about or ignore. (Approximately 50 to 75 percent of the human body is composed of water; water is essential for circulation, urine production, and temperature control.)

As the athlete exercises, heat is produced by the muscles. This heat needs to escape in order for a safe internal body temperature to be maintained. Body heat cannot escape fast enough unless sweat is produced. When sweat evaporates, heat is released from the blood circulating near the skin, and the body is cooled. This water-cooling mechanism is extremely effective in maintaining the necessary body temperature. However, if adequate hydration is not maintained, sweating will diminish or cease entirely. As a result, body temperature quickly rises and heat exhaustion, heat stroke, or even death may result. General signs of thirst should not be relied on to determine when fluids should be consumed during athletic events. Water needs to be consumed prior to the activity and during the activity. The warning signals that occur during severe dehydration are the following:

- Pronounced thirst
- Loss of coordination
- Mental confusion with irritability
- Dry skin
- Decreased urine output

Electrolytes such as sodium, potassium, chloride, and magnesium are all lost in sweat. However, in most cases, electrolytes lost during exercise can be replaced easily by increasing the intake of potassium-rich foods such as citrus fruits, bananas, dark green leafy vegetables, lean meats, legumes, potatoes, and milk. Sports drinks with added electrolytes may be used. Rapid and complete restoration of fluid balance after exercise is an important part of the recovery process. The volume of fluid consumed should be greater than the volume of sweat lost. This can be determined by change in weight. For every 1 pound weight loss during exercise, 2 cups (16 oz) of water need to be consumed. Water alone is adequate for rehydration purposes when solid food is consumed, as this replaces the electrolytes lost in sweat. Continued exercise performance will be impaired if complete rehydration is not achieved (Maughan & Shirreffs, 1997).

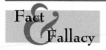
Fact & Fallacy

Fallacy: Salt tablets should be taken by the athlete.

Fact: Salt supplementation is not recommended. Salt tablets can remain whole in the stomach and cause irritation to the stomach lining. Excess salt also draws fluid away from the body cells where it is needed. Thus salt tablets are not necessary and are potentially harmful. Eating foods will naturally replace the amount of sodium lost in sweat from exercise.

Cool or cold water is the ideal fluid, since it empties from the stomach most quickly. Other fluids, such as juices and soda pop, have a high sugar concentration, resulting in a slower gastric emptying time. Athletes should experiment prior to competition to find out what works best for them. Diluted juice may be fine, but generally water is preferred. Commercial sports drinks may be desirable to help maintain blood glucose and electrolyte levels during exercise. Beverages containing caffeine or alcohol cause increased urine production and should not be considered as fluid replacement.

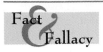

Fallacy: Candy bars are a good source of quick energy before a sports event.

Fact: The fat in the candy bars slows the rate of digestion, and the sugar that is quickly absorbed causes an increase in insulin production, which can lead to hypoglycemia, premature fatigue, and decreased performance.

The Postevent Sports Meal

The athlete should consume carbohydrate foods or drinks as soon as possible after an endurance event. The first several hours after the exercise are most conducive to restoration of glycogen stores. Up to 600 grams of carbohydrate may be needed (American Dietetic Association, 1993). Fruit juice may be most easily consumed, although it would take about a gallon of juice to make up this amount of carbohydrate. This could be achieved by drinking 1 cup of juice every 15 minutes for about 4 or 5 hours after the sports event. When the appetite returns to normal, sandwiches, fruit, and milk—which all contribute carbohydrate—may be appealing to the hungry athlete.

WHAT IS THE ROLE OF THE NURSE OR OTHER HEALTH CARE PROFESSIONAL IN PROMOTING HEALTHY WEIGHT AND PHYSICAL ACTIVITY?

Everyone, from the athlete to the older adult, needs access to reliable nutritional information. The Dietary Guidelines for Americans, the Food Guide Pyramid, and food labels are excellent tools that the health professional can use effectively in teaching individuals to make good food choices for maintaining physical fitness and wellness.

Sports nutrition myths are common, and the health professional has an important responsibility in dispelling misconceptions, such as the unwise belief that protein, vitamin, and mineral supplementation promotes better performance. The school nurse and physician play an important role in advising the coach, who must safeguard the health of students involved in various sports in which optimum performance is necessary.

The nurse or other health care professional can assist persons of all ages to identify appropriate weights for health and effective means to achieve changes in body composition. Female adolescents are particularly vulnerable to the media's representation of underweight models. The nurse or other health care professional can play a positive role in helping to modify unrealistic weight management in sports. There is much to be done to help our nation achieve weight and fitness goals that are positive and sound.

Case Study

Critical Thinking

Kalani had decided he was too young to be carrying so much weight and he wanted to run the marathon, so was swimming in the ocean regularly in an attempt to get fit. He had also reverted to traditional Hawaiian foods because he learned that this type of diet might help him manage his weight. At least that was what his dietitian was encouraging him to do. After all, his grandparents were not overweight at his age. The dietitian had pointed out to him how much sugar was in his favorite beverage, and this concerned him. The weather was hot and he needed to drink something, but when he learned that there was over ¼ cup of pure sugar in every 16-oz bottle of his favorite beverage, he realized he needed to find something else to quench his thirst. He finally decided that bottled carbonated water was tolerable, and he preferred it over tap water.

Applications

1. Research foods that were traditionally eaten in Hawaii.
2. What nutritional advice might you offer Kalani if the next marathon run was to be held in 6 months?
3. What eating behaviors do Americans have that promote the development of obesity? What nutritional suggestions could you make to help a person avoid the development of or correct obesity?
4. How does exercise help with weight management?

Study Questions and Classroom Activities

1. Who requires more kilocalories per kilogram of body weight, a teenaged girl or a teenaged boy? What factors have the greatest effect on energy needs?
2. Determine your body mass index (see Appendix 12). How many kilocalories should you include daily to maintain your current weight?
3. Two slices of whole-wheat bread contain 30 grams of carbohydrate and 6 grams of protein. How many kilocalories do the two slices contain? (*Note:* Count 1 gram of fat for each slice of whole-grain bread.)
4. How might you advise a family to plan meals in order to meet the needs of all family members—overweight adults with growing children? Should you suggest separate meals? Why or why not?

5. Plan a 1200-kilocalorie diet pattern appropriate for weight loss and a 3000-kilocalorie diet to promote weight gain.
6. How many grams of carbohydrate are needed for 500 to 600 kilocalories?
7. Class role-play: One student will play the school nurse, Mrs. Jones, and another will play an overweight teenaged girl. What should the nurse say if the student asks for a diet sheet to follow? How could the nurse discourage an overweight teenager from skipping meals to lose weight? How can the nurse advise students about good weight goals and the means to attain them?

References

American Dietetic Association: Position of The American Dietetic Association and The Canadian Dietetic Association: Nutrition for physical fitness and athletic performance for adults. J Am Diet Assoc. 1993; 93(6):691–695.

Berenson GS, Radhakrishnamurthy B, Bao W, Srinivasan SR: Does adult-onset diabetes mellitus begin in childhood?: The Bogalusa Heart Study. Am J Med Sci. December 1995; 310 (Suppl 1):S77–S82.

Bouchard C: The genetics of obesity: From genetic epidemiology to molecular markers. Mol Med Today. April 1995; 1(1):45–50.

Broussard BA, Sugarman JR, Bachman-Carter K, Booth K, Stephenson L, Strauss K, Gohdes D: Toward comprehensive obesity prevention programs in Native American communities. Obes Res. September 1995; 3 (Suppl 2):289S–297S.

Collier GR, Walder K, Lewandowski P, Sanigorski A, Zimmet P: Leptin and the development of obesity and diabetes in Psammomys obesus. Obes Res. September 1997; 5(5):455–458.

Daluiski A, Rahbar B, Meals RA: Russell's sign. Subtle hand changes in patients with bulimia nervosa. Clin Orthop. October 1997; 343:107–109.

Davis J, Sherer K: Applied Nutrition and Diet Therapy for Nurses, 2nd ed. Philadelphia, WB Saunders, 1994; p. 588.

Dennis SC, Noakes TD, Hawley JA: Nutritional strategies to minimize fatigue during prolonged exercise: Fluid, electrolyte and energy replacement. J Sports Sci. June 1997; 15(3):305–313.

Fujimoto WY, Bergstrom RW, Boyko EJ, Leonetti DL, Newell-Morris LL, Wahl PW: Susceptibility to development of central adiposity among populations. Obes Res. September 1995; 3 (Suppl 2):179S–186S.

HHS News. U.S. Dept. of Health and Human Services. More Americans of all ages are overweight. MMWR; Mar 6, 1997.

Johns Hopkins Medical Letter, "Health After 50." January 1994; 5(11):8.

Kanter MM, Williams MH: Antioxidants, carnitine, and choline as putative ergogenic aids. Int J Sport Nutr. June 1995; 5 (Suppl):S120–S131.

Kiningham RB, Apgar BS, Schwenk TL: Evaluation of amenorrhea. Am Fam Physician. March 1996; 53(4):1185–1194.

Lepke J: Super low-fat diets can't always keep big weight-loss promises. Environmental Nutrition. October 1993; 16(10):6.

Lukaski HC, Bolonchuk WW, Siders WA, Milne DB: Chromium supplementation and resistance training: Effects on body composition, strength, and trace element status of men. Am J Clin Nutr. June 1996; 63(6):954–965.

Mau MK, Grandinetti A, Arakaki RF, Chang HK, Kinney EK, Curb JD: The insulin resistance syndrome in native Hawaiians. Native Hawaiian Health Research (NHHR) Project. Diabetes Care. September 1997; 20(9):1376–1380.

Maughan RJ, Shirreffs SM: Recovery from prolonged exercise: Restoration of water and electrolyte balance. J Sports Sci. June 1997; 15(3):297–303.

McNulty PA: Prevalence and contributing factors of eating disorder behaviors in active duty Navy men. Mil Med. November 1997; 162(11):753–758.

Murphy NJ, Schraer CD, Thiele MC, Boyko EJ, Bulkow LR, Doty BJ, Lanier AP: Dietary change and obesity associated with glucose intolerance in Alaska Natives. J Am Diet Assoc. June 1995; 95(6):676–682.

National Academy of Sciences, National Research Council: Recommended Dietary Allowances, 10th ed. Washington, DC, 1989 and 1997.

Nattiv A, Armsey TD Jr: Stress injury to bone in the female athlete. Clin Sports Med. April 1997; 16(2):197–224.

Noonan SS: Children and obesity: Flunking the fat test. N J Med. June 1997; 94(6):49–51.

Odeleye OE, de Courten M, Pettitt DJ, Ravussin E: Fasting hyperinsulinemia is a predictor of increased body weight gain and obesity in Pima Indian children. Diabetes. August 1997; 48(8):1341–1345.

Otis CL, Drinkwater B, Johnson M, Loucks A, Wilmore J: American College of Sports Medicine position stand. The Female Athlete Triad. Med Sci Sports Exerc. May 1997; 29(5):I–IX.

Parks PS, Read MH: Adolescent male athletes: Body image, diet, and exercise. Adolescence 1997; 32(127):593–602.

Roemmich JN, Sinning WE: Weight loss and wrestling training: Effects on nutrition, growth, maturation, body composition, and strength. J Appl Physiol. June 1997; 82(6):1751–1759.

Rowley KG, Best JD, McDermott R, Green EA, Piers LS, O'Dea K: Insulin resistance syndrome in Australian aboriginal people. Clin Exp Pharmacol Physiol. September 1997; 24(9–10):776–781.

Schonfeld-Warden N, Warden CH: Pediatric obesity. An overview of etiology and treatment. Pediatr Clin North Am. April 1997; 44(2):339–361.

Sobal J, Marquart LF: Vitamin/mineral supplement use among athletes: A review of the literature. Int J Sport Nutr. December 1994; 4(4):320–334.

Timmerman MG: Medical problems of adolescent female athletes. Wis Med J. June 1996; 95(6):351–354.

Toida S, Takahashi M, Shimizu H, Sato N, Shimomura Y, Kobayashi I: Effect of high sucrose feeding on fat accumulation in the male Wistar rat. Obes Res. November 1996; 4(6):561–568.

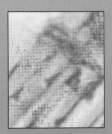

21
Nutrition of the Older Adult

Objectives

After completing this chapter, you should be able to:

- Explain how physiological, economic, and social changes affect nutritional status.
- Discuss how nutrient needs are modified in the aging process.
- Explain how nutritional needs are identified in the elderly population.
- Name and describe nutrition programs for the elderly.
- Name some meal service and food safety considerations for older adults.

Terms to Identify

Aging
Alzheimer's disease
Arthritis
Dementia
DETERMINE Checklist
Geriatrics

Gerontology
Kyphosis
Meals on Wheels
Nutrition Screening
 Initiative
Older Americans Act

Osteoporosis
Over-the-counter
 medications
Pernicious anemia
Polypharmacy

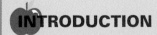

INTRODUCTION

The Bureau of the Census estimates that by the year 2000 the number of people 100 years of age and older will be approximately 100,000. By the year 2050 the number of individuals 80 years and older will increase from 5.9 million to 26 million and those older than 55 years will compose one-third of the population. About 30 years have been added to the average life expectancy since the turn of the century, when life expectancy was only 47 years. This extension of life expectancy has had and will continue to have a profound effect on our society and the health care system.

It is important to recognize the complexity of factors that influence elderly individuals in their selection of foods. These factors include income, household composition, cultural habits and customs, religion, ethnic background, and gender. Elderly persons may be at increased risk of malnutrition in their attempts to lose weight. Because of decreased lean muscle and decreased physical activity, kilocalorie needs also decrease, which can result in inadequate intake of protein, vitamins, and minerals. The older adult needs to have this message reinforced: nutrient-dense foods help prevent the physiological and functional declines found with aging (Blumberg, 1997). Older persons should also be encouraged to walk, because distance walked has been found to be inversely related to mortality (Hakim et al., 1998).

It is important for the health professional to realize that the process of aging diminishes the ability to ingest, digest, absorb, and metabolize nutrients in food. Thus inadequate food choices are of particular concern in the elderly population. **Gerontology** is the study of **geriatrics,** or the health concerns of older people.

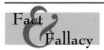

Fallacy: Amino acid supplements will promote longevity.

Fact: The older adult's requirement for protein is essentially the same as that of a younger person, and there is no truth to the notion that amino acid supplements have any effect on the aging process. A wide variety of good protein sources are available, even for individuals who have poor dentition and sore gums. Eggs or egg whites, tuna, cottage cheese, peanut butter, and dried beans and peas are good substitutes for meat if chewing is difficult.

By keeping older adults at good nutritional status, we can help them maintain their health and independence, thereby improving their quality of life and lessening the demands on institutional care. The importance of good nutritional status in maintaining independence among the elderly cannot be overstated. Growing old need not be a burden on society, but increased attention to health is necessary.

WHAT CHANGES OF AGING AFFECT NUTRITIONAL STATUS?

The older adult experiences social, physiological, and economic changes that affect nutrition, but careful consideration can resolve many of the associated concerns. A team approach is important.

Physical Changes

During the aging process, the basal metabolic rate slows and the amount of lean body mass (muscle tissue) is reduced. These changes, combined with a decrease in physical activity, result in a decrease in energy requirements and an increase in fatty tissue. Exercise needs to be part of daily activities. Even bedridden older adults can exercise (Fig. 21–1).

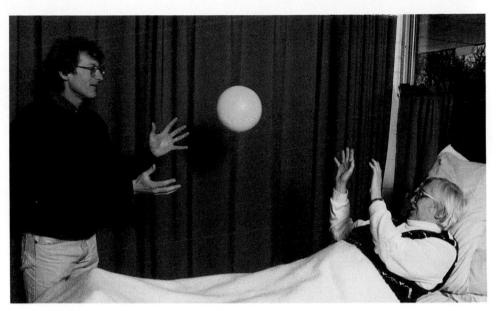

Figure 21–1
Exercise is possible for even bedridden adults.

Perceptual changes may affect eating behavior. Taste may be altered because of a decrease in the number of taste buds that occurs as part of the aging process, or as an effect of disease states, nutritional deficiencies, or medications. A reduced ability to detect odors and impaired hearing and sight may reduce the enjoyment of the social aspects of eating. All these perceptual changes may contribute to a lower intake of food.

Loss of teeth is common in the elderly population. This condition may lead to altered food choices that may decrease the nutritive value of the diet.

If refined foodstuffs are eaten instead of raw fruits and vegetables, constipation may become a problem, because aging is accompanied by a decrease in the body's ability to move waste products through the gastrointestinal tract. Increasing the fiber content of the diet, along with encouraging an adequate fluid intake and exercise, will help control constipation. The use of mineral oil in treating constipation should be discouraged because it reduces the absorption of the fat-soluble vitamins A, D, E, and K.

The kidneys may not function as well as they do in younger individuals. This can result in nutrient loss because the kidneys are not able to conserve and reabsorb some nutrients. The buildup of toxins can also occur when the kidneys lose their ability to filter harmful substances. Because the sense of thirst diminishes with age, it is especially important to be aware of the need for fluids to promote the removal of wastes through the gastrointestinal tract and kidneys.

Decreases in body secretions occur with aging. For example, swallowing may become more difficult because of decreased saliva production, and protein digestion is less efficient because of decreased hydrochloric acid secretion. The body's production of digestive enzymes also decreases with aging.

Even though little is known about an elderly person's nutritional needs, meals should be planned according to the five food group system of the USDA's Food Guide Pyramid as discussed in Chapter 6. Six small meals a day are often more appropriate than three full-sized meals for someone with a small appetite. Beverages that are caffeine-free and alcohol-free can be counted as fluid and should be included with each meal and snack to prevent dehydration.

Economic Changes

For most individuals, advancing age eventually brings retirement from work. This usually results in a decrease in income, which may occur at a time when an increased amount of money is being spent on medical care. As a result less money may be available for food. Protein foods may be consumed in decreased amounts because they are expensive, require preparation, and are difficult to chew and swallow. Older persons may consume excessive amounts of carbohydrate foods, which are inexpensive, easily stored without refrigeration, and simple to prepare.

Social Changes

Losing a spouse, living alone or with the family of a son or daughter, and entering a nursing home are only a few of the social changes that elderly persons may undergo. There is a loss of mobility and independence if physical impairments make driving a car or using public transportation difficult. Isolation from others will result unless there are friends or family on whom the elderly person can rely. The loss of independence that often accompanies these changes in social structure may reduce an elderly person's self-esteem. Such changes may cause the food intake of an elderly individual to suffer if he or she becomes depressed.

Grocery shopping may become more difficult for two reasons. Food labels and prices are hard to read because of visual impairment, and large supermarkets, which are a growing trend, require good mobility and physical stamina.

Table 21–1 summarizes dietary considerations for these physiological, economic, and social changes affecting the older adult. Table 21–2 shows the effect of the physiological changes.

WHAT ARE THE NUTRIENT NEEDS OF THE OLDER ADULT?

The recommended dietary allowances (RDAs) of the Food and Nutrition Board of the National Academy of Sciences do not give any specific recommendation for the adult older than 51 years, as noted in the RDA table on the inside front cover. Table 21–3 gives general recommendations and rationale for nutrient needs of the older adult.

Table 21-1
Dietary Considerations for Physiological, Economic, and Social Changes Affecting the Older Adult

Problem	Comment
Decreased sensation of smell, taste, and sight; diminished appetite and/or eating ability; dry mouth	Provide adequate lighting and comfortable environment Serve food in attractive, colorful, and flavorful manner Encourage adequate mastication, oral hygiene, and smoking cessation to enhance taste perception Experiment with textures, seasonings, and flavorings to promote better intake Use sugarless gum/candy to stimulate salivary flow/relieve discomfort Consider artificial saliva if dryness is severe
Less efficient digestion	Encourage small frequent meals Allow ample time for meal consumption Monitor food intake for possible intolerance
Oral health problems, missing teeth, and/or lack of suitable dentures	Provide appropriate diet texture, e.g., meat: may be chopped, ground or pureed only for individuals who are unable to manage whole or tough pieces (some can masticate well with their gums) Encourage proper oral hygiene and regular check-ups Evaluate dentures for proper fit
Constipation	Provide sufficient fiber and fluids Encourage consumption of fruits, vegetables, whole-grain breads, and cereals Encourage physical activity, adequate rest and relaxation, and regularity of meals and bowel habits Discourage use of mineral oil to avoid fat-soluble vitamin losses
Decreased physical activity; immobility	May result in constipation, pressure ulcer development, weight gain, and loss of ability to shop and prepare food, which can lead to further inactivity May exacerbate osteoporosis by increasing bone calcium loss
Dehydration; fluid retention	May be due to a person's inability to recognize need for fluid, limited access to water, or being afraid to drink to avoid frequent urination Use of laxatives and diarrhea can also lead to dehydration Fluid retention or edema may be affected by the aging kidneys' ability to handle water Immobility and protein deficiency can cause fluid retention
Hearing or vision impairment, memory loss, and short attention span	Can be a problem when giving diet instructions or obtaining nutrition information Short, frequent sessions are preferable Effective communication skills, including clarity and volume of voice, are important Simple, large print instruction materials are more appropriate; if necessary instruct caregiver
Lactose intolerance; osteoporosis	Decreased tolerance to milk and milk products can occur, but many can tolerate small amounts at a time (symptoms of intolerance decrease when lactose content is decreased by 20–30%) and/or when consumed along with other foods

Table continued on following page

Table 21–1
Dietary Considerations for Physiological, Economic, and Social Changes Affecting the Older Adult (*continued*)

Problem	Comment
Lactose intolerance; osteoporosis (*cont.*)	Fermented milk products (e.g., buttermilk, yogurt, cheese) or cooked milk products (e.g., pudding, custard, cream soups) are generally tolerated Lactose-hydrolyzed food products or lactose enzyme tablets or drops may be used to aid in lactose digestion Encourage use of other calcium-rich sources (e.g., hard cheeses, dark-green leafy vegetables, calcium-fortified foods/beverages) to reduce the risk of osteoporosis Encourage weight-bearing exercises and physical activities to slow bone loss
Decreased fat tolerance	Use added fat and fatty foods in moderation Choose lean meats, low-fat or skim milk and milk products Avoid fried foods
Iron deficiency	Can develop with prolonged consumption of low-calorie and/or poor quality diet, low intake of animal protein foods Encourage nutritionally balanced meals, including protein sources Iron-rich foods should be taken in combination with vitamin C foods Encourage congregate or home-delivered meals when resources/food preparation ability is limited Avoid inappropriate supplementation of iron, which can cause gastrointestinal distress and/or excessive iron storage
Low intakes of other vitamins and minerals	Encourage nutritionally balanced meals; consider congregate and home-delivered meals when food access and/or resources are limited Promote healthy eating, using nutrient-dense foods, since fewer calories may be needed while nutrient needs remain high Modify food textures (where appropriate) to ensure adequate consumption Make sure that nutritional supplements, if used, do not interfere with appetite at meals
Modified diets	Same nutritional concerns for the elderly as for younger persons Consider ethnic, religious, social, and economic concerns Consider liberalizing the meal plan when intake is poor
Arthritis	Less efficient manipulation necessitates that food be given in open or easy-to-open containers Finger foods may be more easily managed May want to consider adaptive utensils/equipment Encourage healthy eating for weight control
Economic limitations	Decreased socioeconomic status may be linked to decreased nutrient intake Emphasize economical food buys (e.g., foods in season and special sales) Refer to available community programs (e.g., food stamps, food pantries, congregate meals)

Table 21–1
Dietary Considerations for Physiological, Economic, and Social Changes Affecting the Older Adult (*continued*)

Problem	Comment
Limitation in purchasing, preparation, and/or consumption of adequate diet due to functional deficits	Contact community organizations for transportation, homemaker, home-delivered or congregate meals, therapy service (e.g., physical, occupational, speech), day care, senior centers Provide adaptive utensils/equipment to encourage independent functioning
Need for socialization	Encourage institutionalized persons to eat together Social contact in a pleasant environment may stimulate appetite Noninstitutionalized persons may benefit from community programs (e.g., senior centers, congregate meals, day care). Congregate meals provide important social contacts and at least 1 hot meal per day, 5 times a week; each meal provides at least one third of the RDAs. Home-delivered meals encourage independence. Generally 2 meals are provided, 1 hot and 1 cold, 5 times a week. Some programs offer weekend service.
Drug-nutrient interactions	Can affect appetite, taste perception, and food intake, as well as alter nutrient absorption, metabolism, and excretion; more important in elderly persons because of polypharmacy Monitor appetite, weight changes, and side effects, particularly gastrointestinal distress Encourage checklist for medications used, and review periodically with professional Instruct not to change diet and/or drugs relative to food consumption without medical advice
Food faddism; misinformation	Available income may be spent on unnecessary vitamin or mineral supplements (provide counseling as needed) Because of high prevalence of chronic conditions in this population, the elderly may be especially vulnerable to health-fraud claims or to using supplements
Pressure ulcers	Prevention is the key; early identification and intervention with malnourished individuals help to prevent the development of pressure ulcers Screening for pre-existing nutritional deficits, hydration status, history of weight loss, immobility, bladder and bowel incontinence, altered mental status, and existing medical problems is important Healing pressure ulcers requires attention to all aspects of the individual's care as well as providing appropriate nutrition support

From The Chicago Dietetic Association and The South Suburban Dietetic Association: Manual of Clinical Dietetics, 5th ed. Chicago, The American Dietetic Association, 1996.

Table 21–2
Physiological Changes in the Older Adult

Component	Functional Change	Outcome
Body composition	↓ Muscle mass ↓ Basal metabolic rate ↓ Bone density	↑ Fat tissue in muscle size and strength ↓ Caloric requirements ↑ Risk of osteoporosis
Perceptions	↓ Hearing Slowing of adaptation to darkness ↓ Number of taste buds ↓ Smell	Feeling of isolation Reluctance to eat in public places or at large social affairs Need for brighter light to perform tasks ↓ Ability to taste salt, sweet ↑ Ability to taste bitter and sour ↓ Threshold for odors
Gastrointestinal tract	↓ Motility ↓ Hydrochloric acid ↓ Saliva production	Constipation ↓ Efficiency of protein digestion More prone to food poisoning Difficulty swallowing
Heart	↑ Blood pressure ↓ Ability to use oxygen	↓ Ability to handle physical work and stress
Lungs	↓ Capacity to oxygenate blood	↑ Fatigue ↓ Capacity for exercise
Endocrine	↓ Number of secretory cells ↓ Insulin production	↓ Blood hormone levels ↑ Blood sugar level
Kidney	↓ Renal blood flow	↓ Capacity for filtration and absorption

Energy

We know that energy needs are lower for the older adult because basal metabolism decreases gradually with aging. Food intake generally is lower, and the amount of lean body tissue decreases, whereas the amount of body fat may increase. The relative risk associated with obesity declines with age after age 75 years (Stevens et al., 1998). This finding needs to be considered when the risk of malnutrition from attempting to lose weight may be more detrimental than the actual obesity itself at older ages.

Protein

Protein requirements do not decrease with age, and the RDA remains at 0.8 grams per kilogram of body weight. However, because of the diminishing efficiency of protein utilization in the elderly, a higher intake may be desirable. Factors such as renal health and serum albumin levels can help determine individual protein needs. Also, with any age, protein requirements increase in response to certain physiological stresses such as infection, bone fractures, surgery, and burns.

Table 21–3
Nutrient Guidelines

Nutrient	Recommendations	Rationale
Calories	Age > 50 yr; 30 kcal/kg body weight or Harris-Benedict equation (HBE) for basal energy expenditure × activity factor × injury factor	Based on reference adult engaged in light activity; adjust for physical activity and for body size Requirement for persons older than age 75 is likely to be less as a result of reduced body size, reduced activity, and REE (resting, energy, expenditure) Encourage to maintain physical activity to preserve muscle mass and well-being HBE can be used to more closely estimate basal energy expenditure and then adjust for other factors such as activity level and illness
Protein	0.8–1.0 g/kg body weight or 12–15% of total calories	Necessary for repletion of body proteins because of changes in body composition, protein metabolism, and utilization efficiency This allowance is higher per unit of lean body mass as elderly persons are more likely to have less lean body tissue per kg of body weight than younger persons Need to adjust for illness, surgery, infection, trauma, pressure ulcers, etc.
Fat	≤30% total calories (polyunsaturated fatty acids, 10% of total calories and saturated fatty acids < 10% of total calories). Consider age and risk factors in restricting ≤ 300 mg cholesterol	The result of restricting cholesterol intake in young-olds and old-olds may vary Need to appreciate the balance between possible benefits vs burdens in restricting fats/cholesterol (nutritional requirement depends on desired end result) Low-cholesterol level can be a sensitive predictor of malnutrition
Carbohydrates	Provides remaining needed calories: > 50% or preferably 55–60% of total calories with high intake of complex carbohydrates and low intake of refined sugars	Complex carbohydrates can provide necessary vitamins, minerals, and dietary fiber and add bulk; refined sugar can provide only energy
Calcium	At least 800 mg; higher (1000–1500 mg) for individuals at high risk for osteoporosis (e.g., perimenopausal and post-menopausal women)	Attempt to reduce risk of osteoporosis. May need calcium supplementation and/or use of lactose enzyme if lactose intolerant Encourage physical activities to decrease bone loss. Avoid sedentary lifestyle. Be aware that hypothyroid individuals may develop hypercalcemia from excessive calcium intake due to increased gut absorption
Vitamin D	5 µg/d; some suggest 10–20 µg	Skin synthesis of the vitamin and ability of kidney to convert to active vitamin D decline with age. Decreased exposure to sunlight may occur, especially in winter to housebound persons in more northern states, and due to use of sunscreens or clothing. Avoidance of vitamin D-fortified milk and milk products means decreased intake of vitamin D, which affects calcium absorption, utilization, and bone mass

Table continued on following page

Table 21–3
Nutrient Guidelines (*continued*)

Nutrient	Recommendations	Rationale
Other vitamins and minerals	Nutrients should come from foods first; supplements may need to be medically pre-scribed	To maintain optimal nutritional status; a multivitamin mineral supplement may benefit those who do not consume an adequate diet or those with low-calorie needs
Water	30 mL/kg body weight per day	To facilitate elimination and temperature regulation; as a diluent for medications; to prevent dehydration Be aware of possible diminished sensitivity to thirst/dehydration, purposely restricting fluids due to incontinence or inconvenience, and less efficient kidney function

Note: The Harris-Benedict equation (HBE) is sometimes used by registered dietitions to estimate kilocalorie needs of critically ill patients.
From The Chicago Dietetic Association and The South Suburban Dietetic Association: Manual of Clinical Dietetics, 5th ed. Chicago, The American Dietetic Association, 1996.

Vitamins and Minerals

The RDA for vitamins and minerals is the same for the older adult as it is for the younger adult. The actual nutrient needs of the older adult generally are not well known, however. In particular, there is a general lack of information about mineral nutriture and metabolism in people greater than 85 years of age (Wood et al., 1995). Iron is one mineral that is known to be needed in decreased amounts in the elderly, which the RDA reflects. Women 51 years of age and older need 10 milligrams of iron per day, compared with 15 milligrams of iron per day for younger women.

Good nutritional status has been found to be associated with improved cognitive functioning (La Rue et al., 1997). One study found that higher concentrations of vitamin B_6 were related to better memory (Riggs et al., 1996). Immunity is known to be influenced by nutritional status such as zinc status. There have been conflicting outcomes related to the use of vitamin and mineral supplements. One study showed that 100 milligrams of vitamin E did not affect overall immune responsiveness of elderly subjects (De Waart et al., 1997). Beta-carotene supplementation did not have an enhancing or suppressive effect on the immunity of healthy elderly (Santos et al., 1997).

Drinking vitamin D fortified milk is a good way to ensure adequate vitamin D and calcium in older persons who may be lacking appropriate sun exposure or who have lost the ability to manufacture vitamin D in the skin. Lactose-free milk products are available and may be necessary because the digestive enzyme lactase can become diminished with advancing age.

The elderly do not appear to be at risk for vitamin-mineral toxicity when taking supplements at the RDA level but may be at increased risk when taking large doses because of decreased lean body mass and reduced kidney function. A review of the older adult's vitamin and mineral use by the health care professional can help identify potential toxic amounts of supplements. The general guidelines for all persons also apply to the older population. Use of a vitamin-mineral supplement may be appropriate and safe but should be within 100 to 200 percent of the RDA until safety guidelines establish otherwise. Increased intake of vitamins and minerals is still best achieved via foods in part because of other nutritional factors such as protein, kilocalories, and phytochemicals.

Fluids

Fluids are frequently overlooked in the diets of the elderly. Young adults require an intake of 1 mL/kcal or 30 mL/kg of body weight. The elderly often lose their sense of thirst and may need to be encouraged to consume adequate fluids. It is particularly important for the elderly to meet their fluid needs to help prevent dehydration, which may result in constipation, increased body temperature, low blood pressure, loss of balance with falls, mental confusion, and dental decay.

Fiber

In older adults low intake of fiber is related to chronic disorders such as diverticulosis. The National Cancer Institute recommends consuming 20 to 30 grams of fiber per day, which is reflected in the USDA Food Guide Pyramid's minimum number of servings of fruits, vegetables, and whole grains.

WHAT CONDITIONS ARE COMMON IN THE OLDER ADULT?

Arthritis

There are two major forms of **arthritis:** osteoarthritis and rheumatoid arthritis. In 1992 arthritis was the leading cause of disability in the United States; projections indicate that by 2020 arthritis will affect 18 percent of persons in the United States (MMWR, 1996). Many misconceptions exist concerning the role of nutrition in preventing and managing arthritis. Generally nutrition is felt to play a minor role in the prevention and management of arthritis. The exception is weight control, which helps decrease strain on the joints affected by osteoarthritis. There is some new evidence that links the anti-inflammatory nature of omega-3 fatty acids from fish oil with improved outcomes for rheumatoid arthritis (James & Cleland, 1997). This finding has been reinforced by epidemiological studies that show that women who ate baked or broiled fish one to two times weekly were less likely to develop rheumatoid arthritis (Shapiro et al., 1996).

Rheumatic pain in the right hand has been found to be a prominent symptom among diabetic women. The highest prevalence of most musculoskeletal pains occurred in the highest level of 2-hour oral glucose tolerance test values among women (Qiao et al., 1995). Control of blood sugar levels may have an impact because low blood sugar levels, or the rise and fall in blood sugar levels after eating sweets, can trigger the production of histamine in some individuals. Although histamine production is related to allergies, there is no conclusive evidence that avoiding sugar will help control rheumatoid arthritis. Eating fewer sweets certainly will not cause any physical harm, however, and is part of weight management.

In the medical management of arthritis, there are well-documented nutritional implications. If large amounts of aspirin are used, vitamin C and folate intake needs to be increased. Steroid treatment increases the need for vitamins C and D, pyridoxine, folate, calcium, and phosphorus (Pronsky, 1997).

Gout

Gout resembles arthritis and is characterized by pain in a single joint (often starting with the large toe), followed by complete remission. As the disease progresses, the attacks become more prolonged and more frequent. Eventually degenerative joint changes and deformity take place.

Gout is now recognized to be a strong correlate of the insulin resistance syndrome. As research continues, our understanding of how to prevent and manage gout will be enhanced. For example, a low purine diet is sometimes advocated, which limits the intake of legumes. Legumes, however, which are an example of a high complex carbohydrate food containing soluble fiber and trace minerals, may play a positive role in managing gout by controlling insulin resistance.

Alcohol is to be avoided with gout, as are fatty foods because they may inhibit excretion of urate and hinder weight control. Maintaining sufficient fluid intake as well as ideal body weight is important. Rapid weight loss should be avoided.

It should be noted that drugs are usually more effective in lowering blood uric acid than are dietary modifications. Thus dietary restrictions are usually no longer imposed.

Osteoporosis

Osteoporosis (porous bones) is a major health concern for the older adult, as an estimated 20 million Americans are affected. Osteoporosis develops gradually over a lifetime. Current approaches increasingly focus on prevention. Age-related bone loss begins around the age of 35 to 40 years in both men and women. Physical activity, especially strength training, may delay the progression of osteoporosis and is of paramount importance for maintaining the functional abilities needed to carry out daily tasks of older adults (Taunton et al., 1997).

But for many older adults, osteoporosis has already been diagnosed. With the diagnosis of osteoporosis comes increased risk of bone fractures such that activities of daily living may cause fractures. Estrogen is associated with bone resorption in women, although intake of calcium and vitamin D is also important to control osteoporosis (Nordin, 1997).

Alcohol excess, as well as the use of steroid medications, is an important attributable risk factor for osteoporosis in men. There is no known treatment for osteoporosis in men (Seeman, 1997). Promotion of adequate calcium and vitamin D is still important for men. Elderly people and those who use heavy sun screens should have a dietary intake of 400 to 800 IU of vitamin D per day (Murray, 1996). Calcium intake up to 1500 mg daily has been recommended.

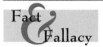

Fallacy: Calcium-based antacid tablets should be taken to prevent osteoporosis.

Fact: Although this message is often advertised as an appropriate strategy to prevent osteoporosis, it is oversimplified and potentially harmful. Individuals who have consumed adequate quantities of milk and milk products over their life span are less prone to the development of osteoporosis in their later years. However, it is still not clear whether the calcium in milk or other combinations of nutrients (such as magnesium) in the milk are of the most benefit. The best approach is to eat or drink foods that are naturally rich in calcium and vitamin D, such as fortified milk. Moderate sun exposure will also help.

Pernicious Anemia

Individuals with **pernicious anemia** lack intrinsic factor and therefore cannot absorb dietary vitamin B_{12}, so vitamin B_{12} is given by injection. This condition increases in prevalence in the elderly but also can occur at any age when diseases of the gastrointestinal tract are involved.

Alzheimer's Disease and Dementia

Alzheimer's disease and **dementia** are diseases that progress in frequency and severity with age. There is some new evidence that the type of dietary fat one consumes influences the development of Alzheimer's disease and dementia. Saturated fat and cholesterol appear to increase risk, whereas fish intake may decrease risk (Kalmijn et al., 1997). Several problems occur with these conditions, including forgetfulness and disorientation, pacing, inability to eat independently, weight gain or weight loss, dysphagia, food behavioral problems, constipation, and pouching. Because of the disorientation, a person with dementia needs to be reminded to chew and swallow. All these problems may affect nutritional status. A low body weight has been implicated as possibly contributing to impaired memory and feeding behavior. The area in the brain where these messages are processed has been shown to be atrophied (reduced in size) when there was low body weight with Alzheimer's disease (Grundman et al., 1996). Interventions might include increasing kilocalories to prevent weight loss, increasing fluid intake for constipation, or offering finger foods to encourage feeding independence.

Pouching (retaining bits of food between the cheeks and gums) is sometimes observed, especially in nursing home patients. If the food retained in the mouth contains fermentable carbohydrate such as fruit, candy, or bread, acid production and plaque will occur, resulting in dental decay. Acidic foods such as oranges may cause erosion of tooth enamel if the food is pouched. Caregivers should inspect the mouth of persons known to pouch.

WHAT ARE SOME CONCERNS RELATED TO FOOD-DRUG INTERACTIONS?

Approximately 30 percent of all prescribed and **over-the-counter medications** (not prescribed) are used by persons over 65 years of age. Older persons often may take three to seven separate drugs at any given time. Organ deterioration, underlying chronic diseases, dietary regimens, an unstable nutritional status, and other factors make the elderly particularly vulnerable to food and drug interactions. Quality of life and health may be affected as a result. **Polypharmacy,** the excessive use of prescription and over-the-counter medications, increases risk for adverse drug reactions and drug-drug interactions. Older women are at highest risk for polypharmacy because of age-related changes in the metabolism of medications (Jones, 1997). Medical nutrition therapy can help individuals avoid, reduce, or discontinue some medications.

HOW IS THE OLDER ADULT'S NUTRITIONAL STATUS ASSESSED?

The nutrition assessment process is discussed in detail in Chapters 2 and 7, but a few important aspects about the older adult need to be mentioned. The nurse is often the first person to discover nutritional problems. In taking a diet history, it is important for the nurse to note any type of food restrictions, ethnic or religious preferences, food aversions, and allergies. Also, certain signs of malnutrition may be noted during the physical examination. For example, low serum albumin is related to edema.

Factors such as bone loss and a shortening of the spinal column during later years indicate the need for current height measurement rather than relying on reported measurements from younger years. Height is frequently difficult to determine because of **kyphosis** (hunched shoulders), although knee height can be used to estimate true height (see Appendix 13).

A calibrated balance beam scale is recommended for weighing ambulatory adults. A calibrated chair or bed scale may be used for those who are in wheelchairs or are bedridden. Weights should be monitored weekly in the hospital and monthly in other health facilities, and the caregiver should keep in mind that fluid retention and dehydration can affect weight status.

What Is the Nutrition Screening Initiative and Its Role in Preventing Malnutrition in Older Adults?

Eighty-five percent of the elderly suffer from chronic diseases that could benefit from dietary interventions. Unfortunately, the warning signs of poor nutritional health are often overlooked.

The **Nutrition Screening Initiative** began in 1990 as a 5-year, multifaceted effort to promote nutrition screening and better nutritional care of older adults. This effort is a project of the American Academy of Family Physicians, the American Dietetic Association, and the National Council on Aging. Many related organizations and health professionals continue to help guide the initiative, which is designed as a direct response to the call of the 1988 Surgeon General's Workshop on Health Promotion and Aging and the U.S. Department of Health and Human Services Report, Healthy People 2000, for increased nutrition screening.

The Level I Screen of the Nutrition Screening Initiative is designed for social service and health professionals to identify older Americans who may need medical or nutritional attention. The Level II Screen provides more specific diagnostic information on nutritional status and is designed for use by health and medical professionals. A public awareness tool that older adults can use to assess their own nutritional risk is called the **DETERMINE Checklist** (Table 21–4).

Many circumstances can negatively affect an elderly person's nutritional status, regardless of income. Warning signals include bereavement, physical or mental disabilities, and poor nutrition knowledge. Care providers can be taught to make observations in the home and then take appropriate steps to prevent the onset of a nutritional crisis. Practical actions can be simple, informal, and inexpensive. For example, one might provide transportation to social activities and assist the older adult in grocery shopping and the preparation of food. However, independence should be encouraged as much as possible in all activities, including eating.

WHAT NUTRITION PROGRAMS ARE AVAILABLE FOR THE OLDER ADULT?

The federal **Older Americans Act** provides the states with money to conduct nutrition programs for the elderly. Under this Title III legislation, a hot noon meal is served to elderly persons 5 days a week in senior centers. This funding also provides transportation for individuals who are otherwise unable to get to the center. Nutrition education, health services, and recreational activities are planned around meals. For homebound elderly persons, up to a week's worth of meals are prepared at the center and delivered. Each of the one or two daily meals provides one-third of the RDA of nutrients. The Title IIIc program is commonly referred to as the Nutrition Program for the Elderly.

Meals on Wheels is a community-sponsored program that provides hot noon meals and cold evening meals to homebound elderly persons. The amount the elderly person is charged for the meals is based on the ability to pay. This program is often operated by local hospitals.

Table 21–4
DETERMINE Checklist

Disease

Any disease, illness, or chronic condition that causes changes in eating habits or makes eating difficult increases nutritional risk. Four of five adults have chronic diseases that are affected by diet. Confusion or memory loss that keeps getting worse is estimated to affect one of five or more of older adults. This can make it hard to remember what, when, or if food has been eaten. Feeling sad or depressed, which happens to about one in eight older adults, can cause big changes in appetite, digestion, energy level, weight, and well-being.

Eating Poorly

Eating too little and eating too much both lead to poor health. Eating the same foods day after day or not eating fruit, vegetables, and milk products daily will also cause poor nutritional health. One in five adults skips meals daily. Only 13 percent of adults eat the minimum amount of fruit and vegetables needed. One in four adults drinks too much alcohol. Many health problems become worse if more than one or two alcoholic beverages are consumed daily.

Tooth Loss or Mouth Pain

A healthy mouth, teeth, and gums are needed to eat. Missing, loose, or rotten teeth or dentures that don't fit well or cause mouth sores make it hard to eat.

Economic Hardship

As many as 40 percent of older Americans have incomes of less than $6000 per year. Having less — or choosing to spend less — than $25 to $30 per week for food makes it very hard to procure adequate foods to stay healthy.

Reduced Social Contact

One-third of all older people live alone. Being with people daily has a positive effect on morale, well-being, and eating habits.

Multiple Medicines

Many older Americans must take medicines for health problems. Almost half of older Americans take multiple medicines daily. Growing old may change the way we respond to drugs. The more medicines used, the greater the chance for side effects such as increased or decreased appetite, change in taste, constipation, weakness, drowsiness, diarrhea, and nausea. When taken in large doses, vitamins and minerals act like drugs and can cause harm. Doctors need to be alerted of all medications taken.

Involuntary Weight Loss or Gain

Losing or gaining a lot of weight when not trying to is an important sign that must not be ignored. Being overweight or underweight also increases the chance of poor health.

Needs Assistance in Self Care

Although most older people are able to eat, one in five has trouble walking, shopping, and buying and cooking food, especially as he or she gets older.

Elder Years Above Age 80

Most older people lead full and productive lives. But as age increases, risk of frailty and health problems increase. Older persons should check their nutritional health regularly.

Modified with permission by the Nutrition Screening Initiative, Washington, DC, a project of the American Academy of Family Physicians, the American Dietetic Association and the National Council on the Aging, Inc. and funded in part by a grant from Ross Laboratories, a division of Abbott Laboratories.

The Food Stamp Program is available to low-income elderly individuals. In some states, food stamps can be used to pay for food provided by the Nutrition Program for the Elderly. Some older adults need to be persuaded that it is acceptable and appropriate for them to use food stamps because of the negative media coverage over the past decade about the use of food stamps.

These nutrition programs have helped improve the nutritional status of the elderly population. Participation in these programs is enhanced by social work agencies that can direct the elderly population to the appropriate programs.

WHAT ARE INSTITUTIONAL MEAL SERVICE CONSIDERATIONS?

The most common nutritional problems facing nursing home residents are weight loss and protein energy undernutrition. Vitamin and mineral deficiencies, especially folate, pyridoxine, and vitamin D deficiencies, frequently develop in nursing home residents (Morley & Silver, 1995).

Mealtimes should be pleasant to help promote adequate intake. Prompt and courteous service is a must. Elderly persons are likely to eat better and enjoy meals more when dining with others, and this habit should be promoted whenever possible.

Food will be more appealing if it is served at the proper temperature (i.e., hot foods hot and cold foods cold) and as soon after preparation as possible to maintain palatability. It may be necessary to cut meat into bite-sized pieces, butter bread, and open containers if the individual is unable to perform those tasks independently because of weakness or pain from arthritis, for example. Certain adaptive equipment may be needed to help maintain independence in feeding oneself. Plates and bowls may need to be stabilized with rubber pads (dycem mats) and suction cups. Soup may be more easily managed if poured into a cup. Foam-covered spoon and fork handles are useful for individuals who have lost some ability to handle silverware easily. See Chapter 18 for a description of various assistive eating devices.

Respect and dignity are important to the elderly. When serving a meal, the health care provider should address the person by his or her last name preceded by Mr., Miss, or Mrs. unless requested to do otherwise. Napkins and a damp cloth should be close at hand for wiping any spilled food from face or clothing. A vision- or hearing-impaired individual will appreciate patience and understanding. Food items and their location on the plate and at the place setting should be identified for a visually impaired person. For the visually impaired person who needs to be fed, it is vital that each bite of food be explained in advance to promote trust in the caregiver and to help the person distinguish the foods being eaten.

WHAT ARE SOME FOOD SAFETY ISSUES FOR OLDER ADULTS?

Food preparation, shopping, and storing food can be very demanding jobs for many elderly persons living alone. The elderly are highly susceptible to food poisoning because of their declining immune systems. Tight budgets and ingrained feelings against waste cause many elderly people to store food longer than is safe. With declining vision and sense of taste, food spoilage may go undetected. Food preparation leads to safety concerns. For instance, an older adult may forget that the stove is turned on. Microwave ovens can be helpful in this regard. The health professional must be alert in identifying problems in household management.

WHAT IS THE ROLE OF THE NURSE OR OTHER HEALTH CARE PROFESSIONAL IN PROMOTING THE NUTRITIONAL HEALTH OF OLDER ADULTS?

Screening and identification of older adults who are at nutritional risk, with referral to appropriate services, is an important role for all health care professionals working with older adults. Use of the tools developed by the Nutrition Screening Initiative is appropriate. Some practical interventions such as promoting a variety of foods from the Food Guide Pyramid; recommending seasonings such as herbs, spices, and lemon juice as alternative methods of flavoring to reduce salt and sugar intake; and advising on the importance of food safety to help prevent food poisoning are appropriate approaches for all health care professionals to take.

Because calorie needs are generally lower while nutrient needs remain high, the use of skim milk and lean meats and the limited use of sauces, gravies, fats, alcohol, and high-calorie desserts can be recommended for those individuals who are overweight. Low-calorie desserts can be encouraged as they enhance the nutritional value of the diet (e.g., canned fruits packed in their own juice, puddings and custard made with skim milk).

If chewing is a problem, tender, ground, or pureed meats; meat or fish loaves; and eggs may provide an acceptable solution. Stewed fruits may be better tolerated than raw ones. Regular foods can be chopped or ground, or even blended, providing a more appealing texture than baby foods. Adding meat to soups will also enhance the protein value of the diet. Breakfast-type foods are generally well accepted because they are easy to chew and swallow. When necessary, these breakfast-type meals can also be eaten for lunch and dinner, but they should include at least three of the food groups from the Food Guide Pyramid—for example, french toast with peach slices, or scrambled eggs made with mostly egg whites and served with lightly toasted whole-grain bread and a side dish of fruit.

Case Study

Critical Thinking

Rita, affectionately known by her family as "Nanna," was having a fabulous time as Sean, whom she had met at her granddaughter's wedding, was getting ready to hit the golf ball. Both were widowed, and they found each other's company enjoyable. Rita's husband had died many years before, but Sean's wife had only recently died after having been in a nursing home due to Alzheimer's disease. Sean in particular seemed to need company. He had talked Rita into playing golf, even though she had never played before.

While they walked the golf course, Sean talked of his former wife and the food she used to prepare. His favorite meal was pork chops cooked with sauerkraut, mashed potatoes, and beets. Rita told him about Pasta Fagioli, and they laughed as she tried to explain how to eat lupini and fava beans by using the teeth to break off the outside membranes, which you would then spit out.

They also talked about how lucky they were now but how difficult it had been when their spouses died. Although both their extended families had recently been beset with health problems, they had all survived. Life was good again. But Rita did worry about what she was going to eat at the golf club. Her stomach didn't seem to handle a lot of greasy foods, especially if they were covered with cheese. But she'd deal with that when the time came. For now she merely wanted to get that golf ball to the next hole.

Applications

1. How might the loss of a loved one affect how a person eats?
2. Describe the grief reaction.
3. Using the Health Belief model (see Chapter 2), describe why Rita and Sean might vary in their eating habits during times of grief and times of joy.
4. How do family members and acquaintances affect eating habits?
5. What might Rita eat if the golf club restaurant offered the following food selections: cheeseburger, hamburger, hot dog, chili dog, french fries, onion rings, and coleslaw?

Study Questions and Classroom Activities

1. Why is it necessary to understand the physiological changes that occur with aging?
2. Why are elderly individuals vulnerable to nutritional deficiencies?
3. How have the nutrition programs for elderly persons helped improve their nutritional status?
4. Observe meal service at a local nursing home. How have the meals been modified to meet individual needs?
5. Take turns feeding a blindfolded classmate and then explain how a visually impaired adult reacts to such an experience. Pureed foods might also be tasted.
6. What dietary advice would be appropriate for an overweight widower who has hypertension and an elevated cholesterol level and relies on convenience foods?

References

Blumberg J: Nutritional needs of seniors. J Am Coll Nutr. December 1997; 16(6):517–523.

De Waart FG, Portengen L, Doekes G, Verwaal CJ, Kok FJ: Effect of 3 months vitamin E supplementation on indices of the cellular and humoral immune response in elderly subjects. Br J Nutr. November 1997; 78(5):761–774.

Factors associated with prevalent self-reported arthritis and other rheumatic conditions—United States, 1989–1991. Morb Mortal Wkly Rep. June 14, 1996; 45(23):487–491.

Grundman M, Corey-Bloom J, Jernigan T, Archibald S, Thal LJ: Low body weight in Alzheimer's disease is associated with mesial temporal cortex. Neurology. June 1996; 46(6):1585–1591.

Hakim AA, Petrovitch H, Burchfiel CM, Ross GW, Rodriguez BL, White LR, Yano K, Curb JD, Abbott RD: Effects of walking on mortality among nonsmoking retired men. N Engl J Med. January 8, 1998; 338(2):94–99.

James MJ, Cleland LG: Dietary n-3 fatty acids and therapy for rheumatoid arthritis. Semin Arthritis Rheum. October 1997; 27(2):85–97.

Jones BA: Decreasing polypharmacy in clients most at risk. AACN Clin Issues. November 1997; 8(4):627–634.

Kalmijn S, Launer LJ, Ott A, Witteman JC, Hofman A, Breteler MM: Dietary fat intake and the risk of incident dementia in the Rotterdam Study. Ann Neurol. November 1997; 42(5):776–782.

La Rue A, Koehler KM, Wayne SJ, Chiulli SJ, Haaland KY, Garry PJ: Nutritional status and cognitive functioning in a normally aging sample: A 6-y reassessment. Am J Clin Nutr. January 1997; 65(1):20–29.

Morley JE, Silver AJ: Nutritional issues in nursing home care. Ann Intern Med. December 1, 1995; 123(11):850–859.

Murray TM: Prevention and management of osteoporosis: Consensus statements from the Scientific Advisory Board of the Osteoporosis Society of Canada. Can Med Assoc J. October 1, 1996; 155(7):935–939.

Nordin BE: Calcium and osteoporosis. Nutrition. July 1997; 13(7–8):664–686.

Pronsky ZM: Powers and Moore's Food Medication Interactions, 10th ed. Published and distributed by Food-Medication Interactions, Pottstown, PA, 1997.

Qiao Q, Keinanen-Kiukaanniemi S, Rajala U, Uusimaki A, Kivela SL: Rheumatic pains of previously undiagnosed diabetic subjects. Scand J Rheumatol. 1995; 24(4):234–237.

Riggs KM, Spiro A 3rd, Tucker K, Rush D: Relations of vitamin B_{12}, vitamin B_6, folate, and homocysteine to cognitive performance in the Normative Aging Study. Am J Clin Nutr. March 1996; 63(3):306–314.

Santos MS, Leka LS, Ribaya-Mercado JD, Russell RM, Meydani M, Hennekens CH, Gaziano JM, Meydani SN: Short- and long-term beta-carotene supplementation do not influence T cell-mediated immunity in healthy elderly persons. Am J Clin Nutr. October 1997; 66(4):917–924.

Seeman E: Do men suffer with osteoporosis? Aust Fam Physician. February 1997; 26(2):135–143.

Shapiro JA, Koepsell TD, Voigt LF, Dugowson CE, Kestin M, Nelson JL: Diet and rheumatoid arthritis in women: A possible protective effect of fish consumption. Epidemiology. May 1996; 7(3):256–263.

Stevens J, Cai J, Pamuk ER, Williamson DF, Thun MJ, Wood JL: The effect of age on the association between body-mass index and mortality. N Engl J Med. January 1, 1998; 338(1):1–7.

Taunton JE, Martin AD, Rhodes EC, Wolski LA, Donelly M, Elliot J: Exercise for the older woman: Choosing the right prescription. Br J Sports Med. March 1997; 31(1):5–10.

Wood RJ, Suter PM, Russell RM: Mineral requirements of elderly people. Am J Clin Nutr. September 1995; 62(3):493–505.

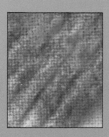

22

National and International Nutrition Programs and Concerns

Objectives

After completing this chapter, you should be able to:

- Identify the basic focus of the various federal community nutrition programs for referral purposes.
- Discuss the importance of controlling food quackery.
- Identify appropriate uses of food additives.
- Describe principles of home-based food sanitation.
- Describe why public health professionals need to be advocates for consumer nutritional and health needs.

Terms to Identify

Ambulatory care
Clostridium botulinum
Clostridium perfringens
Communicable disease
Escherichia coli
Food additives
Food fads

Food quack
Food resource
  management
Generally recognized as
  safe (GRAS) list
Holistic
Hospices

Palliative care
Paraprofessionals
Poverty
Salmonella
Staphylococcus aureus
Thrifty Food Plan

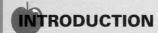 INTRODUCTION

Public health includes the promotion of nutrition in the community. Public health messages are aimed at particular groups or specific conditions. The food label is a public health approach. National initiatives include the Food Guide Pyramid which helps improve food selection and thereby helps reduce obesity and heart disease. Public health programs may provide education, but they may also allow individuals to obtain nourishing food, such as with Food Stamps and the Nutrition Program for the Elderly (see section below and Chapter 21). Iodized salt, vitamin D fortified milk, and the latest folic acid fortification of certain grain products are all designed to improve the health of large segments of the American population. The public health initiative might focus on high-risk populations for a specific disease such as diabetes. This type of initiative has been proposed for minority groups because of their high rate of diabetes (Carter et al., 1996). The WIC program (discussed later in this chapter) was developed in response to high rates of childhood anemia among low-income families. Public health messages are effective at getting simple information to large numbers of individuals. All health care professionals should be promoting public health messages such as the importance of eating less saturated fat. More precise guidance and medical nutrition therapy provided by a registered dietitian is often needed at the individual level for the management of disease states.

WHAT IS OUR NATION'S NUTRITIONAL STATUS?

National Food Consumption Survey

The U.S. Department of Agriculture (USDA) conducts a national food consumption survey approximately every 10 years. The survey that was carried out in 1977/1978 showed evidence of excessive intake of kilocalories, fat, cholesterol, sugar, salt, and alcohol. Generally, the intake of vitamin B_6 (pyridoxine), magnesium, iron, and zinc was shown to be below the recommended dietary allowance (RDA) levels. Furthermore, elderly women were shown to have a significantly low intake of calcium and vitamin B_6. On the other hand, data from this survey revealed that the diet of those with low incomes had improved since the previous USDA survey. This improvement was attributed to various food assistance programs.

Results of the 1987 National Food Consumption Survey (NFCS) showed little positive change in dietary habits since the 1978 survey. The more recent Continuing Survey, 1989–1991, found that one-quarter of all vegetables consumed by children and adolescents were french fries (Krebs et al., 1996). The intake of excessive fat, especially saturated fat, and the inadequate intake of some vitamins and minerals from food sources continue despite major educational efforts. The challenge to alter Americans' eating habits in a positive way appears to demand more than educational messages.

Hunger and Food Insecurity in America

Hunger has always been and will always be with us, but the attempts to control its ravages have changed over the course of history. In this century, the Great Depression of the 1930s led to the establishment of soup kitchens and the Food Stamp Program. During the draft of World War II, poor nutritional status kept many young men from being admitted to the military service. In response to the observations made during World War II, the School Lunch Program was expanded. During the 1960s the issue of domestic hunger received major attention and resulted in the expansion of food programs. But beginning in the 1980s and continuing into the 1990s, underconsumption was again becoming an acute problem. Many early advances taken in the 1960s to combat national hunger were being lost. This was due primarily to political reasons and also a declining U.S. economy. Unemployment and underemployment (part-time work, low wages, or both) increased the demand for public assistance. At the same time, beginning in the Reagan administration, for many families these benefits were being cut back or eliminated. The domestic hunger crisis continues, as reflected in the fact that an estimated 35 to 40 million Americans are eligible for food stamps but fewer than 27 million receive them (Community Nutrition Institute, 1993). And of the number of persons living in **poverty** (lacking the means to meet basic needs such as housing and food), too many are children. For adults, food insufficiency related to poverty has been associated with a low intake of kilocalories, magnesium, and vitamins A, E, C, and B_6. Elderly adults with limited financial access to food were more likely to have low intakes of protein, calcium, and vitamins A and B_6 (Rose & Oliveira, 1997).

Hunger, in the form of a lack of a wide variety of foods that promote health, can be related to food availability issues. A person living in a rural area is relatively dependent on what the local grocery store carries, whether it be in rural Montana or on an Indian Reservation. On one Reservation in Arizona, diets were found to be moderately high in fat (35 percent of energy), saturated fat (12 percent), and sugar (14 percent), with low intakes of zinc, calcium, vitamin A, vitamin B_6, and folate—often less than two-thirds of the RDA. More than half of these individuals were found to consume only food purchased or acquired on the Reservation (Vaughan et al., 1997). In more metropolitan areas, large grocery stores exist with foods from around the world, but these stores are often inaccessible to many because of transportation issues.

WHAT NATIONAL AGENCIES HELP IMPROVE NUTRITION?

Several federal programs give people access to food. In addition to federal programs, there are local soup kitchens, food banks, and food pantries. These volunteer organizations depend on contributions as well as on local, state, and federal grants. These groups help feed the homeless, unemployed, working poor, and developmentally disabled in many states. Some other nutrition programs are as follows.

The Child and Adult Care Feeding Program (CACFP). This program promotes good nutrition through financial reimbursement. Those who qualify are licensed home day care providers and day care centers that serve nutritious meals.

The Expanded Food and Nutrition Education Program (EFNEP). This program is offered by Cooperative Extension associations and is aimed primarily at the nutritional needs of low-income families. Local **paraprofessionals** (people who are trained by professionals) are trained in nutrition to provide free nutrition education at the homes of low-income families (Fig. 22–1). They focus on **food resource management** (strategies to control food costs) and other areas relevant to nutrition, such as breast-feeding support for low-income mothers.

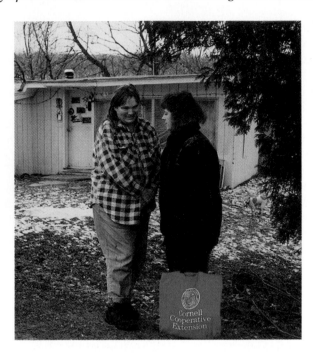

Figure 22–1
A nutrition teaching assistant with EFNEP visits the home of a low-income family.

The Food Stamp Program. This program provides food stamps that can be used to purchase food or seeds to grow food. The allotment is based on the **Thrifty Food Plan,** which is a meal plan designed to meet the lowest possible cost for nutritional adequacy. The Thrifty Food Plan, while beneficial, was not intended to serve long-term nutritional needs. Thus relying on food stamps solely to meet food and nutritional needs is an extreme challenge for even the best-educated person. A disproportionate number of elderly widows live in poverty in the United States. Unless circumstances change, these women need to rely on food stamps to improve nutritional intake (Dodge, 1995).

The Nutrition Program for the Elderly. This program provides nutritious meals through congregate meal settings as well as home-delivered meals for homebound elderly individuals. Nutrition education and counseling on social service needs are provided. Meals on Wheels is a similar program that is often run out of hospitals.

Project Head Start. This program is aimed at children 3 to 5 years old whose parents' income is below the poverty line. The program combines nutrition, social services, parent involvement, and health services within an educational setting. Nutritious meals and snacks are provided. Family-style eating is promoted in that the teachers eat the same foods as the children in order to serve as role models and promote a positive meal environment. Food is served in common dishes and passed around the table so children can take their own portions. This helps build social skills and fine-motor skills and gives children a feeling of control over food choices.

The School Lunch and Breakfast Program. This program provides nutritious foods at reduced cost for children whose families fall within 185 percent

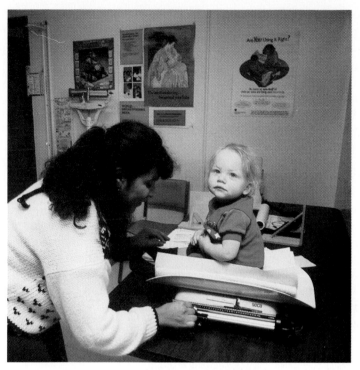

Figure 22–2
Monitoring growth of an infant in the WIC program.

of the poverty line. It further provides free meals for those below the poverty line. Government guidelines for school lunch patterns are provided in Appendix 14.

Women, Infants, and Children Supplemental Nutrition Program (WIC). This program provides nutrition education and vouchers for prescribed supplemental foods. It is aimed at promoting the growth of the young child (Fig. 22–2). Women who are pregnant or breast-feeding, infants, and children up to the age of 5 years are eligible if the family income is within 185 percent of the poverty line. Nutritional risk criteria, such as low hematocrit, poor growth, frequent illness, or other qualifying medical conditions, are specified for enrollment in the WIC program. To further promote child welfare, single fathers, foster parents, or other guardians of children can receive WIC benefits for their children.

WHAT ARE SOME AMBULATORY CARE SERVICES OFFERING NUTRITION GUIDANCE?

Ambulatory care (health care in a noninstitutional setting) is increasing as the costs of hospital-based care continue to rise. Two ambulatory programs are hospices and home health agencies.

Hospices

Hospices offer supportive services for patients who are terminally ill and their families. **Palliative** (noncurative) **care** and supportive care are the general goals of hospices. The services may be provided in an institutional setting or based at home. The hospice movement is probably the best example of the change in attitude toward care of patients through a **holistic** approach (taking into account all aspects of a person's health, such as emotional and spiritual needs in addition to medical and nutritional needs).

In their services for terminally ill patients, emphasizing quality and not quantity of life, hospices have embraced the view espoused by Dr. Elisabeth Kübler-Ross that death is an integral part of life. Kübler-Ross was a pioneer in recognizing that terminally ill patients and their families go through stages of grief. These stages include denial, anger, and acceptance. Nutritional care may need to take into account which stage of grief family members are in. Nutritional goals promote maintaining comfort of the patient over taking a curative approach. Therapeutic diet restrictions may become more lenient. Goals become more short term, such as preventing dehydration or controlling constipation. If a family member is in denial, modifications to the patient's usual diet may not be accepted.

Appropriateness of Nutritional Support for the Terminally Ill

Nutritional support and other life-support measures for terminally ill patients can be viewed as either prolonging life or postponing death. The general philosophy of care for the terminally ill person is palliative care, promoting comfort versus treatment and cure. Thus, most dietary restrictions are lifted unless the comfort of the patient is jeopardized, such as in the case of a patient who is dehydrated or a person with diabetes who may still benefit from controlled blood glucose levels (as physically the person will be expected to feel better with a controlled diet). Nutritional support for the person who is terminally ill generally focuses on oral feedings, but TPN (see Chapter 14) or tube feedings cannot be ruled out. Each patient's case is unique and must be handled individually. The institution should have established, written guidelines for feeding the terminally ill patient. A registered dietitian can assist with the decision as to what form of nutrition intervention is appropriate, based on objective criteria.

Home Health Agencies

Home health agencies are private programs that have nurses and sometimes dietitians on staff to go to patients' homes. Nutritional care of the patient is often provided by the attending nurse. Dietitians generally have limited roles in home health agencies because insurance policies usually do not cover the cost of dietitian services.

WHAT ARE SOME PUBLIC HEALTH CONCERNS THAT HAVE A BEARING ON NUTRITIONAL STATUS?

Nutrition Misinformation

Food fads (a short-term, "quick-fix" diet or supplement) and nutritional quackery have multiplied as the science of nutrition has grown. A trained person can easily differentiate between accurate and unsound information. Unfortunately, the lay person is not always able to do this. In addition, the dramatic manner in which fads and fallacies are presented covers the falseness. Anything that is out of line with current scientific evidence can be considered misinformation.

The **food quack** of today has been likened to the patent medicine man of the past. The food quack uses scientific jargon to sell the product, be it a special food, special food preparation, special diet, regimen, book, magazine, or reducing gadget. It is wise to be suspicious of any writer, lecturer, or TV speaker who makes claims contrary to accepted information. Be aware of (1) those who claim that wholesome food is harmful or undesirable in some way; (2) those who use a scare technique in regard to health or claim to be a scientist or authority; and (3) those who claim association with an unheard-of organization or attack the FDA or medical, public health, or nutrition authorities. One should always be suspicious of any material that comes from an anonymous source.

Authorities on nutrition agree that more widespread and more effective dissemination of sound scientific information on nutrition is necessary to combat food and nutrition misinformation. The FDA has long been concerned about the promotion of food supplements as cure-alls for conditions requiring medical attention. Misleading promotion of food supplements violates federal law. It is carried on in the following ways:

1. So-called health food lecturers who claim, directly or indirectly, that the products they are promoting are of value in preventing and curing disease, when in fact they are ineffective for such purposes.
2. Door-to-door sales agents who pose as experts on nutrition.
3. Pseudoscientific books and journals that frequently recommend some particular food or food combination (the articles are often written by persons with little nutritional background or training). These materials may include advertisements for various products in which the publisher has a commercial interest.

Nutrition authorities agree that the best way to buy vitamins and minerals is in the packages provided by nature: whole-grain and enriched breads and cereals, vegetables, fruits, milk, eggs, meat, and fish. The normal American diet now includes such a variety of foods that most persons can hardly fail to have an ample supply of the essential food constituents if they choose foods wisely. The public should distrust any suggestion of self-medication with vitamins and minerals to cure diseases of the nerves, bones, blood, liver, kidneys, heart, or digestive system.

Food Additives

The 1958 Food Additives Amendment was designed to protect the consumer. Because of this legislation, **food additives** (substances added to foods, generally to make them safer to eat) used in processed food must be proved safe by industry before they can be incorporated into any food product. The **generally recognized as safe (GRAS) list** is another approach used to control the safety of substances used in foods. Additives must meet strict guidelines for inclusion in the GRAS list. Examples of food additives include the use of nitrites to prevent botulism in cured meat products. Ascorbates and other ingredients are added to maintain quality in meat products. Only minute quantities of these additives are used, usually in lower amounts than might exist naturally in many food products. The U.S. Department of Agriculture requires that additives meet the following requirements:

1. They must be approved by the FDA and are limited to specific amounts.
2. They must meet a specific, justifiable need in the product.
3. They must not promote deception as to product freshness, quality, or weight.
4. They must be truthfully and properly listed on the product label.

Table 22–1 lists typical food additives. Table 22–2 lists food and nutrition-related responsibilities of federal agencies.

Food Sanitation

The health of a community depends on safe food and water supplies. Many agencies promote good sanitation practices in order to prevent disease and control **communicable disease** (disease that can spread from person to person, often through water and food). These agencies are concerned with all aspects of food quality, including food preservation and food additives, prevention of both natural and bacterial food poisoning, waterborne diseases, and the dangerous effects of pesticides and other toxic chemicals, such as the heavy metals lead and mercury. The U.S. Public Health Service, which is the principal health agency of the federal government, concerns itself with all factors affecting the health of people, including nutrition.

Food sanitation, although it appears at times unimportant to the general population, can be a matter of life or death, especially for the debilitated or acutely ill patient. Eating can be hazardous to one's health unless three general principles are adhered to: (1) conditions when preparing and consuming food should be clean, clean, clean; (2) when in doubt, throw it out; and (3) keep hot foods hot and cold foods cold.

HOW CAN FOOD POISONING BE PREVENTED?

Lack of sanitation, insufficient cooking, and improper storage can allow bacteria in food to increase to dangerous levels. The Centers for Disease Control (CDC) reported that most foodborne illness results from bacterial growth from food being

Table 22–1
Typical Food Additives, Why and Where Used

Reasons for Use	Substance Used	Foods
To Impart and Maintain Desired Consistency Emulsifiers distribute tiny particles of one liquid in another to improve texture consistency, homogeneity, and quality; stabilizers and thickeners give smooth uniform texture, flavor, and desired consistency	Alginates, lecithin, mono- and diglycerides, agar-agar, methyl cellulose, sodium phosphates, carrageenan	Baked goods, cake mixes, salad dressings, frozen desserts, ice cream, chocolate milk, processed cheese
To Improve Nutritive Value Medical and public health authorities endorse this use to eliminate and prevent certain diseases involving malnutrition; iodized salt has eliminated simple goiter; vitamin D in dairy products and infant foods has virtually eliminated rickets; niacin in bread, cornmeal, and cereals has eliminated pellagra in the southern states	Vitamin A, thiamine, niacin, riboflavin, ascorbic acid, vitamin D, iron, potassium iodide	Wheat flour, bread and biscuits, breakfast cereals, cornmeal, macaroni and noodle products, margarine, milk, iodized salt
To Enhance Flavor Many spices and natural and synthetic flavors give us a desired variety of flavorful foods such as spice cake, gingerbread, and sausage	Cloves, ginger, citrus oils, amyl acetate, benzaldehyde	Ice cream, candy, gingerbread, spice cake, soft drinks, fruit-flavored gelatins, fruit-flavored toppings, sausage
To Provide Desired Texture Leavening agents are used in the baking industry in cakes, biscuits, waffles, muffins, and other baked goods	Sodium bicarbonate, phosphates	Cakes, cookies, crackers
To Impart Tartness to Beverages	Citric acid, lactic acid, phosphates, phosphoric acid	Soft drinks
To Maintain Appearance, Palatability, and Wholesomeness Deterioration due to microbial growth or oxidation is delayed and food spoilage caused by mold, bacteria, and yeast is prevented or slowed by certain additives; antioxidants keep fats from turning rancid and certain fresh fruits from darkening during processing when cut and exposed to air	Propionic acid, sodium and calcium salts of propionic acid, ascorbic acid, butylated hydroxyanisole, butylated hydroxytoluene, benzoates	Bread, cheese, syrup, pie fillings, crackers, frozen and dried fruits, fruit juices, margarine, lard, shortening, potato chips, cake mixes
To Give Desired and Characteristic Color Acceptability and attractiveness are increased by the correction of objectionable natural variations	FDA-approved colors, such as annatto, carotene, cochineal, chlorophyll	Confections, bakery goods, soft drinks, cheeses, ice-cream, jams, and jellies
Other Functions Humectants retain moisture in some foods and keep others, including salts and powders, free flowing	Glycerine, magnesium carbonate	Coconut, table salt

From Chemical Manufacturers Association: Food Additives . . . Who Needs Them? Washington, DC, p. 11.

Table 22–2
Food and Nutrition-Related Responsibilities of Federal Agencies

Agency	Function
Bureau of Alcohol, Tobacco and Firearms (BATF)	Regulation of alcoholic beverages
Consumer Product Safety Commission (CPSC)	Safety of food handling equipment
Department of Agriculture (USDA)	
Economics Research Service (ERS)	Analysis and reporting of food situation and outlook
Food and Nutrition Service (FNS)	Administration of the following programs: Food Stamp; School Lunch; Women, Infants, and Children; and Donated Food
Food Safety and Inspection Service (FSIS)	Inspection and labeling of meat, poultry, and eggs; grading of all foods; controlling nitrite in cured meats and poultry
Human Nutrition Information Service (HNIS)	Food consumption standard tables for nutritive value of food, educational materials
Science and Education Administration (SEA)	Extension Service, Agricultural Research Service Cooperative State Research Service, National Agricultural Library
Department of Health and Human Services (HHS)	
Centers for Disease Control (CDC)	Analysis and reporting of incidence of foodborne diseases
Food and Drug Administration (FDA)	Food labeling, safety of food and food additives, inspection of food processing plants, control of food contaminants, food standards
National Institutes of Health (NIH)	Research related to diet and health
Environmental Protection Agency (EPA)	Standards for drinking water and water pollution, use of pesticides on food crops
Federal Trade Commission (FTC)	Food advertising, competition in food industry
National Marine Fisheries Service (NMFS)	Inspection, standards, and quality of seafood
Occupational Safety and Health Administration (OSHA)	Employee safety in food-processing plants

held at an improper temperature and poor personal hygiene of food handlers (Collins, 1997). Some bacteria produce poisonous substances called toxins that cause illness when contaminated food is eaten. To prevent food poisoning, do the following:

- Serve food soon after cooking or refrigerate promptly. Hot foods may be refrigerated if they do not raise the temperature of the refrigerator to greater than 45° F (7° C).
- Keep food in the refrigerator until served or reheated.
- Speed the cooling of leftovers by refrigerating them in shallow containers.
- Keep hot foods *hot* (at temperatures greater than 140° F or 60° C) and cold foods *cold* (less than 40° F or 4° C). Food may not be safe to eat if held more than 2 or 3 hours at temperatures between 60° F (15° C) and 125° F (52° C), the zone in

which bacteria grow rapidly. Remember to count all time during preparation, storage, and serving.

- Thoroughly clean all dishes, utensils, and work surfaces with soap and water after each use. It is especially important to thoroughly clean equipment and work surfaces that have been used for raw food before you use them for cooked food. This prevents the cooked food from becoming contaminated with bacteria that may have been present in the raw food. Bacteria can be destroyed by rinsing utensils and work surfaces with chlorine laundry bleach in the proportion recommended on the package. Cutting boards, meat grinders, blenders, and can openers particularly need this protection.
- Always wipe up spills with paper towels or other disposable material.
- Thoroughly cook meat to avoid **Escherichia coli** (*E. coli*) contamination.
- *If the odor or color of any food is poor or questionable, do not taste it. Throw it out. The food may be dangerous.*

How Does Personal Hygiene Affect Food Safety?

Anyone who has an infectious disease should not handle, prepare, or serve food. The bacteria in infected cuts or other skin infections may be the source of foodborne illness. Food handlers must always work with clean hands, clean hair, and clean fingernails and must wear clean clothing. Hands must be washed after using the toilet or assisting anyone using the toilet; after cigarette smoking or blowing the nose; after touching raw meat, poultry, or eggs; and before working with other food. Food should be mixed with clean utensils rather than with the hands; however, plastic gloves may be worn if they make it easier to use the hands. Hands should be kept away from the mouth, nose, and hair. It is important to cover coughs and sneezes with disposable tissues and to wash hands afterward. The same spoon should not be used more than once for tasting food while preparing, cooking, or serving.

What Are Some Types of Food Poisoning?

To understand the importance of food poisoning prevention, types of foodborne illnesses must be known. The more common ones are those caused by the following:

- *Salmonella*
- *Staphylococcus aureus* (also referred to as staph poisoning)
- *Clostridium botulinum* (causes botulism)
- *Clostridium perfringens*
- *E. coli*

Specific information on the causes, symptoms, and prevention of these bacterial foodborne illnesses is found in Table 22–3.

Table 22-3
Bacterial Foodborne Illness: Causes, Symptoms, and Prevention

Foods Involved	Symptoms	Characteristics of Illness	Preventive Measures
Salmonellosis: *Salmonella*			
Bacteria widespread in nature, live and grow in intestinal tracts of human beings and animals Foods involved: Poultry Red meats Eggs Dried foods Dairy products	Severe headache, followed by vomiting, diarrhea, abdominal cramps, fever. Infants, elderly, and persons with lower resistance are most susceptible; severe infections cause high fever and may even cause death	Transmitted by eating contaminated food or by contact with infected persons or carriers of the infection; also transmitted by insects, rodents, and pets *Onset:* Usually within 12 to 36 hours *Duration:* 2 to 7 days	Salmonellae are destroyed by heating the food to 140° F and holding for 10 minutes, or to higher temperature for less time (for instance, 155° F for a few seconds) Refrigeration at 40° F inhibits the multiplication of Salmonellae, but they remain alive in foods in the refrigerator or freezer and even in dried food
Perfringens Poisoning: *Clostridium perfringens*			
Spore-forming bacteria that grow in the absence of oxygen; temperatures reached in thorough cooking of most foods are sufficient to destroy vegetative cells, but heat-resistant spores can survive Foods involved: Stews, soups, or gravies made from poultry or red meat	Nausea without vomiting, diarrhea, acute inflammation of stomach and intestines	Transmitted by eating food contaminated with abnormally large numbers of bacteria *Onset:* Usually within 8 to 20 hours *Duration:* May persist for 24 hours	To prevent growth of surviving bacteria in cooked meats, gravies, and meat casseroles that are to be eaten later, cool foods rapidly and refrigerate promptly at 40° F or below, or hold them above 140° F

Staphylococcal Poisoning: Staphylococcus aureus

Bacteria fairly resistant to heat; bacteria growing in food produce a toxin that is extremely resistant to heat Foods involved: Custards Egg salad Potato salad Chicken salad Macaroni salad Ham salad Salami Cheese	Vomiting, diarrhea, prostration, abdominal cramps; generally mild and often attributed to other causes	Transmitted by food handlers who carry the bacteria and by eating food containing the toxin *Onset:* Usually within 3 to 8 hours *Duration:* 1 to 2 days	Growth of bacteria that produce toxin is inhibited by keeping hot foods above 140° F and cold foods at or above 40° F. Toxin is destroyed by boiling for several hours or heating the food in a pressure cooker at 240° F for 30 minutes

Botulism: Clostridium botulinum

Spore-forming organisms that grow and produce toxin in the absence of oxygen, such as in a sealed container Foods involved: Canned low-acid foods Smoked fish	Double vision, inability to swallow, speech difficulty, progressive respiratory paralysis. Fatality rate is high, in the US about 65%	Transmitted by eating food containing the toxin *Onset:* Usually within 12 to 36 hours or longer *Duration:* 3 to 6 days	Bacterial spores in food are destroyed by high temperatures obtained only in the pressure canner.* More than 6 hours is needed to kill the spores at boiling temperature (212° F). The toxin is destroyed by boiling for 10 to 20 minutes; time required depends on type of food.

*For processing times in home canning, see Home and Garden Bulletin No. 8, Home Canning of Fruits and Vegetables, and No. 106, Home Canning of Meat and Poultry. U.S. Department of Agriculture, Washington, DC.

From U.S. Department of Agriculture: Keeping Food Safe to Eat—A Guide for Homemakers. Home and Garden Bulletin No. 162, Washington, DC.

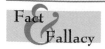

Fallacy: Adding an egg to a milkshake or making eggnog is a good idea for someone who is too ill to eat.

Fact: Raw eggs can contain salmonella (a type of bacteria), which can be deadly for a person who already has a weakened immune system. This is especially true of cracked or soiled eggs. Eggs should be used only in foods that are to be thoroughly cooked, such as baked goods or casseroles. Proper handling of foods with cooked eggs is also important. Set custards and puddings in ice water to cool quickly after their preparation. Then refrigerate promptly until serving time.

WHAT ARE WORLD PROBLEMS IN NUTRITION AND WHAT ARE THE INTERESTED AGENCIES?

In less developed countries, a large number of individuals are undernourished, malnourished, and hungry. The problem is greatest among women and children. Breast milk is an especially important source of energy, protein, and accompanying micronutrients in young children whose family's diet is low in quality. Continued breast-feeding past 1 year of age, in conjunction with table foods, should be encouraged in toddlers living in poor circumstances (Marquis et al., 1997). People in developing countries are hungry primarily because they are too poor to purchase the food that is available, although availability may also be limited. As many as half of the world's children may suffer some degree of malnutrition, temporary or permanent, that causes mental and physical developmental problems. For example, zinc supplementation was found to dramatically reduce the incidence of diarrhea among young, rural Guatemalan children. This may be an effective intervention to improve their health status and growth (Ruel et al., 1997).

Vitamin A deficiency is also a problem worldwide. Millions of children in impoverished countries show signs of moderate vitamin A deficiency and are therefore more vulnerable to infection and blindness. The World Health Organization (WHO) has recommended vitamin A supplementation for children aged 6 months or older in developing countries at the same time that immunization for measles is being provided (Benn et al., 1997).

The four basic ways of dealing with the international hunger problem are through (1) donation of food by various groups; (2) international efforts that direct the food to vulnerable groups, such as women and children; (3) promotion of agricultural production, food technology, and better use of the country's own food resources; and (4) economic assistance.

The United States has developed various programs and campaigns that assist developing countries in combating undernutrition. The U.S. Foreign Aid and Food for Peace programs and activities of the Agency for International Development are coordinated with United Nations agencies. The governments of many nations contribute to the organizations that distribute food or money for the purpose of improving nutritional standards. Some of these agencies are listed in Table 22–4.

Table 22–4
World Organizations for Better Nutrition

Organization	Purposes
United Nations Food and Agriculture Organization (FAO)	Studies aspects of world food problems
	Raises nutrition standards by improving growth, distribution, and storage of food
World Health Organization (WHO)	Focus on worldwide health problems, including nutrition
United National Education, Scientific and Cultural Organization (UNESCO)	Improving the standard of living through science education and elimination of illiteracy
United Nations International Children's Emergency Fund (UNICEF)	Directs the distribution of milk to children worldwide through emergency relief, school feeding, and maternal-child health care centers
Oxford Famine Society (OXFAM-UK)	Donates money and services for agricultural development
CARE	Receives food from the Food for Peace Program for relief activities
World Bank	Sponsors international projects through agricultural and nutritional divisions

WHAT IS THE ROLE OF THE NURSE OR OTHER HEALTH CARE PROFESSIONAL IN NATIONAL AND INTERNATIONAL NUTRITION PROGRAMS?

National Nutrition

Nurses or other health care professionals often provide nutrition education to a variety of groups such as pregnant women and diabetic or hypertensive patients. Information relating to modifications of the Food Guide Pyramid food groups, such as portion sizes and low-sodium, low-fat, or low-sugar alternatives is appropriate. Providing the patient with a rationale for making dietary changes that are in line with physiological needs particularly suits the nurse's skill level. Providing advice on low-cost food shopping is also appropriate (Table 22–5). Consultation should be made with a registered dietitian and physician regarding individual diet needs that go beyond basic nutrition, particularly when good nutrition may be jeopardized.

A health care team approach can help promote good nutritional status. The nurse or other health professional can help combat potentially dangerous nutrition myths and fads by providing correct information and assisting the public in recognizing false nutritional health claims. On a larger scale, the health care professional can help raise society's health consciousness by documenting the health needs of persons such as those with low incomes and those who are homeless. This documentation is necessary in order to justify equitable allocation of resources with legislators and other policy makers.

It is important for the nurse or other health care professional to be aware of programs for referral purposes and direct care. Ambulatory care in particular is a

Table 22–5
Money-Saving Food-Shopping Skills

- Use less tender cuts of meat, which are less expensive. To tenderize, cook slowly with moisture (such as in stews) or grind, cube, or pound the meat. Marinating in an acid such as lemon or tomato juice also helps to tenderize meat.
- Extend meat, poultry, and fish by making casseroles using legumes (dried beans), pasta, rice, or potatoes.
- Include meatless meals once or twice a week using legumes, eggs, cheese, or peanut butter in its place for protein.
- Buy in bulk whenever possible and freeze as needed.
- Study unit pricing to determine the best buy per pound or ounce.
- Take advantage of specials and use coupons.
- Try lower-priced, "generic" store brands, which are often of similar quality to more expensive brands.
- Plan meals to include leftovers.
- Shop for low-cost foods within each food group.
- Use food labels to compare nutritional value for cost to get your money's worth.

growing means of health care, with the nurse often being called on to help patients cope with therapeutic diets and to help prevent the effects of poor food sanitation on the debilitated patient.

International Nutrition

Solving international nutrition concerns is a more complex issue. The health care professional should be aware of programs that can be effectively promoted, such as taking vitamin A tablets to prevent blindness. Food programs meant to help should be closely examined. For example, providing dried milk powder to populations at risk of lactose intolerance is counterproductive. Attempts to solve world hunger must be undertaken in a way that empowers rather than creates dependency. Individuals can have an impact on world hunger by contacting political leaders to express concern. Efforts by credible international agencies, such as the Agency for International Development and the United Nations (see previous discussion), can be supported. For Americans, eating less meat contributes, if only in a small way: it takes about 4 pounds of grain to produce 1 pound of meat; grain grown to feed cattle could be redirected to feed the world's hungry population.

Critical Thinking

Case Study

Pat and Anna were working at the church's food pantry preparing donations for the Indian reservation. They had heard it was becoming very difficult for the people living on the reservation to get enough fresh fruits and vegetables to eat. As Pat continued to pack boxes with canned goods, he wondered about all the salt and sugar listed on the food labels. Pat and Anna had originally met in church when her family first moved here. They were both now keenly aware of hunger issues in their community. Pat's maternal grandmother had taken them to an Indian reservation where she had lived as a young child before going to the Indian school, which had now been long closed.

Pat remembered a college term paper his brother-in-law Joey had written on the cultural origins of food. Many cultures had similar eating habits, including the daily consumption of beans and other foods with a high-fiber content. People from many cultures, such as the Irish, Scottish, and Italian, historically ate a lot of fish, including sardines, which warded off heart disease. Pat thought about all the fish his family ate, such as crawfish and shrimp. Irish and Scottish people also historically ate primarily oats and barley as their grains and many people of British heritage eat baked beans on toast to this day. These ideas made Pat question even more why fruit canned in heavy syrup, donuts, and cookies were often part of food donations to the Indian reservations. Those were certainly not Native American foods.

Applications

1. How might food pantries help or hinder nutritional status. What canned foods would be appropriate for someone with hypertension? How can you include canned fruits into the diabetic diet?
2. Could a person with renal disease and diabetes plan healthy meals with canned foods? How?
3. Do you know of families who might go hungry? How has the new "welfare system" increased the risk of poor nutritional status of low-income families? What might you do to help prevent hunger?

Study Questions and Classroom Activities

1. What community programs might help a low-income family?
2. How has legislation had an impact on public health in relation to food and nutrition issues?
3. What existing programs promote good nutrition?
4. What are the signs of a food faddist?
5. Visit or call your local health department. Learn about any nutrition activities that are conducted under the auspices of the department.
6. Identify other organizations in your area that focus on the promotion of nutrition. Describe who they are and what their programs cover.
7. Contact a federal or state legislator through a letter or a phone call to express your support for legislation on a public health issue.
8. A student volunteer will be assigned to swab the inside of a home refrigerator using a cotton-tipped swab. Students in the class can then rub the swab on a Petri dish and observe bacterial growth.
9. How might you assist a low-income individual who has hypertension and who needs to rely on donated canned foods?

References

Benn CS, Aaby P, Bale C, Olsen J, Michaelsen KF, George E, Whittle H: Randomised trial of effect of vitamin A supplementation on antibody response to measles vaccine in Guinea-Bissau, West Africa. Lancet. July 12, 1997; 350(9071):101–105.

Carter JS, Pugh JA, Monterrosa A: Non-insulin-dependent diabetes mellitus in minorities in the United States. Ann Intern Med. August 1, 1996; 125(3):221–232.

Collins JE: Impact of changing consumer lifestyles on the emergence/reemergence of foodborne pathogens. Emerg Infect Dis. October 1997; 3(4):471–479.

Community Nutrition Institute: Food stamp program points to deep fissures in American economy. Nutrition Week. February 5, 1993; 23(6):2.

Dodge HH: Movements out of poverty among elderly widows. J Gerontol B Psychol Sci Soc Sci. July 1995; 50(4):S240–S249.

Krebs-Smith SM, Cook A, Subar AF, Cleveland L, Friday J, Kahle LL: Fruit and vegetable intakes of children and adolescents in the United States. Arch Pediatr Adolesc Med. January 1996; 150(1):81–86.

Marquis GS, Habicht JP, Lanata CF, Black RE, Rasmussen KM: Breast milk or animal-product foods improve linear growth of Peruvian toddlers consuming marginal diets. Am J Clin Nutr. November 1997; 66(5):1102–1109.

Rose D, Oliveira V: Nutrient intakes of individuals from food-insufficient households in the United States. Am J Public Health. December 1997; 87(12):1956–1961.

Ruel MT, Rivera JA, Santizo MC, Lonnerdal B, Brown KH: Impact of zinc supplementation on morbidity from diarrhea and respiratory infections among rural Guatemalan children. Pediatrics. June 1997; 99(6):808–813.

Vaughan LA, Benyshek DC, Martin JF: Food acquisition habits, nutrient intakes, and anthropometric data of Havasupai adults. J Am Diet Assoc. November 1997; 97(11):1275–1282.

Appendixes

Appendix 1
Sources of Nutrition Information

American Association of Family and Consumer Services
1555 King Street
Alexandria, VA 22314
Tel.: 703–706–4600
Fax.: 703–706–4663

American Dental Association
211 East Chicago Avenue
Chicago, IL 60611
Tel.: 800–621–8099

American Diabetes Association
1660 Duke Street
Alexandria, VA 22314
Tel.: 800–342–2383
Diabetes Forecast (bimonthly)

American Dietetic Association (ADA)
216 West Jackson Boulevard, Suite 800
Chicago, IL 60606–6995
Tel.: 800–877–1600
Journal of the American Dietetic Association (monthly)

American Heart Association (AHA)
7272 Greenville Avenue
Dallas, TX 75231–4596
Tel.: 800–242–8721

American Institute of Nutrition (AIN)
9650 Rockville Pike
Bethesda, MD 20014
Tel.: 301–530–7050
Journal of Nutrition (monthly)

American Medical Association (AMA)
515 N. State Street
Chicago, IL 60610
Tel.: 312–464–4543
Journal of the American Medical Association (weekly)

American Public Health Association (APHA)
1015 16th Street, NW
Washington, DC 20005
Tel.: 202–789–5600
American Journal of Public Health (monthly)
The Nation's Health (monthly newspaper)

American Society of Clinical Nutrition, Inc. (ASCN)
9650 Rockville Pike
Bethesda, MD 20814–3998
Tel.: 301–530–7110
The American Journal of Clinical Nutrition (monthly)

American Society for Nutritional Sciences
9650 Rockville Pike
Bethesda, MD 20814–3990
Journal of Nutrition (monthly)

American Society for Parenteral and Enteral Nutrition (ASPEN)
8630 Fenton, Suite 412
Silver Spring, MD 20910–3805
Tel.: 301–587–6315
Fax.: 301–587–2365
Journal of Parenteral and Enteral Nutrition (bimonthly)
ASPEN Update (monthly newspaper)

Food and Drug Administration (FDA)
Regulatory Affairs
5600 Fishers Lane, No. 1490
Rockville, MD 20857
Tel.: 301–827–3101

Food and Nutrition Board (FNB) of National Research Council (NRC)
2101 Constitution Avenue, NW
Washington, DC 20418
Tel.: 202–334–1738

Food and Nutrition Information Center
USDA/Natl. Agriculture Library, Room 304
10301 Baltimore Boulevard
Beltsville, MD 20715–2315
Tel.: 301–504–5717
Fax.: 301–504–6409

National Dairy Council
10255 W. Itiggins Road, Suite 900
Rosemont, IL 60018–5616
Tel.: 847–803–2000
Dairy Council Digest (bimonthly newsletter)

Nutrition Foundation, Inc.
888 17th Street, NW
Washington, DC 20006
Nutrition Reviews (monthly)

Nutrition Today (published by Williams and Wilkins)
351 West Camden Street
Baltimore, MD 21201–2436
Tel.: 800–638–6423
Nutrition Today (bimonthly)

Society for Nutrition Education (SNE)
2850 Metro Drive, Suite 416
Minneapolis, MN 55425–1412
Tel.: 612–854–0035
Journal of Nutrition Education (quarterly)

U.S. Department of Agriculture
Food, Nutrition and Consumer Services
1400 Independence Avenue, S.W. #240E
Washington, DC 21250
Tel.: 800–205–9953
List of publications available from Office of Information

Appendix 2
Nutrition Materials

American Institute of Baking
1213 Bakers Way
Manhattan, KS 66502
Tel.: 913–537–4750

Armour Food Company
2001 Butterfield Road
Downers Grove, IL 60515–1049
Tel.: 708–512–1840
Fax.: 708–512–1120

Borden, Inc.
Consumer Products Division
108 East Broad Street
Columbus, OH 43215
Tel.: 614–225–4000

California Prune Board
5990 Stonridge Drive, Suite 101
Pleasanton, CA 94588–3234
Tel.: 510–734–5105

Campbell Soup Company
Consumer Products Division Campbell Place
Camden, NJ 08103
Tel.: 609–342–4800 or 800–257–8443 (inquiries)

Del Monte
Consumer Affairs Dept.
P.O. Box 193
San Francisco, CA 94119–3575
Tel.: 800–543–3090
Fax.: 415–242–3080

Florida Department of Citrus
P.O. Box 148
Lakeland, FL 33802
Tel.: 914–499–2500

General Foods Consumer Center
250 North Street
White Plains, NY 10625
Tel.: 914–335–2500

General Mills, Inc.
1 General Mills Boulevard
Minneapolis, MN 55426
Tel.: 612–540–2311
(Maxwell Division: 914–335–2500)

Kellogg Company
One Kellogg Square
Battle Creek, MI 49016–3599
Tel.: 616–961–2000 or 800–961–1413
Fax.: 616–961–2871

Kraft Foods, Inc.
1 Kraft Court
Glenview, IL 60025
Tel.: 800–323–0768

Lacto Milk Products Corporation
Division Johanna
Johanna Farms Road, Box 272
Hemmington, NJ 08822
Tel.: 908–782–1680

McDonald's Corporation
Consumer Products Division
1 McDonald Plaza
Oakbrook, IL 60521
Tel.: 708–575–3000

Mead Johnson Nutritional Division
2400 W. Lloyd Expressway
Evansville, IN 47721
Tel.: 800–457–3550

Metropolitan Life Insurance Company
Health and Welfare Division
1 Madison Avenue
New York, NY 10010

Nabisco Foods Group
Consumer Products Division
7 Campus Drive
Parsipany, NJ 07054
Tel.: 201–682–5000

National Dairy Council
10255 West Hiccins Road, Suite 900
Rosemont, IL 60018–5616
Tel.: 708–803–2000
Fax.: 708–803–2077

National Livestock and Meat Board
Nutrition Research Department
444 N. Michigan Avenue
Chicago, IL 60611
Tel.: 312–467–5520

National Peanut Council (NPC)
1500 King Street, Suite 301
Alexandria, VA 22314
Tel.: 703–838–9500
Fax.: 703–838–9089

Nestlé Food Company (Carnation)
800 North Brand Boulevard
Glendale, CA 91203
Tel.: 800–242–5200 or 818–549–6000

**Nestlé Food Company (Evaporated
 Milk Association)**
800 North Brand Boulevard
Glendale, CA 91203
Tel.: 800–854–8935

**Novartis (previously Sandoz
 Nutrition Corps.)**
5100 Gamble Drive
Saint Louis Park
Minneapolis, MN 55416
Tel.: 800–999–9978

Peanut Association Board
1950 North Park Place, Suite 525
Atlantic, GA 30339
Tel.: 404–933–0357

Peanut Association of America
c/o John Ojala
University of Idaho
1776 Science Center Drive
Idaho Falls, ID 83402
Tel.: 208–529–8376

The Quaker Oats Company
321 N. Clark Street
Quaker Tower
Chicago, IL 60610
Tel.: 312–222–7111

Ralston Purina Company
Checkerboard Square
P.O. Box 618
St. Louis, MO 63188–0618
Tel.: 800–725–7866
Fax.: 314–877–7022

Ross Laboratories
625 Cleveland Avenue
Columbus, OH 43215
Tel.: 800–624–7677

Sunkist Growers
P.O. Box 7888
Van Nuys, CA 91409
Tel.: 818–986–4800

Appendix 3
Metric Conversions and Equivalents

Equivalents

1 oz = 30 g (approximate)	1 c = 16 tbsp = 240 mL
1 lb = 454 g	1 L = 1000 mL
1 g = 1 mL	1 mg = 1000 μg

Metric Measurement Conversions

Symbol	When You Know	Multiply by	To Find	Symbol
Length				
in	inches	2.54	centimeters	cm
ft	feet	30	centimeters	cm
yd	yards	0.9	meters	m
mi	miles	1.6	kilometers	km
mm	millimeters	0.04	inches	in
cm	centimeters	0.4	inches	in
m	meters	3.3	feet	ft
m	meters	1.1	yards	yd
km	kilometers	0.6	miles	mi
Mass (Weight)				
oz	ounces	28	grams	g
lb	pounds	0.45	kilograms	kg
g	grams	0.035	ounce	oz
kg	kilograms	2.2	pounds	lb
	stones (British)	14	pounds	lb
Volume				
tsp	teaspoons	5	milliliters	mL
tbsp	tablespoons	15	milliliters	mL
fl oz	fluid ounces	30	milliliters	mL
c	cups	0.24	liters	L
pt	pints	0.47	liters	L
qt	quarts	0.95	liters	L
gal (U.S.)	gallons (U.S.)	3.8	liters	L
gal (Imp)	gallons (Imperial)	4.5	liters	L
ft^3	cubic feet	0.028	cubic meters	m^3
yd^3	cubic yards	0.76	cubic meters	m^3
mL	milliliters	0.03	fluid ounces	fl oz
L	liters	2.1	pints	pt
L	liters	1.06	quarts	qt
L	liters	0.26	gallons (U.S.)	gal (U.S.)
L	liters	0.22	gallons (Imperial)	gal (Imp)

Temperature

$^\circ C = (^\circ F - 32) \times .555$

$^\circ F = (^\circ C \times 1.8) + 32$

Appendix 4
Nutritive Values for Selected Fast Foods

Burger King

Menu Item	Serving Size (g)	Calories	Total Fat (g)	Saturated Fat (g)	Cholesterol (mg)	Sodium (mg)	Total Carbohydrate (g)	Dietary Fiber (g)	Protein (g)
Burgers									
WHOPPER® Sandwich	270	640	39	11	90	870	45	3	27
WHOPPER® with Cheese Sandwich	294	730	46	16	115	1350	46	3	33
DOUBLE WHOPPER® Sandwich	351	870	56	19	170	940	45	3	46
DOUBLE WHOPPER® with Cheese Sandwich	375	960	63	24	195	1420	46	3	52
WHOPPER JR.® Sandwich	164	420	24	8	60	530	29	2	21
WHOPPER JR.® with Cheese Sandwich	177	460	28	10	75	770	29	2	23
BIG KING Sandwich	226	660	43	18	135	920	29	1	40
Hamburger	126	330	15	6	55	530	28	1	20
Cheeseburger	138	380	19	9	65	770	28	1	23
Double Cheeseburger	210	600	36	17	135	1060	28	1	41
Double Cheeseburger With Bacon	218	640	39	18	145	1240	28	1	44
Sandwiches/Side Orders									
BK BIG FISH® Sandwich	252	720	43	9	80	1180	59	3	23
BK BROILER® Chicken Sandwich	247	530	26	5	105	1060	45	2	29
Chicken Sandwich	229	710	43	9	60	1400	54	2	26
CHICKEN TENDERS® (8 pieces)	123	350	22	7	65	940	17	1	22
Broiled Chicken Salad†	302	190	8	4	75	500	9	3	20
Garden Salad†	215	100	5	3	15	110	7	3	6
Side Salad†	133	60	3	2	5	55	4	2	3
French Fries (Medium, Salted)	116	400	21	8	0	820	50	4	3
Onion Rings	124	310	14	2	0	810	41	6	4
Dutch Apple Pie	113	300	15	3	0	230	39	2	3
Drinks									
Vanilla Shake (Medium)	284	300	6	4	20	230	53	1	9
Chocolate Shake (Medium)	284	320	7	4	20	230	54	3	9
Chocolate Shake (Medium, Syrup Added)	341	440	7	4	20	430	84	2	10
Strawberry Shake (Medium, Syrup Added)	341	420	6	4	20	260	83	1	9
Coca Cola® Classic (Medium)	22 (Fl Oz)	280	0	0	0	@	70	0	0
Diet Coke® (Medium)	22 (Fl Oz)	1	0	0	0	@	<1	0	0
Sprite® (Medium)	22 (Fl Oz)	260	0	0	0	@	66	0	0
Tropicana® Orange Juice	311	140	0	0	0	0	33	0	2
Coffee	355	5	0	0	0	5	1	0	0
Milk—2% Low Fat	244	130	5	3	20	120	12	0	8

Burger King *(continued)*

Menu Item	Serving Size (g)	Calories	Total Fat (g)	Saturated Fat (g)	Cholesterol (mg)	Sodium (mg)	Total Carbohydrate (g)	Dietary Fiber (g)	Protein (g)
Breakfast									
CROISSAN'WICH® w/ Sausage, Egg & Cheese	163	550	42	14	250	1110	22	1	20
CROISSAN'WICH® w/ Sausage & Cheese	106	450	35	12	45	940	21	1	13
Biscuit	93	330	18	4	2	950	37	1	6
Biscuit With Egg	150	420	24	6	205	1110	38	1	13
Biscuit With Sausage	137	530	36	11	35	1350	38	1	13
Biscuit With Bacon, Egg and Cheese	171	510	31	10	225	1530	39	1	19
French Toast Sticks	141	500	27	7	0	490	60	1	4
Hash Browns (Small)	75	240	15	6	0	440	25	2	2
A.M. EXPRESS® Grape Jam	12	30	0	0	0	0	7	0	0
A.M. EXPRESS® Strawberry Jam	12	30	0	0	0	5	8	0	0
Condiments									
Sandwich Condiments/Toppings									
Processed American Cheese (2 slices)	25	90	8	5	25	420	0	0	6
Lettuce	21	0	0	0	0	0	0	0	0
Tomato (2 slices)	28	5	0	0	0	0	1	0	0
Onion	14	5	0	0	0	0	1	0	0
Pickles (4 slices)	14	0	0	0	0	140	0	0	0
Ketchup	14	15	0	0	0	180	4	0	0
King Sauce	14	70	7	1	4	70	2	0	0
Mustard	3	0	0	0	0	40	0	0	0
Mayonnaise	28	210	23	3	20	160	<1	0	0
Tartar Sauce	28	180	19	3	15	220	0	0	0
Land O'Lakes® Whipped Classic Blend	10	65	7	1	0	75	0	0	0
Bull's Eye® Barbecue Sauce	14	20	0	0	0	140	5	0	0
Bacon Bits	3	15	1	0	3	70	0	0	1
Croutons	7	30	1	0	0	90	5	0	<1
Burger King® Salad Dressings									
Thousand Island Dressing	30	140	12	3	15	190	7	<1	0
French Dressing	30	140	10	2	0	190	11	0	0
Ranch Dressing	30	180	19	4	10	170	2	<1	<1
Bleu Cheese Dressing	30	160	16	4	30	260	1	<1	2
Reduced Calorie Light Italian Dressing#	30	15	0.5	0	0	360	3	0	0
Dipping Sauces									
A.M. EXPRESS® Dip	28	80	0	0	0	20	21	0	0
Honey Dipping Sauce	28	90	0	0	0	10	23	0	0
Ranch Dipping Sauce	28	170	17	3	0	200	2	0	0
Barbecue Dipping Sauce	28	35	0	0	0	400	9	0	0
Sweet & Sour Dipping Sauce	28	45	0	0	0	50	11	0	0

† = Without Dressing   @ = Depends on the water supply   # = Regular Italian Dressing – 150 calories – 16 grams (g) Fat.

McDonald's

Menu Item	Serving Size	Calories	Total Fat (g)	Saturated Fat (g)	Cholesterol (mg)	Sodium (mg)	Total Carbohydrate (g)	Dietary Fiber (g)	Protein (g)
Sandwiches									
Hamburger	106 g	260	9	3.5	30	580	34	2	13
Cheeseburger	120 g	320	13	6	40	820	35	2	15
Quarter Pounder®	172 g	420	21	8	70	820	37	2	23
Quarter Pounder® with Cheese	200 g	530	30	13	95	1290	38	2	28
Big Mac®	216 g	560	31	10	85	1070	45	3	26
Arch Deluxe®	239 g	550	31	11	90	1010	39	4	28
Arch Deluxe® with Bacon	247 g	590	34	12	100	1150	39	4	32
Crispy Chicken Deluxe™	223 g	500	25	4	55	1100	43	3	26
Fish Filet Deluxe™	228 g	560	28	6	60	1060	54	4	23
Grilled Chicken Deluxe™	223 g	440	20	3	60	1040	38	3	27
Grilled Chicken Deluxe™ (plain w/o mayo)	205 g	300	5	1	50	930	38	3	27
French Fries									
Small French Fires	68 g	210	10	1.5	0	135	26	2	3
Large French Fries	147 g	450	22	4	0	290	57	5	6
Super Size® French Fries	176 g	540	26	4.5	0	350	68	6	8
Chicken McNuggets®/Sauces									
Chicken McNuggets® (4 piece)	71 g	190	11	2.5	40	340	10	0	12
Chicken McNuggets® (6 piece)	106 g	290	17	3.5	60	510	15	0	18
Chicken McNuggets® (9 piece)	159 g	430	26	5	90	770	23	0	27
Hot Mustard (1 pkg)	28 g	60	3.5	0	5	240	7	<1	1
Barbeque Sauce (1 pkg)	28 g	45	0	0	0	250	10	0	0
Sweet 'N Sour Sauce (1 pkg)	28 g	50	0	0	0	140	11	0	0
Honey (1 pkg)	14 g	45	0	0	0	0	12	0	0
Honey Mustard (1 pkg)	14 g	50	4.5	0.5	10	85	3	0	0
Light Mayonnaise	12 g	40	4	0.5	5	85	<1	0	0
Salads									
Garden Salad	177 g	35	0	0	0	20	7	2	2
Grilled Chicken Salad Deluxe	257 g	120	1.5	0	45	240	7	2	21
Croutons (1 pkg)	12 g	50	1.5	0	0	80	7	<1	2
Salad Dressings									
Caesar (1 pkg)	59.1 ml	160	14	3	20	450	7	0	2
Fat Free Herb Vinaigrette (1 pkg)	59.1 ml	50	0	0	0	330	11	0	0
Ranch (1 pkg)	59.1 ml	230	21	3	20	550	10	0	1
Red French Reduced Calorie (1 pkg)	59.1 ml	160	8	1	0	490	23	0	0

McDonald's *(continued)*

Menu Item	Serving Size	Calories	Total Fat (g)	Saturated Fat (g)	Cholesterol (mg)	Sodium (mg)	Total Carbohydrate (g)	Dietary Fiber (g)	Protein (g)
Breakfast									
Egg McMuffin®	137 g	290	12	4.5	235	710	27	1	17
Sausage McMuffin®	112 g	360	23	8	45	740	26	1	13
Sausage McMuffin® with Egg	163 g	440	28	10	255	810	27	1	19
English Muffin	55 g	140	2	0	0	210	25	1	4
Sausage Biscuit	127 g	470	31	9	35	1080	35	1	11
Sausage Biscuit with Egg	178 g	550	37	10	245	1160	35	1	18
Bacon, Egg & Cheese Biscuit	157 g	470	28	8	235	1250	36	1	18
Biscuit	84 g	290	15	3	0	780	34	1	5
Sausage	43 g	170	16	5	35	290	0	0	6
Scrambled Eggs (2)	102 g	160	11	3.5	425	170	1	0	13
Hash Browns	53 g	130	8	1.5	0	330	14	1	1
Hotcakes (plain)	150 g	310	7	1.5	15	610	53	2	9
Hotcakes (Margarine 2 pats & Syrup)	222 g	570	16	3	15	750	100	2	9
Breakfast Burrito	117 g	320	19	7	195	600	23	1	13
Muffins/Danish									
Lowfat Apple Bran Muffin	114 g	300	3	0.5	0	380	61	3	6
Apple Danish[†]	105 g	360	16	5	40	290	51	1	5
Cheese Danish[†]	105 g	410	22	8	70	340	47	0	7
Cinnamon Roll[†]	95 g	400	20	5	75	340	47	2	7
Desserts/Shakes									
Vanilla Reduced Fat Ice Cream Cone	90 g	150	4.5	3	20	75	23	0	4
Strawberry Sundae	178 g	290	7	5	30	95	50	<1	7
Hot Caramel Sundae	182 g	360	10	6	35	180	61	0	7
Hot Fudge Sundae	179 g	340	12	9	30	170	52	1	8
Nuts (Sundaes)	7 g	40	3.5	0	0	0	2	0	2
Baked Apple Pie	77 g	260	13	3.5	0	200	34	<1	3
Chocolate Chip Cookie	35 g	170	10	6	20	120	22	1	2
McDonaldland® Cookies (1 pkg)	42 g	180	5	1	0	190	32	1	3
Vanilla Shake—Small	414 ml	360	9	6	40	250	59	0	11
Chocolate Shake—Small	414 ml	360	9	6	40	250	60	1	11
Strawberry Shake—Small	414 ml	360	9	6	40	180	60	0	11
Milk/Juices									
1% Lowfat Milk (8 fl oz)	1 crtn.	100	2.5	1.5	10	115	13	0	8
Orange Juice (6 fl oz)	177 ml	80	0	0	0	20	20	0	1

[†]Available at participating McDonald's.

Wendy's

Menu Item	Serving Size	Calories	Total Fat (g)	Saturated Fat (g)	Cholesterol (mg)	Sodium (mg)	Total Carbohydrate (g)	Dietary Fiber (g)	Protein (g)
Sandwiches									
Plain Single	1 ea	360	16	6	65	580	31	2	24
Single with Everything	1 ea	420	20	7	70	920	37	3	25
Big Bacon Classic	1 ea	580	30	12	100	1460	46	3	34
Jr. Hamburger	1 ea	270	10	3.5	30	610	34	2	15
Jr. Cheeseburger	1 ea	320	13	6	45	830	34	2	17
Jr. Bacon Cheeseburger	1 ea	380	19	7	60	850	34	2	20
Jr. Cheeseburger Deluxe	1 ea	360	17	6	50	890	36	3	18
Hamburger, Kids' Meal	1 ea	270	10	3.5	30	610	33	2	15
Cheeseburger, Kids' Meal	1 ea	320	13	6	45	830	33	2	17
Grilled Chicken Sandwich	1 ea	310	8	1.5	65	790	35	2	27
Breaded Chicken Sandwich	1 ea	440	18	3.5	60	840	44	2	28
Chicken Club Sandwich	1 ea	470	20	4	70	970	44	2	31
Spicy Chicken Sandwich	1 ea	410	15	2.5	65	1280	43	2	28
Sandwich Components									
¼ lb Hamburger Patty	¼ lb	200	14	6	65	290	0	0	19
2 oz Hamburger Patty	2 oz	100	7	3	30	150	0	0	9
Grilled Chicken Fillet	1 pc	110	3	1	60	450	0	0	22
Breaded Chicken Fillet	1 pc	230	12	2.5	55	490	10	0	22
Spicy Chicken Fillet	1 pc	210	9	1.5	60	920	10	0	22
Kaiser Bun	1 ea	190	3	0.5	0	340	36	2	6
Sandwich Bun	1 ea	160	2.5	0.5	0	280	29	2	5
American Cheese	1 sl	70	5	3.5	15	320	1	0	3
American Cheese, Jr.	1 sl	45	3.5	2.5	10	220	0	0	2
Bacon	1 pc	20	1.5	0	5	65	0	0	2
Honey Mustard Red. Cal.	1 tsp	25	1.5	0	0	45	2	0	0
Ketchup	1 tsp	10	0	0	0	75	2	0	0
Lettuce	1 leaf	0	0	0	0	0	0	0	0
Mayonnaise	1½ tsp	30	3	0	5	60	1	0	0
Mustard	½ tsp	0	0	0	0	50	0	0	0
Onion	4 rings	5	0	0	0	0	1	0	0
Pickles	4 sl	0	0	0	0	140	0	0	0
Tomatoes	1 sl	5	0	0	0	0	1	0	0

Wendy's *(continued)*

Menu Item	Serving Size	Calories	Total Fat (g)	Saturated Fat (g)	Cholesterol (mg)	Sodium (mg)	Total Carbohydrate (g)	Dietary Fiber (g)	Protein (g)
Fresh Stuffed Pitas™ (with dressing)									
Chicken Caesar	1 ea	490	18	5	65	1320	48	4	34
Classic Greek	1 ea	440	20	8	35	1050	50	4	15
Garden Ranch Chicken	1 ea	480	18	4	70	1180	51	5	30
Garden Veggie	1 ea	400	17	3.5	20	760	52	5	11
Pita Dressings									
Caesar Vinaigrette, Red. Fat, Red. Cal.	1 tbsp	70	7	1	0	170	1	0	0
Garden Ranch Sauce, Red. Fat, Red. Cal.	1 tbsp	50	4.5	1	10	125	1	0	0
Fresh-Salads-to-Go (without dressing)									
Caesar Side Salad	1 ea	100	4	1.5	10	620	8	1	8
Deluxe Garden Salad	1 ea	110	6	1	0	350	9	3	7
Grilled Chicken Salad	1 ea	200	8	1.5	50	720	9	3	25
Grilled Chicken Caesar Salad	1 ea	260	9	3	60	1170	17	2	26
Side Salad	1 ea	60	3	0	0	180	5	2	4
Taco Salad	1 ea	380	19	10	65	1040	28	7	26
Taco Chips	15 ea	210	11	1.5	0	180	24	2	3
Soft Breadstick	1 ea	130	3	0.5	5	250	23	1	4
Salad Dressings									
Blue Cheese	2 tbsp	180	19	3.5	15	180	0	0	1
French	2 tbsp	120	10	1.5	0	330	6	0	0
French, Fat Free	2 tbsp	35	0	0	0	150	8	0	0
Italian Caesar	2 tbsp	150	16	2.5	20	240	1	0	1
Italian, Red. Fat, Red. Cal.	2 tbsp	40	3	0	0	340	2	0	0
Hidden Valley® Ranch	2 tbsp	100	10	1.5	10	220	1	0	1
Hidden Valley® Ranch, Red. Fat, Red. Cal.	2 tbsp	60	5	1	10	240	2	0	1
Salad Oil	1 tbsp	120	14	2	0	0	0	0	0
Thousand Island	2 tbsp	90	8	1.5	10	125	2	0	0
Wine Vinegar	1 tbsp	0	0	0	0	0	0	0	0
Garden Spot® Salad Bar									
Applesauce	2 tbsp	30	0	0	0	0	7	0	0
Bacon Bits	2 tbsp	45	2	1	10	550	0	0	6
Bananas & Strawberry Glaze	¼ c	30	0	0	0	0	8	1	0
Broccoli	¼ c	0	0	0	0	0	1	0	0

Table continued on following page

Wendy's *(continued)*

Menu Item	Serving Size	Calories	Total Fat (g)	Saturated Fat (g)	Cholesterol (mg)	Sodium (mg)	Total Carbohydrate (g)	Dietary Fiber (g)	Protein (g)
Cantaloupe, sliced	1 pc	15	0	0	0	0	4	0	0
Carrots	¼ c	5	0	0	0	5	2	0	0
Cauliflower	¼ c	0	0	0	0	0	1	0	0
Cheese, shredded (imitation)	2 tbsp	50	4	0.5	0	260	1	0	3
Chicken Salad	2 tbsp	70	5	1	0	135	2	0	4
Cottage Cheese	2 tbsp	30	1.5	1	5	125	1	0	4
Croutons	2 tbsp	25	1	0	0	65	4	0	1
Cucumbers	2 sl	0	0	0	0	0	0	0	0
Eggs, hard cooked	2 tbsp	40	3	1	110	30	0	0	3
Green Peas	2 tbsp	15	0	0	0	25	3	1	1
Green Peppers	2 pc	0	0	0	0	0	1	0	0
Lettuce (Iceberg/Romaine)	1 c	10	0	0	0	5	2	1	0
Mushrooms	¼ c	0	0	0	0	0	1	0	0
Orange, sliced	2 sl	15	0	0	0	0	4	1	0
Parmesan Blend, grated	2 tbsp	70	4	2	10	290	5	0	4
Pasta Salad	2 tbsp	35	1.5	0	0	180	4	1	1
Peaches, sliced	1 pc	15	0	0	0	0	4	0	0
Pepperoni, sliced	6 sl	30	3	1	5	70	0	0	1
Potato Salad	2 tbsp	80	7	2.5	5	180	5	0	0
Pudding, Chocolate	¼ c	70	3	0.5	0	60	10	0	0
Red Onions	3 rings	0	0	0	0	0	1	0	0
Sunflower Seeds & Raisins	2 tbsp	80	5	0.5	0	0	5	1	0
Tomato, wedged	1 pc	5	0	0	0	0	1	0	0
Turkey Ham, diced	2 tbsp	50	4	1	25	280	0	0	3
Watermelon, wedged	1 pc	20	0	0	0	0	4	0	0

Potatoes, Chili & Nuggets

French Fries

Small	3.2 oz	270	13	2	0	85	35	3	4
Medium	4.6 oz	390	19	3	0	120	50	5	5
Biggie	5.6 oz	470	23	3.5	0	150	61	6	7
Great Biggie	6.7 oz	570	27	4	0	180	73	7	8

Baked Potato

Plain	10 oz	310	0	0	0	25	71	7	7
Bacon & Cheese	1 ea	530	18	4	20	1390	78	7	17
Broccoli & Cheese	1 ea	470	14	2.5	5	470	80	9	9

Wendy's *(continued)*

Menu Item	Serving Size	Calories	Total Fat (g)	Saturated Fat (g)	Cholesterol (mg)	Sodium (mg)	Total Carbohydrate (g)	Dietary Fiber (g)	Protein (g)
Cheese	1 ea	570	23	8	30	640	78	7	14
Chili & Cheese	1 ea	630	24	9	40	770	83	9	20
Sour Cream & Chives	1 ea	380	6	4	15	40	74	8	8
Sour Cream	1 pkt	60	6	3.5	10	15	1	0	1
Whipped Margarine	1 pkt	60	7	1.5	0	115	0	0	0
Chili									
Small	8 oz	210	7	2.5	30	800	21	5	15
Large	12 oz	310	10	3.5	45	1190	32	7	23
Cheddar Cheese, shredded	2 tbsp	70	6	3.5	15	110	1	0	4
Saltine Crackers	2 ea	25	0.5	0	0	80	4	0	1
Chicken Nuggets									
5 Piece	5	230	16	3	30	470	11	0	11
4 Piece Kids' Meal	4	190	13	2.5	25	380	9	0	9
Barbecue Sauce	1 pkt	45	0	0	0	160	10	0	1
Honey Mustard Sauce	1 pkt	130	12	2	10	220	6	0	0
Spicy Buffalo Wing Sauce	1 pkt	25	1	0	0	210	4	0	0
Sweet & Sour Sauce	1 pkt	50	0	0	0	120	12	0	0
Desserts, Beverages									
Desserts									
Chocolate Chip Cookie	1 ea	270	13	6	30	120	36	1	3
Frosty™ Dairy Dessert									
Small, 12 oz cup	1 ea	330	8	5	35	200	56	0	8
Medium, 16 oz cup	1 ea	440	11	7	50	260	73	0	11
Large, 20 oz cup	1 ea	540	14	9	60	320	91	0	14
Beverages									
Cola Soft Drink	11 oz	130	0	0	0	0	36	0	0
Diet Cola Soft Drink	11 oz	0	0	0	0	15	0	0	0
Lemon-Lime Soft Drink	11 oz	130	0	0	0	30	36	0	0
Lemonade	11 oz	130	0	0	0	0	37	0	0
Coffee	6 oz	0	0	0	0	0	1	0	0
Decaffeinated Coffee	6 oz	0	0	0	0	0	1	0	0
Hot Chocolate	6 oz	80	3	0	0	135	15	0	1
Tea, Hot	6 oz	0	0	0	0	0	0	0	0
Tea, Iced	6 oz	0	0	0	0	0	0	0	0
Milk, 2%	8 oz	110	4	2.5	15	115	11	0	8

Arby's

Menu Item	Serving Size (oz)	Calories	Total Fat (g)	Saturated Fat (g)	Cholesterol (mg)	Sodium (mg)	Total Carbohydrate (g)	Dietary Fiber (g)	Protein (g)
Roast Beef Sandwiches									
Arby's Melt with Cheddar	5.2	368	18	6	31	937	36	2	18
Arby-Q	6.4	431	18	6	37	1,321	48	3	20
Bac'n Cheddar Deluxe	8.1	539	34	10	44	1,140	38	3	22
Beef'n Cheddar	6.7	507	28	9	50	1,216	40	2	25
Big Montana	11.0	686	35	14.5	121	2,295	47	3	48
Giant Roast Beef	8.1	555	28	11	71	1,561	43	5	35
Junior Roast Beef	4.4	324	14	5	30	779	35	2	17
Regular Roast Beef	5.4	388	19	7	43	1,009	33	3	23
Super Roast Beef	8.7	523	27	9	43	1,189	50	5	25
Chicken									
Breaded Chicken Fillet	7.2	536	28	5	45	1,016	46	5	28
Chicken Cordon Bleu	8.5	623	33	8	77	1,594	46	5	38
Chicken Fingers (2 Pieces)	3.6	290	16	2	32	677	20	0.5	16
Grilled Chicken BBQ	7.1	388	13	3	43	1,002	47	2	23
Grilled Chicken Deluxe	8.1	430	20	4	61	848	41	3	23
Roast Chicken Club	8.5	546	31	9	58	1,103	37	2	31
Roast Chicken Deluxe	7.6	433	22	5	34	763	36	2	24
Roast Chicken Santa Fe	6.4	463	22	6	54	818	38	1	29
Sub Roll Sandwiches									
French Dip	6.8	475	22	8	55	1,411	40	3	30
Hot Ham 'n Swiss	9.3	500	23	7	68	1,664	43	2	30
Italian Sub	10.1	633	36	13	83	2,089	46	2	30
Philly Beef 'n Swiss	10.4	755	47	15	91	2,025	48	3	39
Roast Beef Sub	10.8	700	42	14	84	2,034	44	4	38
Triple Cheese Melt	8.4	720	45	16	91	1,797	46	2	37
Turkey Sub	9.8	550	27	7	65	2,084	47	2	31
Light Menu									
Roast Beef Deluxe	6.4	296	10	3	42	826	33	6	18
Roast Chicken Deluxe	6.8	276	6	2	33	777	33	4	20
Roast Turkey Deluxe	6.8	260	7	2	33	1,262	33	4	20
Garden Salad	11.9	61	0.5	0	0	40	12	5	3
Roast Chicken Salad	14.4	149	2	0.5	29	418	12	5	20
Side Salad	5	23	0.3	0	0	15	4	2	1

Arby's *(continued)*

Menu Item	Serving Size (oz)	Calories	Total Fat (g)	Saturated Fat (g)	Cholesterol (mg)	Sodium (mg)	Total Carbohydrate (g)	Dietary Fiber (g)	Protein (g)
Other Sandwiches									
Fish Fillet	7.7	529	27	7	43	864	50	2	23
Ham 'n Cheese	5.9	359	14	5	53	1,283	34	2	24
Ham 'n Cheese Melt	4.9	329	13	4	40	1,013	34	2	20
Potatoes									
Cheddar Curly Fries	4.25	333	18	4	3	1,016	40	0	5
Curly Fries	3.5	300	15	3	0	853	38	0	4
Homestyle Fries	2.5	212	10	2	0	414	29	2	2.5
Homestyle Fries	4	340	15.5	3	0	665	46	3	4
Homestyle Fries	5	423	19	3.5	0	828	57	4	5.5
Potato Cakes	3	204	12	2	0	397	20	0	2
Baked Potato (Plain)	11.5	355	0.3	0	0	26	82	7	7
Baked Potato with Margarine & Sour Cream	14	578	24	9	25	209	85	7	9
Broccoli 'n Cheddar Baked Potato	15.7	571	20	5	12	565	89	9	14
Deluxe Baked Potato	15.3	736	36	16	59	499	86	7	19
Soups									
Boston Clam Chowder	8	190	9	3	25	965	18	1	9
Cream of Broccoli	8	160	8	4	25	1,005	15	2	7
Lumberjack Mixed Vegetable	8	90	4	2	5	1,150	10	1	2
Old Fashion Chicken Noodle	8	80	2	0	20	850	11	1	6
Potato with Bacon	8	170	7	3	20	905	23	2	6
Timberline Chili	8	220	10	4	30	1,130	17	7	18
Wisconsin Cheese	8	280	18	7	35	1,065	20	2	10
Desserts									
Apple Turnover	3.2	330	14	7	0	180	48	0	4
Cherry Turnover	3.2	320	13	5	0	190	46	0	4
Cheesecake (Plain)	3	320	23	14	95	240	23	0	5
Chocolate Chip Cookie	1	125	6	2	10	85	16	0	2
Chocolate Shake	12	451	12	3	36	341	76	0	15
Jamocha Shake	12	384	10	3	36	262	62	0	15
Vanilla Shake	12	360	12	4	36	281	50	0	15
Butterfinger Polar Swirl	11.6	457	18	8	28	318	62	0	15
Heath Polar Swirl	11.6	543	22	5	39	346	76	0	15
Oreo Polar Swirl	11.6	482	22	10	35	521	66	0	15

Table continued on following page

Arby's *(continued)*

Menu Item	Serving Size (oz)	Calories	Total Fat (g)	Saturated Fat (g)	Cholesterol (mg)	Sodium (mg)	Total Carbohydrate (g)	Dietary Fiber (g)	Protein (g)
Peanut Butter Cup Polar Swirl	11.6	517	24	8	34	385	61	1	20
Snickers Polar Swirl	11.6	511	19	7	33	351	73	1	15
Drinks									
2% Milk	8	112	4	3	20	113	11	0	7
Coca Cola Classic	12	140	0	0	0	50	39	0	0
Coffee	8	3	0	0	0	3	0	0	0
Diet Coke	12	0	0	0	0	40	0	0	0
Diet Pepsi	12	0	0	0	0	35	0	0	0
Diet Seven Up	12	0	0	0	0	35	0	0	0
Dr. Pepper	12	160	0	0	0	55	40	0	0
Hot Chocolate	8	110	1	0.7	0	120	23	0	2
Iced Tea	16	6	0	0	0	12	1	0	0
Nehi Orange	12	195	0	0	0	52	52	0	0
Orange Juice	6	82	0	0	0	2	20	0	0
Pepsi Cola	12	150	0	0	0	35	41	0	0
RC Cola	12	165	0	0	0	52	43	0	0
RC Diet Rite	12	1	0	0	0	10	0	0	0
Seven Up	12	144	0	0	0	34	38	0	0
Upper Ten	12	169	0	0	0	40	42	0	0
Sauces and Dressings									
Arby's Sauce	0.5	15	0.2	0	0	113	4	0	0.1
Beef Stock Au Jus	2	10	0	0	0	440	1	0	0
Barbeque Sauce	0.5	30	0	0	0	185	7	0	0
Blue Cheese Dressing	2	290	31	6	50	580	2	0	2
Cheddar Cheese Sauce	0.75	35	3	1	4	139	1	0	1
Honey French Dressing	2	280	23	3	0	400	18	0	0
Horsey Sauce	0.5	60	5	1	5	150	2	0	0
Ketchup	0.5	16	0	0	0	143	4	0	0.3
Light Cholesterol Free Mayonnaise	0.25	12	1	0	0	64	0.5	0.5	0
Mayonnaise	0.5	110	12	7	5	80	0	0	0
Mustard, German Style	0.16	5	0	0	0	70	1	0	0
Non-Separating Italian Sub Sauce	0.5	70	7	1	0	240	1	0	0
Parmesan Cheese Sauce	0.5	70	7	1	5	130	2	0	1
Red Ranch Dressing	0.5	75	6	1	0	115	5	0	0

Arby's *(continued)*

Menu Item	Serving Size (oz)	Calories	Total Fat (g)	Saturated Fat (g)	Cholesterol (mg)	Sodium (mg)	Total Carbohydrate (g)	Dietary Fiber (g)	Protein (g)
Reduced Calorie Honey Mayonnaise	0.5	70	7	1	20	135	1	0	0
Reduced Calorie Italian Dressing	2	20	1	0	0	1,000	3	0	0
Reduced Calorie Buttermilk Ranch Dressing	2	50	0	0	0	710	12	0	0
Tartar Sauce	1	140	15	2	30	220	0	0	0
Thousand Island Dressing	2	260	26	4	30	420	7	0	0
Breakfast Items									
Bacon	0.53	90	7	3	15	220	0	0	5
Biscuit (Plain)	2.9	280	15	3	0	730	34	1	6
Blueberry Muffin	2.3	230	9	2	25	290	35	0	2
Cinnamon Nut Danish	3.5	360	11	1	0	105	60	1	6
Croissant (Plain)	2	220	12	7	25	230	25	0	4
Egg Portion	1.6	95	8	2	180	54	0.5	0	0.5
French-Toastix	4.4	430	21	5	0	550	52	3	10
Ham	1.5	45	1	0.5	20	405	0	0	7
Sausage	1.3	163	15	6	25	321	0	0	7
Swiss	0.5	45	3	2	12	175	0.5	0	4
Table Syrup	1	100	0	0	0	30	25	0	0

KFC

Menu Item	Serving Size (oz)	Calories	Total Fat (g)	Saturated Fat (g)	Cholesterol (mg)	Sodium (mg)	Total Carbohydrate (g)	Dietary Fiber (g)	Protein (g)
Original Recipe® Chicken									
Whole Wing	1.6	140	10	2.5	55	414	5	0	9
Breast	5.4	400	24	6	135	1,116	16	1	29
Drumstick	2.2	140	9	2	75	422	4	0	13
Thigh	3.2	250	18	4.5	95	747	6	1	16
Tender Roast® Chicken with Skin									
Wing with Skin	1.8	121	7.7	2.1	74	331	1	0	12.2
Breast with Skin	4.9	251	10.8	3	151	830	2	0	37
Thigh with Skin	3.2	207	12	3.8	120	504	<2	0	18.4
Drumstick with Skin	1.9	97	4.3	1.2	85	271	<1	0	14.5
Tender Roast® Chicken without Skin									
Breast without Skin	4.2	169	4.3	1.2	112	797	1	0	31.4
Thigh without Skin	2.1	106	5.5	1.7	84	312	<1	0	12.9
Drumstick without Skin	1.2	67	2.4	.7	63	259	<1	0	11
Hot & Spicy Chicken									
Whole Wing	1.9	210	15	4	50	340	9	<1	10
Breast	6.5	530	35	8	110	1,110	23	2	32
Drumstick	2.3	190	11	3	50	300	10	<1	13
Thigh	3.8	370	27	7	90	570	13	1	18
Extra Tasty Crispy™ Chicken									
Whole Wing	1.9	200	13	4	45	290	10	<1	10
Breast	5.9	470	28	7	80	930	25	1	31
Drumstick	2.4	190	11	3	60	260	8	<1	13
Thigh	4.2	370	25	6	70	540	18	2	19
Crispy Strips									
Colonel's Crispy Strips® (3)	3.25	261	15.8	3.7	40	658	10	3	19.8
Spicy Buffalo Crispy Strips™ (3)	4.2	350	19	4	35	1,110	22	2	22
Pot Pie									
Chunky Chicken Pot Pie	13.0	770	42	13	70	2,160	69	5	29

KFC *(continued)*

Menu Item	Serving Size (oz)	Calories	Total Fat (g)	Saturated Fat (g)	Cholesterol (mg)	Sodium (mg)	Total Carbohydrate (g)	Dietary Fiber (g)	Protein (g)
Sandwiches & More									
Hot Wings™ Pieces (6)	4.8	471	33	8	150	1,230	18	2	27
Original Recipe® Chicken Sandwich	7.3	497	22.3	4.8	52	1,213	45.5	3	28.6
Value BBQ Flavored Chicken Sandwich	5.3	256	8	1	57	782	28	2	17
Salads									
Cole Slaw	5.0	180	9	1.5	5	280	21	3	2
Potato Salad	5.6	230	14	2	15	540	23	23	4
Breads									
1 Biscuit	2.0	180	10	2.5	0	560	20	<1	4
1 Cornbread	2.0	228	13	2	42	194	25	1	3
Potatoes & Specials									
Mashed Potatoes with Gravy	4.8	120	6	1	<1	440	17	2	1
Potato Wedges	4.8	180	13	4	5	750	28	5	5
Macaroni & Cheese	5.4	180	8	3	10	860	21	2	7
Vegetables									
Corn on the Cob	5.7	150	1.5	0	0	20	35	2	5
Green Beans	4.7	45	1.5	0.5	5	730	7	3	1
BBQ Baked Beans	5.5	190	3	1	5	760	33	6	6
Mean Greens®	5.4	70	3	1	10	650	11	5	4

Appendix 5
Nutritive Value of the Edible Part of Food

Foods, approximate measures, units, and weight (weight of edible portion only)		Grams	Water (g)	Food energy (Calories)	Pro-tein (g)	Fat (g)	Fatty Acids		
							Satu-rated (g)	Mono-unsatu-rated (g)	Poly-unsatu-rated (g)
Beverages									
Alcoholic									
Beer									
Regular	12 fl oz	360	92	150	1	0	0.0	0.0	0.0
Light	12 fl oz	355	95	95	1	0	0.0	0.0	0.0
Gin, rum, vodka, whiskey 80-proof	1½ fl oz	42	67	95	0	0	0.0	0.0	0.0
Table wine									
Red	3½ fl oz	102	88	75	tr	0	0.0	0.0	0.0
White	3½ fl oz	102	87	80	tr	0	0.0	0.0	0.0
Carbonated[2]									
Club soda	12 fl oz	355	100	0	0	0	0.0	0.0	0.0
Cola type									
Regular	12 fl oz	369	89	160	0	0	0.0	0.0	0.0
Diet, artificially sweetened	12 fl oz	355	100	tr	0	0	0.0	0.0	0.0
Ginger ale	12 fl oz	366	91	125	0	0	0.0	0.0	0.0
Coffee									
Brewed	6 fl oz	180	100	tr	tr	tr	tr	tr	tr
Instant, prepared (2 tsp powder plus 6 fl oz water)	6 fl oz	182	99	tr	tr	tr	tr	tr	tr
Fruit drinks, noncarbonated									
Canned									
Fruit punch drink	6 fl oz	190	88	85	tr	0	0.0	0.0	0.0
Tea									
Brewed	8 fl oz	240	100	tr	tr	tr	tr	tr	tr
Instant, powder, prepared:									
Unsweetened (1 tsp powder plus 8 fl oz water)	8 fl oz	241	100	tr	tr	tr	tr	tr	tr
Sweetened (3 tsp powder plus 8 fl oz water)	8 fl oz	262	91	85	tr	tr	tr	tr	tr
Dairy Products									
Butter. See Fats and Oils									
Cheese									
Natural									
Blue	1 oz	28	42	100	6	8	5.3	2.2	0.2
Camembert (3 wedges per 4-oz container)	1 wedge	38	52	115	8	9	5.8	2.7	0.3
Cheddar									
Cut pieces	1 oz	28	37	115	7	9	6.0	2.7	0.3
	1 in[3]	17	37	70	4	6	3.6	1.6	0.2
Shredded	1 c	113	37	455	28	37	23.8	10.6	1.1

tr = nutrient present in trace amounts.

[1]Value not determined.

[2]Mineral content varies depending on water source.

502

							Vitamin A value					
Cho-les-terol (mg)	Carbo-hydrate (g)	Calcium (mg)	Phos-phorus (mg)	Iron (mg)	Potas-sium (mg)	Sodium (mg)	IU	RE	Thiamin (mg)	Ribo-flavin (mg)	Niacin (mg)	Ascorbic acid (mg)

NUTRIENTS IN INDICATED QUANTITY

Cho-les-terol (mg)	Carbo-hydrate (g)	Calcium (mg)	Phos-phorus (mg)	Iron (mg)	Potas-sium (mg)	Sodium (mg)	IU	RE	Thiamin (mg)	Ribo-flavin (mg)	Niacin (mg)	Ascorbic acid (mg)
0	13	14	50	0.1	115	18	0	0	0.02	0.09	1.8	0
0	5	14	43	0.1	64	11	0	0	0.03	0.11	1.4	0
0	tr	tr	tr	tr	1	tr	0	0	tr	tr	tr	0
0	3	8	18	0.4	113	5	(^{1})	(^{1})	0.00	0.03	0.1	0
0	3	9	14	0.3	83	5	(^{1})	(^{1})	0.00	0.01	0.1	0
0	0	18	0	tr	0	78	0	0	0.00	0.00	0.0	0
0	41	11	52	0.2	7	18	0	0	0.00	0.00	0.0	0
0	tr	14	39	0.2	7	[3]32	0	0	0.00	0.00	0.0	0
0	32	11	0	0.1	4	29	0	0	0.00	0.00	0.0	0
0	tr	4	2	tr	124	2	0	0	0.00	0.02	0.4	0
0	1	2	6	0.1	71	tr	0	0	0.00	0.03	0.6	0
0	22	15	2	0.4	48	15	20	2	0.03	0.04	tr	[4]61
0	tr	0	2	tr	36	1	0	0	0.00	0.03	tr	0
0	1	1	4	tr	61	1	0	0	0.00	0.02	0.1	0
0	22	1	3	tr	49	tr	0	0	0.00	0.04	0.1	0
21	1	150	110	0.1	73	396	200	65	0.01	0.11	0.3	0
27	tr	147	132	0.1	71	320	350	96	0.01	0.19	0.2	0
30	tr	204	145	0.2	28	176	300	86	0.01	0.11	tr	0
18	tr	123	87	0.1	17	105	180	52	tr	0.06	tr	0
119	1	815	579	0.8	111	701	1,200	342	0.03	0.42	0.1	0

[3]Blend of aspartame and saccharin; if only sodium saccharin is used, sodium is 75 mg; if only aspartame is used, sodium is 23 mg.
[4]With added ascorbic acid.

Foods, approximate measures, units, and weight (weight of edible portion only)		Grams	Water (g)	Food energy (Calories)	Pro-tein (g)	Fat (g)	Fatty Acids		
							Satu-rated (g)	Mono-unsatu-rated (g)	Poly-unsatu-rated (g)
Dairy Products (*cont.*)									
Cottage (curd not pressed down)									
Creamed (cottage cheese, 4% fat)									
Large curd	1 c	225	79	235	28	10	6.4	2.9	0.3
Small curd	1 c	210	79	215	26	9	6.0	2.7	0.3
With fruit	1 c	226	72	280	22	8	4.9	2.2	0.2
Lowfat (2%)	1 c	226	79	205	31	4	2.8	1.2	0.1
Uncreamed (cottage cheese dry curd, less than ½% fat)	1 c	145	80	125	25	1	0.4	0.2	tr
Cream	1 oz	28	54	100	2	10	6.2	2.8	0.4
Feta	1 oz	28	55	75	4	6	4.2	1.3	0.2
Mozzarella, made with									
Whole milk	1 oz	28	54	80	6	6	3.7	1.9	0.2
Part skim milk (low moisture)	1 oz	28	49	80	8	5	3.1	1.4	0.1
Muenster	1 oz	28	42	105	7	9	5.4	2.5	0.2
Parmesan, grated									
Cup, not pressed down	1 c	100	18	455	42	30	19.1	8.7	0.7
Tablespoon	1 tbsp	5	18	25	2	2	1.0	0.4	tr
Ounce	1 oz	28	18	130	12	9	5.4	2.5	0.2
Provolone	1 oz	28	41	100	7	8	4.8	2.1	0.2
Ricotta, made with									
Whole milk	1 c	246	72	430	28	32	20.4	8.9	0.9
Part skim milk	1 c	246	74	340	28	19	12.1	5.7	0.6
Swiss	1 oz	28	37	105	8	8	5.0	2.1	0.3
Pasteurized process cheese									
American	1 oz	28	39	105	6	9	5.6	2.5	0.3
Swiss	1 oz	28	42	95	7	7	4.5	2.0	0.2
Pasteurized process cheese food, American	1 oz	28	43	95	6	7	4.4	2.0	0.2
Pasteurized process cheese spread, American	1 oz	28	48	80	5	6	3.8	1.8	0.2
Cream, sweet									
Half-and-half (cream and milk)	1 c	242	81	315	7	28	17.3	8.0	1.0
	1 tbsp	15	81	20	tr	2	1.1	0.5	0.1
Light, coffee, or table	1 c	240	74	470	6	46	28.8	13.4	1.7
	1 tbsp	15	74	30	tr	3	1.8	0.8	0.1
Whipping, unwhipped (volume about double when whipped)									
Light	1 c	239	64	700	5	74	46.2	21.7	2.1
	1 tbsp	15	64	45	tr	5	2.9	1.4	0.1
Heavy	1 c	238	58	820	5	88	54.8	25.4	3.3
	1 tbsp	15	58	50	tr	6	3.5	1.6	0.2
Whipped topping, (pressurized)	1 c	60	61	155	2	13	8.3	3.9	0.5
	1 tbsp	3	61	10	tr	1	0.4	0.2	tr
Cream, sour	1 c	230	71	495	7	48	30.0	13.9	1.8
	1 tbsp	12	71	25	tr	3	1.6	0.7	0.1

tr = nutrient present in trace amounts.

NUTRIENTS IN INDICATED QUANTITY

Cholesterol (mg)	Carbohydrate (g)	Calcium (mg)	Phosphorus (mg)	Iron (mg)	Potassium (mg)	Sodium (mg)	Vitamin A value		Thiamin (mg)	Riboflavin (mg)	Niacin (mg)	Ascorbic acid (mg)
							IU	RE				
34	6	135	297	0.3	190	911	370	108	0.05	0.37	0.3	tr
31	6	126	277	0.3	177	850	340	101	0.04	0.34	0.3	tr
25	30	108	236	0.2	151	915	280	81	0.04	0.29	0.2	tr
19	8	155	340	0.4	217	918	160	45	0.05	0.42	0.3	tr
10	3	46	151	0.3	47	19	40	12	0.04	0.21	0.2	0
31	1	23	30	0.3	34	84	400	124	tr	0.06	tr	0
25	1	140	96	0.2	18	316	130	36	0.04	0.24	0.3	0
22	1	147	105	0.1	19	106	220	68	tr	0.07	tr	0
15	1	207	149	0.1	27	150	180	54	0.01	0.10	tr	0
27	tr	203	133	0.1	38	178	320	90	tr	0.09	tr	0
79	4	1,376	807	1.0	107	1,861	700	173	0.05	0.39	0.3	0
4	tr	69	40	tr	5	93	40	9	tr	0.02	tr	0
22	1	390	229	0.3	30	528	200	49	0.01	0.11	0.1	0
20	1	214	141	0.1	39	248	230	75	0.01	0.09	tr	0
124	7	509	389	0.9	257	207	1,210	330	0.03	0.48	0.3	0
76	13	669	449	1.1	307	307	1,060	278	0.05	0.46	0.2	0
26	1	272	171	tr	31	74	240	72	0.01	0.10	tr	0
27	tr	174	211	0.1	46	406	340	82	0.01	0.10	tr	0
24	1	219	216	0.2	61	338	230	65	tr	0.08	tr	0
18	2	163	130	0.2	79	337	260	62	0.01	0.13	tr	0
16	2	159	202	0.1	69	381	220	54	0.01	0.12	tr	0
89	10	254	230	0.2	314	98	1,050	259	0.08	0.36	0.2	2
6	1	16	14	tr	19	6	70	16	0.01	0.02	tr	tr
159	9	231	192	0.1	292	95	1,730	437	0.08	0.36	0.1	2
10	1	14	12	tr	18	6	110	27	tr	0.02	tr	tr
265	7	166	146	0.1	231	82	2,690	705	0.06	0.30	0.1	1
17	tr	10	9	tr	15	5	170	44	tr	0.02	tr	tr
326	7	154	149	0.1	179	89	3,500	1,002	0.05	0.26	0.1	1
21	tr	10	9	tr	11	6	220	63	tr	0.02	tr	tr
46	7	61	54	tr	88	78	550	124	0.02	0.04	tr	0
2	tr	3	3	tr	4	4	30	6	tr	tr	tr	0
102	10	268	195	0.1	331	123	1,820	448	0.08	0.34	0.2	2
5	1	14	10	tr	17	6	90	23	tr	0.02	tr	tr

Foods, approximate measures, units, and weight (weight of edible portion only)		Grams	Water (g)	Food energy (Calories)	Pro-tein (g)	Fat (g)	Fatty Acids		
							Satu-rated (g)	Mono-unsaturated (g)	Poly-unsaturated (g)
Dairy Products (*cont.*)									
Milk									
Fluid									
Whole (3.3% fat)	1 c	244	88	150	8	8	5.1	2.4	0.3
Lowfat (2%)									
No milk solids added	1 c	244	89	120	8	5	2.9	1.4	0.2
Milk solids added, label claim less									
than 10 g of protein per cup	1 c	245	89	125	9	5	2.9	1.4	0.2
Lowfat (1%)									
No milk solids added	1 c	244	90	100	8	3	1.6	0.7	0.1
Milk solids added, label claim less									
than 10 g of protein per cup	1 c	245	90	105	9	2	1.5	0.7	0.1
Nonfat (skim)									
No milk solids added	1 c	245	91	85	8	tr	0.3	0.1	tr
Milk solids added, label claim less									
than 10 g of protein per cup	1 c	245	90	90	9	1	0.4	0.2	tr
Buttermilk	1 c	245	90	100	8	2	1.3	0.6	0.1
Milk desserts, frozen									
Ice cream, vanilla									
Regular (about 11% fat)									
Hardened	½ gal	1,064	61	2,155	38	115	71.3	33.1	4.3
	1 c	133	61	270	5	14	8.9	4.1	0.5
	3 fl oz	50	61	100	2	5	3.4	1.6	0.2
Soft serve (frozen custard)	1 c	173	60	375	7	23	13.5	6.7	1.0
Rich (about 16% fat), hardened	½ gal	1,188	59	2,805	33	190	118.3	54.9	7.1
	1 c	148	59	350	4	24	14.7	6.8	0.9
Ice milk, vanilla									
Hardened (about 4% fat)	½ gal	1,048	69	1,470	41	45	28.1	13.0	1.7
	1 c	131	69	185	5	6	3.5	1.6	0.2
Soft serve (about 3% fat)	1 c	175	70	225	8	5	2.9	1.3	0.2
Sherbet (about 2% fat)	½ gal	1,542	66	2,160	17	31	19.0	8.8	1.1
	1 c	193	66	270	2	4	2.4	1.1	0.1
Eggs									
Eggs, large (24 oz per dozen)									
Raw									
Whole, without shell	1 egg	50	75	80	6	6	1.7	2.2	0.7
White	1 white	33	88	15	3	tr	0.0	0.0	0.0
Yolk	1 yolk	17	49	65	3	6	1.7	2.2	0.7
Fats and Oils									
Butter (4 sticks per lb)									
Stick	½ c	113	16	810	1	92	57.1	26.4	3.4
Tablespoon (⅛ stick)	1 tbsp	14	16	100	tr	11	7.1	3.3	0.4
Pat (1 in square, ⅓ in high; 90 per lb)	1 pat	5	16	35	tr	4	2.5	1.2	0.2

tr = nutrient present in trace amounts.

[5]For salted butter; unsalted butter contains 12 mg sodium per stick, 2 mg per tbsp, or 1 mg per pat.

NUTRIENTS IN INDICATED QUANTITY

Cholesterol (mg)	Carbohydrate (g)	Calcium (mg)	Phosphorus (mg)	Iron (mg)	Potassium (mg)	Sodium (mg)	Vitamin A value		Thiamin (mg)	Riboflavin (mg)	Niacin (mg)	Ascorbic acid (mg)
							IU	RE				
33	11	291	228	0.1	370	120	310	76	0.09	0.40	0.2	2
18	12	297	232	0.1	377	122	500	139	0.10	0.40	0.2	2
18	12	313	245	0.1	397	128	500	140	0.10	0.42	0.2	2
10	12	300	235	0.1	381	123	500	144	0.10	0.41	0.2	2
10	12	313	245	0.1	397	128	500	145	0.10	0.42	0.2	2
4	12	302	247	0.1	406	126	500	149	0.09	0.34	0.2	2
5	12	316	255	0.1	418	130	500	149	0.10	0.43	0.2	2
9	12	285	219	0.1	371	257	80	20	0.08	0.38	0.1	2
476	254	1,406	1,075	1.0	2,052	929	4,340	1,064	0.42	2.63	1.1	6
59	32	176	134	0.1	257	116	540	133	0.05	0.33	0.1	1
22	12	66	51	tr	96	44	200	50	0.02	0.12	0.1	tr
153	38	236	199	0.4	338	153	790	199	0.8	0.45	0.2	1
703	256	1,213	927	0.8	1,771	868	7,200	1,758	0.36	2.27	0.9	5
88	32	151	115	0.1	221	108	900	219	0.04	0.28	0.1	1
146	232	1,409	1,035	1.5	2,117	836	1,710	419	0.61	2.78	0.9	6
18	29	176	129	0.2	265	105	210	52	0.08	0.35	0.1	1
13	38	274	202	0.3	412	163	175	44	0.12	0.54	0.2	1
113	469	827	594	2.5	1,585	706	1,480	308	0.26	0.71	1.0	31
14	59	103	74	0.3	198	88	190	39	0.03	0.09	0.1	4
274	1	28	90	1.0	65	69	260	78	0.04	0.15	tr	0
0	tr	4	4	tr	45	50	0	0	tr	0.09	tr	0
272	tr	26	86	0.9	15	8	310	94	0.04	0.07	tr	0
247	tr	27	26	0.2	29	[5]933	[6]13,460	[6]852	0.01	0.04	tr	0
31	tr	3	3	tr	4	[5]116	[6]430	[6]106	tr	tr	tr	0
11	tr	1	1	tr	1	[5]41	[6]150	[6]38	tr	tr	tr	0

[6]Values for vitamin A are year-round average.

Foods, approximate measures, units, and weight (weight of edible portion only)		Grams	Water (g)	Food energy (Calories)	Pro-tein (g)	Fat (g)	Fatty Acids		
							Satu-rated (g)	Mono-unsatu-rated (g)	Poly-unsatu-rated (g)
ats and Oils (*cont.*)									
Fats, cooking (vegetable shortenings)	1 c	205	0	1,810	0	205	51.3	91.2	53.5
	1 tbsp	13	0	115	0	13	3.3	5.8	3.4
Lard	1 c	205	0	1,850	0	205	80.4	92.5	23.0
	1 tbsp	13	0	115	0	13	5.1	5.9	1.5
Oils, salad or cooking									
Corn	1 c	218	0	1,925	0	218	27.7	52.8	128.0
	1 tbsp	14	0	125	0	14	1.8	3.4	8.2
Olive	1 c	216	0	1,910	0	216	29.2	159.2	18.1
	1 tbsp	14	0	125	0	14	1.9	10.3	1.2
Peanut	1 c	216	0	1,910	0	216	36.5	99.8	69.1
	1 tbsp	14	0	125	0	14	2.4	6.5	4.5
Safflower	1 c	218	0	1,925	0	218	19.8	26.4	162.4
	1 tbsp	14	0	125	0	14	1.3	1.7	10.4
Soybean oil, hydrogenated (partially hardened)	1 c	218	0	1,925	0	218	32.5	93.7	82.0
	1 tbsp	14	0	125	0	14	2.1	6.0	5.3
Soybean-cottonseed oil blend, hydrogenated	1 c	218	0	1,925	0	218	39.2	64.3	104.9
	1 tbsp	14	0	125	0	14	2.5	4.1	6.7
Sunflower	1 c	218	0	1,925	0	218	22.5	42.5	143.2
	1 tbsp	14	0	125	0	14	1.4	2.7	9.2
Salad dressings									
Commercial									
Blue cheese	1 tbsp	15	32	75	1	8	1.5	1.8	4.2
French									
Regular	1 tbsp	16	35	85	tr	9	1.4	4.0	3.5
Low calorie	1 tbsp	16	75	25	tr	2	0.2	0.3	1.0
Italian									
Regular	1 tbsp	15	34	80	tr	9	1.3	3.7	3.2
Low calorie	1 tbsp	15	86	5	tr	tr	tr	tr	tr
Mayonnaise									
Regular	1 tbsp	14	15	100	tr	11	1.7	3.2	5.8
Imitation	1 tbsp	15	63	35	tr	3	0.5	0.7	1.6
Prepared from home recipe									
Cooked type[7]	1 tbsp	16	69	25	1	2	0.5	0.6	0.3
Vinegar and oil	1 tbsp	16	47	70	0	8	1.5	2.4	3.9
Fish and Shellfish									
Clams									
Raw, meat only	3 oz	85	82	65	11	1	0.3	0.3	0.3
Canned, drained solids	3 oz	85	77	85	13	2	0.5	0.5	0.4
Crabmeat, canned	1 c	135	77	135	23	3	0.5	0.8	1.4
Fish sticks, frozen, reheated, (stick, 4 by 1 by ½ in)	1 fish stick	28	52	70	6	3	0.8	1.4	0.8

tr = nutrient present in trace amounts.

[7]Fatty acid values apply to product made with regular margarine.

NUTRIENTS IN INDICATED QUANTITY

Cho-les-terol (mg)	Carbo-hydrate (g)	Calcium (mg)	Phos-phorus (mg)	Iron (mg)	Potas-sium (mg)	Sodium (mg)	Vitamin A value		Thiamin (mg)	Ribo-flavin (mg)	Niacin (mg)	Ascorbic acid (mg)
							IU	RE				
0	0	0	0	0.0	0	0	0	0	0.00	0.00	0.0	0
0	0	0	0	0.0	0	0	0	0	0.00	0.00	0.0	0
195	0	0	0	0.0	0	0	0	0	0.00	0.00	0.0	0
12	0	0	0	0.0	0	0	0	0	0.00	0.00	0.0	0
0	0	0	0	0.0	0	0	0	0	0.00	0.00	0.0	0
0	0	0	0	0.0	0	0	0	0	0.00	0.00	0.0	0
0	0	0	0	0.0	0	0	0	0	0.00	0.00	0.0	0
0	0	0	0	0.0	0	0	0	0	0.00	0.00	0.0	0
0	0	0	0	0.0	0	0	0	0	0.00	0.00	0.0	0
0	0	0	0	0.0	0	0	0	0	0.00	0.00	0.0	0
0	0	0	0	0.0	0	0	0	0	0.00	0.00	0.0	0
0	0	0	0	0.0	0	0	0	0	0.00	0.00	0.0	0
0	0	0	0	0.0	0	0	0	0	0.00	0.00	0.0	0
0	0	0	0	0.0	0	0	0	0	0.00	0.00	0.0	0
0	0	0	0	0.0	0	0	0	0	0.00	0.00	0.0	0
0	0	0	0	0.0	0	0	0	0	0.00	0.00	0.0	0
0	0	0	0	0.0	0	0	0	0	0.00	0.00	0.0	0
0	0	0	0	0.0	0	0	0	0	0.00	0.00	0.0	0
3	1	12	11	tr	6	164	30	10	tr	0.02	tr	tr
0	1	2	1	tr	2	188	tr	tr	tr	tr	tr	tr
0	2	6	5	tr	3	306	tr	tr	tr	tr	tr	tr
0	1	1	1	tr	5	162	30	3	tr	tr	tr	tr
0	2	1	1	tr	4	136	tr	tr	tr	tr	tr	tr
8	tr	3	4	0.1	5	80	40	12	0.00	0.00	tr	0
4	2	tr	tr	0.0	2	75	0	0	0.00	0.00	0.0	0
9	2	13	14	0.1	19	117	70	20	0.01	0.02	tr	tr
0	tr	0	0	0.0	1	tr	0	0	0.00	0.00	0.0	0
43	2	59	138	2.6	154	102	90	26	0.09	0.15	1.1	9
54	2	47	116	3.5	119	102	90	26	0.01	0.09	0.9	3
135	1	61	246	1.1	149	1,350	50	14	0.11	0.11	2.6	0
26	4	11	58	0.3	94	53	20	5	0.03	0.05	0.6	0

Fish and Shellfish (*cont.*)

Foods, approximate measures, units, and weight (weight of edible portion only)		Grams	Water (g)	Food energy (Calories)	Pro-tein (g)	Fat (g)	Fatty Acids		
							Satu-rated (g)	Mono-unsatu-rated (g)	Poly-unsatu-rated (g)
Flounder or Sole, baked, with lemon juice									
With butter	3 oz	85	73	120	16	6	3.2	1.5	0.5
With margarine	3 oz	85	73	120	16	6	1.2	2.3	1.9
Without added fat	3 oz	85	78	80	17	1	0.3	0.2	0.4
Haddock, breaded, fried[8]	3 oz	85	61	175	17	9	2.4	3.9	2.4
Halibut, broiled, with butter and lemon juice	3 oz	85	67	140	20	6	3.3	1.6	0.7
Herring, pickled	3 oz	85	59	190	17	13	4.3	4.6	3.1
Ocean perch, breaded, fried[8]	1 fillet	85	59	185	16	11	2.6	4.6	2.8
Oysters									
Raw, meat only (13–19 medium Selects)	1 c	240	85	160	20	4	1.4	0.5	1.4
Breaded, fried[8]	1 oyster	45	65	90	5	5	1.4	2.1	1.4
Salmon									
Canned (pink), solids and liquid	3 oz	85	71	120	17	5	0.9	1.5	2.1
Baked (red)	3 oz	85	67	140	21	5	1.2	2.4	1.4
Smoked	3 oz	85	59	150	18	8	2.6	3.9	0.7
Sardines, Atlantic, canned in oil, drained solids	3 oz	85	62	175	20	9	2.1	3.7	2.9
Scallops, breaded, frozen, reheated	6 scallops	90	59	195	15	10	2.5	4.1	2.5
Shrimp									
Canned, drained solids	3 oz	85	70	100	21	1	0.2	0.2	0.4
French fried (7 medium)[10]	3 oz	85	55	200	16	10	2.5	4.1	2.6
Trout, broiled, with butter and lemon juice	3 oz	85	63	175	21	9	4.1	2.9	1.6
Tuna, canned, drained solids									
Oil pack, chunk light	3 oz	85	61	165	24	7	1.4	1.9	3.1
Water pack, solid white	3 oz	85	63	135	30	1	0.3	0.2	0.3
Tuna salad[11]	1 c	205	63	375	33	19	3.3	4.9	9.2
Fruits and Fruit Juices									
Apples									
Raw									
Unpeeled, without cores									
2¾-in diam. (about 3 per lb with cores)	1 apple	138	84	80	tr	tr	0.1	tr	0.1
3¼-in diam. (about 2 per lb with cores)	1 apple	212	84	125	tr	1	0.1	tr	0.2
Peeled, sliced	1 c	110	84	65	tr	tr	0.1	tr	0.1
Dried, sulfured	10 rings	64	32	155	1	tr	tr	tr	0.1
Apple juice, bottled or canned[13]	1 c	248	88	115	tr	tr	tr	tr	0.1
Applesauce, canned									
Sweetened	1 c	255	80	195	tr	tr	0.1	tr	0.1
Unsweetened	1 c	244	88	105	tr	tr	tr	tr	tr

tr = nutrient present in trace amounts.

[8]Dipped in egg, milk, and breadcrumbs; fried in vegetable shortening.

[9]If bones are discarded, value for calcium will be greatly reduced.

[10]Dipped in egg, breadcrumbs, and flour; fried in vegetable shortening.

NUTRIENTS IN INDICATED QUANTITY

Cholesterol (mg)	Carbohydrate (g)	Calcium (mg)	Phosphorus (mg)	Iron (mg)	Potassium (mg)	Sodium (mg)	Vitamin A value		Thiamin (mg)	Riboflavin (mg)	Niacin (mg)	Ascorbic acid (mg)
							IU	RE				
68	tr	13	187	0.3	272	145	210	54	0.05	0.08	1.6	1
55	tr	14	187	0.3	273	151	230	69	0.05	0.08	1.6	1
59	tr	13	197	0.3	286	101	30	10	0.05	0.08	1.7	1
75	7	34	183	1.0	270	123	70	20	0.06	0.10	2.9	0
62	tr	14	206	0.7	441	103	610	174	0.06	0.07	7.7	1
85	0	29	128	0.9	85	850	110	33	0.04	0.18	2.8	0
66	7	31	191	1.2	241	138	70	20	0.10	0.11	2.0	0
120	8	226	343	15.6	290	175	740	223	0.34	0.43	6.0	24
35	5	49	73	3.0	64	70	150	44	0.07	0.10	1.3	4
34	0	[9]167	243	0.7	307	443	60	18	0.03	0.15	6.8	0
60	0	26	269	0.5	305	55	290	87	0.18	0.14	5.5	0
51	0	12	208	0.8	327	1,700	260	77	0.17	0.17	6.8	0
85	0	[9]371	424	2.6	349	425	190	56	0.03	0.17	4.6	0
70	10	39	203	2.0	369	298	70	21	0.11	0.11	1.6	0
128	1	98	224	1.4	104	1,955	50	15	0.01	0.03	1.5	0
168	11	61	154	2.0	189	384	90	26	0.06	0.09	2.8	0
71	tr	26	259	1.0	297	122	230	60	0.07	0.07	2.3	1
55	0	7	199	1.6	298	303	70	20	0.04	0.09	10.1	0
48	0	17	202	0.6	255	468	110	32	0.03	0.10	13.4	0
80	19	31	281	2.5	531	877	230	53	0.06	0.14	13.3	6
0	21	10	10	0.2	159	tr	70	7	0.02	0.02	0.1	8
0	32	15	15	0.4	244	tr	110	11	0.04	0.03	0.2	12
0	16	4	8	0.1	124	tr	50	5	0.02	0.01	0.1	4
0	42	9	24	0.9	288	[12]56	0	0	0.00	0.10	0.6	2
0	29	17	17	0.9	295	7	tr	tr	0.05	0.04	0.2	[14]2
0	51	10	18	0.9	156	8	30	3	0.03	0.07	0.5	[14]4
0	28	7	17	0.3	183	5	70	7	0.03	0.06	0.5	[14]3

[11]Made with drained chunk light tuna, celery, onion, pickle relish, and mayonnaise-type salad dressing.

[12]Sodium bisulfite used to preserve color; unsulfited product would contain less sodium.

[13]Also applies to pasteurized apple cider.

[14]Without added ascorbic acid. For value with added ascorbic acid, refer to label.

Fruits and Fruit Juices (*cont.*)

Foods, approximate measures, units, and weight (weight of edible portion only)		Grams	Water (g)	Food energy (Calories)	Pro-tein (g)	Fat (g)	Satu-rated (g)	Mono-unsatu-rated (g)	Poly-unsatu-rated (g)
								Fatty Acids	
Apricots									
Raw, without pits (about 12 per lb with pits)	3 apricots	106	86	50	1	tr	tr	0.2	0.1
Canned (fruit and liquid)									
Heavy syrup pack	1 c	258	78	215	1	tr	tr	0.1	tr
	3 halves	85	78	70	tr	tr	tr	tr	tr
Juice pack	1 c	248	87	120	2	tr	tr	tr	tr
	3 halves	84	87	40	1	tr	tr	tr	tr
Dried									
Uncooked (28 large or 37 medium halves per cup)	1 c	130	31	310	5	1	tr	0.3	0.1
Cooked, unsweetened, fruit and liquid	1 c	250	76	210	3	tr	tr	0.2	0.1
Apricot nectar, canned	1 c	251	85	140	1	tr	tr	0.1	tr
Avocados, raw, whole, without skin and seed									
California (about 2 per lb with skin and seed)	1 avocado	173	73	305	4	30	4.5	19.4	3.5
Florida (about 1 per lb with skin and seed)	1 avocado	304	80	340	5	27	5.3	14.8	4.5
Bananas, raw, without peel									
Whole (about 2½ per lb with peel)	1 banana	114	74	105	1	1	0.2	tr	0.1
Sliced	1 c	150	74	140	2	1	0.3	0.1	0.1
Blackberries, raw	1 c	144	86	75	1	1	0.2	0.1	0.1
Blueberries									
Raw	1 c	145	85	80	1	1	tr	0.1	0.3
Frozen, sweetened	10-oz container	284	77	230	1	tr	tr	0.1	0.2
	1 c	230	77	185	1	tr	tr	tr	0.1
Cantaloup. See Melons									
Cherries									
Sour, red, pitted, canned, water pack	1 c	244	90	90	2	tr	0.1	0.1	0.1
Sweet, raw, without pits and stems	10 cherries	68	81	50	1	1	0.1	0.2	0.2
Cranberry juice cocktail, bottled, sweetened	1 c	253	85	145	tr	tr	tr	tr	0.1
Cranberry sauce, sweetened, canned, strained	1 c	277	61	420	1	tr	tr	0.1	0.2
Dates									
Whole, without pits	10 dates	83	23	230	2	tr	0.1	0.1	tr
Chopped	1 c	178	23	490	4	1	0.3	0.2	tr
Figs, dried	10 figs	187	28	475	6	2	0.4	0.5	1.0

tr = nutrient present in trace amounts.

[14]Without added ascorbic acid. For value with added ascorbic acid, refer to label.

NUTRIENTS IN INDICATED QUANTITY

Cho-les-terol (mg)	Carbo-hydrate (g)	Calcium (mg)	Phos-phorus (mg)	Iron (mg)	Potas-sium (mg)	Sodium (mg)	Vitamin A value		Thiamin (mg)	Ribo-flavin (mg)	Niacin (mg)	Ascorbic acid (mg)
							IU	RE				
0	12	15	20	0.6	314	1	2,770	277	0.03	0.04	0.6	11
0	55	23	31	0.8	361	10	3,170	317	0.05	0.06	1.0	8
0	18	8	10	0.3	119	3	1,050	105	0.02	0.02	0.3	3
0	31	30	50	0.7	409	10	4,190	419	0.04	0.05	0.9	12
0	10	10	17	0.3	139	3	1,420	142	0.02	0.02	0.3	4
0	80	59	152	6.1	1,791	13	9,410	941	0.01	0.20	3.9	3
0	55	40	103	4.2	1,222	8	5,910	591	0.02	0.08	2.4	4
0	36	18	23	1.0	286	8	3,300	330	0.02	0.04	0.7	[14]2
0	12	19	73	2.0	1,097	21	1,060	106	0.19	0.21	3.3	14
0	27	33	119	1.6	1,484	15	1,860	186	0.33	0.37	5.8	24
0	27	7	23	0.4	451	1	90	9	0.05	0.11	0.6	10
0	35	9	30	0.5	594	2	120	12	0.07	0.15	0.8	14
0	18	46	30	0.8	282	tr	240	24	0.04	0.06	0.6	30
0	20	9	15	0.2	129	9	150	15	0.07	0.07	0.5	19
0	62	17	20	1.1	170	3	120	12	0.06	0.15	0.7	3
0	50	14	16	0.9	138	2	100	10	0.05	0.12	0.6	2
0	22	27	24	3.3	239	17	1,840	184	0.04	0.10	0.4	5
0	11	10	13	0.3	152	tr	150	15	0.03	0.04	0.3	5
0	38	8	3	0.4	61	10	10	1	0.01	0.04	0.1	[15]108
0	108	11	17	0.6	72	80	60	6	0.04	0.06	0.3	6
0	61	27	33	1.0	541	2	40	4	0.07	0.08	1.8	0
0	131	57	71	2.0	1,161	5	90	9	0.16	0.18	3.9	0
0	122	269	127	4.2	1,331	21	250	25	0.13	0.16	1.3	1

[15]With added ascorbic acid.

Fruits and Fruit Juices (*cont.*)

Foods, approximate measures, units, and weight (weight of edible portion only)		Grams	Water (g)	Food energy (Calories)	Protein (g)	Fat (g)	Fatty Acids		
							Saturated (g)	Mono-unsaturated (g)	Poly-unsaturated (g)
Fruit cocktail, canned, fruit and liquid									
Heavy syrup pack	1 c	255	80	185	1	tr	tr	tr	0.1
Juice pack	1 c	248	87	115	1	tr	tr	tr	tr
Grapefruit									
Raw, without peel, membrane and seeds (3¾-in diam., 1 lb 1 oz, whole, with refuse)	½ grapefruit	120	91	40	1	tr	tr	tr	tr
Canned, sections with syrup	1 c	254	84	150	1	tr	tr	tr	0.1
Grapefruit juice									
Raw	1 c	247	90	95	1	tr	tr	tr	0.1
Canned									
Unsweetened	1 c	247	90	95	1	tr	tr	tr	0.1
Sweetened	1 c	250	87	115	1	tr	tr	tr	0.1
Frozen concentrate, unsweetened									
Undiluted	6-fl-oz can	207	62	300	4	1	0.1	0.1	0.2
Diluted with 3 parts water by volume	1 c	247	89	100	1	tr	tr	tr	0.1
Grapes, European type (adherent skin), raw									
Thompson Seedless	10 grapes	50	81	35	tr	tr	0.1	tr	0.1
Tokay and Emperor, seeded types	10 grapes	57	81	40	tr	tr	0.1	tr	0.1
Grape juice									
Canned or bottled	1 c	253	84	155	1	tr	0.1	tr	0.1
Frozen concentrate, sweetened									
Undiluted	6-fl-oz can	216	54	385	1	1	0.2	tr	0.2
Diluted with 3 parts water by volume	1 c	250	87	125	tr	tr	0.1	tr	0.1
Kiwifruit, raw, without skin (about 5 per lb with skin)	1 kiwifruit	76	83	45	1	tr	tr	0.1	0.1
Lemons, raw, without peel and seeds (about 4 per lb with peel and seeds)	1 lemon	58	89	15	1	tr	tr	tr	0.1
Lemon juice									
Raw	1 c	244	91	60	1	tr	tr	tr	tr
Canned or bottled, unsweetened	1 c	244	92	50	1	1	0.1	tr	0.2
	1 tbsp	15	92	5	tr	tr	tr	tr	tr
Frozen, single-strength, unsweetened	6-fl-oz can	244	92	55	1	1	0.1	tr	0.2
Lime juice									
Raw	1 c	246	90	65	1	tr	tr	tr	0.1
Canned, unsweetened	1 c	246	93	50	1	1	0.1	0.1	0.2
Mangos, raw, without skin and seed (about 1½ per lb with skin and seed)	1 mango	207	82	135	1	1	0.1	0.2	0.1

tr = nutrient present in trace amounts.

[14]Without added ascorbic acid. For value with added ascorbic acid, refer to label.

[15]With added ascorbic acid.

NUTRIENTS IN INDICATED QUANTITY

Cho-les-terol (mg)	Carbo-hydrate (g)	Calcium (mg)	Phos-phorus (mg)	Iron (mg)	Potas-sium (mg)	Sodium (mg)	Vitamin A value		Thiamin (mg)	Ribo-flavin (mg)	Niacin (mg)	Ascorbic acid (mg)
							IU	RE				
0	48	15	28	0.7	224	15	520	52	0.05	0.05	1.0	5
0	29	20	35	0.5	236	10	760	76	0.03	0.04	1.0	7
0	10	14	10	0.1	167	tr	[16]10	[16]1	0.04	0.02	0.3	41
0	39	36	25	1.0	328	5	tr	tr	0.10	0.05	0.6	54
0	23	22	37	0.5	400	2	20	2	0.10	0.05	0.5	94
0	22	17	27	0.5	378	2	20	2	0.10	0.05	0.6	72
0	28	20	28	0.9	405	5	20	2	0.10	0.06	0.8	67
0	72	56	101	1.0	1,002	6	60	6	0.30	0.16	1.6	248
0	24	20	35	0.3	336	2	20	2	0.10	0.05	0.5	83
0	9	6	7	0.1	93	1	40	4	0.05	0.03	0.2	5
0	10	6	7	0.1	105	1	40	4	0.05	0.03	0.2	6
0	38	23	28	0.6	334	8	20	2	0.07	0.09	0.7	[14]tr
0	96	28	32	0.8	160	15	60	6	0.11	0.20	0.9	[15]179
0	32	10	10	0.3	53	5	20	2	0.04	0.07	0.3	[15]60
0	11	20	30	0.3	252	4	130	13	0.02	0.04	0.4	74
0	5	15	9	0.3	80	1	20	2	0.02	0.01	0.1	31
0	21	17	15	0.1	303	2	50	5	0.07	0.02	0.2	112
0	16	27	22	0.3	249	[17]51	40	4	0.10	0.02	0.5	61
0	1	2	1	tr	15	[17]3	tr	tr	0.01	tr	tr	4
0	16	20	20	0.3	217	2	30	3	0.14	0.03	0.3	77
0	22	22	17	0.1	268	2	20	2	0.05	0.02	0.2	72
0	16	30	25	0.6	185	[17]39	40	4	0.08	0.01	0.4	16
0	35	21	23	0.3	323	4	8,060	806	0.12	0.12	1.2	57

[16]For white grapefruit; pink grapefruit have about 310 IU or 31 RE.
[17]Sodium benzoate and sodium bisulfite added as preservatives.

							Fatty Acids		
Foods, approximate measures, units, and weight (weight of edible portion only)		Grams	Water (g)	Food energy (Calories)	Pro-tein (g)	Fat (g)	Satu-rated (g)	Mono-unsatu-rated (g)	Poly-unsatu-rated (g)

Fruits and Fruit Juices (*cont.*)

Melons, raw, without rind and cavity contents									
Cantaloup, orange-fleshed (5-in diam., 2⅓ lb, whole, with rind and cavity contents)	½ melon	267	90	95	2	1	0.1	0.1	0.3
Honeydew (6½-in diam., 5¼ lb, whole, with rind and cavity contents)	¹⁄₁₀ melon	129	90	45	1	tr	tr	tr	0.1
Nectarines, raw, without pits (about 3 per lb with pits)	1 nectarine	136	86	65	1	1	0.1	0.2	0.3
Oranges, raw									
Whole, without peel and seeds (2⅝-in diam., about 2½ per lb, with peel and seeds)	1 orange	131	87	60	1	tr	tr	tr	tr
Sections without membranes	1 c	180	87	85	2	tr	tr	tr	tr
Orange juice									
Raw, all varieties	1 c	248	88	110	2	tr	0.1	0.1	0.1
Canned, unsweetened	1 c	249	89	105	1	tr	tr	0.1	0.1
Chilled	1 c	249	88	110	2	1	0.1	0.1	0.2
Frozen concentrate									
Undiluted	6-fl-oz can	213	58	340	5	tr	0.1	0.1	0.1
Diluted with 3 parts water by volume	1 c	249	88	110	2	tr	tr	tr	tr
Orange and grapefruit juice, canned	1 c	247	89	105	1	tr	tr	tr	tr
Papayas, raw, ½-in cubes	1 c	140	86	65	1	tr	0.1	0.1	tr
Peaches									
Raw									
Whole, 2½-in diam., peeled, pitted (about 4 per lb with peels and pits)	1 peach	87	88	35	1	tr	tr	tr	tr
Sliced	1 c	170	88	75	1	tr	tr	0.1	0.1
Canned, fruit and liquid									
Heavy syrup pack	1 c	256	79	190	1	tr	tr	0.1	0.1
	1 half	81	79	60	tr	tr	tr	tr	tr
Juice pack	1 c	248	87	110	2	tr	tr	tr	tr
	1 half	77	87	35	tr	tr	tr	tr	tr
Dried									
Uncooked	1 c	160	32	380	6	1	0.1	0.4	0.6
Cooked, unsweetened, fruit and liquid	1 c	258	78	200	3	1	0.1	0.2	0.3
Frozen, sliced, sweetened	10-oz container	284	75	265	2	tr	tr	0.1	0.2
	1 c	250	75	235	2	tr	tr	0.1	0.2

tr = nutrient present in trace amounts.

NUTRIENTS IN INDICATED QUANTITY

Cho-les-terol (mg)	Carbo-hydrate (g)	Calcium (mg)	Phos-phorus (mg)	Iron (mg)	Potas-sium (mg)	Sodium (mg)	Vitamin A value		Thiamin (mg)	Ribo-flavin (mg)	Niacin (mg)	Ascorbic acid (mg)
							IU	RE				
0	22	29	45	0.6	825	24	8,610	861	0.10	0.06	1.5	113
0	12	8	13	0.1	350	13	50	5	0.10	0.02	0.8	32
0	16	7	22	0.2	288	tr	1,000	100	0.02	0.06	1.3	7
0	15	52	18	0.1	237	tr	270	27	0.11	0.05	0.4	70
0	21	72	25	0.2	326	tr	370	37	0.16	0.07	0.5	96
0	26	27	42	0.5	496	2	500	50	0.22	0.07	1.0	124
0	25	20	35	1.1	436	5	440	44	0.15	0.07	0.8	86
0	25	25	27	0.4	473	2	190	19	0.28	0.05	0.7	82
0	81	68	121	0.7	1,436	6	590	59	0.60	0.14	1.5	294
0	27	22	40	0.2	473	2	190	19	0.20	0.04	0.5	97
0	25	20	35	1.1	390	7	290	29	0.14	0.07	0.8	72
0	17	35	12	0.3	247	9	400	40	0.04	0.04	0.5	92
0	10	4	10	0.1	171	tr	470	47	0.01	0.04	0.9	6
0	19	9	20	0.2	335	tr	910	91	0.03	0.07	1.7	11
0	51	8	28	0.7	236	15	850	85	0.03	0.06	1.6	7
0	16	2	9	0.2	75	5	270	27	0.01	0.02	0.5	2
0	29	15	42	0.7	317	10	940	94	0.02	0.04	1.4	9
0	9	5	13	0.2	99	3	290	29	0.01	0.01	0.4	3
0	98	45	190	6.5	1,594	11	3,460	346	tr	0.34	7.0	8
0	51	23	98	3.4	826	5	510	51	0.01	0.05	3.9	10
0	68	9	31	1.1	369	17	810	81	0.04	0.10	1.9	[15]268
0	60	8	28	0.9	325	15	710	71	0.03	0.09	1.6	[15]236

[15]With added ascorbic acid.

Foods, approximate measures, units, and weight (weight of edible portion only)		Grams	Water (g)	Food energy (Calories)	Pro-tein (g)	Fat (g)	Fatty Acids		
							Satu-rated (g)	Mono-unsatu-rated (g)	Poly-unsatu-rated (g)

Fruits and Fruit Juices (*cont.*)

Pears									
Raw, with skin, cored									
Bartlett, 2½-in diam. (about 2½ per lb with cores and stems)	1 pear	166	84	100	1	1	tr	0.1	0.2
Bosc, 2½-in diam. (about 3 per lb with cores and stems)	1 pear	141	84	85	1	1	tr	0.1	0.1
D'Anjou, 3-in diam. (about 2 per lb with cores and stems)	1 pear	200	84	120	1	1	tr	0.2	0.2
Canned, fruit and liquid									
Heavy syrup pack	1 c	255	80	190	1	tr	tr	0.1	0.1
	1 half	79	80	60	tr	tr	tr	tr	tr
Juice pack	1 c	248	86	125	1	tr	tr	tr	tr
	1 half	77	86	40	tr	tr	tr	tr	tr
Pineapple									
Raw, diced	1 c	155	87	75	1	1	tr	0.1	0.2
Canned, fruit and liquid									
Heavy syrup pack									
Crushed, chunks, tidbits	1 c	255	79	200	1	tr	tr	tr	0.1
Slices	1 slice	58	79	45	tr	tr	tr	tr	tr
Juice pack									
Chunks or tidbits	1 c	250	84	150	1	tr	tr	tr	0.1
Slices	1 slice	58	84	35	tr	tr	tr	tr	tr
Pineapple juice, unsweetened, canned	1 c	250	86	140	1	tr	tr	tr	0.1
Plantains, without peel									
Raw	1 plantain	179	65	220	2	1	0.3	0.1	0.1
Cooked, boiled, sliced	1 c	154	67	180	1	tr	0.1	tr	0.1
Plums, without pits									
Raw									
2⅛-in diam. (about 6½ per lb with pits)	1 plum	66	85	35	1	tr	tr	0.3	0.1
1½-in diam. (about 15 per lb with pits)	1 plum	28	85	15	tr	tr	tr	0.1	tr
Canned, purple, fruit and liquid									
Heavy syrup pack	1 c	258	76	230	1	tr	tr	0.2	0.1
	3 plums	133	76	120	tr	tr	tr	0.1	tr
Juice pack	1 c	252	84	145	1	tr	tr	tr	tr
	3 plums	95	84	55	tr	tr	tr	tr	tr
Prunes, dried									
Uncooked	4 extra large or 5 large prunes	49	32	115	1	tr	tr	0.2	0.1
Cooked, unsweetened, fruit and liquid	1 c	212	70	225	2	tr	tr	0.3	0.1
Prune juice, canned or bottled	1 c	256	81	180	2	tr	tr	0.1	tr
Raisins, seedless									
Cup, not pressed down	1 c	145	15	435	5	1	0.2	tr	0.2
Packet, ½ oz (1½ tbsp)	1 packet	14	15	40	tr	tr	tr	tr	tr

tr = nutrient present in trace amounts.

NUTRIENTS IN INDICATED QUANTITY

Cho-les-terol (mg)	Carbo-hydrate (g)	Calcium (mg)	Phos-phorus (mg)	Iron (mg)	Potas-sium (mg)	Sodium (mg)	Vitamin A value		Thiamin (mg)	Ribo-flavin (mg)	Niacin (mg)	Ascorbic acid (mg)
							IU	RE				
0	25	18	18	0.4	208	tr	30	3	0.03	0.07	0.2	7
0	21	16	16	0.4	176	tr	30	3	0.03	0.06	0.1	6
0	30	22	22	0.5	250	tr	40	4	0.04	0.08	0.2	8
0	49	13	18	0.6	166	13	10	1	0.03	0.06	0.6	3
0	15	4	6	0.2	51	4	tr	tr	0.01	0.02	0.2	1
0	32	22	30	0.7	238	10	10	1	0.03	0.03	0.5	4
0	10	7	9	0.2	74	3	tr	tr	0.01	0.01	0.2	1
0	19	11	11	0.6	175	2	40	4	0.14	0.06	0.7	24
0	52	36	18	1.0	265	3	40	4	0.23	0.06	0.7	19
0	12	8	4	0.2	60	1	10	1	0.05	0.01	0.2	4
0	39	35	15	0.7	305	3	100	10	0.24	0.05	0.7	24
0	9	8	3	0.2	71	1	20	2	0.06	0.01	0.2	6
0	34	43	20	0.7	335	3	10	1	0.14	0.06	0.6	27
0	57	5	61	1.1	893	7	2,020	202	0.09	0.10	1.2	33
0	48	3	43	0.9	716	8	1,400	140	0.07	0.08	1.2	17
0	9	3	7	0.1	114	tr	210	21	0.03	0.06	0.3	6
0	4	1	3	tr	48	tr	90	9	0.01	0.03	0.1	3
0	60	23	34	2.2	235	49	670	67	0.04	0.10	0.8	1
0	31	12	17	1.1	121	25	340	34	0.02	0.05	0.4	1
0	38	25	38	0.9	388	3	2,540	254	0.06	0.15	1.2	7
0	14	10	14	0.3	146	1	960	96	0.02	0.06	0.4	3
0	31	25	39	1.2	365	2	970	97	0.04	0.08	1.0	2
0	60	49	74	2.4	708	4	650	65	0.05	0.21	1.5	6
0	45	31	64	3.0	707	10	10	1	0.04	0.18	2.0	10
0	115	71	141	3.0	1,089	17	10	1	0.23	0.13	1.2	5
0	11	7	14	0.3	105	2	tr	tr	0.02	0.01	0.1	tr

Foods, approximate measures, units, and weight (weight of edible portion only)		Grams	Water (g)	Food energy (Calories)	Protein (g)	Fat (g)	Fatty Acids		
							Saturated (g)	Monounsaturated (g)	Polyunsaturated (g)

Fruits and Fruit Juices (*cont.*)

Raspberries									
Raw	1 c	123	87	60	1	1	tr	0.1	0.4
Frozen, sweetened	10-oz container	284	73	295	2	tr	tr	tr	0.3
	1 c	250	73	255	2	tr	tr	tr	0.2
Rhubarb, cooked, added sugar	1 c	240	68	280	1	tr	tr	tr	0.1
Strawberries									
Raw, capped, whole	1 c	149	92	45	1	1	tr	0.1	0.3
Frozen, sweetened, sliced	10-oz container	284	73	275	2	tr	tr	0.1	0.2
	1 c	255	73	245	1	tr	tr	tr	0.2
Tangerines									
Raw, without peel and seeds (2⅜-in diam., about 4 per lb, with peel and seeds)	1 tangerine	84	88	35	1	tr	tr	tr	tr
Canned, light syrup, fruit and liquid	1 c	252	83	155	1	tr	tr	tr	0.1
Tangerine juice, canned, sweetened	1 c	249	87	125	1	tr	tr	tr	0.1
Watermelon, raw, without rind and seeds									
Piece (4 by 8 in wedge with rind and seeds; ¹⁄₁₆ of 32⅔-lb melon, 10 by 16 in)	1 piece	482	92	155	3	2	0.3	0.2	1.0
Diced	1 c	160	92	50	1	1	0.1	0.1	0.3
Grain Products									
Bagels, plain or water, enriched, 3½-in diam.[18]	1 bagel	68	29	200	7	2	0.3	0.5	0.7
Barley, pearled, light, uncooked	1 c	200	11	700	16	2	0.3	0.2	0.9
Biscuits, baking powder, 2-in diam. (enriched flour, vegetable shortening)									
From home recipe	1 biscuit	28	28	100	2	5	1.2	2.0	1.3
From mix	1 biscuit	28	29	95	2	3	0.8	1.4	0.9
From refrigerated dough	1 biscuit	20	30	65	1	2	0.6	0.9	0.6
Breadcrumbs, enriched									
Dry, grated	1 c	100	7	390	13	5	1.5	1.6	1.0
Soft. See White bread									
Breads									
Boston brown bread, canned, slice, 3¼ in by ½ in[19]	1 slice	45	45	95	2	1	0.3	0.1	0.1
Cracked-wheat bread (¾ enriched wheat flour, ¼ cracked wheat flour)[19]									
Loaf, 1 lb	1 loaf	454	35	1,190	42	16	3.1	4.3	5.7
Slice (18 per loaf)	1 slice	25	35	65	2	1	0.2	0.2	0.3
Toasted	1 slice	21	26	65	2	1	0.2	0.2	0.3

tr = nutrient present in trace amounts.

[18]Egg bagels have 44 mg cholesterol and 22 IU or 7 RE vitamin A per bagel.

NUTRIENTS IN INDICATED QUANTITY

Cholesterol (mg)	Carbohydrate (g)	Calcium (mg)	Phosphorus (mg)	Iron (mg)	Potassium (mg)	Sodium (mg)	Vitamin A value		Thiamin (mg)	Riboflavin (mg)	Niacin (mg)	Ascorbic acid (mg)
							IU	RE				
0	14	27	15	0.7	187	tr	160	16	0.04	0.11	1.1	31
0	74	43	48	1.8	324	3	170	17	0.05	0.13	0.7	47
0	65	38	43	1.6	285	3	150	15	0.05	0.11	0.6	41
0	75	348	19	0.5	230	2	170	17	0.04	0.06	0.5	8
0	10	21	28	0.6	247	1	40	4	0.03	0.10	0.3	84
0	74	31	37	1.7	278	9	70	7	0.05	0.14	1.1	118
0	66	28	33	1.5	250	8	60	6	0.04	0.13	1.0	106
0	9	12	8	0.1	132	1	770	77	0.09	0.02	0.1	26
0	41	18	25	0.9	197	15	2,120	212	0.13	0.11	1.1	50
0	30	45	35	0.5	443	2	1,050	105	0.15	0.05	0.2	55
0	35	39	43	0.8	559	10	1,760	176	0.39	0.10	1.0	46
0	11	13	14	0.3	186	3	590	59	0.13	0.03	0.3	15
0	38	29	46	1.8	50	245	0	0	0.26	0.20	2.4	0
0	158	32	378	4.2	320	6	0	0	0.24	0.10	6.2	0
tr	13	47	36	0.7	32	195	10	3	0.08	0.08	0.8	tr
tr	14	58	128	0.7	56	262	20	4	0.12	0.11	0.8	tr
1	10	4	79	0.5	18	249	0	0	0.08	0.05	0.7	0
5	73	122	141	4.1	152	736	0	0	0.35	0.35	4.8	0
3	21	41	72	0.9	131	113	[20]0	[20]0	0.06	0.04	0.7	0
0	227	295	581	12.1	608	1,966	tr	tr	1.73	1.73	15.3	tr
0	12	16	32	0.7	34	106	tr	tr	0.10	0.09	0.8	tr
0	12	16	32	0.7	34	106	tr	tr	0.07	0.09	0.8	tr

[19]Made with vegetable shortening.

[20]Made with white cornmeal. If made with yellow cornmeal, value is 32 IU or 3 RE.

522   Appendix 5: Nutritive Value of the Edible Part of Food

Foods, approximate measures, units, and weight (weight of edible portion only)		Grams	Water (g)	Food energy (Calories)	Pro-tein (g)	Fat (g)	Fatty Acids		
							Satu-rated (g)	Mono-unsatu-rated (g)	Poly-unsatu-rated (g)
Grain Products (cont.)									
Breads (cont.)									
French or Vienna bread, enriched[19]									
Loaf, 1 lb	1 loaf	454	34	1,270	43	18	3.8	5.7	5.9
Slice									
French, 5 by 2½ by 1 in	1 slice	35	34	100	3	1	0.3	0.4	0.5
Vienna, 4¾ by 4 by ½ in	1 slice	25	34	70	2	1	0.2	0.3	0.3
Italian bread, enriched									
Loaf, 1 lb	1 loaf	454	32	1,255	41	4	0.6	0.3	1.6
Slice, 4½ by 3¼ by ¾ in	1 slice	30	32	85	3	tr	tr	tr	0.1
Mixed grain bread, enriched[19]									
Loaf, 1 lb	1 loaf	454	37	1,165	45	17	3.2	4.1	6.5
Slice (18 per loaf)	1 slice	25	37	65	2	1	0.2	0.2	0.4
Toasted	1 slice	23	27	65	2	1	0.2	0.2	0.4
Oatmeal bread, enriched[19]									
Loaf, 1 lb	1 loaf	454	37	1,145	38	20	3.7	7.1	8.2
Slice (18 per loaf)	1 slice	25	37	65	2	1	0.2	0.4	0.5
Toasted	1 slice	23	30	65	2	1	0.2	0.4	0.5
Pita bread, enriched, white, 6½-in diam.	1 pita	60	31	165	6	1	0.1	0.1	0.4
Pumpernickel (⅔ rye flour, ⅓ enriched wheat flour)[19]									
Loaf, 1 lb	1 loaf	454	37	1,160	42	16	2.6	3.6	6.4
Slice, 5 by 4 by ⅜ in	1 slice	32	37	80	3	1	0.2	0.3	0.5
Toasted	1 slice	29	28	80	3	1	0.2	0.3	0.5
Raisin bread, enriched[19]									
Loaf, 1 lb	1 loaf	454	33	1,260	37	18	4.1	6.5	6.7
Slice (18 per loaf)	1 slice	25	33	65	2	1	0.2	0.3	0.4
Toasted	1 slice	21	24	65	2	1	0.2	0.3	0.4
Rye bread, light (⅔ enriched wheat flour, ⅓ rye flour)[19]									
Loaf, 1lb	1 loaf	454	37	1,190	38	17	3.3	5.2	5.5
Slice, 4¾ by 3¾ by 7/16 in	1 slice	25	37	65	2	1	0.2	0.3	0.3
Toasted	1 slice	22	28	65	2	1	0.2	0.3	0.3
Wheat bread, enriched[19]									
Loaf, 1 lb	1 loaf	454	37	1,160	43	19	3.9	7.3	4.5
Slice (18 per loaf)	1 slice	25	37	65	2	1	0.2	0.4	0.3
Toasted	1 slice	23	28	65	3	1	0.2	0.4	0.3
White bread, enriched[19]									
Loaf, 1 lb	1 loaf	454	37	1,210	38	18	5.6	6.5	4.2
Slice (18 per loaf)	1 slice	25	37	65	2	1	0.3	0.4	0.2
Toasted	1 slice	22	28	65	2	1	0.3	0.4	0.2
Slice (22 per loaf)	1 slice	20	37	55	2	1	0.2	0.3	0.2
Toasted	1 slice	17	28	55	2	1	0.2	0.3	0.2
Cubes	1 c	30	37	80	2	1	0.4	0.4	0.3
Crumbs, soft	1 c	45	37	120	4	2	0.6	0.6	0.4

tr = nutrient present in trace amounts.

NUTRIENTS IN INDICATED QUANTITY

Cho-lesterol (mg)	Carbo-hydrate (g)	Calcium (mg)	Phos-phorus (mg)	Iron (mg)	Potas-sium (mg)	Sodium (mg)	Vitamin A value		Thiamin (mg)	Ribo-flavin (mg)	Niacin (mg)	Ascorbic acid (mg)
							IU	RE				
0	230	499	386	14.0	409	2,633	tr	tr	2.09	1.59	18.2	tr
0	18	39	30	1.1	32	203	tr	tr	0.16	0.12	1.4	tr
0	13	28	21	0.8	23	145	tr	tr	0.12	0.09	1.0	tr
0	256	77	350	12.7	336	2,656	0	0	1.80	1.10	15.0	0
0	17	5	23	0.8	22	176	0	0	0.12	0.07	1.0	0
0	212	472	962	14.8	990	1,870	tr	tr	1.77	1.73	18.9	tr
0	12	27	55	0.8	56	106	tr	tr	0.10	0.10	1.1	tr
0	12	27	55	0.8	56	106	tr	tr	0.08	0.10	1.1	tr
0	212	267	563	12.0	707	2,231	0	0	2.09	1.20	15.4	0
0	12	15	31	0.7	39	124	0	0	0.12	0.07	0.9	0
0	12	15	31	0.7	39	124	0	0	0.09	0.07	0.9	0
0	33	49	60	1.4	71	339	0	0	0.27	0.12	2.2	0
0	218	322	990	12.4	1,966	2,461	0	0	1.54	2.36	15.0	0
0	16	23	71	0.9	141	177	0	0	0.11	0.17	1.1	0
0	16	23	71	0.9	141	177	0	0	0.09	0.17	1.1	0
0	239	463	395	14.1	1,058	1,657	tr	tr	1.50	2.81	18.6	tr
0	13	25	22	0.8	59	92	tr	tr	0.08	0.15	1.0	tr
0	13	25	22	0.8	59	92	tr	tr	0.06	0.15	1.0	tr
0	218	363	658	12.3	926	3,164	0	0	1.86	1.45	15.0	0
0	12	20	36	0.7	51	175	0	0	0.10	0.08	0.8	0
0	12	20	36	0.7	51	175	0	0	0.08	0.08	0.8	0
0	213	572	835	15.8	627	2,447	tr	tr	2.09	1.45	20.5	tr
0	12	32	47	0.9	35	138	tr	tr	0.12	0.08	1.2	tr
0	12	32	47	0.9	35	138	tr	tr	0.10	0.08	1.2	tr
0	222	572	490	12.9	508	2,334	tr	tr	2.13	1.41	17.0	tr
0	12	32	27	0.7	28	129	tr	tr	0.12	0.08	0.9	tr
0	12	32	27	0.7	28	129	tr	tr	0.09	0.08	0.9	tr
0	10	25	21	0.6	22	101	tr	tr	0.09	0.06	0.7	tr
0	10	25	21	0.6	22	101	tr	tr	0.07	0.06	0.7	tr
0	15	38	32	0.9	34	154	tr	tr	0.14	0.09	1.1	tr
0	22	57	49	1.3	50	231	tr	tr	0.21	0.14	1.7	tr

[19]Made with vegetable shortening.

Foods, approximate measures, units, and weight (weight of edible portion only)		Grams	Water (g)	Food energy (Calories)	Pro- tein (g)	Fat (g)	Fatty Acids		
							Satu- rated (g)	Mono- unsatu- rated (g)	Poly- unsatu- rated (g)
Grain Products (*cont.*)									
Breads (*cont.*)									
Whole-wheat bread[19]									
Loaf, 1 lb	1 loaf	454	38	1,110	44	20	5.8	6.8	5.2
Slice (16 per loaf)	1 slice	28	38	70	3	1	0.4	0.4	0.3
Toasted	1 slice	25	29	70	3	1	0.4	0.4	0.3
Bread stuffing (from enriched bread), prepared from mix									
Dry type	1 c	140	33	500	9	31	6.1	13.3	9.6
Moist type	1 c	203	61	420	9	26	5.3	11.3	8.0
Buckwheat flour, light, sifted	1 c	98	12	340	6	1	0.2	0.4	0.4
Bulgur, uncooked	1 c	170	10	600	19	3	1.2	0.3	1.2
Cakes prepared from cake mixes with enriched flour[21]									
Angelfood									
Whole cake, 9¾-in diam. tube cake	1 cake	635	38	1,510	38	2	0.4	0.2	1.0
Piece, 1/12 of cake	1 piece	53	38	125	3	tr	tr	tr	0.1
Coffeecake, crumb									
Whole cake, 7¾ by 5⅝ by 1¼ in	1 cake	430	30	1,385	27	41	11.8	16.7	9.6
Piece, 1/6 of cake	1 piece	72	30	230	5	7	2.0	2.8	1.6
Devil's food with chocolate frosting									
Whole, 2-layer cake, 8- or 9-in diam.	1 cake	1,107	24	3,755	49	136	55.6	51.4	19.7
Piece, 1/16 of cake	1 piece	69	24	235	3	8	3.5	3.2	1.2
Cupcake, 2½-in diam.	1 cupcake	35	24	120	2	4	1.8	1.6	0.6
Gingerbread									
Whole cake, 8 in square	1 cake	570	37	1,575	18	39	9.6	16.4	10.5
Piece, 1/9 of cake	1 piece	63	37	175	2	4	1.1	1.8	1.2
Cheesecake									
Whole cake, 9-in diam.	1 cake	1,110	46	3,350	60	213	119.9	65.5	14.4
Piece, 1/12 of cake	1 piece	92	46	280	5	18	9.9	5.4	1.2
Cookies made with enriched flour									
Brownies with nuts									
Commercial, with frosting, 1½ by 1¾ by ⅞ in	1 brownie	25	13	100	1	4	1.6	2.0	0.6
From home recipe, 1¾ by 1¾ by ⅞ in[22]	1 brownie	20	10	95	1	6	1.4	2.8	1.2
Chocolate chip									
Commercial, 2¼-in diam., ⅜ in thick	4 cookies	42	4	180	2	9	2.9	3.1	2.6
Cornmeal									
Whole-ground, unbolted, dry form	1 c	122	12	435	11	5	0.5	1.1	2.5
Bolted (nearly whole-grain), dry form	1 c	122	12	440	11	4	0.5	0.9	2.2
Degermed, enriched									
Dry form	1 c	138	12	500	11	2	0.2	0.4	0.9
Cooked	1 c	240	88	120	3	tr	tr	0.1	0.2

tr = nutrient present in trace amounts.

[20]Made with white cornmeal. If made with yellow cornmeal, value is 32 IU or 3 RE.

[21]Excepting angelfood cake, cakes were made from mixes containing vegetable shortening and frostings were made with margarine.

NUTRIENTS IN INDICATED QUANTITY

Cholesterol (mg)	Carbohydrate (g)	Calcium (mg)	Phosphorus (mg)	Iron (mg)	Potassium (mg)	Sodium (mg)	Vitamin A value		Thiamin (mg)	Riboflavin (mg)	Niacin (mg)	Ascorbic acid (mg)
							IU	RE				
0	206	327	1,180	15.5	799	2,887	tr	tr	1.59	0.95	17.4	tr
0	13	20	74	1.0	50	180	tr	tr	0.10	0.06	1.1	tr
0	13	20	74	1.0	50	180	tr	tr	0.08	0.06	1.1	tr
0	50	92	136	2.2	126	1,254	910	273	0.17	0.20	2.5	0
67	40	81	134	2.0	118	1,023	850	256	0.10	0.18	1.6	0
0	78	11	86	1.0	314	2	0	0	0.08	0.04	0.4	0
0	129	49	575	9.5	389	7	0	0	0.48	0.24	7.7	0
0	342	527	1,086	2.7	845	3,226	0	0	0.32	1.27	1.6	0
0	29	44	91	0.2	71	269	0	0	0.03	0.11	0.1	0
279	225	262	748	7.3	469	1,853	690	194	0.82	0.90	7.7	1
47	38	44	125	1.2	78	310	120	32	0.14	0.15	1.3	tr
598	645	653	1,162	22.1	1,439	2,900	1,660	498	1.11	1.66	10.0	1
37	40	41	72	1.4	90	181	100	31	0.07	0.10	0.6	tr
19	20	21	37	0.7	46	92	50	16	0.04	0.05	0.3	tr
6	291	513	570	10.8	1,562	1,733	0	0	0.86	1.03	7.4	1
1	32	57	63	1.2	173	192	0	0	0.09	0.11	0.8	tr
2053	317	622	977	5.3	1,088	2,464	2,820	833	0.33	1.44	5.1	56
170	26	52	81	0.4	90	204	230	69	0.03	0.12	0.4	5
14	16	13	26	0.6	50	59	70	18	0.08	0.07	0.3	tr
18	11	9	26	0.4	35	51	20	6	0.05	0.05	0.3	tr
5	28	13	41	0.8	68	140	50	15	0.10	0.23	1.0	tr
0	90	24	312	2.2	346	1	620	62	0.46	0.13	2.4	0
0	91	21	272	2.2	303	1	590	59	0.37	0.10	2.3	0
0	108	8	137	5.9	166	1	610	61	0.61	0.36	4.8	0
0	26	2	34	1.4	38	0	140	14	0.14	0.10	1.2	0

[22]Made with vegetable oil.

Foods, approximate measures, units, and weight (weight of edible portion only)		Grams	Water (g)	Food energy (Calories)	Pro- tein (g)	Fat (g)	Fatty Acids		
							Satu- rated (g)	Mono- unsatu- rated (g)	Poly- unsatu- rated (g)
Grain Products (*cont.*)									
Crackers[23]									
Cheese									
Plain, 1 in square	10 crackers	10	4	50	1	3	0.9	1.2	0.3
Sandwich type									
(peanut butter)	1 sandwich	8	3	40	1	2	0.4	0.8	0.3
Graham, plain, 2½ in square	2 crackers	14	5	60	1	1	0.4	0.6	0.4
Melba toast, plain	1 piece	5	4	20	1	tr	0.1	0.1	0.1
Rye wafers, whole-grain, 1⅞ by 3½ in	2 wafers	14	5	55	1	1	0.3	0.4	0.3
Saltines[24]	4 crackers	12	4	50	1	1	0.5	0.4	0.2
Snack-type, standard	1 round cracker	3	3	15	tr	1	0.2	0.4	0.1
Wheat, thin	4 crackers	8	3	35	1	1	0.5	0.5	0.4
Whole-wheat wafers	2 crackers	8	4	35	1	2	0.5	0.6	0.4
Croissants, made with enriched flour, 4½ by 4 by 1¾ in	1 croissant	57	22	235	5	12	3.5	6.7	1.4
Danish pastry, made with enriched flour									
Plain without fruit or nuts									
Packaged ring, 12 oz	1 ring	340	27	1,305	21	71	21.8	28.6	15.6
Round piece, about 4¼-in diam., 1 in high	1 pastry	57	27	220	4	12	3.6	4.8	2.6
Ounce	1 oz	28	27	110	2	6	1.8	2.4	1.3
Fruit, round piece	1 pastry	65	30	235	4	13	3.9	5.2	2.9
Doughnuts, made with enriched flour									
Cake type, plain, 3¼-in diam., 1 in high	1 doughnut	50	21	210	3	12	2.8	5.0	3.0
Yeast-leavened, glazed, 3¾-in diam., 1¼ in high	1 doughnut	60	27	235	4	13	5.2	5.5	0.9
English muffins, plain, enriched	1 muffin	57	42	140	5	1	0.3	0.2	0.3
Toasted	1 muffin	50	29	140	5	1	0.3	0.2	0.3
Pies, piecrust made with enriched flour, vegetable shortening, 9-in diam.									
Apple									
Whole	1 pie	945	48	2,420	21	105	27.4	44.4	26.5
Piece, ⅙ of pie	1 piece	158	48	405	3	18	4.6	7.4	4.4
Blueberry									
Whole	1 pie	945	51	2,285	23	102	25.5	44.4	27.4
Piece, ⅙ of pie	1 piece	158	51	380	4	17	4.3	7.4	4.6
Cherry									
Whole	1 pie	945	47	2,465	25	107	28.4	46.3	27.4
Piece, ⅙ of pie	1 piece	158	47	410	4	18	4.7	7.7	4.6
Creme									
Whole	1 pie	910	43	2,710	20	139	90.1	23.7	6.4
Piece, ⅙ of pie	1 piece	152	43	455	3	23	15.0	4.0	1.1

tr = nutrient present in trace amounts.

[23]Crackers made with enriched flour except for rye wafers and whole-wheat wafers.

NUTRIENTS IN INDICATED QUANTITY

Cho-les-terol (mg)	Carbo-hydrate (g)	Calcium (mg)	Phos-phorus (mg)	Iron (mg)	Potas-sium (mg)	Sodium (mg)	Vitamin A value		Thiamin (mg)	Ribo-flavin (mg)	Niacin (mg)	Ascorbic acid (mg)
							IU	RE				
6	6	11	17	0.3	17	112	20	5	0.05	0.04	0.4	0
1	5	7	25	0.3	17	90	tr	tr	0.04	0.03	0.6	0
0	11	6	20	0.4	36	86	0	0	0.02	0.03	0.6	0
0	4	6	10	0.1	11	44	0	0	0.01	0.01	0.1	0
0	10	7	44	0.5	65	115	0	0	0.06	0.03	0.5	0
4	9	3	12	0.5	17	165	0	0	0.06	0.05	0.6	0
0	2	3	6	0.1	4	30	tr	tr	0.01	0.01	0.1	0
0	5	3	15	0.3	17	69	tr	tr	0.04	0.03	0.4	0
0	5	3	22	0.2	31	59	0	0	0.02	0.03	0.4	0
13	27	20	64	2.1	68	452	50	13	0.17	0.13	1.3	0
292	152	360	347	6.5	316	1,302	360	99	0.95	1.02	8.5	tr
49	26	60	58	1.1	53	218	60	17	0.16	0.17	1.4	tr
24	13	30	29	0.5	26	109	30	8	0.08	0.09	0.7	tr
56	28	17	80	1.3	57	233	40	11	0.16	0.14	1.4	tr
20	24	22	111	1.0	58	192	20	5	0.12	0.12	1.1	tr
21	26	17	55	1.4	64	222	tr	tr	0.28	0.12	1.8	0
0	27	96	67	1.7	331	378	0	0	0.26	0.19	2.2	0
0	27	96	67	1.7	331	378	0	0	0.23	0.19	2.2	0
0	360	76	208	9.5	756	2,844	280	28	1.04	0.76	9.5	9
0	60	13	35	1.6	126	476	50	5	0.17	0.13	1.6	2
0	330	104	217	12.3	945	2,533	850	85	1.04	0.85	10.4	38
0	55	17	36	2.1	158	423	140	14	0.17	0.14	1.7	6
0	363	132	236	9.5	992	2,873	4,160	416	1.13	0.85	9.5	0
0	61	22	40	1.6	166	480	700	70	0.19	0.14	1.6	0
46	351	273	919	6.8	796	2,207	1,250	391	0.36	0.89	6.4	0
8	59	46	154	1.1	133	369	210	65	0.06	0.15	1.1	0

[24]Made with lard.

Foods, approximate measures, units, and weight (weight of edible portion only)		Grams	Water (g)	Food energy (Calories)	Pro-tein (g)	Fat (g)	Fatty Acids		
							Satu-rated (g)	Mono-unsatu-rated (g)	Poly-unsatu-rated (g)
Grain Products (*cont.*)									
Pies (*cont.*)									
Custard									
Whole	1 pie	910	58	1,985	56	101	33.7	40.0	19.1
Piece, ⅙ of pie	1 piece	152	58	330	9	17	5.6	6.7	3.2
Lemon meringue									
Whole	1 pie	840	47	2,140	31	86	26.0	34.4	17.6
Piece, ⅙ of pie	1 piece	140	47	355	5	14	4.3	5.7	2.9
Peach									
Whole	1 pie	945	48	2,410	24	101	24.6	43.5	26.5
Piece, ⅙ of pie	1 piece	158	48	405	4	17	4.1	7.3	4.4
Pecan									
Whole	1 pie	825	20	3,450	42	189	28.1	101.5	47.0
Piece, ⅙ of pie	1 piece	138	20	575	7	32	4.7	17.0	7.9
Pumpkin									
Whole	1 pie	910	59	1,920	36	102	38.2	40.0	18.2
Piece, ⅙ of pie	1 piece	152	59	320	6	17	6.4	6.7	3.0
Pies, fried									
Apple	1 pie	85	43	255	2	14	5.8	6.6	0.6
Cherry	1 pie	85	42	250	2	14	5.8	6.7	0.6
Popcorn, popped									
Air-popped, unsalted	1 c	8	4	30	1	tr	tr	0.1	0.2
Popped in vegetable oil, salted	1 c	11	3	55	1	3	0.5	1.4	1.2
Sugar syrup coated	1 c	35	4	135	2	1	0.1	0.3	0.6
Pretzels, made with enriched flour									
Stick, 2¼ in long	10 pretzels	3	3	10	tr	tr	tr	tr	tr
Twisted, dutch, 2¾ by 2⅝ in	1 pretzel	16	3	65	2	1	0.1	0.2	0.2
Twisted, thin, 3¼ by 2¼ by ¼ in	10 pretzels	60	3	240	6	2	0.4	0.8	0.6
Rice									
Brown, cooked, served hot	1 c	195	70	230	5	1	0.3	0.3	0.4
White, enriched									
Commercial varieties, all types									
Raw	1 c	185	12	670	12	1	0.2	0.2	0.3
Cooked, served hot	1 c	205	73	225	4	tr	0.1	0.1	0.1
Wheat flours									
All-purpose or family flour, enriched									
Sifted, spooned	1 c	115	12	420	12	1	0.2	0.1	0.5
Unsifted, spooned	1 c	125	12	455	13	1	0.2	0.1	0.5
Cake or pastry flour, enriched, sifted, spooned	1 c	96	12	350	7	1	0.1	0.1	0.3
Self-rising, enriched, unsifted, spooned	1 c	125	12	440	12	1	0.2	0.1	0.5
Whole-wheat, from hard wheats, stirred	1 c	120	12	400	16	2	0.3	0.3	1.1

tr = nutrient present in trace amounts.

NUTRIENTS IN INDICATED QUANTITY

Cho-les-terol (mg)	Carbo-hydrate (g)	Calcium (mg)	Phos-phorus (mg)	Iron (mg)	Potas-sium (mg)	Sodium (mg)	Vitamin A value		Thiamin (mg)	Ribo-flavin (mg)	Niacin (mg)	Ascorbic acid (mg)
							IU	RE				
1010	213	874	1,028	9.1	1,247	2,612	2,090	573	0.82	1.91	5.5	0
169	36	146	172	1.5	208	436	350	96	0.14	0.32	0.9	0
857	317	118	412	8.4	420	2,369	1,430	395	0.59	0.84	5.0	25
143	53	20	69	1.4	70	395	240	66	0.10	0.14	0.8	4
0	361	95	274	11.3	1,408	2,533	6,900	690	1.04	0.95	14.2	28
0	60	16	46	1.9	235	423	1,150	115	0.17	0.16	2.4	5
569	423	388	850	27.2	1,015	1,823	1,320	322	1.82	0.99	6.6	0
95	71	65	142	4.6	170	305	220	54	0.30	0.17	1.1	0
655	223	464	628	8.2	1,456	1,947	22,480	2,493	0.82	1.27	7.3	0
109	37	78	105	1.4	243	325	3,750	416	0.14	0.21	1.2	0
14	31	12	34	0.9	42	326	30	3	0.09	0.06	1.0	1
13	32	11	41	0.7	61	371	190	19	0.06	0.06	0.6	1
0	6	1	22	0.2	20	tr	10	1	0.03	0.01	0.2	0
0	6	3	31	0.3	19	86	20	2	0.01	0.02	0.1	0
0	30	2	47	0.5	90	tr	30	3	0.13	0.02	0.4	0
0	2	1	3	0.1	3	48	0	0	0.01	0.01	0.1	0
0	13	4	15	0.3	16	258	0	0	0.05	0.04	0.7	0
0	48	16	55	1.2	61	966	0	0	0.19	0.15	2.6	0
0	50	23	142	1.0	137	0	0	0	0.18	0.04	2.7	0
0	149	44	174	5.4	170	9	0	0	0.81	0.06	6.5	0
0	50	21	57	1.8	57	0	0	0	0.23	0.02	2.1	0
0	88	18	100	5.1	109	2	0	0	0.73	0.46	6.1	0
0	95	20	109	5.5	119	3	0	0	0.80	0.50	6.6	0
0	76	16	70	4.2	91	2	0	0	0.58	0.38	5.1	0
0	93	331	583	5.5	113	1,349	0	0	0.80	0.50	6.6	0
0	85	49	446	5.2	444	4	0	0	0.66	0.14	5.2	0

Foods, approximate measures, units, and weight (weight of edible portion only)		Grams	Water (g)	Food energy (Calories)	Pro-tein (g)	Fat (g)	Fatty Acids		
							Satu-rated (g)	Mono-unsatu-rated (g)	Poly-unsatu-rated (g)
Legumes, Nuts, and Seeds									
Almonds, shelled									
Slivered, packed	1 c	135	4	795	27	70	6.7	45.8	14.8
Whole	1 oz	28	4	165	6	15	1.4	9.6	3.1
Beans, dry									
Cooked, drained									
Black	1 c	171	66	225	15	1	0.1	0.1	0.5
Great Northern	1 c	180	69	210	14	1	0.1	0.1	0.6
Lima	1 c	190	64	260	16	1	0.2	0.1	0.5
Pea (navy)	1 c	190	69	225	15	1	0.1	0.1	0.7
Pinto	1 c	180	65	265	15	1	0.1	0.1	0.5
Canned, solids and liquid									
White with									
Frankfurters (sliced)	1 c	255	71	365	19	18	7.4	8.8	0.7
Pork and tomato sauce	1 c	255	71	310	16	7	2.4	2.7	0.7
Pork and sweet sauce	1 c	255	66	385	16	12	4.3	4.9	1.2
Red kidney	1 c	255	76	230	15	1	0.1	0.1	0.6
Black-eyed peas, dry, cooked									
(with residual cooking liquid)	1 c	250	80	190	13	1	0.2	tr	0.3
Brazil nuts, shelled	1 oz	28	3	185	4	19	4.6	6.5	6.8
Carob flour	1 c	140	3	255	6	tr	tr	0.1	0.1
Cashew nuts, salted									
Dry roasted	1 c	137	2	785	21	63	12.5	37.4	10.7
	1 oz	28	2	165	4	13	2.6	7.7	2.2
Roasted in oil	1 c	130	4	750	21	63	12.4	36.9	10.6
	1 oz	28	4	165	5	14	2.7	8.1	2.3
Chestnuts, European (Italian),									
roasted, shelled	1 c	143	40	350	5	3	0.6	1.1	1.2
Chickpeas, cooked, drained	1 c	163	60	270	15	4	0.4	0.9	1.9
Coconut									
Raw									
Piece, about 2 by 2 by ½ in	1 piece	45	47	160	1	15	13.4	0.6	0.2
Shredded or grated	1 c	80	47	285	3	27	23.8	1.1	0.3
Dried, sweetened, shredded	1 c	93	13	470	3	33	29.3	1.4	0.4
Filberts (hazelnuts), chopped	1 c	115	5	725	15	72	5.3	56.5	6.9
	1 oz	28	5	180	4	18	1.3	13.9	1.7
Lentils, dry, cooked	1 c	200	72	215	16	1	0.1	0.2	0.5
Macadamia nuts, roasted in									
oil, salted	1 c	134	2	960	10	103	15.4	80.9	1.8
	1 oz	28	2	205	2	22	3.2	17.1	0.4
Mixed nuts, with peanuts, salted									
Dry roasted	1 oz	28	2	170	5	15	2.0	8.9	3.1
Roasted in oil	1 oz	28	2	175	5	16	2.5	9.0	3.8
Peanuts, roasted in oil, salted	1 c	145	2	840	39	71	9.9	35.5	22.6
	1 oz	28	2	165	8	14	1.9	6.9	4.4

tr = nutrient present in trace amounts.

[25]Cashews without salt contain 21 mg sodium per cup or 4 mg per oz.

[26]Cashews without salt contain 22 mg sodium per cup or 5 mg per oz.

NUTRIENTS IN INDICATED QUANTITY

Cholesterol (mg)	Carbohydrate (g)	Calcium (mg)	Phosphorus (mg)	Iron (mg)	Potassium (mg)	Sodium (mg)	Vitamin A value		Thiamin (mg)	Riboflavin (mg)	Niacin (mg)	Ascorbic acid (mg)
							IU	RE				
0	28	359	702	4.9	988	15	0	0	0.28	1.05	4.5	1
0	6	75	147	1.0	208	3	0	0	0.06	0.22	1.0	tr
0	41	47	239	2.9	608	1	tr	tr	0.43	0.05	0.9	0
0	38	90	266	4.9	749	13	0	0	0.25	0.13	1.3	0
0	49	55	293	5.9	1,163	4	0	0	0.25	0.11	1.3	0
0	40	95	281	5.1	790	13	0	0	0.27	0.13	1.3	0
0	49	86	296	5.4	882	3	tr	tr	0.33	0.16	0.7	0
30	32	94	303	4.8	668	1,374	330	33	0.18	0.15	3.3	tr
10	48	138	235	4.6	536	1,181	330	33	0.20	0.08	1.5	5
10	54	161	291	5.9	536	969	330	33	0.15	0.10	1.3	5
0	42	74	278	4.6	673	968	10	1	0.13	0.10	1.5	0
0	35	43	238	3.3	573	20	30	3	0.40	0.10	1.0	0
0	4	50	170	1.0	170	1	tr	tr	0.28	0.03	0.5	tr
0	126	390	102	5.7	1,275	24	tr	tr	0.07	0.07	2.2	tr
0	45	62	671	8.2	774	[25]877	0	0	0.27	0.27	1.9	0
0	9	13	139	1.7	160	[25]181	0	0	0.06	0.06	0.4	0
0	37	53	554	5.3	689	[26]814	0	0	0.55	0.23	2.3	0
0	8	12	121	1.2	150	[26]177	0	0	0.12	0.05	0.5	0
0	76	41	153	1.3	847	3	30	3	0.35	0.25	1.9	37
0	45	80	273	4.9	475	11	tr	tr	0.18	0.09	0.9	0
0	7	6	51	1.1	160	9	0	0	0.03	0.01	0.2	1
0	12	11	90	1.9	285	16	0	0	0.05	0.02	0.4	3
0	44	14	99	1.8	313	244	0	0	0.03	0.02	0.4	1
0	18	216	359	3.8	512	3	80	8	0.58	0.13	1.3	1
0	4	53	88	0.9	126	1	20	2	0.14	0.03	0.3	tr
0	38	50	238	4.2	498	26	40	4	0.14	0.12	1.2	0
0	17	60	268	2.4	441	[27]348	10	1	0.29	0.15	2.7	0
0	4	13	57	0.5	93	[27]74	tr	tr	0.06	0.03	0.6	0
0	7	20	123	1.0	169	[28]190	tr	tr	0.06	0.06	1.3	0
0	6	31	131	0.9	165	[28]185	10	1	0.14	0.06	1.4	tr
0	27	125	734	2.8	1,019	[29]626	0	0	0.42	0.15	21.5	0
0	5	24	143	0.5	199	[29]122	0	0	0.08	0.03	4.2	0

[27]Macadamia nuts without salt contain 9 mg sodium per cup or 2 mg per oz.

[28]Mixed nuts without salt contain 3 mg sodium per oz.

[29]Peanuts without salt contain 22 mg sodium per cup or 4 mg per oz.

Foods, approximate measures, units, and weight (weight of edible portion only)		Grams	Water (g)	Food energy (Calories)	Protein (g)	Fat (g)	Fatty Acids		
							Saturated (g)	Mono-unsaturated (g)	Poly-unsaturated (g)
Legumes, Nuts, and Seeds (*cont.*)									
Peanut butter	1 tbsp	16	1	95	5	8	1.4	4.0	2.5
Peas, split, dry, cooked	1 c	200	70	230	16	1	0.1	0.1	0.3
Pecans, halves	1 c	108	5	720	8	73	5.9	45.5	18.1
	1 oz	28	5	190	2	19	1.5	12.0	4.7
Pine nuts (pinyons), shelled	1 oz	28	6	160	3	17	2.7	6.5	7.3
Pistachio nuts, dried, shelled	1 oz	28	4	165	6	14	1.7	9.3	2.1
Pumpkin and squash kernels, dry, hulled	1 oz	28	7	155	7	13	2.5	4.0	5.9
Refried beans, canned	1 c	290	72	295	18	3	0.4	0.6	1.4
Sesame seeds, dry, hulled	1 tbsp	8	5	45	2	4	0.6	1.7	1.9
Soybeans, dry, cooked, drained	1 c	180	71	235	20	10	1.3	1.9	5.3
Soy products									
Miso	1 c	276	53	470	29	13	1.8	2.6	7.3
Tofu, piece 2½ by 2¾ by 1 in	1 piece	120	85	85	9	5	0.7	1.0	2.9
Sunflower seeds, dry, hulled	1 oz	28	5	160	6	14	1.5	2.7	9.3
Tahini	1 tbsp	15	3	90	3	8	1.1	3.0	3.5
Walnuts									
Black, chopped	1 c	125	4	760	30	71	4.5	15.9	46.9
	1 oz	28	4	170	7	16	1.0	3.6	10.6
English or Persian, pieces or chips	1 c	120	4	770	17	74	6.7	17.0	47.0
	1 oz	28	4	180	4	18	1.6	4.0	11.1
Meat and Meat Products									
Beef, cooked[30]									
Cuts braised, simmered, or pot roasted									
Relatively fat such as chuck blade									
Lean and fat, piece,									
2½ by 2½ by ¾ in	3 oz	85	43	325	22	26	10.8	11.7	0.9
Lean only	2.2 oz	62	53	170	19	9	3.9	4.2	0.3
Relatively lean, such as bottom round									
Lean and fat, piece,									
4⅛ by 2¼ by ½ in	3 oz	85	54	220	25	13	4.8	5.7	0.5
Lean only	2.8 oz	78	57	175	25	8	2.7	3.4	0.3
Ground beef, broiled, patty, 3 by ⅝ in									
Lean	3 oz	85	56	230	21	16	6.2	6.9	0.6
Regular	3 oz	85	54	245	20	18	6.9	7.7	0.7
Heart, lean, braised	3 oz	85	65	150	24	5	1.2	0.8	1.6
Liver, fried, slice, 6½ by 2⅜ by ⅜ in[31]	3 oz	85	56	185	23	7	2.5	3.6	1.3
Roast, oven cooked, no liquid added									
Relatively fat, such as rib									
Lean and fat, 2 pieces,									
4⅛ by 2¼ by ¼ in	3 oz	85	46	315	19	26	10.8	11.4	0.9
Lean only	2.2 oz	61	57	150	17	9	3.6	3.7	0.3

tr = nutrient present in trace amounts.

[30]Outer layer of fat was removed to within approximately ½ in of the lean. Deposits of fat within the cut were not removed.

NUTRIENTS IN INDICATED QUANTITY

Cho- les- terol (mg)	Carbo- hydrate (g)	Calcium (mg)	Phos- phorus (mg)	Iron (mg)	Potas- sium (mg)	Sodium (mg)	Vitamin A value		Thiamin (mg)	Ribo- flavin (mg)	Niacin (mg)	Ascorbic acid (mg)
							IU	RE				
0	3	5	60	0.3	110	75	0	0	0.02	0.02	2.2	0
0	42	22	178	3.4	592	26	80	8	0.30	0.18	1.8	0
0	20	39	314	2.3	423	1	140	14	0.92	0.14	1.0	2
0	5	10	83	0.6	111	tr	40	4	0.24	0.04	0.3	1
0	5	2	10	0.9	178	20	10	1	0.35	0.06	1.2	1
0	7	38	143	1.9	310	2	70	7	0.23	0.05	0.3	tr
0	5	12	333	4.2	229	5	110	11	0.06	0.09	0.5	tr
0	51	141	245	5.1	1,141	1,228	0	0	0.14	0.16	1.4	17
0	1	11	62	0.6	33	3	10	1	0.06	0.01	0.4	0
0	19	131	322	4.9	972	4	50	5	0.38	0.16	1.1	0
0	65	188	853	4.7	922	8,142	110	11	0.17	0.28	0.8	0
0	3	108	151	2.3	50	8	0	0	0.07	0.04	0.1	0
0	5	33	200	1.9	195	1	10	1	0.65	0.07	1.3	tr
0	3	21	119	0.7	69	5	10	1	0.24	0.02	0.8	1
0	15	73	580	3.8	655	1	370	37	0.27	0.14	0.9	tr
0	3	16	132	0.9	149	tr	80	8	0.06	0.03	0.2	tr
0	22	113	380	2.9	602	12	150	15	0.46	0.18	1.3	4
0	5	27	90	0.7	142	3	40	4	0.11	0.04	0.3	1
87	0	11	163	2.5	163	53	tr	tr	0.06	0.19	2.0	0
66	0	8	146	2.3	163	44	tr	tr	0.05	0.17	1.7	0
81	0	5	217	2.8	248	43	tr	tr	0.06	0.21	3.3	0
75	0	4	212	2.7	240	40	tr	tr	0.06	0.20	3.3	0
74	0	9	134	1.8	256	65	tr	tr	0.04	0.18	4.4	0
76	0	9	144	2.1	248	70	tr	tr	0.03	0.16	4.9	0
164	0	5	213	6.4	198	54	tr	tr	0.12	1.31	3.4	5
410	7	9	392	5.3	309	90	[32]30,690	[32]9,120	0.18	3.52	12.3	23
72	0	8	145	2.0	246	54	tr	tr	0.06	0.16	3.1	0
49	0	5	127	1.7	218	45	tr	tr	0.05	0.13	2.7	0

[31]Fried in vegetable shortening.
[32]Value varies widely.

Foods, approximate measures, units, and weight (weight of edible portion only)		Grams	Water (g)	Food energy (Calories)	Pro-tein (g)	Fat (g)	Fatty Acids		
							Satu-rated (g)	Mono-unsatu-rated (g)	Poly-unsatu-rated (g)
Meat and Meat Products (*cont.*)									
Beef, cooked (*cont.*)									
Relatively lean, such as eye of round									
Lean and fat, 2 pieces,									
2½ by 2½ by ⅜ in	3 oz	85	57	205	23	12	4.9	5.4	0.5
Lean only	2.6 oz	75	63	135	22	5	1.9	2.1	0.2
Steak									
Sirloin, broiled									
Lean and fat, piece,									
2½ by 2½ by ¾ in	3 oz	85	53	240	23	15	6.4	6.9	0.6
Lean only from item 587	2.5 oz	72	59	150	22	6	2.6	2.8	0.3
Beef, canned, corned	3 oz	85	59	185	22	10	4.2	4.9	0.4
Beef, dried, chipped	2.5 oz	72	48	145	24	4	1.8	2.0	0.2
Lamb, cooked									
Chops, (3 per lb with bone)									
Arm, braised									
Lean and fat	2.2 oz	63	44	220	20	15	6.9	6.0	0.9
Lean only	1.7 oz	48	49	135	17	7	2.9	2.6	0.4
Loin, broiled									
Lean and fat	2.8 oz	80	54	235	22	16	7.3	6.4	1.0
Lean only	2.3 oz	64	61	140	19	6	2.6	2.4	0.4
Leg, roasted									
Lean and fat, 2 pieces,									
4⅛ by 2¼ by ¼ in	3 oz	85	59	205	22	13	5.6	4.9	0.8
Lean only	2.6 oz	73	64	140	20	6	2.4	2.2	0.4
Rib, roasted									
Lean and fat, 3 pieces,									
2½ by 2½ by ¼ in	3 oz	85	47	315	18	26	12.1	10.6	1.5
Lean only	2 oz	57	60	130	15	7	3.2	3.0	0.5
Pork, cured, cooked									
Bacon									
Regular	3 medium slices	19	13	110	6	9	3.3	4.5	1.1
Canadian-style	2 slices	46	62	85	11	4	1.3	1.9	0.4
Ham, light cure, roasted									
Lean and fat, 2 pieces,									
4⅛ by 2¼ by ¼ in	3 oz	85	58	205	18	14	5.1	6.7	1.5
Lean only	2.4 oz	68	66	105	17	4	1.3	1.7	0.4
Ham, canned, roasted,									
2 pieces, 4⅛ by 2¼ by ¼ in	3 oz	85	67	140	18	7	2.4	3.5	0.8
Luncheon meat									
Canned, spiced or unspiced,									
slice, 3 by 2 by ½ in	2 slices	42	52	140	5	13	4.5	6.0	1.5
Chopped ham (8 slices per									
6-oz pkg)	2 slices	42	64	95	7	7	2.4	3.4	0.9
Cooked ham (8 slices per 8-oz pkg)									
Regular	2 slices	57	65	105	10	6	1.9	2.8	0.7
Extra lean	2 slices	57	71	75	11	3	0.9	1.3	0.3

tr = nutrient present in trace amounts.

NUTRIENTS IN INDICATED QUANTITY

Cho-les-terol (mg)	Carbo-hydrate (g)	Calcium (mg)	Phos-phorus (mg)	Iron (mg)	Potas-sium (mg)	Sodium (mg)	Vitamin A value		Thiamin (mg)	Ribo-flavin (mg)	Niacin (mg)	Ascorbic acid (mg)
							IU	RE				
62	0	5	177	1.6	308	50	tr	tr	0.07	0.14	3.0	0
52	0	3	170	1.5	297	46	tr	tr	0.07	0.13	2.8	0
77	0	9	186	2.6	306	53	tr	tr	0.10	0.23	3.3	0
64	0	8	176	2.4	290	48	tr	tr	0.09	0.22	3.1	0
80	0	17	90	3.7	51	802	tr	tr	0.02	0.20	2.9	0
46	0	14	287	2.3	142	3,053	tr	tr	0.05	0.23	2.7	0
77	0	16	132	1.5	195	46	tr	tr	0.04	0.16	4.4	0
59	0	12	111	1.3	162	36	tr	tr	0.03	0.13	3.0	0
78	0	16	162	1.4	272	62	tr	tr	0.09	0.21	5.5	0
60	0	12	145	1.3	241	54	tr	tr	0.08	0.18	4.4	0
78	0	8	162	1.7	273	57	tr	tr	0.09	0.24	5.5	0
65	0	6	150	1.5	247	50	tr	tr	0.08	0.20	4.6	0
77	0	19	139	1.4	224	60	tr	tr	0.08	0.18	5.5	0
50	0	12	111	1.0	179	46	tr	tr	0.05	0.13	3.5	0
16	tr	2	64	0.3	92	303	0	0	0.13	0.05	1.4	6
27	1	5	136	0.4	179	711	0	0	0.38	0.09	3.2	10
53	0	6	182	0.7	243	1,009	0	0	0.51	0.19	3.8	0
37	0	5	154	0.6	215	902	0	0	0.46	0.17	3.4	0
35	tr	6	188	0.9	298	908	0	0	0.82	0.21	4.3	[33]19
26	1	3	34	0.3	90	541	0	0	0.15	0.08	1.3	tr
21	0	3	65	0.3	134	576	0	0	0.27	0.09	1.6	[33]8
32	2	4	141	0.6	189	751	0	0	0.49	0.14	3.0	[33]16
27	1	4	124	0.4	200	815	0	0	0.53	0.13	2.8	[33]15

[33]Contains added sodium ascorbate. If sodium ascorbate is not added, ascorbic acid content is negligible.

Foods, approximate measures, units, and weight (weight of edible portion only)	Grams	Water (g)	Food energy (Calories)	Pro- tein (g)	Fat (g)	Fatty Acids		
						Satu- rated (g)	Mono- unsatu- rated (g)	Poly- unsatu- rated (g)
Meat and Meat Products (*cont.*)								
Pork, fresh, cooked								
Chop, loin (cut 3 per lb with bone)								
Broiled								
Lean and fat	3.1 oz	87	50	275	24	19	7.0	8.8	2.2
Lean only	2.5 oz	72	57	165	23	8	2.6	3.4	0.9
Pan fried								
Lean and fat	3.1 oz	89	45	335	21	27	9.8	12.5	3.1
Lean only	2.4 oz	67	54	180	19	11	3.7	4.8	1.3
Ham (leg), roasted								
Lean and fat, piece, 2½ by 2½ by ¾ in	3 oz	85	53	250	21	18	6.4	8.1	2.0
Lean only	2.5 oz	72	60	160	20	8	2.7	3.6	1.0
Rib, roasted								
Lean and fat, piece, 2½ by ¾ in	3 oz	85	51	270	21	20	7.2	9.2	2.3
Lean only	2.5 oz	71	57	175	20	10	3.4	4.4	1.2
Shoulder cut, braised								
Lean and fat, 3 pieces, 2½ by 2½ by ¼ in	3 oz	85	47	295	23	22	7.9	10.0	2.4
Lean only	2.4 oz	67	54	165	22	8	2.8	3.7	1.0
Sausages (See also Luncheon meats)								
Bologna, slice (8 per 8-oz pkg)	2 slices	57	54	180	7	16	6.1	7.6	1.4
Braunschweiger, slice (6 per 6-oz pkg)	2 slices	57	48	205	8	18	6.2	8.5	2.1
Brown and serve (10–11 per 8-oz pkg), browned	1 link	13	45	50	2	5	1.7	2.2	0.5
Frankfurter (10 per 1-lb pkg), cooked (reheated)	1 frankfurter	45	54	145	5	13	4.8	6.2	1.2
Pork link (16 per 1-lb pkg), cooked[34]	1 link	13	45	50	3	4	1.4	1.8	0.5
Salami								
Cooked type, slice (8 per 8-oz pkg)	2 slices	57	60	145	8	11	4.6	5.2	1.2
Dry type, slice (12 per 4-oz pkg)	2 slices	20	35	85	5	7	2.4	3.4	0.6
Sandwich spread (pork, beef)	1 tbsp	15	60	35	1	3	0.9	1.1	0.4
Vienna sausage (7 per 4-oz can)	1 sausage	16	60	45	2	4	1.5	2.0	0.3
Veal, medium fat, cooked, bone removed								
Cutlet, 4⅛ by 2¼ by ½ in, braised or broiled	3 oz	85	60	185	23	9	4.1	4.1	0.6
Rib, 2 pieces, 4⅛ by 2¼ by ¼ in, roasted	3 oz	85	55	230	23	14	6.0	6.0	1.0

tr = nutrient present in trace amounts.

[33]Contains added sodium ascorbate. If sodium ascorbate is not added, ascorbic acid content is negligible.

NUTRIENTS IN INDICATED QUANTITY

Cho-les-terol (mg)	Carbo-hydrate (g)	Calcium (mg)	Phos-phorus (mg)	Iron (mg)	Potas-sium (mg)	Sodium (mg)	Vitamin A value		Thiamin (mg)	Ribo-flavin (mg)	Niacin (mg)	Ascorbic acid (mg)
							IU	RE				
84	0	3	184	0.7	312	61	10	3	0.87	0.24	4.3	tr
71	0	4	176	0.7	302	56	10	1	0.83	0.22	4.0	tr
92	0	4	190	0.7	323	64	10	3	0.91	0.24	4.6	tr
72	0	3	178	0.7	305	57	10	1	0.84	0.22	4.0	tr
79	0	5	210	0.9	280	50	10	2	0.54	0.27	3.9	tr
68	0	5	202	0.8	269	46	10	1	0.50	0.25	3.6	tr
69	0	9	190	0.8	313	37	10	3	0.50	0.24	4.2	tr
56	0	8	182	0.7	300	33	10	2	0.45	0.22	3.8	tr
93	0	6	162	1.4	286	75	10	3	0.46	0.26	4.4	tr
76	0	5	151	1.3	271	68	10	1	0.40	0.24	4.0	tr
31	2	7	52	0.9	103	581	0	0	0.10	0.08	1.5	[33]12
89	2	5	96	5.3	113	652	8,010	2,405	0.14	0.87	4.8	[33]6
9	tr	1	14	0.1	25	105	0	0	0.05	0.02	0.4	0
23	1	5	39	0.5	75	504	0	0	0.09	0.05	1.2	[33]12
11	tr	4	24	0.2	47	168	0	0	0.10	0.03	0.6	tr
37	1	7	66	1.5	113	607	0	0	0.14	0.21	2.0	[33]7
16	1	2	28	0.3	76	372	0	0	0.12	0.06	1.0	[33]5
6	2	2	9	0.1	17	152	10	1	0.03	0.02	0.3	0
8	tr	2	8	0.1	16	152	0	0	0.01	0.02	0.3	0
109	0	9	196	0.8	258	56	tr	tr	0.06	0.21	4.6	0
109	0	10	211	0.7	259	57	tr	tr	0.11	0.26	6.6	0

[34]One patty (8 per pound) of bulk sausage is equivalent to 2 links.

Foods, approximate measures, units, and weight (weight of edible portion only)	Grams	Water (g)	Food energy (Calories)	Pro-tein (g)	Fat (g)	Fatty Acids		
						Satu-rated (g)	Mono-unsatu-rated (g)	Poly-unsatu-rated (g)
Poultry and Poultry Products								
Chicken								
Fried, flesh, with skin[35]								
Batter dipped								
Breast, ½ breast								
(5.6 oz with bones) 4.9 oz	140	52	365	35	18	4.9	7.6	4.3
Drumstick (3.4 oz with bones) 2.5 oz	72	53	195	16	11	3.0	4.6	2.7
Flour coated								
Breast, ½ breast								
(4.2 oz with bones) 3.5 oz	98	57	220	31	9	2.4	3.4	1.9
Drumstick (2.6 oz with bones) 1.7 oz	49	57	120	13	7	1.8	2.7	1.6
Roasted, flesh only								
Breast, ½ breast (4.2 oz with bones and skin) 3.0 oz	86	65	140	27	3	0.9	1.1	0.7
Drumstick, (2.9 oz with bones and skin) 1.6 oz	44	67	75	12	2	0.7	0.8	0.6
Stewed, flesh only, light and dark meat, chopped or diced 1 c	140	67	250	38	9	2.6	3.3	2.2
Chicken liver, cooked 1 liver	20	68	30	5	1	0.4	0.3	0.2
Duck, roasted, flesh only ½ duck	221	46	445	52	25	9.2	8.2	3.2
Turkey, roasted, flesh only								
Dark meat, piece, 2½ by 1⅝ by ¼ in 4 pieces	85	63	160	24	6	2.1	1.4	1.8
Light meat, piece, 4 by 2 by ¼ in 2 pieces	85	66	135	25	3	0.9	0.5	0.7
Light and dark meat								
Chopped or diced 1 c	140	65	240	41	7	2.3	1.4	2.0
Pieces (1 slice white meat, 4 by 2 by ¼ in and 2 slices dark meat, 2½ by 1⅝ by ¼ in) 3 pieces	85	65	145	25	4	1.4	0.9	1.2
Poultry food products								
Chicken								
Canned, boneless 5 oz	142	69	235	31	11	3.1	4.5	2.5
Frankfurter (10 per 1-lb pkg) 1 frankfurter	45	58	115	6	9	2.5	3.8	1.8
Roll, light (6 slices per 6 oz pkg) 2 slices	57	69	90	11	4	1.1	1.7	0.9
Turkey								
Gravy and turkey, frozen 5-oz package	142	85	95	8	4	1.2	1.4	0.7
Ham, cured turkey thigh meat (8 slices per 8-oz pkg) 2 slices	57	71	75	11	3	1.0	0.7	0.9
Loaf, breast meat (8 slices per 6-oz pkg) 2 slices	42	72	45	10	1	0.2	0.2	0.1
Patties, breaded, battered, fried (2.25 oz) 1 patty	64	50	180	9	12	3.0	4.8	3.0
Roast, boneless, frozen, seasoned, light and dark meat, cooked 3 oz	85	68	130	18	5	1.6	1.0	1.4

tr = nutrient present in trace amounts.

[35]Fried in vegetable shortening.

[36]If sodium ascorbate is used, product contains 11 mg ascorbic acid.

NUTRIENTS IN INDICATED QUANTITY

Cho-les-terol (mg)	Carbo-hydrate (g)	Calcium (mg)	Phos-phorus (mg)	Iron (mg)	Potas-sium (mg)	Sodium (mg)	Vitamin A value		Thiamin (mg)	Ribo-flavin (mg)	Niacin (mg)	Ascorbic acid (mg)
							IU	RE				
119	13	28	259	1.8	281	385	90	28	0.16	0.20	14.7	0
62	6	12	106	1.0	134	194	60	19	0.08	0.15	3.7	0
87	2	16	228	1.2	254	74	50	15	0.08	0.13	13.5	0
44	1	6	86	0.7	112	44	40	12	0.04	0.11	3.0	0
73	0	13	196	0.9	220	64	20	5	0.06	0.10	11.8	0
41	0	5	81	0.6	108	42	30	8	0.03	0.10	2.7	0
116	0	20	210	1.6	252	98	70	21	0.07	0.23	8.6	0
126	tr	3	62	1.7	28	10	3,270	983	0.03	0.35	0.9	3
197	0	27	449	6.0	557	144	170	51	0.57	1.04	11.3	0
72	0	27	173	2.0	246	67	0	0	0.05	0.21	3.1	0
59	0	16	186	1.1	259	54	0	0	0.05	0.11	5.8	0
106	0	35	298	2.5	417	98	0	0	0.09	0.25	7.6	0
65	0	21	181	1.5	253	60	0	0	0.05	0.15	4.6	0
88	0	20	158	2.2	196	714	170	48	0.02	0.18	9.0	3
45	3	43	48	0.9	38	616	60	17	0.03	0.05	1.4	0
28	1	24	89	0.6	129	331	50	14	0.04	0.07	3.0	0
26	7	20	115	1.3	87	787	60	18	0.03	0.18	2.6	0
32	tr	6	108	1.6	184	565	0	0	0.03	0.14	2.0	0
17	0	3	97	0.2	118	608	0	0	0.02	0.05	3.5	[36]0
40	10	9	173	1.4	176	512	20	7	0.06	0.12	1.5	0
45	3	4	207	1.4	253	578	0	0	0.04	0.14	5.3	0

Foods, approximate measures, units, and weight (weight of edible portion only)		Grams	Water (g)	Food energy (Calories)	Pro-tein (g)	Fat (g)	Fatty Acids		
							Satu-rated (g)	Mono-unsatu-rated (g)	Poly-unsatu-rated (g)
Sugars and Sweets									
Sugars									
Brown, pressed down	1 c	220	2	820	0	0	0.0	0.0	0.0
White									
Granulated	1 c	200	1	770	0	0	0.0	0.0	0.0
	1 tbsp	12	1	45	0	0	0.0	0.0	0.0
	1 packet	6	1	25	0	0	0.0	0.0	0.0
Powdered, sifted, spooned into cup	1 c	100	1	385	0	0	0.0	0.0	0.0
Syrups									
Chocolate-flavored syrup or topping									
Thin type	2 tbsp	38	37	85	1	tr	0.2	0.1	0.1
Fudge type	2 tbsp	38	25	125	2	5	3.1	1.7	0.2
Molasses, cane, blackstrap	2 tbsp	40	24	85	0	0	0.0	0.0	0.0
Table syrup (corn and maple)	2 tbsp	42	25	122	0	0	0.0	0.0	0.0
Vegetables and Vegetable Products									
Alfalfa seeds, sprouted, raw	1 c	33	91	10	1	tr	tr	tr	0.1
Artichokes, globe or French, cooked, drained	1 artichoke	120	87	55	3	tr	tr	tr	0.1
Asparagus, green									
Cooked, drained									
From raw									
Cuts and tips	1 c	180	92	45	5	1	0.1	tr	0.2
Spears, ½-in diam. at base	4 spears	60	92	15	2	tr	tr	tr	0.1
From frozen									
Cuts and tips	1 c	180	91	50	5	1	0.2	tr	0.3
Spears, ½-in diam. at base	4 spears	60	91	15	2	tr	0.1	tr	0.1
Canned, spears, ½-in diam. at base	4 spears	80	95	10	1	tr	tr	tr	0.1
Bamboo shoots, canned, drained	1 c	131	94	25	2	1	0.1	tr	0.2
Beans									
Lima, immature seeds, frozen, cooked, drained									
Thick-seeded types (Ford-hooks)	1 c	170	74	170	10	1	0.1	tr	0.3
Thin-seeded types (baby limas)	1 c	180	72	190	12	1	0.1	tr	0.3
Snap									
Cooked, drained									
From raw (cut and French style)	1 c	125	89	45	2	tr	0.1	tr	0.2
From frozen (cut)	1 c	135	92	35	2	tr	tr	tr	0.1
Canned, drained solids (cut)	1 c	135	93	25	2	tr	tr	tr	0.1

tr = nutrient present in trace amounts.

[37]For regular pack; special dietary pack contains 3 mg sodium.

[38]For green varieties; yellow varieties contain 101 IU or 10 RE.

NUTRIENTS IN INDICATED QUANTITY

Cho-les-terol (mg)	Carbo-hydrate (g)	Calcium (mg)	Phos-phorus (mg)	Iron (mg)	Potas-sium (mg)	Sodium (mg)	Vitamin A value		Thiamin (mg)	Ribo-flavin (mg)	Niacin (mg)	Ascorbic acid (mg)
							IU	RE				
0	212	187	56	4.8	757	97	0	0	0.02	0.07	0.2	0
0	199	3	tr	0.1	7	5	0	0	0.00	0.00	0.0	0
0	12	tr	tr	tr	tr	tr	0	0	0.00	0.00	0.0	0
0	6	tr	tr	tr	tr	tr	0	0	0.00	0.00	0.0	0
0	100	1	tr	tr	4	2	0	0	0.00	0.00	0.0	0
0	22	6	49	0.8	85	36	tr	tr	tr	0.02	0.1	0
0	21	38	60	0.5	82	42	40	13	0.02	0.08	0.1	0
0	22	274	34	10.1	1,171	38	0	0	0.04	0.08	0.8	0
0	32	1	4	tr	7	19	0	0	0.00	0.00	0.0	0
0	1	11	23	0.3	26	2	50	5	0.03	0.04	0.2	3
0	12	47	72	1.6	316	79	170	17	0.07	0.06	0.7	9
0	8	43	110	1.2	558	7	1,490	149	0.18	0.22	1.9	49
0	3	14	37	0.4	186	2	500	50	0.06	0.07	0.6	16
0	9	41	99	1.2	392	7	1,470	147	0.12	0.19	1.9	44
0	3	14	33	0.4	131	2	490	49	0.04	0.06	0.6	15
0	2	11	30	0.5	122	[37]278	380	38	0.04	0.07	0.7	13
0	4	10	33	0.4	105	9	10	1	0.03	0.03	0.2	1
0	32	37	107	2.3	694	90	320	32	0.13	0.10	1.8	22
0	35	50	202	3.5	740	52	300	30	0.13	0.10	1.4	10
0	10	58	49	1.6	374	4	[38]830	[38]83	0.09	0.12	0.8	12
0	8	61	32	1.1	151	18	[39]710	[39]71	0.06	0.10	0.6	11
0	6	35	26	1.2	147	[40]339	[41]470	[41]47	0.02	0.08	0.3	6

[39]For green varieties; yellow varieties contain 151 IU or 15 RE.
[40]For regular pack; special dietary pack contains 3 mg sodium.
[41]For green varieties; yellow varieties contain 142 IU or 14 RE.

Vegetables and Vegetable Products (*cont.*)

Foods, approximate measures, units, and weight (weight of edible portion only)		Grams	Water (g)	Food energy (Calories)	Pro-tein (g)	Fat (g)	Fatty Acids		
							Satu-rated (g)	Mono-unsatu-rated (g)	Poly-unsatu-rated (g)
Beans, mature. See Beans, dry and Black-eyed peas, dry.									
Bean sprouts (mung)									
Raw	1 c	104	90	30	3	tr	tr	tr	0.1
Cooked, drained	1 c	124	93	25	3	tr	tr	tr	tr
Beets									
Cooked, drained									
Diced or sliced	1 c	170	91	55	2	tr	tr	tr	tr
Whole beets, 2-in diam.	2 beets	100	91	30	1	tr	tr	tr	tr
Canned, drained solids, diced or sliced	1 c	170	91	55	2	tr	tr	tr	0.1
Beet greens, leaves and stems, cooked, drained	1 c	144	89	40	4	tr	tr	0.1	0.1
Black-eyed peas, immature seeds, cooked and drained									
From raw	1 c	165	72	180	13	1	0.3	0.1	0.6
From frozen	1 c	170	66	225	14	1	0.3	0.1	0.5
Broccoli									
Raw	1 spear	151	91	40	4	1	0.1	tr	0.3
Cooked, drained									
From raw									
Spear, medium	1 spear	180	90	50	5	1	0.1	tr	0.2
Spears, cut into ½-in pieces	1 c	155	90	45	5	tr	0.1	tr	0.2
From frozen									
Piece, 4½ to 5 in long	1 piece	30	91	10	1	tr	tr	tr	tr
Chopped	1 c	185	91	50	6	tr	tr	tr	0.1
Brussels sprouts, cooked, drained									
From raw, 7-8 sprouts, 1¼- to 1½-in diam.	1 c	155	87	60	4	1	0.2	0.1	0.4
From frozen	1 c	155	87	65	6	1	0.1	tr	0.3
Cabbage, common varieties									
Raw, coarsely shredded or sliced	1 c	70	93	15	1	tr	tr	tr	0.1
Cooked, drained	1 c	150	94	30	1	tr	tr	tr	0.2
Cabbage, Chinese									
Pak-choi, cooked, drained	1 c	170	96	20	3	tr	tr	tr	0.1
Pe-tsai, raw, 1-in pieces	1 c	76	94	10	1	tr	tr	tr	0.1
Cabbage, red, raw, coarsely shredded or sliced	1 c	70	92	20	1	tr	tr	tr	0.1
Cabbage, savoy, raw, coarsely shredded or sliced	1 c	70	91	20	1	tr	tr	tr	tr
Carrots									
Raw, without crowns and tips, scraped									
Whole, 7½ by 1⅛ in, or strips, 2½ to 3 in long	1 carrot or 18 strips	72	88	30	1	tr	tr	tr	0.1
Grated	1 c	110	88	45	1	tr	tr	tr	0.1
Cooked, sliced, drained									
From raw	1 c	156	87	70	2	tr	0.1	tr	0.1
From frozen	1 c	146	90	55	2	tr	tr	tr	0.1
Canned, sliced, drained solids	1 c	146	93	35	1	tr	0.1	tr	0.1

tr = nutrient present in trace amounts.

[42]For regular pack; special dietary pack contains 78 mg sodium.

Cho-lesterol (mg)	Carbo-hydrate (g)	Calcium (mg)	Phos-phorus (mg)	Iron (mg)	Potas-sium (mg)	Sodium (mg)	Vitamin A value		Thiamin (mg)	Ribo-flavin (mg)	Niacin (mg)	Ascorbic acid (mg)
							IU	RE				
0	6	14	56	0.9	155	6	20	2	0.09	0.13	0.8	14
0	5	15	35	0.8	125	12	20	2	0.06	0.13	1.0	14
0	11	19	53	1.1	530	83	20	2	0.05	0.02	0.5	9
0	7	11	31	0.6	312	49	10	1	0.03	0.01	0.3	6
0	12	26	29	3.1	252	[42]466	20	2	0.02	0.07	0.3	7
0	8	164	59	2.7	1,309	347	7,340	734	0.17	0.42	0.7	36
0	30	46	196	2.4	693	7	1,050	105	0.11	0.18	1.8	3
0	40	39	207	3.6	638	9	130	13	0.44	0.11	1.2	4
0	8	72	100	1.3	491	41	2,330	233	0.10	0.18	1.0	141
0	10	205	86	2.1	293	20	2,540	254	0.15	0.37	1.4	113
0	9	177	74	1.8	253	17	2,180	218	0.13	0.32	1.2	97
0	2	15	17	0.2	54	7	570	57	0.02	0.02	0.1	12
0	10	94	102	1.1	333	44	3,500	350	0.10	0.15	0.8	74
0	13	56	87	1.9	491	33	1,110	111	0.17	0.12	0.9	96
0	13	37	84	1.1	504	36	910	91	0.16	0.18	0.8	71
0	4	33	16	0.4	172	13	90	9	0.04	0.02	0.2	33
0	7	50	38	0.6	308	29	130	13	0.09	0.08	0.3	36
0	3	158	49	1.8	631	58	4,370	437	0.05	0.11	0.7	44
0	2	59	22	0.2	181	7	910	91	0.03	0.04	0.3	21
0	4	36	29	0.3	144	8	30	3	0.04	0.02	0.2	40
0	4	25	29	0.3	161	20	700	70	0.05	0.02	0.2	22
0	7	19	32	0.4	233	25	20,250	2,025	0.07	0.04	0.7	7
0	11	30	48	0.6	355	39	30,940	3,094	0.11	0.06	1.0	10
0	16	48	47	1.0	354	103	38,300	3,830	0.05	0.09	0.8	4
0	12	41	38	0.7	231	86	25,850	2,585	0.04	0.05	0.6	4
0	8	37	35	0.9	261	[43]352	20,110	2,011	0.03	0.04	0.8	4

[43]For regular pack; special dietary pack contains 61 mg sodium.

Foods, approximate measures, units, and weight (weight of edible portion only)		Grams	Water (g)	Food energy (Calories)	Protein (g)	Fat (g)	Fatty Acids		
							Saturated (g)	Monounsaturated (g)	Polyunsaturated (g)
Vegetables and Vegetable Products (*cont.*)									
Cauliflower									
Raw (flowerets)	1 c	100	92	25	2	tr	tr	tr	0.1
Cooked, drained									
From raw (flowerets)	1 c	125	93	30	2	tr	tr	tr	0.1
From frozen (flowerets)	1 c	180	94	35	3	tr	0.1	tr	0.2
Celery, pascal type, raw									
Stalk, large outer, 8 by 1½ in									
(at root end)	1 stalk	40	95	5	tr	tr	tr	tr	tr
Pieces, diced	1 c	120	95	20	1	tr	tr	tr	0.1
Collards, cooked, drained									
From raw (leaves without stems)	1 c	190	96	25	2	tr	0.1	tr	0.2
From frozen (chopped)	1 c	170	88	60	5	1	0.1	0.1	0.4
Corn, sweet									
Cooked, drained									
From raw, ear 5 by 1¾ in	1 ear	77	70	85	3	1	0.2	0.3	0.5
From frozen									
Ear, trimmed to about 3½ in long	1 ear	63	73	60	2	tr	0.1	0.1	0.2
Kernels	1 c	165	76	135	5	tr	tr	tr	0.1
Canned									
Cream style	1 c	256	79	185	4	1	0.2	0.3	0.5
Whole kernel, vacuum pack	1 c	210	77	165	5	1	0.2	0.3	0.5
Cowpeas. See Black-eyed peas, immature, mature									
Cucumber, with peel, slices, ⅛ in thick (large, 2⅛-in diam.; small, 1¾-in diam.)	6 large or 8 small slices	28	96	5	tr	tr	tr	tr	tr
Dandelion greens, cooked, drained	1 c	105	90	35	2	1	0.1	tr	0.3
Eggplant, cooked, steamed	1 c	96	92	25	1	tr	tr	tr	0.1
Endive, curly (including escarole), raw, small pieces	1 c	50	94	10	1	tr	tr	tr	tr
Jerusalem-artichoke, raw, sliced	1 c	150	78	115	3	tr	0.0	tr	tr
Kale, cooked, drained									
From raw, chopped	1 c	130	91	40	2	1	0.1	tr	0.3
From frozen, chopped	1 c	130	91	40	4	1	0.1	tr	0.3
Kohlrabi, thickened bulb-like stems, cooked, drained, diced	1 c	165	90	50	3	tr	tr	tr	0.1
Lettuce, raw									
Butterhead, as Boston types									
Head, 5-in diam	1 head	163	96	20	2	tr	tr	tr	0.2
Leaves	1 outer or 2 inner leaves	15	96	tr	tr	tr	tr	tr	tr
Crisphead, as iceberg									
Head, 6-in diam	1 head	539	96	70	5	1	0.1	tr	0.5
Wedge, ¼ of head	1 wedge	135	96	20	1	tr	tr	tr	0.1
Pieces, chopped or shredded	1 c	55	96	5	1	tr	tr	tr	0.1

tr = nutrient present in trace amounts.

[44]For yellow varieties; white varieties contain only a trace of vitamin A.

NUTRIENTS IN INDICATED QUANTITY

Cho-les-terol (mg)	Carbo-hydrate (g)	Calcium (mg)	Phos-phorus (mg)	Iron (mg)	Potas-sium (mg)	Sodium (mg)	Vitamin A value		Thiamin (mg)	Ribo-flavin (mg)	Niacin (mg)	Ascorbic acid (mg)
							IU	RE				
0	5	29	46	0.6	355	15	20	2	0.08	0.06	0.6	72
0	6	34	44	0.5	404	8	20	2	0.08	0.07	0.7	69
0	7	31	43	0.7	250	32	40	4	0.07	0.10	0.6	56
0	1	14	10	0.2	144	35	50	5	0.01	0.01	0.1	3
0	4	43	31	0.6	341	106	150	15	0.04	0.04	0.4	8
0	5	148	19	0.8	177	36	4,220	422	0.03	0.08	0.4	19
0	12	357	46	1.9	427	85	10,170	1,017	0.08	0.20	1.1	45
0	19	2	79	0.5	192	13	[44]170	[44]17	0.17	0.06	1.2	5
0	14	2	47	0.4	158	3	[46]130	[46]13	0.11	0.04	1.0	3
0	34	3	78	0.5	229	8	[46]410	[46]41	0.11	0.12	2.1	4
0	46	8	131	1.0	343	[45]730	[46]250	[46]25	0.06	0.14	2.5	12
0	41	11	134	0.9	391	[46]571	[46]510	[46]51	0.09	0.15	2.5	17
0	1	4	5	0.1	42	1	10	1	0.01	0.01	0.1	1
0	7	147	44	1.9	244	46	12,290	1,229	0.14	0.18	0.5	19
0	6	6	21	0.3	238	3	60	6	0.07	0.02	0.6	1
0	2	26	14	0.4	157	11	1,030	103	0.04	0.04	0.2	3
0	26	21	117	5.1	644	6	30	3	0.30	0.09	2.0	6
0	7	94	36	1.2	296	30	9,620	962	0.07	0.09	0.7	53
0	7	179	36	1.2	417	20	8,260	826	0.06	0.15	0.9	33
0	11	41	74	0.7	561	35	60	6	0.07	0.03	0.6	89
0	4	52	38	0.5	419	8	1,580	158	0.10	0.10	0.5	13
0	tr	5	3	tr	39	1	150	15	0.01	0.01	tr	1
0	11	102	108	2.7	852	49	1,780	178	0.25	0.16	1.0	21
0	3	26	27	0.7	213	12	450	45	0.06	0.04	0.3	5
0	1	10	11	0.3	87	5	180	18	0.03	0.02	0.1	2

[45]For regular pack; special dietary pack contains 8 mg sodium.
[46]For regular pack; special dietary pack contains 6 mg sodium.

						Fatty Acids		
Foods, approximate measures, units, and weight (weight of edible portion only)	Grams	Water (g)	Food energy (Calories)	Pro-tein (g)	Fat (g)	Satu-rated (g)	Mono-unsatu-rated (g)	Poly-unsatu-rated (g)

Vegetables and Vegetable Products (*cont.*)

Lettuce, raw (*cont.*)								
Looseleaf (bunching varieties including romaine or cos), chopped or shredded pieces	1 c	56	94	10	1	tr	tr	tr	0.1
Mushrooms								
Raw, sliced or chopped	1 c	70	92	20	1	tr	tr	tr	0.1
Cooked, drained	1 c	156	91	40	3	1	0.1	tr	0.3
Canned, drained solids	1 c	156	91	35	3	tr	0.1	tr	0.2
Mustard greens, without stems and midribs, cooked, drained	1 c	140	94	20	3	tr	tr	0.2	0.1
Okra pods, 3 by ⅝ in, cooked	8 pods	85	90	25	2	tr	tr	tr	tr
Onions								
Raw								
Chopped	1 c	160	91	55	2	tr	0.1	0.1	0.2
Sliced	1 c	115	91	40	1	tr	0.1	tr	0.1
Cooked (whole or sliced), drained	1 c	210	92	60	2	tr	0.1	tr	0.1
Onions, spring, raw, bulb (⅜-in diam.) and white portion of top	6 onions	30	92	10	1	tr	tr	tr	tr
Onion rings, breaded, pan-fried, frozen, prepared	2 rings	20	29	80	1	5	1.7	2.2	1.0
Parsley								
Raw	10 sprigs	10	88	5	tr	tr	tr	tr	tr
Freeze-dried	1 tbsp	0.4	2	tr	tr	tr	tr	tr	tr
Parsnips, cooked (diced or 2 in lengths), drained	1 c	156	78	125	2	tr	0.1	0.2	0.1
Peas, edible pod, cooked, drained	1 c	160	89	65	5	tr	0.1	tr	0.2
Peas, green								
Canned, drained solids	1 c	170	82	115	8	1	0.1	0.1	0.3
Frozen, cooked, drained	1 c	160	80	125	8	tr	0.1	tr	0.2
Peppers								
Hot chili, raw	1 pepper	45	88	20	1	tr	tr	tr	tr
Sweet (about 5 per lb, whole), stem and seeds removed								
Raw	1 pepper	74	93	20	1	tr	tr	tr	0.2
Cooked, drained	1 pepper	73	95	15	tr	tr	tr	tr	0.1
Potatoes, cooked								
Baked (about 2 per lb, raw)								
With skin	1 potato	202	71	220	5	tr	0.1	tr	0.1
Flesh only	1 potato	156	75	145	3	tr	tr	tr	0.1
Boiled (about 3 per lb, raw)								
Peeled after boiling	1 potato	136	77	120	3	tr	tr	tr	0.1
Peeled before boiling	1 potato	135	77	115	2	tr	tr	tr	0.1

tr = nutrient present in trace amounts.

[47]For regular pack; special dietary pack contains 3 mg sodium.

[48]For red peppers; green peppers contain 350 IU or 35 RE.

[49]For green peppers; red peppers contain 4,220 IU or 422 RE.

NUTRIENTS IN INDICATED QUANTITY

Cho-les-terol (mg)	Carbo-hydrate (g)	Calcium (mg)	Phos-phorus (mg)	Iron (mg)	Potas-sium (mg)	Sodium (mg)	Vitamin A value		Thiamin (mg)	Ribo-flavin (mg)	Niacin (mg)	Ascorbic acid (mg)
							IU	RE				
0	2	38	14	0.8	148	5	1,060	106	0.03	0.04	0.2	10
0	3	4	73	0.9	259	3	0	0	0.07	0.31	2.9	2
0	8	9	136	2.7	555	3	0	0	0.11	0.47	7.0	6
0	8	17	103	1.2	201	663	0	0	0.13	0.03	2.5	0
0	3	104	57	1.0	283	22	4,240	424	0.06	0.09	0.6	35
0	6	54	48	0.4	274	4	490	49	0.11	0.05	0.7	14
0	12	40	46	0.6	248	3	0	0	0.10	0.02	0.2	13
0	8	29	33	0.4	178	2	0	0	0.07	0.01	0.1	10
0	13	57	48	0.4	319	17	0	0	0.09	0.02	0.2	12
0	2	18	10	0.6	77	1	1,500	150	0.02	0.04	0.1	14
0	8	6	16	0.3	26	75	50	5	0.06	0.03	0.7	tr
0	1	13	4	0.6	54	4	520	52	0.01	0.01	0.1	9
0	tr	1	2	0.2	25	2	250	25	tr	0.01	tr	1
0	30	58	108	0.9	573	16	0	0	0.13	0.08	1.1	20
0	11	67	88	3.2	384	6	210	21	0.20	0.12	0.9	77
0	21	34	114	1.6	294	[47]372	1,310	131	0.21	0.13	1.2	16
0	23	38	144	2.5	269	139	1,070	107	0.45	0.16	2.4	16
0	4	8	21	0.5	153	3	[48]4,840	[48]484	0.04	0.04	0.4	109
0	4	4	16	0.9	144	2	[49]390	[49]39	0.06	0.04	0.4	[50]95
0	3	3	11	0.6	94	1	[51]280	[51]28	0.04	0.03	0.3	[52]81
0	51	20	115	2.7	844	16	0	0	0.22	0.07	3.3	26
0	34	8	78	0.5	610	8	0	0	0.16	0.03	2.2	20
0	27	7	60	0.4	515	5	0	0	0.14	0.03	2.0	18
0	27	11	54	0.4	443	7	0	0	0.13	0.03	1.8	10

[50]For green peppers; red peppers contain 141 mg ascorbic acid.
[51]For green peppers; red peppers contain 2,740 IU or 274 RE.
[52]For green peppers; red peppers contain 121 mg ascorbic acid.

Foods, approximate measures, units, and weight (weight of edible portion only)		Grams	Water (g)	Food energy (Calories)	Pro- tein (g)	Fat (g)	Fatty Acids		
							Satu- rated (g)	Mono- unsatu- rated (g)	Poly- unsatu- rated (g)
Vegetables and Vegetable Products (*cont.*)									
Potatoes, cooked (*cont.*)									
French fried, strip, 2 to 3½ in long, frozen									
Oven heated	10 strips	50	53	110	2	4	2.1	1.8	0.3
Fried in vegetable oil	10 strips	50	38	160	2	8	2.5	1.6	3.8
Potato products, prepared									
Au gratin									
From dry mix	1 c	245	79	230	6	10	6.3	2.9	0.3
From home recipe	1 c	245	74	325	12	19	11.6	5.3	0.7
Hashed brown, from frozen	1 c	156	56	340	5	18	7.0	8.0	2.1
Mashed									
From home recipe									
Milk added	1 c	210	78	160	4	1	0.7	0.3	0.1
Milk and margarine added	1 c	210	76	225	4	9	2.2	3.7	2.5
From dehydrated flakes (without milk), water, milk, butter, and salt added	1 c	210	76	235	4	12	7.2	3.3	0.5
Potato salad, made with mayonnaise	1 c	250	76	360	7	21	3.6	6.2	9.3
Scalloped									
From dry mix	1 c	245	79	230	5	11	6.5	3.0	0.5
From home recipe	1 c	245	81	210	7	9	5.5	2.5	0.4
Potato chips	10 chips	20	3	105	1	7	1.8	1.2	3.6
Pumpkin									
Cooked from raw, mashed	1 c	245	94	50	2	tr	0.1	tr	tr
Canned	1 c	245	90	85	3	1	0.4	0.1	tr
Radishes, raw, stem ends, rootlets cut off	4 radishes	18	95	5	tr	tr	tr	tr	tr
Sauerkraut, canned, solids and liquid	1 c	236	93	45	2	tr	0.1	tr	0.1
Seaweed									
Kelp, raw	1 oz	28	82	10	tr	tr	0.1	tr	tr
Spirulina, dried	1 oz	28	5	80	16	2	0.8	0.2	0.6
Southern peas. See Black-eyed peas, immature, mature									
Spinach									
Raw, chopped	1 c	55	92	10	2	tr	tr	tr	0.1
Cooked, drained									
From raw	1 c	180	91	40	5	tr	0.1	tr	0.2
From frozen (leaf)	1 c	190	90	55	6	tr	0.1	tr	0.2
Canned, drained solids	1 c	214	92	50	6	1	0.2	tr	0.4
Spinach souffle	1 c	136	74	220	11	18	7.1	6.8	3.1
Squash, cooked									
Summer (all varieties), sliced, drained	1 c	180	94	35	2	1	0.1	tr	0.2
Winter (all varieties), baked, cubes	1 c	205	89	80	2	1	0.3	0.1	0.5
Sunchoke. See Jerusalem-artichoke									

tr = nutrient present in trace amounts.

NUTRIENTS IN INDICATED QUANTITY

Cho-les-terol (mg)	Carbo-hydrate (g)	Calcium (mg)	Phos-phorus (mg)	Iron (mg)	Potas-sium (mg)	Sodium (mg)	Vitamin A value		Thiamin (mg)	Ribo-flavin (mg)	Niacin (mg)	Ascorbic acid (mg)
							IU	RE				
0	17	5	43	0.7	229	16	0	0	0.06	0.02	1.2	5
0	20	10	47	0.4	366	108	0	0	0.09	0.01	1.6	5
12	31	203	233	0.8	537	1,076	520	76	0.05	0.20	2.3	8
56	28	292	277	1.6	970	1,061	650	93	0.16	0.28	2.4	24
0	44	23	112	2.4	680	53	0	0	0.17	0.03	3.8	10
4	37	55	101	0.6	628	636	40	12	0.18	0.08	2.3	14
4	35	55	97	0.5	607	620	360	42	0.18	0.08	2.3	13
29	32	103	118	0.5	489	697	380	44	0.23	0.11	1.4	20
170	28	48	130	1.6	635	1,323	520	83	0.19	0.15	2.2	25
27	31	88	137	0.9	497	835	360	51	0.05	0.14	2.5	8
29	26	140	154	1.4	926	821	330	47	0.17	0.23	2.6	26
0	10	5	31	0.2	260	94	0	0	0.03	tr	0.8	8
0	12	37	74	1.4	564	2	2,650	265	0.08	0.19	1.0	12
0	20	64	86	3.4	505	12	54,040	5,404	0.06	0.13	0.9	10
0	1	4	3	0.1	42	4	tr	tr	tr	0.01	0.1	4
0	10	71	47	3.5	401	1,560	40	4	0.05	0.05	0.3	35
0	3	48	12	0.8	25	66	30	3	0.01	0.04	0.1	(¹)
0	7	34	33	8.1	386	297	160	16	0.67	1.04	3.6	3
0	2	54	27	1.5	307	43	3,690	369	0.04	0.10	0.4	15
0	7	245	101	6.4	839	126	14,740	1,474	0.17	0.42	0.9	18
0	10	277	91	2.9	566	163	14,790	1,479	0.11	0.32	0.8	23
0	7	272	94	4.9	740	[53]683	18,780	1,878	0.03	0.30	0.8	31
184	3	230	231	1.3	201	763	3,460	675	0.09	0.30	0.5	3
0	8	49	70	0.6	346	2	520	52	0.08	0.07	0.9	10
0	18	29	41	0.7	896	2	7,290	729	0.17	0.05	1.4	20

[53]With added salt; if none is added, sodium content is 58 mg.

Foods, approximate measures, units, and weight (weight of edible portion only)		Grams	Water (g)	Food energy (Calories)	Pro-tein (g)	Fat (g)	Fatty Acids		
							Satu-rated (g)	Mono-unsatu-rated (g)	Poly-unsatu-rated (g)
Vegetables and Vegetable Products (*cont.*)									
Sweet potatoes									
Cooked (raw, 5 by 2 in; about 2½ per lb)									
Baked in skin, peeled	1 potato	114	73	115	2	tr	tr	tr	0.1
Boiled, without skin	1 potato	151	73	160	2	tr	0.1	tr	0.2
Candied, 2½ by 2-in piece	1 piece	105	67	145	1	3	1.4	0.7	0.2
Canned									
Solid pack (mashed)	1 c	255	74	260	5	1	0.1	tr	0.2
Vacuum pack, piece 2¾ by 1 in	1 piece	40	76	35	1	tr	tr	tr	tr
Tomatoes									
Raw, 2⅗-in diam. (3 per 12 oz pkg.)	1 tomato	123	94	25	1	tr	tr	tr	0.1
Canned, solids and liquid	1 c	240	94	50	2	1	0.1	0.1	0.2
Tomato juice, canned	1 c	244	94	40	2	tr	tr	tr	0.1
Tomato products, canned									
Paste	1 c	262	74	220	10	2	0.3	0.4	0.9
Puree	1 c	250	87	105	4	tr	tr	tr	0.1
Sauce	1 c	245	89	75	3	tr	0.1	0.1	0.2
Turnips, cooked, diced	1 c	156	94	30	1	tr	tr	tr	0.1
Turnip greens, cooked, drained									
From raw (leaves and stems)	1 c	144	93	30	2	tr	0.1	tr	0.1
From frozen (chopped)	1 c	164	90	50	5	1	0.2	tr	0.3
Vegetable juice cocktail, canned	1 c	242	94	45	2	tr	tr	tr	0.1
Vegetables, mixed									
Canned, drained solids	1 c	163	87	75	4	tr	0.1	tr	0.2
Frozen, cooked, drained	1 c	182	83	105	5	tr	0.1	tr	0.1
Waterchestnuts, canned	1 c	140	86	70	1	tr	tr	tr	tr

[54]For regular pack; special dietary pack contains 31 mg sodium.
[55]With added salt; if none is added, sodium content is 24 mg.
[56]With no added salt; if salt is added, sodium content is 2,070 mg.

NUTRIENTS IN INDICATED QUANTITY

Cho-les-terol (mg)	Carbo-hydrate (g)	Calcium (mg)	Phos-phorus (mg)	Iron (mg)	Potas-sium (mg)	Sodium (mg)	Vitamin A value		Thiamin (mg)	Ribo-flavin (mg)	Niacin (mg)	Ascorbic acid (mg)
							IU	RE				
0	28	32	63	0.5	397	11	24,880	2,488	0.08	0.14	0.7	28
0	37	32	41	0.8	278	20	25,750	2,575	0.08	0.21	1.0	26
8	29	27	27	1.2	198	74	4,400	440	0.02	0.04	0.4	7
0	59	77	133	3.4	536	191	38,570	3,857	0.07	0.23	2.4	13
0	8	9	20	0.4	125	21	3,190	319	0.01	0.02	0.3	11
0	5	9	28	0.6	255	10	1,390	139	0.07	0.06	0.7	22
0	10	62	46	1.5	530	[54]391	1,450	145	0.11	0.07	1.8	36
0	10	22	46	1.4	537	[55]881	1,360	136	0.11	0.08	1.6	45
0	49	92	207	7.8	2,442	[56]170	6,470	647	0.41	0.50	8.4	111
0	25	38	100	2.3	1,050	[57]50	3,400	340	0.18	0.14	4.3	88
0	18	34	78	1.9	909	[58]1,482	2,400	240	0.16	0.14	2.8	32
0	8	34	30	0.3	211	78	0	0	0.04	0.04	0.5	18
0	6	197	42	1.2	292	42	7,920	792	0.06	0.10	0.6	39
0	8	249	56	3.2	367	25	13,080	1,308	0.09	0.12	0.8	36
0	11	27	41	1.0	467	883	2,830	283	0.10	0.07	1.8	67
0	15	44	68	1.7	474	243	18,990	1,899	0.08	0.08	0.9	8
0	24	46	93	1.5	308	64	7,780	778	0.13	0.22	1.5	6
0	17	6	27	1.2	165	11	10	1	0.02	0.03	0.5	2

[57]With no added salt; if salt is added, sodium content is 998 mg.
[58]With salt added.
From Nutritive Value of Foods, U.S. Department of Agriculture, Home and Garden Bulletin No. 72.

Appendix 6
Dietary Fiber Content and Composition of Typical Servings of U.S. Foods

Food	SERVING SIZE Household	Wt	Soluble HC	P	Total	Insoluble C	HC	P	KL	Total	Total
Fruits											
Category 1											
Apple pie filling, canned	⅛ of 9-in pie	71	0.1	0.1	0.2	0.2	0.1	0.1	tr	0.5	0.7
Cantaloupe, fresh	½ c cubed	80	tr	0.1	0.1	0.3	0.1	0.1	tr	0.5	0.6
Cherries, tart, canned	½ c	89	0.1	0.1	0.2	0.1	0.1	0.2	0.2	0.6	0.8
Cherry pie filling, canned	⅛ of 9-in pie	106	0.5	tr	0.5	0.1	0.1	0.1	0.1	0.4	0.9
Cranberry sauce, canned	¼ c	69	tr	0.1	0.2	0.2	0.1	tr	0.2	0.5	0.7
Fruit cocktail, canned	½ c	84	0.1	0.1	0.2	0.2	0.2	0.1	0.2	0.7	0.9
Grapes, fresh, black, red, Thompson (3)	10	50	tr	tr	tr	0.1	0.1	0.1	0.2	0.5	0.5
Honeydew melon, fresh	½ c cubed	85	tr	0.1	0.1	0.2	0.1	0.1	tr	0.4	0.5
Lemon, fresh, peeled	1 wedge (¼ fruit)	15	tr	tr	tr	0.1	tr	0.1	tr	0.2	0.2
Lemonade, with pulp	1 c	244	0.0	0.0	0.0	0.0	0.0	0.0	0.0	0.0	0.0
Orange, mandarin, canned	½ c	107	tr	tr	tr	tr	0.1	0.1	tr	0.2	0.3
Pineapple, canned or fresh (2)	2 slices (3-in diameter, 5⁄16-in thick) or ½ c diced	78	tr	tr	0.1	0.3	0.3	tr	tr	0.6	0.7
Plum, Friar, fresh, unpeeled	1 (2⅛-in diameter)	66	0.1	0.2	0.3	0.2	0.1	0.1	0.1	0.5	0.8
Plum, prune, fresh, unpeeled	1 (1½-in diameter)	28	tr	0.1	0.1	0.1	0.1	0.1	0.1	0.4	0.5
Plum, canned	*3*	*65*	*0.1*	*0.3*	*0.4*	*0.3*	*0.3*	*0.1*	*0.1*	*0.8*	*1.2*
Watermelon, fresh	½ c cubed	80	tr	tr	tr	0.1	0.1	0.1	tr	0.3	0.3
Category 2											
Applesauce, canned	½ c	122	0.1	0.2	0.3	0.5	0.4	0.2	0.1	1.2	1.5
Apricot, canned or fresh, unpeeled (2)	4 halves canned or 2 fresh	75	0.1	0.3	0.4	0.4	0.3	0.1	0.1	0.9	1.3
Apricot, dried	*4 halves*	*14*	*0.1*	*0.2*	*0.3*	*0.3*	*0.2*	*0.1*	*0.1*	*0.7*	*1.0*
Banana	1 (8¾-in long)	114	0.2	0.3	0.5	0.3	0.2	0.2	0.6	1.3	1.8
Grapefruit, fresh, with membrane (4)	½ (3 9⁄16 in diameter)	100	0.1	0.2	0.3	0.3	0.3	0.5	tr	1.1	1.4
Grapefruit, fresh, without membrane (3)	*½ (3 9⁄16 in diameter)*	*100*	*0.1*	*0.1*	*0.1*	*0.1*	*0.1*	*0.1*	*tr*	*0.3*	*0.4*
Kiwi fruit	1 medium	76	0.1	0.2	0.3	0.3	0.2	0.1	0.6	1.2	1.5

Food	SERVING SIZE			DIETARY FIBER COMPONENTS (G/SERVING FRESH WT)								
				Soluble			Insoluble					
	Household	Wt		HC	P	Total	C	HC	P	KL	Total	To-tal
Fruits (cont.)												
Nectarine, fresh, unpeeled	1 (2½-in diameter)	136		0.2	0.3	0.6	0.4	0.3	0.2	0.1	1.0	1.6
Papaya, fresh	½ c cubed	70		tr	tr	0.1	0.6	0.3	0.5	tr	1.4	1.5
Peach, canned or fresh, peeled (2)	2 halves canned or 1 fresh (2½-in diameter)	100		0.2	0.3	0.5	0.3	0.2	0.1	0.1	0.8	1.3
Peach, fresh, unpeeled	1	100		0.2	0.4	0.6	0.5	0.4	0.1	0.1	1.1	1.7
Raisins, seedless	¼ c	37		0.1	0.1	0.2	0.3	0.2	0.2	0.7	1.4	1.6
Rhubarb, fresh, cooked with sugar	½ c	135		tr	0.2	0.2	0.5	0.2	0.1	0.1	0.9	1.1
Strawberries, fresh or frozen (2)	½ c	75		0.1	0.2	0.3	0.3	0.2	0.1	0.4	1.0	1.3
Tangerine, fresh	1 medium (2⅜-in diameter)	84		0.1	0.2	0.3	0.4	0.3	0.4	0.1	1.2	1.5
Category 3												
Apple, unpeeled, Granny Smith, McIntosh, Red Delicious (3)	1 (2¾-in diameter)	138		0.1	0.3	0.4	1.0	0.8	0.5	0.3	2.6	3.0
Apple, fresh, peeled	*1 (2¾-in diameter)*	*128*		*tr*	*0.2*	*0.2*	*0.7*	*0.5*	*0.4*	*0.1*	*1.7*	*1.9*
Blueberries, fresh or frozen (2)	½ c	73		0.1	0.1	0.2	0.4	0.5	0.3	0.7	1.9	2.1
Orange, fresh, Florida, navel, Temple, Valencia (4)	1 (2⅝-in diameter)	131		0.2	0.3	0.5	0.5	0.5	0.6	0.1	1.7	2.2
Raspberries, red, fresh	½ c	62		0.1	0.2	0.3	0.4	0.4	0.1	1.4	2.3	2.6
Category 4												
Avocado (2)	½	95		0.4	0.8	1.2	1.3	0.9	0.3	0.1	2.6	3.8
Blackberries, frozen	½ c	76		0.1	0.3	0.4	0.9	0.9	0.4	2.3	4.5	4.9
Dates, dried	3	25		0.0	0.1	0.1	0.9	0.9	0.4	2.0	4.2	4.3
Figs, dried	3	62		0.2	0.3	0.5	1.0	0.8	1.1	1.5	4.4	4.9
Pear, Bartlett, fresh, unpeeled	1 (2½-in diameter, 3½-in long)	166		0.3	0.4	0.7	1.2	1.4	0.7	0.6	3.9	4.6
Pear, canned	*2 halves*	*102*		*0.1*	*0.2*	*0.3*	*0.6*	*0.6*	*0.1*	*0.2*	*1.5*	*1.8*
Prunes, dried	5	42		0.4	0.7	1.1	0.5	0.7	0.3	0.5	2.0	3.1
Vegetables												
Category 1												
Bamboo shoots, canned	½ c sliced	66		0.1	tr	0.1	0.5	0.3	tr	0.1	0.9	1.0
Bean sprouts, mung, raw, canned or cooked (3)	½ c	60		tr	tr	tr	0.3	0.3	0.1	0.1	0.8	0.8
Cabbage, Chinese, fresh	½ c shredded	38		tr	tr	tr	0.2	0.1	0.1	tr	0.4	0.4
Cabbage, green or red, raw (2)	½ c shredded	35		tr	tr	tr	0.3	0.2	0.2	tr	0.7	0.7
Cabbage, green, cooked	*½ c shredded*	*73*		*tr*	*0.1*	*0.1*	*0.6*	*0.5*	*0.4*	*0.1*	*1.6*	*1.7*
Cucumber, unpeeled	½ c	52		tr	tr	tr	0.2	0.1	0.1	0.1	0.5	0.5
Cucumber, peeled	½ c	70		tr	tr	tr	0.2	0.1	0.1	tr	0.4	0.4
Endive, fresh	½ c chopped	25		tr	tr	tr	0.2	0.1	0.3	0.1	0.7	0.7

Food	SERVING SIZE Household	Wt	Soluble HC	Soluble P	Soluble Total	Insoluble C	Insoluble HC	Insoluble P	Insoluble KL	Insoluble Total	To-tal
Vegetables (*cont.*)											
Escarole, fresh	½ c pieces	25	tr	tr	tr	0.1	0.1	0.1	0.1	0.4	0.4
Ketchup	2½ oz packets or 2 tbsp	14	tr	tr	0.1	0.1	tr	tr	tr	0.1	0.2
Lettuce, fresh, leaf, romaine or iceberg (4)	1 c shredded or 4 to 6 leaves	56	tr	tr	tr	0.3	0.1	0.2	0.1	0.7	0.7
Mushrooms, fresh	½ c pieces or 2	35	0.1	tr	0.1	0.1	tr	tr	0.1	0.2	0.3
Mushrooms, canned	¼ c	39	0.1	tr	0.1	0.7	0.1	0.1	tr	0.9	1.0
Olives, green with pimento, or black (2)	5 large	20	tr	tr	tr	0.1	0.1	0.1	0.1	0.4	0.4
Onion, green, raw	1 stalk (10½-in long) or 2 tbsp chopped	13	tr	tr	tr	0.1	0.1	0.1	tr	0.3	0.3
Pickle, dill or bread and butter chips (2)	2 slices (1½-in diameter, ¼-in thick)	13	tr	tr	tr	0.1	tr	tr	tr	0.1	0.1
Pickle relish	1 tbsp	15	tr	tr	tr	0.1	tr	tr	tr	0.2	0.2
Radish, red or white, fresh (2)	10 (¾- to 1-in diameter) or ½ c sliced	50	tr	tr	tr	0.3	0.1	0.2	tr	0.6	0.6
Soup, cream of mushroom, canned	1 c prepared	244	0.1	tr	0.2	0.2	0.1	tr	0.0	0.3	0.5
Soup, cream of tomato, canned	1 c prepared	244	0.1	0.1	0.2	0.4	0.2	tr	0.1	0.7	0.9
Squash, yellow zucchini, cooked or raw (2)	½ c sliced	80	tr	tr	0.1	0.2	0.2	0.2	tr	0.6	0.7
Tomato, canned or fresh (3)	½ c or 1 whole (2⅗-in diameter)	100	tr	0.1	0.2	0.3	0.1	0.1	0.1	0.6	0.8
Water chestnuts, canned	½ c sliced	70	tr	tr	tr	0.5	0.3	tr	tr	0.8	0.8
Category 2											
Asparagus, canned or fresh, cooked (2)	½ c or 6 spear (6½-in long, ½-in diameter)	100	0.2	0.1	0.3	0.5	0.5	0.2	0.2	1.4	1.7
Beans, green, or yellow wax, canned, cooked, or raw (5)	½ c	65	0.1	0.1	0.3	0.5	0.4	0.3	0.1	1.2	1.5
Beets, canned or fresh, cooked (2)	½ c sliced	85	0.2	0.3	0.5	0.6	0.4	0.2	tr	1.2	1.6
Beet greens, fresh, cooked	½ c (1-in pieces)	72	0.1	0.2	0.3	0.6	0.4	0.2	0.1	1.3	1.6
Bok choy, fresh, cooked	½ c shredded	85	tr	tr	0.1	0.4	0.2	0.4	0.1	1.1	1.2
Broccoli, cooked or raw or frozen (3)	2 stalks (4½- to 5-in long)	60	0.1	0.1	0.2	0.6	0.5	0.4	0.1	1.7	1.8
Carrot, canned, cooked, or raw (3)	1 (1⅛-in diameter, 7½-in long) or ½ c sliced	70	0.2	0.2	0.4	0.6	0.4	0.4	0.1	1.5	1.9
Cauliflower, cooked or raw (2)	½ c (1-in pieces)	55	0.1	0.1	0.2	0.4	0.4	0.2	tr	1.0	1.2
Celery, cooked or raw (2)	½ c diced or 3 stalks (5-in long, ¾-in diameter)	62	tr	tr	0.1	0.5	0.2	0.3	tr	1.0	1.1
Corn, creamed, canned	½ c	128	0.4	tr	0.4	0.4	0.6	tr	0.2	1.2	1.6

Food	SERVING SIZE		DIETARY FIBER COMPONENTS (G/SERVING FRESH WT)									
			Soluble			Insoluble					To-tal
	Household	Wt	HC	P	Total	C	HC	P	KL	Total	
Vegetables (*cont.*)											
Corn, whole kernel, canned or frozen (2)	½ c	82	0.1	tr	0.1	0.5	0.7	0.2	0.1	1.5	1.6
Corn, cooked on cob	*1 ear (3½-in diameter)*	*77*	*tr*	*tr*	*0.1*	*0.3*	*0.5*	*0.1*	*tr*	*0.9*	*1.0*
Eggplant, fresh, cooked	½ c cubed	48	0.1	0.2	0.2	0.4	0.3	0.1	0.1	0.9	1.2
Kohlrabi, fresh, cooked	½ c sliced	82	0.1	0.1	0.2	0.6	0.4	0.3	tr	1.4	1.6
Onion rings, frozen, cooked	7 rings	70	0.2	0.2	0.4	0.7	0.4	0.1	0.1	1.3	1.7
Onion, red, white, or yellow, raw or cooked (4)	½ c chopped	80	tr	0.1	0.1	0.4	0.4	0.3	tr	1.1	1.2
Pea pods, fresh, cooked	½ c	80	0.1	0.2	0.2	0.8	0.4	0.4	0.1	1.6	1.8
Pepper, green or chili, canned or raw (2)	1 green or 2 canned chilis or ½ c chopped	62	tr	0.1	0.1	0.3	0.2	0.1	0.1	0.8	0.9
Potato Chips	*1 bag*	*28*	*0.1*	*0.1*	*0.2*	*0.3*	*0.4*	*0.1*	*0.0*	*0.8*	*0.9*
Potato, french fries	10 strips	50	0.1	0.1	0.2	0.5	0.3	0.1	tr	0.9	1.1
Potato, red, peeled, boiled	1 (2½-in diameter)	135	0.2	0.2	0.4	0.4	0.3	0.1	tr	0.8	1.2
Potato, red, unpeeled, boiled	*1 (2½-in diameter)*	*150*	*0.3*	*0.3*	*0.6*	*0.8*	*0.6*	*0.2*	*0.2*	*1.8*	*2.4*
Potato, white, peeled, boiled, or baked without skin (6)	1 (2½-in diameter)	135	0.2	0.2	0.4	0.8	0.6	0.3	tr	1.7	2.1
Potato, white, unpeeled, baked	*1 (2½-in diameter)*	*170*	*0.6*	*0.4*	*1.0*	*1.7*	*0.8*	*0.2*	*0.5*	*3.1*	*4.1*
Potato hash, with corned beef, canned	1 c	225	0.5	0.2	0.7	0.9	0.2	0.1	0.1	1.3	2.0
Potato salad, American, peeled	½ c	125	0.2	0.2	0.4	0.6	0.3	0.1	tr	1.1	1.5
Potato, scalloped, frozen, cooked	*½ c*	*122*	*0.1*	*0.1*	*0.2*	*0.4*	*0.2*	*0.1*	*tr*	*0.7*	*0.9*
Rutabaga, fresh, cooked	½ c cubed	85	0.1	0.2	0.3	0.6	0.4	0.5	0.1	1.6	1.9
Sauerkraut, canned	½ c	73	0.1	0.1	0.2	0.7	0.4	0.5	tr	1.7	1.9
Soup, vegetable and beef, canned	1 c prepared	251	0.3	0.1	0.4	0.7	0.2	0.1	0.2	1.1	1.6
Squash, acorn or butternut, cooked (2)	½ c cubed	102	0.1	0.3	0.3	0.9	0.3	0.3	tr	1.6	1.9
Sweet potato, canned or baked, peeled (2)	½ c or 1 whole (5-in long, 2-in diameter)	106	0.2	0.3	0.5	0.8	0.4	0.2	0.1	1.4	1.9
Category 3											
Collard, frozen, cooked	½ c chopped	85	0.1	0.1	0.2	1.0	0.7	0.8	0.2	2.7	2.9
Kale, fresh, cooked	½ c	65	0.1	0.2	0.3	0.7	0.7	0.7	0.2	2.2	2.5
Mustard greens, frozen, cooked	½ c chopped	75	tr	0.2	0.2	0.8	0.5	0.6	0.1	2.0	2.2
Okra, frozen, cooked	½ c sliced	92	0.3	0.3	0.6	0.4	0.3	0.2	0.6	1.5	2.1
Parsnip, fresh, cooked	½ c sliced	78	0.2	0.4	0.6	0.9	0.9	0.5	0.1	2.4	3.0
Soup, vegetarian vegetable, canned	1 c prepared	241	0.3	0.2	0.6	0.9	0.4	0.1	0.1	1.6	2.1
Spaghetti sauce, meatless	½ c	125	0.1	0.4	0.6	0.9	0.4	0.3	0.8	2.4	3.0

Food	SERVING SIZE Household	Wt	Soluble HC	Soluble P	Soluble Total	Insoluble C	Insoluble HC	Insoluble P	Insoluble KL	Insoluble Total	To-tal
Vegetables (*cont.*)											
Spinach, canned, cooked or raw (3)	½ c canned or cooked, or 2 c raw	100	0.1	0.2	0.3	0.8	0.5	0.3	0.3	2.0	2.3
Swiss chard, fresh, cooked	½ c chopped	88	0.1	0.2	0.3	0.7	0.5	0.3	0.2	1.8	2.1
Turnip greens, frozen	½ c chopped	82	tr	0.1	0.1	0.7	0.5	0.6	0.1	1.9	2.1
Category 4											
Artichoke, fresh, cooked	1 medium	120	3.0	0.5	3.5	1.2	1.0	0.7	0.1	2.9	6.4
Brussels sprout, frozen, cooked	½ c	78	0.1	0.3	0.4	1.0	1.2	0.6	0.1	2.8	3.2
Pumpkin, canned	½ c	122	0.2	0.5	0.6	1.8	0.4	0.5	0.2	2.9	3.5
Grain Products											
Category 1											
Biscuit, baking powder (2)	1 (2-in diameter, 1¼-in high)	28	0.1	tr	0.1	0.1	0.2	tr	tr	0.4	0.5
Bread, French	2 small slices (2½-in wide, 2-in high, ½-in thick)	30	0.2	tr	0.2	0.3	0.2	tr	tr	0.6	0.8
Bread, raisin without icing	1 slice	25	0.1	tr	0.2	0.1	0.1	tr	0.2	0.5	0.7
Bread, white or Italian (4)	1 slice	25	0.2	tr	0.2	0.2	0.2	tr	0.2	0.6	0.8
Bread, rye	1 slice	25	0.2	tr	0.2	0.1	0.3	tr	0.1	0.5	0.7
Brownie, plain	1 (1¾-in square)	20	0.1	tr	0.1	tr	0.1	tr	0.2	0.3	0.4
Brownie, with nuts	1 (1¾-in square)	20	0.1	tr	0.1	0.1	0.1	tr	0.3	0.5	0.6
Bun, hamburger	1	40	0.3	tr	0.3	0.3	0.3	tr	0.1	0.7	1.0
Cake, pound or sponge (3)	1/15 of 1-lb loaf	30	0.1	tr	0.1	0.1	0.1	tr	0.1	0.2	0.4
Cake, gingerbread	1 piece (2¾-in square)	63	0.2	tr	0.2	0.2	0.3	tr	0.2	0.6	0.9
Cake, coffee (2)	⅛ of 8-in round cake	58	0.2	tr	0.2	0.1	0.3	tr	0.1	0.5	0.8
Cake, white or yellow (4)	3-in square sheet cake or 1/12 of 9-in 2-layer cake	80	0.3	tr	0.3	0.2	0.2	tr	0.1	0.5	0.8
Cake, coconut, frozen	1/10 of 6-in square, 3-layer cake	48	0.1	tr	0.1	tr	0.3	tr	tr	0.3	0.4
Cake, Twinkies	1 piece	42	0.1	tr	0.1	0.1	0.1	tr	tr	0.2	0.3
Cereal, Corn Chex	1 c	28	tr	tr	tr	0.3	0.1	tr	0.4	0.8	0.8
Cereal, Total, cornflakes	1 c	28	tr	0.0	tr	0.3	0.1	tr	0.5	0.8	0.9
Cereal, Golden Grahams	1 c	28	0.1	tr	0.1	0.3	0.3	tr	0.1	0.7	0.8
Cereal, puffed rice	1 c	14	tr	0.0	tr	tr	tr	tr	0.1	0.1	0.2
Cereal, puffed wheat	1 c	14	0.3	tr	0.3	0.2	0.3	tr	0.1	0.6	0.9
Cereal, Rice Krispies	1 c	28	0.1	tr	0.1	0.1	0.1	tr	0.2	0.4	0.5
Cereal, Special K	1 c	28	tr	tr	0.1	0.2	0.2	tr	0.2	0.7	0.7
Cereal, Smacks	¾ c	28	0.2	tr	0.2	0.2	0.2	tr	tr	0.5	0.7
Cereal, sugar-frosted cornflakes	¾ c	28	tr	tr	tr	0.3	0.1	tr	0.1	0.5	0.5
Cookies, gingersnap	4	28	0.2	tr	0.2	0.1	0.2	0.0	0.1	0.4	0.5

Food	SERVING SIZE		DIETARY FIBER COMPONENTS (G/SERVING FRESH WT)								
			Soluble			Insoluble					
	Household	Wt	HC	P	Total	C	HC	P	KL	Total	To-tal
Grain Products (*cont.*)											
Cookies, oatmeal (2)	1 large	28	0.1	tr	0.3	0.1	0.2	tr	0.2	0.6	0.9
Cookies, oatmeal and raisin (2)	2	24	0.1	tr	0.3	0.1	0.2	tr	0.2	0.6	1.0
Cookies, peanut	1 large	26	0.1	tr	0.1	0.2	0.3	0.1	tr	0.5	0.6
Cookies, plain sugar	1	20	0.1	0.0	0.1	tr	0.1	tr	tr	0.1	0.2
Cookies, macaroon	2	30	0.1	tr	0.1	0.1	0.3	tr	tr	0.3	0.5
Cookies, shortbread (2)	4	30	0.2	tr	0.2	0.1	0.2	tr	0.0	0.3	0.4
Cookies, sugar wafer, cream filled	8	28	0.1	tr	0.1	0.1	0.1	tr	tr	0.2	0.3
Crackers, cheese, snack	13 small	14	0.1	tr	0.1	0.1	0.1	tr	tr	0.2	0.3
Crackers, graham	2 pieces (2½-in square)	14	0.1	tr	o.1	0.1	0.1	tr	0.1	0.3	0.4
Crackers, peanut butter and cheese squares	2 sandwiches	14	0.1	tr	0.1	0.2	0.2	tr	0.1	0.4	0.5
Crackers, Ritz	4 crackers	14	0.1	0.0	0.1	tr	0.1	0.0	tr	0.2	0.3
Crackers, saltine	4	11	0.1	tr	0.1	0.1	0.1	tr	0.1	0.2	0.3
Crackers, Waverly	4	14	0.1	tr	0.1	0.1	0.1	tr	tr	0.2	0.3
Croutons, seasoned	¼ c	8	0.1	0.0	0.1	0.1	0.1	0.0	tr	0.1	0.2
Doughnut, jelly	1	65	0.3	tr	0.3	0.1	0.2	tr	0.1	0.4	0.7
Doughnut, plain (2)	1	25	0.1	tr	0.1	0.1	0.1	tr	tr	0.2	0.3
Flour, white, wheat, all purpose	1 tbsp	8	0.1	tr	0.1	tr	0.1	0.0	tr	0.2	0.2
Hominy, white, cooked	½ c	80	tr	tr	tr	0.4	0.1	tr	tr	0.5	0.5
Ice cream cone, Comet cup	1	5	tr	0.0	tr	tr	0.1	0.0	tr	0.1	0.1
Muffin, blueberry (2)	1 small	40	0.2	tr	0.2	0.2	0.2	tr	0.3	0.6	0.8
Muffin, plain (2)	1 small	40	0.2	tr	0.2	0.1	0.2	tr	0.1	0.4	0.6
Pancake	2 (4-in diameter)	54	0.2	tr	0.2	0.3	0.3	tr	0.1	0.7	0.8
Pancake, buckwheat	*2 (4-in diameter)*	*54*	*0.3*	*tr*	*0.3*	*0.8*	*0.7*	*tr*	*0.9*	*2.3*	*2.6*
Piecrust (3)	⅛ of 9-in pie	23	0.1	tr	0.1	0.1	0.2	tr	0.1	0.4	0.5
Rice, medium grain, regular, cooked	½ c	102	tr	tr	tr	0.1	0.1	tr	0.1	0.3	0.4
Roll, dinner (3)	1 small	28	0.3	tr	0.3	0.2	0.2	tr	0.1	0.5	0.8
Roll, hard	1 small	25	0.2	0.0	0.2	0.1	0.2	tr	0.3	0.6	0.8
Taco shell	1	11	tr	tr	tr	0.3	0.3	tr	0.1	0.7	0.7
Tortilla, flour	1	30	0.1	0.0	0.1	0.1	0.1	0.0	0.1	0.3	0.4
Waffle (3)	1 (4½-in square)	50	0.2	tr	0.2	0.1	0.2	tr	0.2	0.5	0.7
Category 2											
Cake, devil's food	3-in square sheet cake or ¹⁄₁₂ of 9-in 2-layer cake	81	0.2	0.1	0.2	0.3	0.2	0.1	0.8	1.3	1.6
Cereal, Product 19	¾ c	28	0.1	tr	0.1	0.5	0.4	0.1	0.4	1.4	1.5
Cereal, Cream of Wheat, quick, cooked	¾ c	179	0.3	tr	0.3	0.5	0.4	tr	0.2	1.1	1.4
Cereal, cornflakes	1 c	28	0.1	tr	0.1	0.6	0.3	tr	0.2	1.1	1.2
Cereal, Grapenuts	¼ c	28	0.4	tr	0.4	0.4	0.9	tr	0.2	1.6	2.0

Food	SERVING SIZE Household	Wt	Soluble HC	Soluble P	Soluble Total	Insoluble C	Insoluble HC	Insoluble P	Insoluble KL	Insoluble Total	To-tal
Grain Products (*cont.*)											
Cereal, granola	¼ c	28	0.2	tr	0.5	0.3	0.9	0.1	0.1	1.4	1.9
Cookies, date (2)	2	30	0.1	tr	0.1	0.2	0.2	0.1	0.5	1.0	1.1
Cookies, fig	2	30	0.2	0.2	0.4	0.2	0.2	0.3	0.3	1.0	1.4
Crackers, Triscuits	3	14	0.1	tr	0.1	0.4	0.7	tr	0.1	1.2	1.3
Cream puff, fresh, without filling	1	50	0.2	tr	0.2	0.3	0.4	0.0	0.3	1.0	1.2
Doughnut, glazed	1	64	0.3	tr	0.3	0.2	0.3	tr	0.3	0.8	1.1
Éclair, frozen	1	100	0.7	tr	0.7	0.2	0.2	tr	0.5	1.0	1.7
Hush puppies, fresh	3	45	0.2	tr	0.2	0.3	0.5	0.1	0.2	1.1	1.3
Muffin, English	1	57	0.3	tr	0.3	0.5	0.5	tr	0.4	1.3	1.7
Noodles, chow mein	1 c	45	0.4	tr	0.4	0.4	0.6	tr	tr	1.1	1.5
Pasta, macaroni, spaghetti, shells, egg noodles, or vermicelli (8)	1 c	130	0.4	tr	0.4	0.5	0.7	tr	0.3	1.6	2.0
Pie, apple	⅛ of 9-in pie	118	0.5	0.1	0.5	0.3	0.4	0.1	0.1	0.9	1.5
Pie, cherry	⅛ of 9-in pie	118	0.6	tr	0.6	0.2	0.2	0.1	0.1	0.6	1.2
Pie, pecan	⅛ of 9-in pie	103	0.2	tr	0.3	0.2	0.4	0.1	0.2	0.9	1.2
Pie, rhubarb	⅛ of 9-in pie	118	0.3	0.2	0.6	0.6	0.4	0.1	0.1	1.1	1.7
Pie, strawberry	⅛ of 9-in pie	93	0.4	0.1	0.5	0.2	0.2	tr	0.2	0.6	1.1
Roll, submarine	½ of 11½-in roll	68	0.5	tr	0.5	0.3	0.5	tr	0.6	1.4	1.9
Roll, sweetened, cinnamon (2)	1	56	0.3	tr	0.3	0.3	0.3	tr	0.2	0.8	1.1
Roll, sweetened, with raisins	1	53	0.3	tr	0.3	0.2	0.3	tr	0.3	0.8	1.1
Roll, sweetened, with nuts (2)	1	73	0.4	tr	0.4	0.4	0.4	0.1	0.2	1.0	1.4
Stuffing, cornbread	½ c	90	0.2	tr	0.2	0.5	0.2	0.1	0.1	0.9	1.1
Category 3											
Bread, whole wheat	1 slice	28	0.3	tr	0.3	0.6	1.2	tr	0.4	2.2	2.5
Cereal, Frosted Mini Wheats	4 biscuits	31	0.2	0.0	0.2	0.8	1.2	0.1	0.3	2.3	2.5
Cereal, Grape Nut Flakes	⅛ c	28	0.4	tr	0.4	0.6	1.0	tr	0.2	1.9	2.3
Cereal, Life	⅔ c	28	0.2	tr	0.7	0.2	0.6	tr	0.5	1.4	2.2
Cereal, oatmeal, cooked	¾ c	175	0.2	tr	1.2	0.2	0.5	tr	0.6	1.5	2.7
Cereal, shredded wheat	1 large	24	0.2	tr	0.3	0.8	1.4	tr	0.2	2.4	2.7
Cereal, Wheat Chex	⅔ c	28	0.5	tr	0.5	0.9	1.2	0.1	0.1	2.3	2.8
Cornbread	1 piece (2½-in square)	78	0.2	tr	0.2	1.0	0.8	tr	0.3	2.1	2.3
Muffin, wheat bran, home prepared	1 small	40	0.3	tr	0.3	0.6	1.1	tr	0.3	2.0	2.3
Muffin, wheat bran commercial	1 small	40	0.2	tr	0.2	0.5	0.8	P	0.2	1.5	1.8
Category 4											
Cereal, 40% bran flakes	¾ c	28	0.5	tr	0.6	1.3	3.0	0.1	0.4	4.9	5.5
Cereal, All Bran	⅓ c	28	0.7	tr	0.7	2.0	4.4	0.2	0.8	7.4	8.1
Cereal, oat bran, uncooked	⅓ c	31	0.5	tr	2.0	0.3	1.1	0.1	1.1	3.3	5.3
Cereal, Wheaties	1 c	28	0.5	tr	0.5	0.8	1.4	0.1	0.4	2.7	3.2

| Food | SERVING SIZE | | DIETARY FIBER COMPONENTS (G/SERVING FRESH WT) | | | | | | | | |
| | | | Soluble | | | Insoluble | | | | | To-tal |
	Household	Wt	HC	P	Total	C	HC	P	KL	Total	
Grain Products (*cont.*)											
Lasagna, with meat sauce, frozen	½ of package	298	0.4	0.3	0.7	1.4	0.9	0.3	0.8	3.4	4.1
Wheat germ	¼ c	28	0.3	tr	0.3	1.0	2.1	0.2	0.3	3.6	3.9
Legumes											
Category 3											
Beans, black, dry, cooked	½ c	86	0.1	tr	0.1	1.2	0.9	0.2	0.4	2.7	2.8
Lentils, dry, cooked	½ c	99	0.1	tr	0.1	1.5	0.9	0.2	0.2	2.8	2.9
Peas, black-eyed, dry, cooked	½ c	82	0.1	0.1	0.2	1.4	0.6	0.3	0.3	2.6	2.8
Peas, crowder, canned	½ c	86	0.3	0.1	0.4	0.9	0.5	0.2	0.3	1.9	2.3
Peas, green, canned, or frozen (3)	½ c	85	0.1	0.1	0.3	1.9	0.5	0.3	0.1	2.8	3.0
Peas, prepared pea soup	1 c	244	0.7	0.1	0.8	1.2	0.4	0.2	0.4	2.2	3.0
Category 4											
Baked beans, canned with pork	½ c	126	1.3	0.4	1.7	2.0	1.1	0.4	0.3	3.8	5.5
Beans, great northern, dry, cooked	½ c	88	0.2	0.1	0.3	5.1	2.0	0.6	0.1	7.9	8.2
Beans, lima, canned or dry, cooked (3)	½ c	87	0.3	0.1	0.5	1.5	1.1	0.2	0.1	2.9	3.4
Beans, kidney, canned	½ c	88	0.8	0.2	1.0	1.9	1.0	0.3	0.3	3.5	4.5
Beans, navy, dry, canned	½ c	91	0.2	0.1	0.2	1.2	1.2	0.3	0.1	2.9	3.1
Peas, pigeon, canned	½ c	77	0.1	0.1	0.2	1.9	0.6	0.2	0.8	3.5	3.7
Nuts and Seeds											
Category 1											
Coconut, shredded, sweetened	2 tbsp	9	tr	tr	tr	0.1	0.5	tr	0.0	0.6	0.6
Popcorn, white or yellow, popped (2)	1 c	6	tr	tr	tr	0.2	0.4	tr	0.1	0.8	0.8
Pumpkin seeds	1 tbsp	5	tr	tr	tr	0.2	0.1	tr	0.4	0.7	0.8
Category 2											
Cashews, roasted	18 medium	28	tr	tr	0.1	0.4	0.3	0.2	0.3	1.2	1.3
Peanut butter, chunky	2 tbsp	32	tr	tr	0.1	0.5	0.6	0.3	0.1	1.5	1.6
Peanuts, Spanish or Virginia (2)	30 to 40 whole	28	tr	tr	0.1	0.6	0.8	0.4	0.1	1.9	1.9
Pecans	15 halves	28	0.1	tr	0.1	0.4	0.5	0.3	0.4	1.6	1.7
Walnuts, English	14 halves	28	tr	tr	tr	0.3	0.2	0.2	0.2	1.0	1.1
Category 3											
Almonds, roasted, with skin	22 whole	28	tr	tr	0.1	0.5	0.9	0.5	0.5	2.4	2.5

From Marlette JA, Cheung T: Database and quick methods of assessing typical dietary fiber intakes using data for 228 commonly consumed foods. JADA, October 1997; 97(10):1142–1147.

Appendix 7
Nutritive Value of Selected Ethnic Foods

Food	Quantity	Grams per Serving	Kcal	Pro (g)	Fat (g)	Cho (g)	Na (mg)	K (mg)	Chol (mg)	Sat Fatty Acids (g)	Mono Fatty Acids (g)	Poly Fatty Acids (g)	Total Dietary Fiber (g)
Navajo													
Starch/bread													
Blue corn mush with ash*	¾ c	180	94	2.5	0.5	21.2	32	288	0	—	—	—	—
Flour tortilla, 8-in diameter†‡	¼	34	87	2.5	0.2	19.3	211	29	0	—	—	—	—
Steamed corn hominy, ck†	½ c	115	70	1.8	1.0	13.3	18	108	0	—	—	—	—
Lean meat													
Mutton, flesh, lean only, ck without added fat§	1 oz	28	58	7.9	2.7¶	0	21	96	26	1.0	1.2	0.2	0
High-fat meat													
Mutton, flesh, lean and fat, ck without added fat§	1 oz	28	82	6.7	5.9¶	0	20	87	27	2.5	2.5	0.4	0
Fat													
Piñon nuts in shell	1 tbsp (25 nuts)	9	60	1.3	5.8	0.7	7	67	0	0.8	2.1	2.3	0.4
Alaskan Native													
Starch/bread													
Pilot bread, 4-in diameter	1	25	104	2.1	2.0	18.2	142	57	—	—	—	—	—
Lean meats													
Caribou, ck	1 oz	28	47	8.3	1.2	0	17	87	31	0.5	0.4	0.2	—
Gumboots (leathery chiton)	2 oz	56	46	9.6	0.9	0	—	—	—	—	—	—	—
Halibut, ck	1 oz	28	39	7.5	0.8	0	20	164	12	0.1	0.3	0.3	—
Herring eggs, plain	0.5 c	85	48	8.2	0.8	3.7	52	—	—	—	—	—	—
Moose, ck	1 oz	28	38	8.2	0.3	0	19	94	22	0.1	0.1	0.1	—
Pike, ck	1 oz	28	33	6.9	0.2	0	13	93	14	0.04	0.1	0.1	—
Seal meat, raw	1 oz	28	41	8.9	0.6	0	—	—	—	0.1	0.1	—	—
Venison, ck	1 oz	28	44	8.5	0.9	0	15	94	31	0.4	0.3	0.2	—
Walrus, raw	1 oz	28	56	5.4	3.9	0	—	—	22	0.7	2.4	0.7	—
Whale, bowhead, raw	1 oz	28	37	7.3	0.7	0	17	—	—	0.2	0.4	0.1	—
Medium-fat meats													
Dried fish (king salmon)	0.5 oz	14	60	7.1	5.3	0	—	—	—	—	—	0.1	—
Muskrat, ck	1 oz	28	67	8.5	3.3	0	27	91	—	—	—	0.7	—
Salmon, sockeye, ck	1 oz	28	60	7.6	3.1	0	18	105	24	0.5	1.5	0.7	—

	Serving size												
High-fat meat													
Hooligan (eulachon), smoked	1 oz	28	86	5.7	6.9	0	—	—	—	—	—	—	—
High-fat meat + 1 fat													
Muktuk, skin and fat	1 × 1 × 2 in	38	138	8	12	0	—	—	—	—	—	—	—
Vegetables													
Fiddlehead fern, raw	1 c	180	34	3.2	0.2	5.0	84	—	—	0.1	0.1	—	0.8
Seaweed, dried black	1 c	13	39	3.7	0.3	5.3	40	—	—	0.4	0.1	—	3.5
Willow greens, ck	0.5 c	28	28	1.7	0.4	5.8	—	—	—	0.4	0.2	—	3.5
Sour dock, ck	0.5 c	55	19	1.3	0.4	3.6	—	—	—	0.8	1.3	—	0.9
Fruits													
Highbush cranberries	1.25 c	119	58	0.5	0.2	15	1	8	0	0	—	—	—
Huckleberries	1 c	150	56	0.6	0.2	13	15	—	—	—	—	—	—
Salmonberries	1.25 c	181	55	1.3	0.1	13	52	—	—	—	—	—	—
Fat													
Seal oil	1 tsp	5	45	0	5	0	—	—	8	0.6	3.0	1.4	—
Free													
Beach asparagus	1 c	55	15	1	0.2	2.4	23	—	—	—	—	—	—
Mexican American													
Starch/bread													
Bolillo, large, 4.5–5-in long	¼	30	87	2.8	0.9	16.6	174	27	0	—	—	—	0.8
Frijoles cocidos	⅓ c	56	77	4.6	0.3	14.4	1	262	0	0.1	0.1	0.1	3.5
Frijoles refritos, cn	⅓ c	83	89	5.2	0.9	15.9	365	338	0	0.4	0.4	0.1	3.5
Tortilla, corn, 7.5 in across, ready to bake/fry	1	30	69	1.7	0.8	12.8	7	46	0	0.1	0.2	0.5	0.9
Tortilla, flour, 7 in across, ready to bake/fry (Starch/bread 1½)	1	40	118	3.5	2.7	22	164	52	0	0.8	1.3	0.8	0.9
Tortilla, flour, 9 in across, ready to bake/fry	⅓	22	65	1.9	1.5	12	90	28.7	0	0.4	0.7	0.4	0.5
Starch/bread prepared with fat													
Taco shell, 5 in across (corn tortilla, ready to use)	2	24	109	2.0	4.7	15.8	42	58	0	0.7	2.6	1.0	1.2
Lean meat													
Menudo	½ c	—	55	8	1.5	1.8	431	24.5	25	—	—	—	—
Medium-fat meat													
Queso fresco	2 oz or ¼ c	57	80	6.4	4.6	3.0	72	72	18	2.8	1.3	0.1	0
High-fat meat													
Chorizo (High-fat meat 1 + Fat 1)	1 oz	28.5	132	7.2	11.5	—	(367)	(58)	(30)	4.3	5.7	1.0	0
Vegetable													
Chayote, boiled, drained	½ c	80	19	0.5	0.4	4.1	1	138	0	(0)	(0)	(0.2)	(0.6)
Jicama, ck	½ c	(50)	23	0.6	0	5.2	3	90	0	0	0	0	—
Jicama, raw	½ c	60	23	0.8	0.1	5.2	4	105	0	0	0	0	0.4
Nopales, raw	½ c	59	24	0.4	0.3	5.6	3	130	0	0.1	0.1	0.1	2.1

Table continued on following page

Food	Quantity	Grams per Serving	Kcal	Pro (g)	Fat (g)	Cho (g)	Na (mg)	K (mg)	Chol (mg)	Sat Fatty Acids (g)	Mono Fatty Acids (g)	Poly Fatty Acids (g)	Total Dietary Fiber (g)
Mexican American (*cont.*)													
Fruit													
Mango, raw	½ small	104	68	0.5	0.3	17.6	2	161	0	0	0	0	1.5
Papaya, raw	1 c	140	54	0.9	0.2	13.7	4	359	0	0	0	0	1.7
Fat													
Avocado	⅛ medium	25	40	0.5	3.8	1.9	3	150	0	0.6	2.4	0.5	0.5
Free													
Cilantro	¼ c	4	1	0	0	0	1	22	0	0	0	0	—
Jalapeño chili, cn, s + l, chopped	½ c	68	17	0.5	0.4	3.3	995	92	0	(0)	(0)	(0.2)	(1.2)
Salsa de chile	2 tbsp	34	13	0.3	0	3.1	167	46	0	0	0	0	0.7
Verdolagas, ck	½ c	58	10	0.9	0.1	2.1	26	283	0	0	0	0	(1.2)
Occasional													
Pan dulce, 4.5 in across (no frosting or fruit) (Starch/bread 4 + Fat 1)	1	100	384	9.1	11.6	60.8	389	124	?	?	?	?	?
Chinese American													
Starch/bread													
Cellophane or mung bean noodles, ck	¾ c	93	73	—	—	18	—	—	—	—	—	—	—
Ginkgo seeds, cn	½ c	76	86	1.8	1.2	17.1	238	139	—	0.24	0.46	0.46	—
Lotus root, ¼-in thick, 2½-in diameter, raw	10 slices	81	45	2.1	0.1	14	33	450	—	—	—	—	—
Mung beans or green gram beans, ck	⅓ c	67	71	4.7	0.3	12.7	1	177	—	0.08	0.36	0.08	—
Red beans, ck	⅓ c	58	61	4.1	0.3	11.0	0.9	153	—	0.08	0.36	0.08	—
Rice congee or soup	¾ c	180	69	1.5	—	15	—	20	—	—	—	—	—
Rice noodles, fresh	½ c	49	99	1.3	0.1	23	—	—	—	—	—	—	—
Rice vermicelli, ck	½ c	64	56	1	0	13	—	—	—	—	—	—	—
Taro, ck	⅓ c	44	62	0.2	0.1	15	7	210	—	—	—	—	—
Lean meat or substitute													
Beef jerky, 3½-in × 1-in piece	½ oz	14	44	6.98	1.3	0.7	(610)	—	—	—	—	—	—
Dried scallop, large	1	13	44	8.6	0.3	1.1	—	205	—	—	—	—	—
Dried shrimp, medium	1 tbsp or 10 shrimp	11	40	6.9	0.4	1.7	—	—	—	—	—	—	—
Soybeans, ck	3 tbsp	32	56	5.4	3	3.2	0	166	0	0.42	0.64	1.62	—
Squid, raw	2 oz	57	52	8.8	0.8	1.8	26	140	132	0.20	0.06	0.24	—
Tripe, beef, raw	2 oz	57	56	8.2	2.2	0	26	154	54	1.16	0.74	0.04	—

	Serving												
Medium-fat meat or substitute													
Beef tongue	1 oz	28	81	6.3	5.9	0.1	17	51	30	2.54	2.70	0.22	—
Tofu or soybean curd, 2½ × 2¾ × 1 in	4 oz or ½ c	124	94	10	5.9	2.3	9	150	0	0.86	1.31	3.35	1.5
High-fat meat or substitute													
Salted duck egg	1 whole	68	137	9.8	10.3	0.5	—	171	—	—	—	—	—
Thousand-year-old or preserved limed duck egg	1 whole	63	114	8.8	7.3	2.6	—	323	—	—	—	—	—
High-fat meat + 1 fat													
Chinese sausage (pork and spices)	1 (2 oz)	56	199	11.9	16.4	3.7	493	—	—	6.1	7.5	1.8	—
Chinese sausage (pork, liver, and spices)	1 (2 oz)	56	205	14.9	15.7	—	560	—	—	5.8	7.2	1.7	—
Vegetable													
Amaranth or Chinese spinach, ck	½ c	61	14	1.4	0.1	2.7	14	423	—	—	—	—	—
Arrowheads, or fresh corms, large, 3½-in diameter, raw	1	25	25	1.2	0.2	5.0	6	470	—	—	—	—	—
Baby corn, cn	½ c	64	13	1.9	0.3	1.9	730	117	—	—	—	—	—
Bamboo shoots, cn	½ c	66	25	2.3	0.5	4.2	9	104	—	—	—	—	—
Bitter melon or bitter gourd, raw	1 c	146	28	1.2	0.2	6.6	6	394	—	—	—	—	—
Chayote, raw	1 c	124	32	1.2	0.4	7.2	4	198	—	—	—	—	—
Chinese celery, raw	1 c	120	26	1.6	0.4	5.0	116	392	—	—	—	—	—
Chinese eggplant, white, ck	½ c	87	20	0.9	0.1	4.9	—	—	—	—	—	—	—
Chinese eggplant, purple, ck	½ c	72	17	0.7	0.1	4.0	—	—	—	—	—	—	—
Chinese or black mushrooms, medium, dried	2	8	22	0.7	0.1	5.6	1	115	—	—	—	—	—
Hairy melon or hairy cucumber, raw	2	156	22	1.0	—	5.4	—	—	—	—	—	—	—
Leeks, ck	1 c	52	16	0.4	0.1	4.0	6	46	—	—	—	—	—
Luffa, angled, raw	½ c	178	30	1.2	0.2	7.2	2	252	—	—	—	—	—
Luffa, smooth or sponge, raw	1 c	178	34	2.0	0.4	8.0	6	274	—	—	—	—	—
Mung bean sprouts, seed attached, raw	1 c	104	32	3.2	0.2	6.2	6	144	—	—	—	—	—
Mung bean sprouts, seed attached, ck	½ c	62	13	1.3	0.1	2.6	6	63	—	—	—	—	—
Mustard greens, ck	½ c	70	11	1.6	0.2	1.5	11	141	—	—	—	—	—
Peapods or sugar peas, ck	½ c	80	34	2.6	0.2	5.6	3	192	—	—	—	—	—
Soybean sprouts, seed attached, raw	½ c	35	45	4.6	2.4	3.9	5	169	—	0.25	0.26	1.30	—

Table continued on following page

563

Chinese American (cont.)

Food	Quantity	Grams per Serving	Kcal	Pro (g)	Fat (g)	Cho (g)	Na (mg)	K (mg)	Chol (mg)	Sat Fatty Acids (g)	Mono Fatty Acids (g)	Poly Fatty Acids (g)	Total Dietary Fiber (g)
Soybean sprouts, seed attached, ck	½ c	47	38	4.0	2.1	3.1	10	334	—	0.45	0.47	2.32	—
Straw mushroms, cn	½ c	66	20	1.5	0.1	3.8	172	47	—	—	—	—	—
Turnip, raw	1 c	110	36	1.2	0.2	8.0	88	248	—	—	—	—	—
Water chestnuts, 1¼–2-in diameter, raw	4 whole	36	38	0.5	0	8.6	5	210	—	—	—	—	—
Water chestnuts, cn (s + l)	½ c	70	35	0.6	0.0	8.7	6	82	—	—	—	—	(1.3)
Winter melon or waxed gourd, raw	1 c	132	17	0.5	0.3	4.0	8	14.7	—	—	—	—	—
Yard-long beans, raw	1 c	90	44	2.6	0.4	7.6	4	218	—	—	—	—	—
Yard-long beans, ck	½ c	52	24	1.3	—	4.8	2	151	—	—	—	—	—
Fruit													
Carambola or star fruit, medium, raw	1½	191	63	1.0	0.6	14.8	2.5	230	—	—	—	—	—
Chinese banana, dwarf, raw	1	100	72	1.8	0.2	18.0	18	435	—	—	—	—	—
Guava, medium, raw	1½	135	69	1.2	0.9	15.9	3	384	—	—	—	—	—
Kumquat, medium, raw	5	100	60	1.0	—	16.0	5	220	—	—	—	—	—
Litchi or lychee, raw	10	96	60	0.7	0.4	16.0	0	144	—	—	—	—	—
Litchi or lychee, cn	½ c	77	57	0.2	0.3	14.9	27	52	—	—	—	—	—
Longan, raw	30	96	60	1.2	0	14.4	0	27	—	—	—	—	—
Longan, cn	¾ c	100	68	0.4	0.3	17.6	54	41	—	—	—	—	—
Mango, small, raw	½	104	68	0.5	0.3	17.6	2	161	—	—	—	—	—
Papaya, ripe, 3½-in diameter, 5⅛-in high, raw	½	152	59	0.9	0.2	14.9	4	389	—	—	—	—	—
Persimmon, Japanese (soft type), raw	½	84	59	0.5	0.2	15.6	2.0	135	—	—	—	—	—
Pummelo, raw	¾ c	142	58	1.0	0.4	14.2	1	352	—	—	—	—	—
Milk													
Soybean milk, unsweetened	1 c	240	78	6.6	4.6	4.4	30	338	0	0.52	0.78	2.0	—
Fat													
Coconut milk*	1 tbsp	15	35	0.3	3.6	0.8	2	39	0	3.17	0.15	0.04	—
Sesame paste	1½ tsp	8	48	1.4	4.0	2.0	1	46	0	0.57	1.54	1.78	—
Sesame seeds, whole, dried	1 tbsp	9	52	1.6	4.5	2.1	1	42	0	0.63	1.69	1.96	0.8

Food	Amount													
Free														
Amaranth or Chinese spinach, raw	1 c	28	7	0.7	0.1	1.1	5	171	—	—	—	—	—	—
Bok choy, raw	1 c	70	10	1.1	0.1	1.5	46	176	—	—	—	—	—	—
Bok choy, ck	½ c	85	10	1.3	0.1	1.5	29	315	—	—	—	—	—	—
Chili pepper, raw	1	45	18	0.9	0.1	4.3	3	153	—	—	—	—	—	—
Chinese or Peking cabbage, raw	1 c	76	12	0.9	0.2	2.5	7	181	—	—	—	—	—	—
Chinese or Peking cabbage, ck	½ c	60	8	0.9	0.1	1.4	6	134	—	—	—	—	—	—
Choy sum or Chinese flowering cabbage, raw	1 c	56	9	1.2	—	1.6	—	—	—	—	—	—	—	—
Coriander, raw	½ c	8	2	—	—	0.2	2	44	—	—	—	—	—	—
Garland chrysanthemum, raw	1 c	25	4	0.4	0	1.1	13	143	—	—	—	—	—	—
Gingerroot, raw	¼ c	24	17	0.4	0.2	3.6	3	100	—	—	—	—	—	—
Mustard greens, salted and soured	2 tbsp	23	14	0.5	0.1	4.0	—	—	—	—	—	—	—	—
Oriental radish or daikon, raw	1 c	88	16	0.6	0	1.8	9	—	—	—	—	—	—	—
Watercress, raw	1 c	34	4	0.8	0	0.4	14	112	—	—	—	—	—	—
Combination														
Mock duck or wheat gluten, cn	½ c	74	88	14	—	10	—	28	—	—	—	—	—	—
Hmong American														
Starch/bread														
Cellophane or mung bean noodles, ck	¾ c	93	73	—	—	18	—	—	—	—	—	—	—	—
Rice noodles, fresh	½ c	49	99	1.3	0.1	23	—	—	—	—	—	—	—	—
Rice soup	¾ c	180	69	1.5	—	15	—	20	—	—	—	—	—	—
Yard-long beans, pod and seeds, ck	½ c	86	102	7.1	0.4	18.1	4	271	0	0.10	0.03	0.17	—	—
Medium-fat meat or substitute														
Pig's feet	2½ oz (= 2 exchanges)	71	138	13.6	8.8	0	71	—	0	3.04	4.13	0.96	—	0
Tofu or soybean curd, 2½ × 2¾ × 1 in	4 oz or ½ c	124	94	10	5.9	2.3	9	150	0	0.86	1.31	3.35	—	1.5
Vegetables														
Bamboo shoots, cn, drained	½ c	66	13	1.1	0.3	2.1	4	52	0	0.06	0.01	0.11	—	0.43
Bitter melon, raw	1 c	146	28	1.2	0.2	6.6	6	394	—	—	—	—	—	—
Cucuzzi squash (spaghetti squash), ck	½ c	78	23	0.5	0.2	5.0	14	91	0	0.05	0.02	0.10	—	1.09
Luffa gourd/squash, angled, raw	1 c	178	30	1.2	0.2	7.2	2	252	—	—	—	—	—	—
Luffa gourd/smooth or sponge, raw	1 c	178	34	2	0.4	8	6	274	—	—	—	—	—	—
Mung bean sprouts, seeds attached, ck	½ c	62	13	1.3	0.1	2.6	6	63	—	—	—	—	—	—
Pumpkin, ck	½ c	122	24	0.9	0.1	6.0	2	281	0	0.04	0.01	0.00	—	1.01

Table continued on following page

Hmong American (*cont.*)

Food	Quantity	Grams per Serving	Kcal	Pro (g)	Fat (g)	Cho (g)	Na (mg)	K (mg)	Chol (mg)	Sat Fatty Acids (g)	Mono Fatty Acids (g)	Poly Fatty Acids (g)	Total Dietary Fiber (g)
Fruits													
Apple pear, raw, 2¼-in high, 2½-in diameter	1	122	51	0.6	0.3	13	0	148	0	0	0	0	—
Guava, medium, raw	1½	135	69	1.2	0.8	15.9	3	384	—	—	0	—	—
Jackfruit	½ c	90	85	1	0.3	22	3	273	0	—	—	—	—
Fats													
Beef tallow	1 tsp	4.3	39	0	4.3	0	0	0	5	2.13	1.77	0.17	0
Chicken fat	1 tsp	4.3	38	0	4.3	0	—	—	4	1.27	1.9	0.9	0
Coconut cream	1 tbsp	19	36	0.5	3.4	1.6	10	19	0	2.99	0.14	0.04	—
Coconut milk, raw	1 tbsp	15	35	0.3	3.6	0.8	2	39	0	3.17	0.15	0.04	—
Coconut milk, cn	1 tbsp	15	30	0.3	3.2	0.9	2	33	0	2.89	0.14	0.04	—
Pork lard	1 tsp	4.2	39	0	4.3	0	0	0	4	1.67	1.93	0.47	0
Free													
Coriander (Chinese parsley), raw	1 c	16	4	0.3	0.1	0.4	4	88	—	—	—	—	—
Fish sauce	1 tbsp	16	4	0.8	0.1	0	1088	—	—	—	—	—	0
Pumpkin blossom, ck	1 c	134	20	1.5	0.1	4.4	8	142	0	0.05	0.02	0.01	—
Tender vines and leaves of pumpkin, squash, luffa gourd, and pea plant, ck	1 c	70	14	2	0	2	6	306	0	—	0	0	—
Vinespinach, raw	1 c	56	11	1	0.2	1.9	—	—	0	—	—	—	—
Occasional													
Condensed milk, sweetened	1 fl oz	38.2	123	3.0	3.3	20.8	49	142	13	2.10	0.93	0.13	0

Jewish

Food	Quantity	Grams per Serving	Kcal	Pro (g)	Fat (g)	Cho (g)	Na (mg)	K (mg)	Chol (mg)	Sat Fatty Acids (g)	Mono Fatty Acids (g)	Poly Fatty Acids (g)	Total Dietary Fiber (g)
Starch/bread													
Bagel or bialy	½ sm (1 oz)	28.5	82	3.0	0.7	15.4	99	20	0	0.1	0.3	0.3	0.8
Bulgur, ck	½ c	91	76	2.8	0.2	16.9	4	62	0	0.0	0.0	0.1	(0.5)
Bulke	½ med	28.5	76	2.4	0.9	14	142	29	0	0.2	0.3	0.3	0.4
Farfel, dry	½ c	37.5	90	3.4	0.4	(20.5)	1	42	0	0	0	0.8	(1.2)
Hallah	1 slice	28.5	85	2.6	1.8	14.0	140	30	26	0.5	0.9	0.3	0.7
Kasha, ck	½ c	99	91	3.3	0.6	19.7	4	88	0	0.1	0.2	0.2	(2.0)
Kasha, raw	2 tbsp	20.5	71	2.4	0.6	15.4	5	66	0	0.1	0.2	0.2	(1.3)

Food	Measure												
Lentils	⅓ c	66	77	6.0	0.2	13.3	1 (160)	244	0	0	0	0.1	2.4
Matzoh	¾ oz	21	86	2.2	1.4	16.5	135	26	0	—	—	—	(0.8)
Matzoh meal	2½ tbsp	22.5	86	2.2	18.2	0.2	1	25	0	0	0	0.2	(0.8)
Potato starch (flour)	2 tbsp	22.5	79	1.8	0.2	18.0	8	357	0	0.0	0.0	0.1	(0.4)
Pumpernickel bread	1 sl, 5 × 4 × ⅜ in	28	69	2.5	0.4	14.9	159	127	0	—	—	—	3.8
Rye bread	1 sl, 4¾ × 3¾ × 7/16 in	28	68	2.6	0.3	14.6	156	40	0	—	—	—	1.0
Split peas, ck	⅓ c	65	77	5.4	0.2	13.7	1	237	0	0.0	0.1	0.1	3.4
Starch/bread prepared with fat													
Matzoh ball (Starch/bread 1 + Fat 1)	3 balls (1½ oz)	42	134	6	4.6	17	469	62	165	1.3	1.8	0.9	0.7
Potato pancake (Starch/bread 1 + Fat 1)	½ pancake	38	119	2.3	6.3	13.2	194	269	47	1.7	2.7	1.3	(0.4)
Lean meat													
Flanken	1 oz	28.5	57	9.6	1.8	0	18	127	22	0.6	0.8	0.1	0
Gefilte fish (in broth)	2 oz	57	48	5.2	1	4	299	52	17	0.2	0.5	0.2	0
Herring, smoked	1 oz	28.5	61	7	3.5	0	260	127	23	0.8	1.5	0.8	0
Lox (smoked salmon)	1 oz	28.5	33	5.2	1.2	0	397	50	7	0.3	0.6	0.3	0
Sardines, cn, drained	2 med, 3 × 1 × ½ in	24	50	6	2.8	0	121	95	34	0.4	0.9	1.2	0
Smelts	1 oz	28.5	35	6.4	0.9	0	22	106	26	0.2	0.2	0.3	0
Medium-fat meat													
Beef tongue	1 oz	28.5	81	6.3	5.9	0.1	17	51	30	2.5	2.7	0.2	0
Brisket, beef	1 oz	28.5	69	8.4	3.7	0	21	82	27	1.3	1.6	0.1	0
Chopped liver	¼ c	57	75	7	4.2	3	33	100	195	1.3	1.5	0.7	0.8
Corned beef	1 oz	28.5	72	5.2	5.4	0.1	323	41	28	1.8	2.6	0.2	0
Sablefish, smoked	1 oz	28.5	73	5.0	5.7	0	210	134	18	1.2	3.0	0.8	0
Salmon, cn	¼ c	57	79	11.3	3.4	0	43 (316)	186	(20)	0.9	1.0	1.2	0
High-fat meat													
Pastrami	1 oz	28.5	99	4.9	8.3	0.9	350	65	26	3.0	4.1	0.3	0
Vegetable													
Borscht, beet (no sugar or sour cream)	½ c	—	38	2.0	1.5	4.5	200	173	0	0.3	0.7	0.4	1.4
Sorrel, ck	½ c	72	14	1.3	0.5	2.1	2	231	0	—	—	0.2	2.4
Cream cheese	1 tbsp	14	49	1.1	4.9	0.4	41	17	15	3.1	1.4	0.2	0
Nondairy liquid creamer	2 tbsp	30	40	0.3	3.0	3.4	24	58	0	variable	variable	variable	0
Nondairy powdered creamer	4 tsp	8	44	0.4	2.8	4.4	16	64	0	2.6	0.1	0	0
Schmaltz	1 tsp	5	31	0.2	3.4	0	2	3	3	1.0	1.5	0.7	0
Sour Cream	2 tbsp	24	52	0.8	5.0	1.0	12	34	10	3.1	1.5	0.2	0

Table continued on following page

Food	Quantity	Grams per Serving	Kcal	Pro (g)	Fat (g)	Cho (g)	Na (mg)	K (mg)	Chol (mg)	Sat Fatty Acids (g)	Mono Fatty Acids (g)	Poly Fatty Acids (g)	Total Dietary Fiber (g)
Jewish (cont.)													
Free													
Horseradish	1 tbsp	15	6	0.2	0	4.4	14	44	0	0	0	0	1.6
Pickle, dill	1 med	65	7	0.5	0.1	1.4	928	130	0	0.1	0	0.1	0.9
Occasional													
Sweet wine (fat 2)	½ c	118	83	0.2	0	1.7	76	140	0	0	0	0	0
Soul													
Starch/breads													
Hominy	¾ c	120	86	1.8	1.1	17.1	252	11	0	0.2	0.3	0.5	3.0
Succotash	½ c	85	79	3.7	0.8	17.0	38	225	0	0.1	0.2	0.4	4.6
Lean meat													
Hog maw	1 oz	28	45	4.7	2.7	0	15	57	55	—	—	—	0
Pork brains	1 oz	28	39	3.5	2.7	0	26	56	727	0.6	0.5	0.4	0
Pig ear	1 oz (¼ ear)	28	47	4.5	3.1	0	48	11	26	—	—	—	0
Tripe	2 oz	57	56	8.3	2.2	0	26	154	54	1.2	0.7	0.0	0
Opossum	1 oz	28	63	8.6	2.9	0	(27)	(91)	(23)	—	—	—	0
Medium-fat meat													
Neck bones, pork	1 oz	28	66	6.9	4.1	0	20	97	24	1.5	1.8	0.4	0
Pig foot	½ foot	35	68	6.7	4.3	0	(58)	(14)	35	1.5	2.0	0.5	0
Sousemeat (headcheese)	1 oz or 1 sl 4 × 4 × ⅒ in	28	60	4.6	4.5	0.1	357	9	23	1.4	2.3	0.5	0
Tongue, pork	1 oz (⅓ tongue)	28	77	6.9	5.3	0	31	68	42	1.8	2.5	0.6	0
Pork skin (rind) fried (packaged snack pack or vendor purchased)	1 c medium pieces, not crushed	12	68	7.7	4.3	0	231	—	17	1.7	—	—	0
Oxtail	1 oz	28	72	8.9	3.7	0	20	75	30	1.4	1.6	0.1	0

Food	Portion	g	kcal	Pro (g)	Fat (g)	CHO (g)	K (mg)	Na (mg)	Chol (mg)	Sat.	Mono.	Poly.	Fiber
High-fat meats													
Pig tail	1 oz (⅓ tail)	28	113	4.8	10.2	0	(11)	(48)	37	3.6	4.8	1.1	0
Ham hock	1 oz	28	90	5.7	6.7	1.7	98	383	18	2.0	(1.69)	(0.34)	0
Vienna sausage	2 small 2 × ⅞ in diameter	32	90	3.3	8.1	0.7	32	304	16	3.0	4.0	0.5	0
Vegetables													
Kale, ck	½ c	65	21	1.2	0.3	3.7	148	15	0	0.0	0.0	0.1	1.3
Poke salad, ck	½ c	82	16	1.9	0.3	2.5	—	—	0	—	—	—	1.2
Fruits													
Muscadines	17	85	60	0.6	0.5	15.0	156	2	0	0.2	0.0	0.1	0.7
Saturated fats													
Pork cracklings (Hormel)	1 tbsp	8	57	2.3	5.1	0	—	18	9	1.7	(2.3)	(0.6)	0
Fatback, raw	¼ oz	7	58	0.2	6.3	0	5	1	4	2.3	3.0	0.7	0
Hog jowl	1 oz	28	(54)	1.8	4.8	0	(41)	(7)	(9)	1.6	2.4	0.6	0
Lard	1 tsp	4	38	0	4.3	0	0	0	4	1.7	1.9	0.5	0

*The addition of ash significantly increases the potassium content.

†Although data for flour tortillas and hominy are available from USDA sources, they reflect preparation techniques from other parts of the country. This database contains information from a Navajo-specific study.

‡The 8-inch diameter of the tortilla was chosen to represent the size that is commonly eaten.

§Because of the lack of published data on mutton, the National Live Stock and Meat Board and the New Mexico Cooperative Extension Service recommend substituting lamb nutrient values for mutton, as has been done in this data base. However, everyday observation on the Navajo reservation suggests that the untrimmed mutton eaten by many clients is considerably higher in fat than the published data for lean and fat lamb. Thus, trimming mutton might reduce fat and kilocalories beyond the estimates given here.

ǁTotal fat value includes fatty acids and glycerol.

**Raw liquid expressed from mixture of grated coconut meat and water.

KEY: CHO = carbohydrate; Chol = cholesterol; ck = cooked; cn = canned; K = potassium; Mono. = monounsaturated; Na = sodium; Poly. = polyunsaturated; Pro = protein; Sat. = saturated; s + l = small and large.

From Ethnic and Regional Food Practices, A Series. Navaho (1991), Alaskan Native (1991), Mexican American (1993), Chinese American (1989), Chinese American (1990), and Hmong American (1992) Food Practices, Customs, and Holidays. The American Dietetic Association and American Diabetes Association, Inc.

Appendix 8
Enteral Supplements

		NUTRIENT SOURCE		
Product	Manufacturer	Protein Source	Fat Source	Calories/mL
Nutritional Supplements, Ready to Drink				
RESOURCE® Fruit Beverage	Novartis Nutrition	Whey protein concentrate	Not applicable	0.76
RESOURCE® Standard	Novartis Nutrition	Sodium and calcium caseinates, soy protein isolate	High-oleic sunflower oil, soybean oil, corn oil	1.06
RESOURCE® Plus	Novartis Nutrition	Sodium and calcium caseinates, soy protein isolate	High-oleic sunflower oil, soybean oil, corn oil	1.5
RESOURCE® Yogurt Flavored Beverage	Novartis Nutrition	Whey protein concentrate, sodium and calcium caseinates, dehydrated lowfat yogurt	Corn oil	1.06
Ensure®	Ross Laboratories	Sodium and calcium caseinates, soy protein isolate, whey protein concentrate	High-oleic safflower oil, soy oil, canola oil, corn oil	1.06
Ensure Plus®	Ross Laboratories	Sodium and calcium caseinates, soy protein isolate	Corn oil	1.5
Ensure Plus® HN	Ross Laboratories	Sodium and calcium caseinates, soy protein isolate	Corn oil	1.5
Ensure® with Fiber	Ross Laboratories	Sodium and calcium caseinates, soy protein isolate	Corn oil	1.1
NuBasics®	Nestle Nutrition	Calcium-potassium caseinates	Canola oil, corn oil, soy lecithin	1.0
NuBasics® Plus	Nestle Nutrition	Calcium-potassium caseinates	Canola oil, corn oil, soy lecithin	1.5
NuBasics® Juice Drink	Nestle Nutrition	Whey protein isolate	Not applicable	1.0
Sustacal® Basic™	Mead Johnson	Sodium caseinate, calcium caseinate, soy protein isolate	Canola oil, high oleic sunflower oil, corn oil	1.06
Sustacal® Plus	Mead Johnson	Calcium and sodium caseinate	Corn oil	1.52
Suscatal® with Fiber	Mead Johnson	Calcium and sodium caseinate, soy protein isolate	Corn oil	1.06

*Value listed equal 8 oz.

| NUTRITIONAL PROFILE | | | | | NUTRIENT PER SERVING | | | | |
Calories* per serving	Protein (g/serving)	Carbohydrate (g/serving)	Fat (g/serving)	Osmolality (mOsm/kg Water)	Sodium mg (mEq)	Potassium mg (mEq)	Calcium mg (mEq)	Phosphorus mg (mmol)	Fiber (g)
180	8.8	36	0	700	<70 (<3.0)	<22 (<0.6)	135 (6.7)	160* (5.2)	—
250	9	40	6	650	220 (9.6)	340 (9.6)	300 (15)	250 (8.1)	—
360	13	52	11	870	310 (13.5)	460 (11.8)	300 (15)	250 (8.1)	—
250	8.8	44.4	4.2	800	65 (2.8)	200 (5.1)	250 (12.5)	180 (5.8)	—
250	8.8	40	6.1	555	200 (9)	370 (10)	300 (15)	300 (9.7)	—
355	13	47.3	12.6	690	250 (11)	460 (12)	167 (8)	167 (5)	—
355	14.8	47.3	11.8	650	280 (12)	430 (11)	250 (13)	250 (8)	—
260	9.4	38.3	8.8	480	200 (9)	400 (10)	170 (9)	170 (6)	3.4
250	8.75	33.1	9.2	500–520	219 (10)	312 (8)	125 (6)	125 (4)	—
375	13.1	44.1	16.2	620–650	292 (13)	467 (12)	187 (9)	187 (6)	—
163	6.5	34	0.1	1000	50 (2.2)	50 (1.3)	83 (4)	166 (5.4)	—
250	9	34	9	500	200 (8.7)	370 (9.5)	125 (6)	125 (4)	—
360	14.4	45	13.6	630	200 (8.7)	350 (9.0)	200 (10)	200 (7)	<1
250	11	33	8	480	170 (7.4)	330 (8.4)	200 (10)	167 (5)	2.5

Table continued on following page

Product	Manufacturer	NUTRIENT SOURCE	
		Protein Source	Fat Source
Standard Formulas			
IsoSource® Standard	Novartis Nutrition	Soy protein isolate	Canola oil, MCT
IsoSource® HN	Novartis Nutrition	Soy protein isolate	Canola oil, MCT
Comply®	Mead Johnson	Sodium caseinate, calcium caseinate	Canola oil, high-oleic sunflower oil, MCT, corn oil
Isocal®	Mead Johnson	Calcium caseinate, sodium caseinate, soy protein isolate	Soy oil, MCT
Isocal® HN	Mead Johnson	Calcium caseinate, sodium caseinate, soy protein isolate	Soy oil, MCT
Nutren® 1.0	Nestle Nutrition	Calcium-potassium caseinate	Canola oil, MCT oil, corn oil, soy lecithin
Nutren® 1.5	Nestle Nutrition	Calcium-potassium caseinate	MCT, canola oil, corn oil, soy lecithin
Osmolite®	Ross Laboratories	Sodium and calcium caseinates, soy protein isolate	High-oleic safflower oil, canola oil, MCT, lecithin
Osmolite® HN	Ross Laboratories	Sodium and calcium caseinates, soy protein isolate	High-oleic safflower oil, canola oil, MCT, lecithin
Osmolite® HN Plus	Ross Laboratories	Sodium and calcium caseinates	High-oleic safflower oil, canola oil, MCT, lecithin
Standard Fiber Containing Formulas			
FiberSource™	Novartis Nutrition	Soy protein isolate, soy protein concentrate	Canola oil, MCT
FiberSource™ HN	Novartis Nutrition	Soy protein isolate, soy protein concentrate	Canola oil, MCT
IsoSource® 1.5 Cal	Novartis Nutrition	Sodium and calcium caseinates	Canola oil, MCT, soybean oil
Jevity®	Ross Laboratories	Sodium and calcium caseinates	High-oleic safflower oil, canola oil, MCT, lecithin
Jevity® Plus	Ross Laboratories	Sodium and calcium caseinates	High-oleic safflower oil, canola oil, MCT, lecithin
Nutren® 1.0 with Fiber	Nestle Nutrition	Calcium-potassium caseinates	Canola oil, MCT oil, corn oil, soy lecithin
ProBalance™	Nestle Nutrition	Calcium-potassium caseinates	Canola oil, MCT oil, corn oil, soy lecithin
Ultracal®	Mead Johnson	Calcium and sodium caseinates	Canola oil, MCT

	NUTRITIONAL PROFILE				NUTRIENT PER LITER				
Calories/mL	Protein (g/L)	Carbohydrate (g/L)	Fat (g/L)	Osmolality (mOsm/kg Water)	Sodium mg (mEq)	Potassium mg (mEq)	Calcium mg (mEq)	Phosphorus mg (mmol)	Fiber (g)
1.2	43	170	39	490	1100 (48)	1700 (43)	1200 (60)	1100 (36)	—
1.2	53	160	39	490	1100 (48)	1700 (43)	1200 (60)	1200 (39)	—
1.5	60	180	61	460	1200 (52)	1850 (47)	1200 (60)	1200 (39)	—
1.06	34	135	44	270	530 (23)	1320 (34)	630 (32)	530 (17)	—
1.06	44	123	45	270	930 (40)	1610 (41)	850 (42)	850 (27)	—
1.0	40	127	38	300–350	876 (38.1)	1248 (32)	668 (33)	668 (22)	—
1.5	60	169.2	67.6	430–530	1170 (50.9)	1872 (48)	1000 (50)	1000 (32)	—
1.06	37.1	151.1	34.7	300	640 (28)	1020 (26)	530 (26)	530 (17)	—
1.06	44.3	143.9	34.7	300	930 (40)	1570 (40)	758 (38)	758 (25)	—
1.2	55.5	157.5	39.3	360	1420 (62)	1940 (50)	1200 (60)	1200 (39)	—
1.2	43	170	39	490	1100 (48)	1800 (46)	1000 (33)	940 (30)	10
1.2	53	160	39	490	1100 (48)	1800 (46)	1000 (33)	1000 (32)	10
1.5	68	170	65	650	1300 (57)	2100 (54)	1100 (55)	1100 (35)	8
1.06	44.3	154.4	34.7	300	930 (40)	1570 (40)	909 (45)	758 (25)	14.4
1.2	55.5	174.6	39.3	450	1350 (59)	1850 (47)	1200 (60)	1200 (39)	12
1.0	40	127	38	310–370	876 (38.1)	1248 (32)	668 (33)	668 (22)	14
1.2	54	156	40.6	350–450	763 (33)	1560 (40)	1250 (62)	1000 (32)	10
1.06	44	123	45	310	930 (40)	1610 (41)	850 (42)	850 (27)	14.4

Table continued on following page

Product	Manufacturer	NUTRIENT SOURCE	
		Protein Source	Fat Source
Blenderized Formulas			
COMPLEAT® Modified	Novartis Nutrition	Beef, calcium caseinate	Canola oil, beef
COMPLEAT® Pediatric	Novartis Nutrition	Sodium and calcium caseinates, beef	High oleic sunflower oil, soybean oil, MCT, beef
Very High Protein/Wound Healing Formulas			
IsoSource® VHN	Novartis Nutrition	Sodium and calcium caseinates	MCT, canola oil
Promote®	Ross Laboratories	Sodium and calcium caseinates, soy protein isolate	High-oleic safflower oil, canola oil, MCT, lecithin
Promote® With Fiber	Ross Laboratories	Sodium and calcium caseinates	High-oleic safflower oil, canola oil, MCT, lecithin
Protain XL®	Mead Johnson	Sodium and calcium caseinate	Canola oil, high oleic sunflower oil, MCT oil, corn oil
TraumaCal®	Mead Johnson	Sodium caseinate, calcium caseinate	Soybean oil, MCT
Replete®	Nestle Nutrition	Calcium-potassium caseinate	Canola oil, MCT oil, soy lecithin
Replete® with Fiber	Nestle Nutrition	Calcium-potassium caseinate	Canola oil, MCT oil, soy lecithin
Elemental and Semi-elemental Formulas			
SandoSource® Peptide	Novartis Nutrition	Casein hydrolysate, free amino acids, sodium caseinate (26% free amino acids, 34% peptide chain length 2–4 amino acids, 40% peptide chain length > 4 amino acids)	MCT, soybean oil, hydroxylated lecithin
TOLEREX®	Novartis Nutrition	Free amino acids (16.8% BCAA, 17.1% glutamine, 8.9% arginine)	Safflower oil
VIVONEX® PLUS	Novartis Nutrition	Free amino acids (30% BCAA, 22% glutamine, 11% arginine)	Soybean oil
VIVONEX® T.E.N.	Novartis Nutrition	Free amino acids (33.2% BCAA, 12.9% glutamine, 7.6% arginine)	Safflower oil
Criticare HN®	Mead Johnson	Hydrolyzed casein, amino acids	Safflower oil, emulsifiers
Crucial™	Nestle Nutrition	Enzymatically hydrolyzed casein, L-arginine	MCT oil, fish oil, soybean oil, soy lecithin

	NUTRITIONAL PROFILE				NUTRIENT PER LITER				
Calories/mL	Protein (g/L)	Carbohydrate (g/L)	Fat (g/L)	Osmolality (mOsm/kg Water)	Sodium mg (mEq)	Potassium mg (mEq)	Calcium mg (mEq)	Phosphorus mg (mmol)	Fiber (g)
1.07	43	140	37	300	1000 (43)	1400 (36)	670 (33)	870 (28)	4.3
1.0	38	130	39	380	680 (30)	1500 (38)	1000 (50)	1000 (32)	4.4
1.0	62	130	29	300	1300 (57)	1600 (41)	800 (40)	800 (26)	10
1.0	62.5	130	26	340	1000 (43)	1980 (51)	1200 (60)	1200 (39)	—
1.0	62.5	139.4	28.2	370	1300 (57)	1980 (51)	1200 (60)	1200 (39)	14.4
1.0	57	129	30	340	920 (40)	1760 (45)	800 (40)	800 (26)	9.1
1.5	82	142	68	490	1180 (51)	1390 (36)	750 (38)	750 (24)	—
1.0	62.5	113	34	300–350	876 (38.1)	1500 (38.5)	1000 (50)	1000 (32)	—
1.0	62.5	113	34	310–390	876 (38.1)	1500 (38.5)	1000 (50)	1000 (32)	14
1.0	50	160	17	490	1200 (52)	1600 (41)	570 (28)	570 (18)	—
1.0	21	230	1.5	550	470 (20)	1170 (30)	560 (28)	560 (18)	—
1.0	45	190	6.7	650	610 (27)	1060 (27)	560 (28)	560 (18)	—
1.0	38	210	2.8	630	460 (20)	780 (20)	500 (25)	500 (16)	—
1.06	38	220	5.3	650	630 (27)	1320 (34)	530 (26)	530 (17)	—
1.5	94	135	68	490	1168 (50.8)	1872 (47.9)	1000 (50)	1000 (32)	—

Table continued on following page

Product	Manufacturer	NUTRIENT SOURCE	
		Protein Source	**Fat Source**
Peptamen®	Nestle Nutrition	Enzymatically hydrolyzed whey protein	MCT, sunflower oil, soy lecithin
Peptamen VHP™	Nestle Nutrition	Enzymatically hydrolyzed whey protein	MCT, soy oil, soy lecithin
Reabilan® HN	Nestle Nutrition	Casein peptides, whey peptides	MCT, soy oil, canola oil, soy lecithin
Perative®	Ross Laboratories	Partially hydrolyzed sodium caseinate, lactalbumin hydrolysate, L-arginine	Canola oil, MCT, corn oil, lecithin
Vital® High Nitrogen	Ross Laboratories	Partially hydrolyzed whey, meat and soy, free amino acids	Safflower oil, MCT
Renal Formulas			
NovaSource™ Renal	Novartis Nutrition	Sodium and calcium caseinates, L-arginine	High-oleic sunflower oil, corn oil, MCT
Nepro®	Ross Laboratories	Calcium, magnesium and sodium caseinates, milk protein isolate	High-oleic safflower oil, canola oil, soy lecithin
Magnacal® Renal	Mead Johnson	Calcium and sodium caseinates	Canola oil, high-oleic sunflower oil, MCT oil, corn oil
Glucose Intolerance Formulas			
DiabetiSource®	Novartis Nutrition	Calcium caseinate, beef	High-oleic sunflower oil, canola oil, beef fat, emulsifiers
RESOURCE® Diabetic	Novartis Nutrition	Sodium and calcium caseinates, soy protein isolate	High-oleic sunflower oil, soybean oil, soy lecithin
Choice dm™	Mead Johnson	Milk protein concentrate, soy fiber	Canola, high oleic sunflower, corn and MCT oil
Glytrol™	Nestle Nutrition	Calcium-potassium caseinate	Canola oil, high oleic safflower oil, MCT oil, soy lecithin
Glucerna®	Ross Laboratories	Sodium and calcium caseinates	High-oleic safflower oil, canola oil, soy lecithin
Immune Enhancing Formulas			
IMPACT®	Novartis Nutrition	Sodium and calcium caseinates, L-arginine	Structured lipid from palm kernal and sunflower oil, menhaden fish oil
IMPACT® 1.5	Novartis Nutrition	Sodium and calcium caseinates, L-arginine	MCT, structured lipid from palm kernal and sunflower oil, menhaden fish oil
IMPACT® with Fiber	Novartis Nutrition	Sodium and calcium caseinates, L-arginine	Structured lipid from palm kernal and sunflower oil, menhaden fish oil
Immun-Aid®	McGaw	Lactalbumin, L-arginine, L-glutamine, BCAA	Canola oil, MCT

	NUTRITIONAL PROFILE				NUTRIENT PER LITER				
Calories/mL	Protein (g/L)	Carbohydrate (g/L)	Fat (g/L)	Osmolality (mOsm/kg Water)	Sodium mg (mEq)	Potassium mg (mEq)	Calcium mg (mEq)	Phosphorus mg (mmol)	Fiber (g)
1.0	40	127	39	270–380	500 (22)	1250 (32)	800 (40)	700 (23)	—
1.0	62.5	104.5	39	300–430	560 (24)	1500 (38)	800 (40)	700 (23)	—
1.33	58.2	158	54	490	1000 (43)	1662 (43)	665 (33)	665 (22)	—
1.3	66.6	177.2	37.4	385	1040 (45)	1730 (44)	867 (43)	867 (28)	—
1.0	41.7	185	10.8	500	566 (25)	1400 (36)	667 (33)	667 (22)	—
2	74	200	100	700	1000 (43)	810 (21)	1300 (65)	650 (21)	—
2	70	222.3	95.6	665	842 (37)	1053 (27)	1308 (68)	695 (22)	—
2	75	200	101	570	800 (35)	1270 (33)	1010 (50)	800 (26)	—
1.0	50	90	49	360	930 (40)	1400 (36)	670 (33)	800 (26)	4.3
1.06	63	99	47	450	970 (42)	1100 (29)	930 (46)	930 (30)	13
1.06	45	106	51	300–440	850 (37)	1820 (47)	1060 (53)	1060 (34)	14.4
1.0	45	100	47.5	380	740 (32.2)	1400 (35.9)	720 (36)	720 (23)	15
1.0	41.8	95.8	54.4	355	930 (40)	1570 (40)	704 (35)	704 (23)	14.4
1.0	56	130	28	375	1100 (48)	1400 (36)	800 (40)	800 (26)	—
1.5	80	140	69	550	1280 (56)	1680 (43)	960 (48)	960 (31)	—
1.0	56	140	28	375	1100 (48)	1400 (36)	800 (40)	800 (26)	10
1.0	80	120	22	460	580 (25)	1060 (27)	500 (25)	500 (16)	—

Table continued on following page

Product	Manufacturer	NUTRIENT SOURCE	
		Protein Source	Fat Source
Pediatric Formulas			
COMPLEAT® Pediatric	Novartis Nutrition	Sodium and calcium caseinates, beef	High oleic sunflower oil, soybean oil, MCT, beef
RESOURCE® Just for Kids	Novartis Nutrition	Sodium and calcium caseinates, whey protein concentrate	High oleic sunflower oil, soybean oil, MCT
VIVONEX® PEDIATRIC	Novartis Nutrition	Free amino acids (12.9% glutamine, 6.2% arginine, 21.6% BCAA)	MCT, soybean oil
Kindercal®	Mead Johnson	Calcium caseinate, sodium caseinate, milk protein concentrate	Canola oil, MCT, corn oil, high oleic sunflower oil
Neocate One +	SHS North America	Free amino acids	Fractionated coconut oil, canola oil, safflower oil
PediaSure®	Ross Laboratories	Sodium caseinate, whey protein concentrate	High oleic safflower oil, soy oil, MCT, lecithin
PediaSure® With Fiber	Ross Laboratories	Sodium caseinate, whey protein concentrate	High oleic safflower oil, soy oil, MCT, lecithin
Peptamen Junior™	Nestle Nutrition	Enzymatically hydrolyzed whey protein	MCT oil, soy oil, canola oil, soy lecithin

| | NUTRITIONAL PROFILE | | | | NUTRIENT PER LITER | | | | |
Calories/mL	Protein (g/L)	Carbohydrate (g/L)	Fat (g/L)	Osmolality (mOsm/kg Water)	Sodium mg (mEq)	Potassium mg (mEq)	Calcium mg (mEq)	Phosphorus mg (mmol)	Fiber (g)
1.0	38	130	39	380	680 (30)	1500 (38)	1000 (50)	1000 (32)	4.4
1.0	30	110	50	390	380 (17)	1300 (33)	1140 (57)	800 (26)	—
0.8	24	130	24	360	400 (17)	1200 (31)	970 (48)	800 (26)	—
1.06	34	135	44	310	370 (16)	1310 (33.5)	850 (42)	850 (27)	6.3
1.0	25	146	35	610	200 (8.7)	930 (23.8)	620 (31)	620 (20)	—
1.0	30	109.7	49.7	345	380 (17)	1310 (33.5)	970 (48)	800 (26)	—
1.0	30	113.5	49.7	345	380 (17)	1310 (33.5)	970 (48)	800 (26)	5
1.0	30	137.5	38.5	260–360	460 (20)	1320 (33.8)	1000 (50)	800 (26)	—

Appendix 9
The Exchange System

"This material has been modified from Exchange Lists for Meal Planning, which is the basis of a meal planning system designed by a committee of the American Diabetes Association and the American Dietetic Association. While designed primarily for people with diabetes and others who must follow special diets, the Exchange Lists are based on principles of good nutrition that apply to everyone."
© 1995 American Diabetes Association, The American Dietetic Association.

Groups/Lists	Carbohydrate (g)	Protein (g)	Fat (g)	Calories
Carbohydrate Group				
Starch	15	3	1 or less	80
Fruit	15	—	—	60
Milk				
Skim	12	8	0–3	90
Low-fat	12	8	5	120
Whole	12	8	8	150
Other carbohydrates	15	varies	varies	varies
Vegetables	5	2	—	25
Meat and Meat Substitute Group				
Very lean	—	7	0–1	35
Lean	—	7	3	55
Medium-fat	—	7	5	75
High-fat	—	7	8	100
Fat Group	—	—	5	45

Starch List

Bread

Bagel	½ (1 oz)
Bread, reduced-calorie	2 slices (1½ oz)
Bread, white, whole-wheat, pumpernickel, rye	1 slice (1 oz)
Bread sticks, crisp, 4 in. long × ½ in.	2 (⅔ oz)
English muffin	½
Hot dog or hamburger bun	½ (1 oz)
Pita, 6 in. across	½
Roll, plain, small	1 (1 oz)
Raisin bread, unfrosted	1 slice (1 oz)
Tortilla, corn, 6 in. across	1
Tortilla, flour, 7–8 in. across	1
Waffle, 4½ in. square, reduced-fat	1

Cereals and Grains

Bran cereals	½ cup
Bulgur	½ cup
Cereals	½ cup
Cereals, unsweetened, ready-to-eat	¾ cup
Cornmeal (dry)	3 tbsp
Couscous	⅓ cup
Flour (dry)	3 tbsp
Granola, low-fat	¼ cup
Grape-Nuts	¼ cup
Grits	½ cup
Kasha	½ cup
Millet	¼ cup
Muesli	¼ cup
Oats	½ cup
Pasta	½ cup
Puffed cereal	1½ cups
Rice milk	½ cup
Rice, white or brown	⅓ cup
Shredded Wheat	½ cup
Sugar-frosted cereal	½ cup
Wheat germ	3 tbsp

Starchy Vegetables

Baked beans	⅓ cup
Corn	½ cup
Corn on cob, medium	1 (5 oz)
Mixed vegetables with corn, peas, or pasta	1 cup
Peas, green	½ cup
Plantain	½ cup
Potato, baked or boiled	1 small (3 oz)
Potato, mashed	½ cup
Squash, winter (acorn, butternut)	1 cup
Yam, sweet potato, plain	½ cup

Crackers and Snacks

Animal crackers	8
Graham crackers, 2½ in. square	3
Matzoh	¾ oz
Melba toast	4 slices
Oyster crackers	24
Popcorn (popped, no fat added or low-fat microwave)	3 cups
Pretzels	¾ oz
Rice cakes, 4 in. across	2
Saltine-type crackers	6
Snack chips, fat-free (tortilla, potato)	15–20 (¾ oz)
Whole-wheat crackers, no fat added	2–5 (¾ oz)

Dried Beans, Peas, and Lentils*

Beans and peas (garbanzo, pinto, kidney, white, split, black-eyed)	½ cup
Lima beans	⅔ cup
Lentils	½ cup
Miso[†]	3 tbsp

Starchy Foods Prepared with Fat[‡]

Biscuit, 2½ in. across	1
Chow mein noodles	½ cup
Corn bread, 2 in. cube	1 (2 oz)
Crackers, rounded butter type	6
Croutons	1 cup
French-fried potatoes	16–25 (3 oz)
Granola	¼ cup
Muffin, small	1 (1½ oz)
Pancake, 4 in. across	2
Popcorn, microwave	3 cups
Sandwich crackers, cheese or peanut butter filling	3
Stuffing, bread (prepared)	⅓ cup
Taco shell, 6 in. across	2
Waffle, 4½ in. square	1
Whole-wheat crackers, fat added	4–6 (1 oz)

*Count as 1 starch exchange, plus 1 very lean meat exchange.
[†]Contains 400 mg or more of sodium per serving.
[‡]Count as 1 starch exchange, plus 1 fat exchange.

Fruit List

Fruit

Apple, unpeeled, small	1 (4 oz)	Papaya	½ fruit (8 oz) or 1 cup cubes
Applesauce, unsweetened	½ cup	Peach, medium, fresh	1 (6 oz)
Apples, dried	4 rings	Peaches, canned	½ cup
Apricots, fresh	4 whole (5½ oz)	Pear, large, fresh	½ (4 oz)
Apricots, dried	8 halves	Pears, canned	½ cup
Apricots, canned	½ cup	Pineapple, fresh	¾ cup
Banana, small	1 (4 oz)	Pineapple, canned	½ cup
Blackberries	¾ cup	Plums, small	2 (5 oz)
Blueberries	¾ cup	Plums, canned	½ cup
Cantaloupe, small	⅓ melon (11 oz) or 1 cup cubes	Prunes, dried	3
Cherries, sweet, fresh	12 (3 oz)	Raisins	2 tbsp
Cherries, sweet, canned	½ cup	Raspberries	1 cup
Dates	3	Strawberries	1¼ cup whole berries
Figs, fresh	1½ large or 2 medium (3½ oz)	Tangerines, small	2 (8 oz)
Figs, dried	1½	Watermelon	1 slice (13½ oz) or 1¼ cup cubes
Fruit cocktail	½ cup		
Grapefruit, large	½ (11 oz)		

Fruit Juice

Grapefruit sections, canned	¾ cup	Apple juice/cider	½ cup
Grapes, small	17 (3 oz)	Cranberry juice cocktail	⅓ cup
Honeydew melon	1 slice (10 oz) or 1 cup cubes	Cranberry juice cocktail, reduced-calorie	1 cup
Kiwi	1 (3½ oz)	Fruit juice blends, 100% juice	⅓ cup
Mandarin oranges, canned	¾ cup	Grape juice	⅓ cup
Mango, small	½ fruit (5½ oz) or ½ cup	Grapefruit juice	½ cup
Nectarine, small	1 (5 oz)	Orange juice	½ cup
Orange, small	1 (6½ oz)	Pineapple juice	½ cup
		Prune juice	⅓ cup

Milk List

Skim and Very Low-Fat Milk*

Skim milk	1 cup
½% milk	1 cup
1% milk	1 cup
Nonfat or low-fat buttermilk	1 cup
Evaporated skim milk	½ cup
Nonfat dry milk	⅓ cup dry
Plain nonfat yogurt	¾ cup
Nonfat or low-fat fruit-flavored yogurt sweetened with aspartame or with a nonnutritive sweetener	1 cup

Low-Fat†

2% milk	1 cup
Plain low-fat yogurt	¾ cup
Sweet acidophilus milk	1 cup

Whole Milk‡

Whole milk	1 cup
Evaporated whole milk	½ cup
Goat's milk	1 cup
Kefir	1 cup

*0–3 grams fat per serving.
†5 grams fat per serving.
‡8 grams of fat per serving.

Other Carbohydrates

Food	Serving Size	Exchanges per Serving
Angel food cake, unfrosted	1/12 cake	2 carbohydrates
Brownie, small, unfrosted	2 in. square	1 carbohydrate, 1 fat
Cake, unfrosted	2 in. square	1 carbohydrate, 1 fat
Cake, frosted	2 in. square	2 carbohydrates, 1 fat
Cookie, fat-free	2 small	1 carbohydrate
Cookie or sandwich cookie with creme filling	2 small	1 carbohydrate, 1 fat
Cupcake, frosted	1 small	2 carbohydrates, 1 fat
Cranberry sauce, jellied	¼ cup	2 carbohydrates
Doughnut, plain cake	1 medium (1½ oz)	1½ carbohydrates, 2 fats
Doughnut, glazed	3¾ in. across (2 oz)	2 carbohydrates, 2 fats
Fruit juice bars, frozen, 100% juice	1 bar (3 oz)	1 carbohydrate
Fruit snacks, chewy (pureed fruit concentrate)	1 roll (¾ oz)	1 carbohydrate
Fruit spreads, 100% fruit	1 tbsp	1 carbohydrate
Gelatin, regular	½ cup	1 carbohydrate
Gingersnaps	3	1 carbohydrate
Granola bar	1 bar	1 carbohydrate, 1 fat
Granola bar, fat-free	1 bar	2 carbohydrates
Hummus	⅓ cup	1 carbohydrate, 1 fat
Ice cream	½ cup	1 carbohydrate, 2 fats
Ice cream, light	½ cup	1 carbohydrate, 1 fat
Ice cream, fat-free, no sugar added	½ cup	1 carbohydrate
Jam or jelly, regular	1 tbsp	1 carbohydrate
Milk, chocolate, whole	1 cup	2 carbohydrates, 1 fat
Pie, fruit, 2 crusts	⅙ pie	3 carbohydrates, 2 fats
Pie, pumpkin or custard	⅛ pie	1 carbohydrate, 2 fats
Potato chips	12–18 (1 oz)	1 carbohydrate, 2 fats
Pudding, regular (made with low-fat milk)	½ cup	2 carbohydrates
Pudding, sugar-free (made with low-fat milk)	½ cup	1 carbohydrate
Salad dressing, fat-free*	¼ cup	1 carbohydrate
Sherbet, sorbet	½ cup	2 carbohydrates
Spaghetti or pasta sauce, canned*	½ cup	1 carbohydrate, 1 fat
Sweet roll or Danish	1 (2½ oz)	2½ carbohydrates, 2 fats
Syrup, light	2 tbsp	1 carbohydrate
Syrup, regular	1 tbsp	1 carbohydrate
Syrup, regular	¼ cup	4 carbohydrates
Tortilla chips	6–12 (1 oz)	1 carbohydrate, 2 fats
Yogurt, frozen, low-fat, fat-free	⅓ cup	1 carbohydrate, 0–1 fat
Yogurt, frozen, fat-free, no sugar added	½ cup	1 carbohydrate
Yogurt, low-fat with fruit	1 cup	3 carbohydrates, 0–1 fat
Vanilla wafers	5	1 carbohydrate, 1 fat

*Contains 400 mg or more sodium per exchange.

Vegetable List

Artichoke	Eggplant	Salad greens (endive, escarole,
Artichoke hearts	Green onions or scallions	lettuce, romaine, spinach)
Asparagus	Greens (collard, kale, mustard, turnip)	Sauerkraut*
Beans (green, wax, Italian)	Kohlrabi	Spinach
Bean sprouts	Leeks	Summer squash
Beets	Mixed vegetables (without corn, peas,	Tomato
Broccoli	or pasta)	Tomatoes, canned
Brussels sprouts	Mushrooms	Tomato sauce*
Cabbage	Okra	Tomato/vegetable juice*
Carrots	Onions	Turnips
Cauliflower	Pea pods	Water chestnuts
Celery	Peppers (all varieties)	Watercress
Cucumber	Radishes	Zucchini

*Contains 400 mg or more sodium per exchange.

Meat and Meat Substitutes List

Very Lean Meat and Substitutes List

Poultry	Chicken or turkey (white meat, no skin), Cornish hen (no skin)	1 oz
Fish	Fresh or frozen cod, flounder, haddock, halibut, trout; tuna fresh or canned in water	1 oz
Shellfish	Clams, crab, lobster, scallops, shrimp, imitation shellfish	1 oz
Game	Duck or pheasant (no skin), venison, buffalo, ostrich	1 oz
Cheese	Nonfat or low-fat cottage cheese	¼ cup
	Fat-free cheese	1 oz
Other	Processed sandwich meats with 1 gram or less fat per ounce, such as deli thin, shaved meats, chipped beef,* turkey ham	1 oz
	Egg whites	2
	Egg substitutes, plain	¼ cup
	Hot dogs with 1 gram or less fat per ounce*	1 oz
	Kidney (high in cholesterol)	1 oz
	Sausage with 1 gram or less fat per ounce	1 oz
	Dried beans, peas, lentils (cooked)⁺	½ cup

Lean Meat and Substitutes List

Beef	USDA Select or Choice grades of lean beef trimmed of fat, such as round, sirloin, and flank steak; tenderloin; roast (rib, chuck, rump); steak (T-bone, porterhouse, cubed), ground round	1 oz
Pork	Lean pork, such as fresh ham; canned, cured, or boiled ham; Canadian bacon*; tenderloin, center loin chop	1 oz
Lamb	Roast, chop, leg	1 oz
Veal	Lean chop, roast	1 oz
Poultry	Chicken, turkey (dark meat, no skin), chicken white meat (with skin), domestic duck or goose (well-drained of fat, no skin)	1 oz

Meat and Meat Substitutes List *(continued)*

Fish	Herring (uncreamed or smoked)	1 oz
	Oysters	6 medium
	Salmon (fresh or canned), catfish	1 oz
	Sardines (canned)	2 medium
	Tuna (canned in oil, drained)	1 oz
Game	Goose (no skin), rabbit	1 oz
Cheese	4.5%–fat cottage cheese	¼ cup
	Grated Parmesan	2 tbsp
	Cheeses with 3 grams or less fat per ounce	1 oz
Other	Hot dogs with 3 grams or less fat per ounce*	1½ oz
	Processed sandwich meat with 3 grams or less fat per ounce, such as turkey pastrami or kielbasa	1 oz
	Liver, heart (high in cholesterol)	1 oz

Medium-Fat Meat and Substitutes List

Beef	Most beef products fall into this category (ground beef, meatloaf, corned beef, short ribs, Prime grades of meat trimmed of fat, such as prime rib)	1 oz
Pork	Top loin, chop, Boston butt, cutlet	1 oz
Lamb	Rib roast, ground	1 oz
Veal	Cutlet (ground or cubed, unbreaded)	1 oz
Poultry	Chicken dark meat (with skin), ground turkey or ground chicken, fried chicken (with skin)	1 oz
Fish	Any fried fish product	1 oz
Cheese	With 5 grams or less fat per ounce	
	Feta	1 oz
	Mozzarella	1 oz
	Ricotta	¼ cup (2 oz)
Other	Egg (high in cholesterol, limit to 3 per week)	1
	Sausage with 5 grams or less fat per ounce	1 oz
	Soy milk	1 cup
	Tempeh	¼ cup
	Tofu	4 oz or ½ cup

High-Fat Meat and Substitutes List

Pork	Spareribs, ground pork, pork sausage	1 oz
Cheese	All regular cheeses, such as American,* cheddar, Monterey Jack, Swiss	1 oz
Other	Processed sandwich meats with 8 grams or less fat per ounce, such as bologna, pimento loaf, salami	1 oz
	Sausage, such as bratwurst, Italian, knockwurst, Polish, smoked	1 oz
	Hot dog (turkey or chicken)*	1 (10/lb)
	Bacon	3 slices (20 slices/lb)
	Hot dog (beef, pork, or combination)*‡	1 (10/lb)
	Peanut butter (contains unsaturated fat)‡	2 tbsp

*Contains 400 mg or more sodium per exchange.
†Count as one very lean meat and one starch exchange.
‡Count as one high-fat meat plus one fat exchange.

Fat List

Monounsaturated Fats List

Avocado, medium	⅛ (1 oz)
Oil (canola, olive, peanut)	1 tsp
Olives	
Ripe (black)	8 large
Green, stuffed	10 large
Nuts	
Almonds, cashews	6 nuts
Mixed (50% peanuts)	6 nuts
Peanuts	10 nuts
Pecans	4 halves
Peanut butter, smooth or crunchy	2 tsp
Sesame seeds	1 tbsp
Tahini paste	2 tsp

Polyunsaturated Fats List

Margarine	
Stick, tub, or squeeze	1 tsp
Lower-fat (30% to 50% vegetable oil)	1 tbsp
Mayonnaise	
Regular	1 tsp
Reduced-fat	1 tbsp
Nuts, walnuts, English	4 halves
Oil (corn, safflower, soybean)	1 tsp
Salad dressing	
Regular*	1 tbsp
Reduced-fat	2 tbsp

*Contains 400 mg or more sodium per exchange.

Miracle Whip Salad Dressing®	
Regular	2 tsp
Reduced-fat	1 tbsp
Seeds	
Pumpkin, sunflower	1 tbsp

Saturated Fats List

Bacon, cooked	1 slice (20 slices/lb)
Bacon, grease	1 tsp
Butter	
Stick	1 tsp
Whipped	2 tsp
Reduced-fat	1 tbsp
Chitterlings, boiled	2 tbsp (½ oz)
Coconut, sweetened, shredded	2 tbsp
Cream, half and half	2 tbsp
Cream cheese	
Regular	1 tbsp (½ oz)
Reduced-fat	2 tbsp (1 oz)
Fatback or salt pork	
Shortening or lard	1 tsp
Sour cream	
Regular	2 tbsp
Reduced-fat	3 tbsp

Free Foods List

Fat-Free or Reduced-Fat Foods

Cream cheese, fat-free	1 tbsp
Creamers, nondairy, liquid	1 tbsp
Creamers, nondairy, powdered	2 tsp
Mayonnaise, fat-free	1 tbsp
Mayonnaise, reduced-fat	1 tsp
Margarine, fat-free	4 tbsp
Margarine, reduced-fat	1 tsp
Miracle Whip®, nonfat	1 tbsp
Miracle Whip®, reduced-fat	1 tsp
Nonstick cooking spray	
Salad dressing, fat-free	1 tbsp
Salad dressing, fat-free Italian	2 tbsp
Salsa	¼ cup
Sour cream, fat-free, reduced-fat	1 tbsp
Whipped topping, regular or light	2 tbsp

Sugar-Free or Low-Sugar Foods

Candy, hard, sugar-free	1 candy
Gelatin dessert, sugar-free	
Gelatin, unflavored	
Gum, sugar-free	
Jam or jelly, low-sugar or light	2 tsp
Sugar substitutes	
Syrup, sugar-free	2 tbsp

Drinks

Bouillon, broth, consommé*	
Bouillon or broth, low-sodium	

*Contains 400 mg or more of sodium per choice.

Carbonated or mineral water	
Cocoa powder, unsweetened	1 tbsp
Coffee	
Club soda	
Diet soft drinks, sugar-free	
Drink mixes, sugar-free	
Tea	
Tonic water, sugar-free	

Condiments

Catsup	1 tbsp
Horseradish	
Lemon juice	
Lime juice	
Mustard	
Pickles, dill*	1½ large
Soy sauce, regular or light*	
Taco sauce	1 tbsp
Vinegar	

Seasonings

Flavoring extracts	
Garlic	
Herbs, fresh or dried	
Pimento	
Spices	
Tabasco® or hot pepper sauce	
Wine, used in cooking	
Worcestershire sauce	

Combination Foods List

Food	Serving Size	Exchanges per Serving
Entrees		
Tuna noodle casserole, lasagna, spaghetti with meatballs, chili with beans, macaroni and cheese*	1 cup (8 oz)	2 carbohydrates, 2 medium-fat meats
Chow mein (without noodles or rice)	2 cups (16 oz)	1 carbohydrate, 2 lean meats
Pizza, cheese, thin crust*	¼ of 10 in. (5 oz)	2 carbohydrates, 2 medium-fat meats, 1 fat
Pizza, meat topping, thin crust*	¼ of 10 in. (5 oz)	2 carbohydrates, 2 medium-fat meats, 2 fats
Pot pie*	1 (7 oz)	2 carbohydrates, 1 medium-fat meat, 4 fats
Frozen Entrees		
Salisbury steak with gravy, mashed potato*	1 (11 oz)	2 carbohydrates, 3 medium-fat meats, 3–4 fats
Turkey with gravy, mashed potato, dressing*	1 (11 oz)	2 carbohydrates, 2 medium-fat meats, 2 fats
Entree with less than 300 calories*	1 (8 oz)	2 carbohydrates, 3 lean meats
Soups		
Bean*	1 cup	1 carbohydrate, 1 very lean meat
Cream (made with water)*	1 cup (8 oz)	1 carbohydrate, 1 fat
Split pea (made with water)*	½ cup (4 oz)	1 carbohydrate
Tomato (made with water)*	1 cup (8 oz)	1 carbohydrate
Vegetable beef, chicken noodle, or other broth type*	1 cup (8 oz)	1 carbohydrate

*Contains 400 mg or more sodium per exchange.

Appendix 10
Growth Charts for Boys and Girls from Birth to 18 Years of Age

Take all measurements with the child nude or with minimal clothing and without shoes. Measure length with the infant (under 3 years; use "Birth to 36 months" chart) lying on his or her back fully extended. Two people are needed to measure recumbent length properly. Measure stature with the child (at least 2 years of age; use "2 to 18 years" chart) standing. Use a beam balance to measure weight.

From the Department of Health, Education, and Welfare, Public Health Service, Health Resource Administration, National Center for Health Statistics, and Centers for Disease Control and Prevention.

BOYS FROM BIRTH TO 36 MONTHS

LENGTH FOR AGE

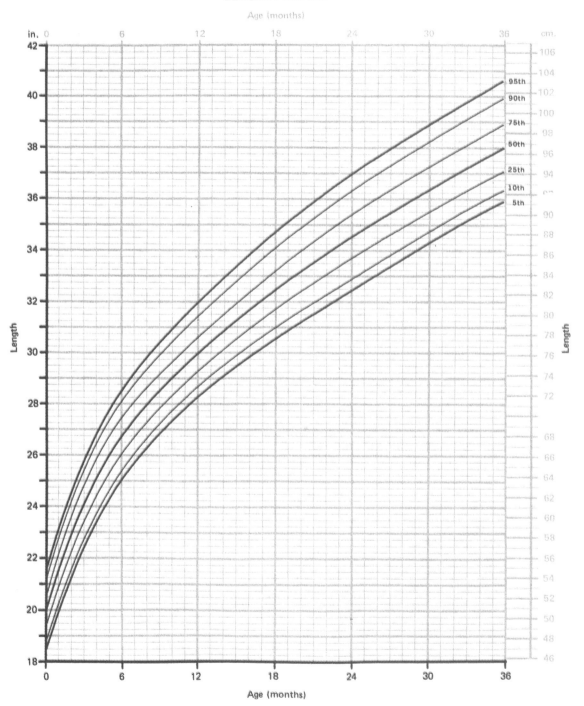

BOYS FROM BIRTH TO 36 MONTHS

WEIGHT FOR AGE

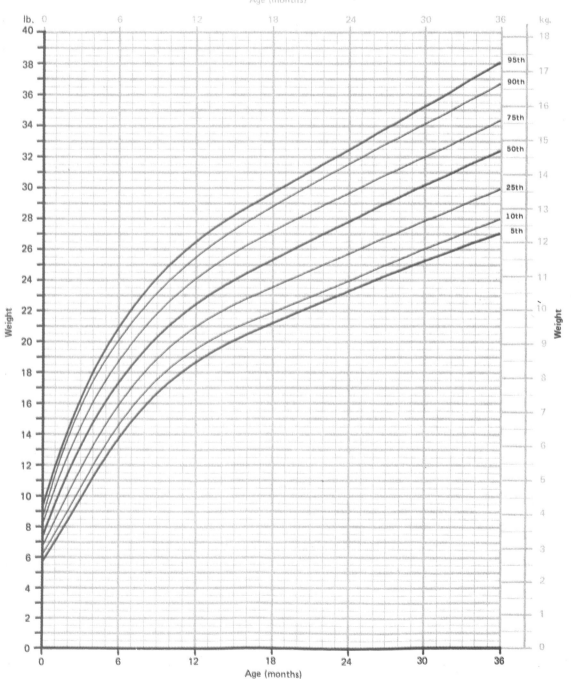

BOYS FROM BIRTH TO 36 MONTHS

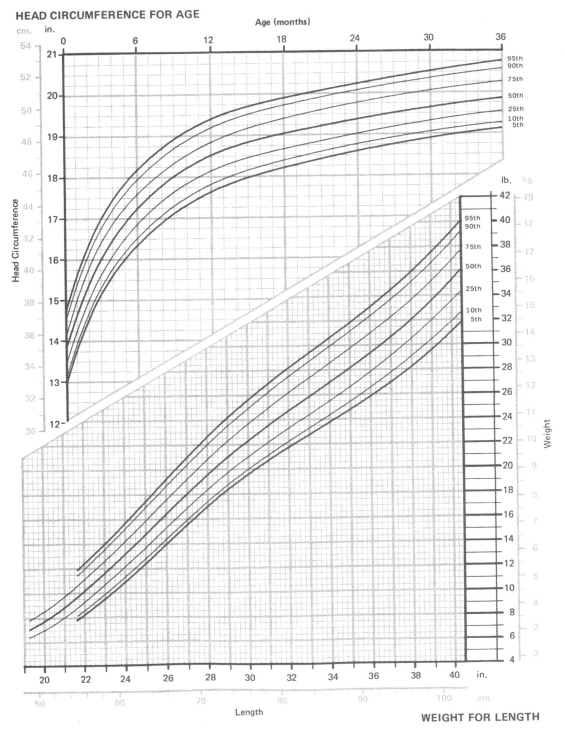

HEAD CIRCUMFERENCE FOR AGE

WEIGHT FOR LENGTH

GIRLS FROM BIRTH TO 36 MONTHS

LENGTH FOR AGE

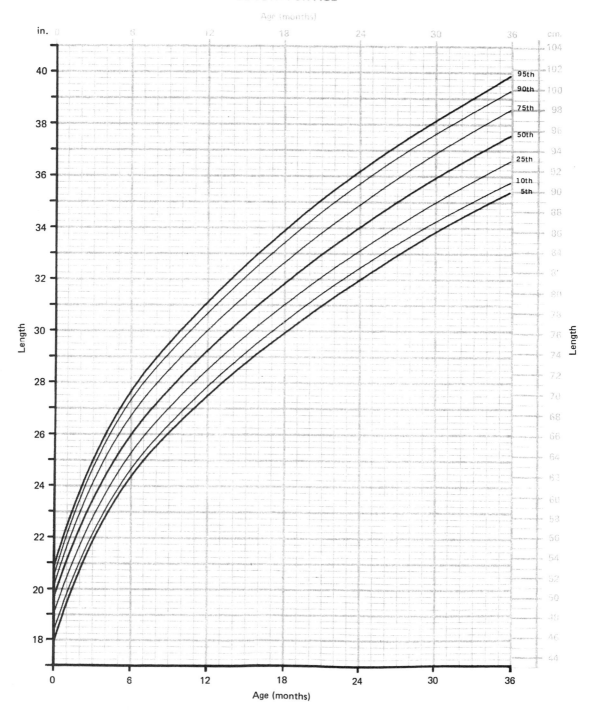

GIRLS FROM BIRTH TO 36 MONTHS

WEIGHT FOR AGE

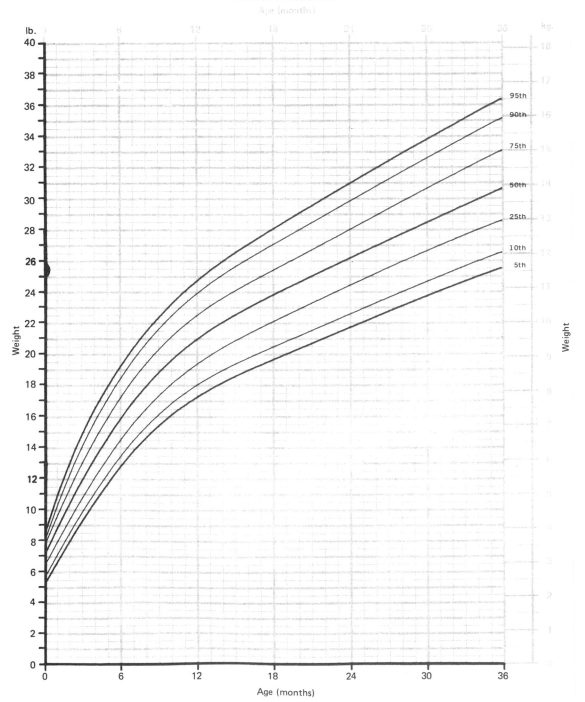

GIRLS FROM BIRTH TO 36 MONTHS

HEAD CIRCUMFERENCE FOR AGE

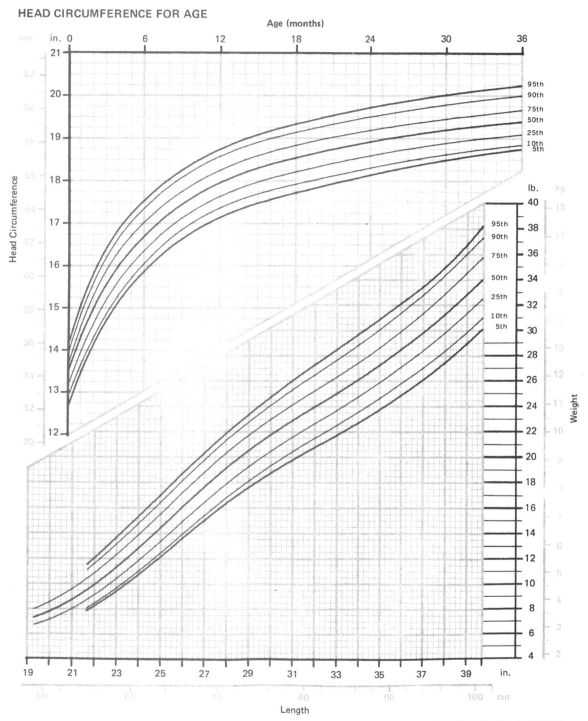

WEIGHT FOR LENGTH

BOYS FROM 2 TO 18 YEARS

STATURE FOR AGE

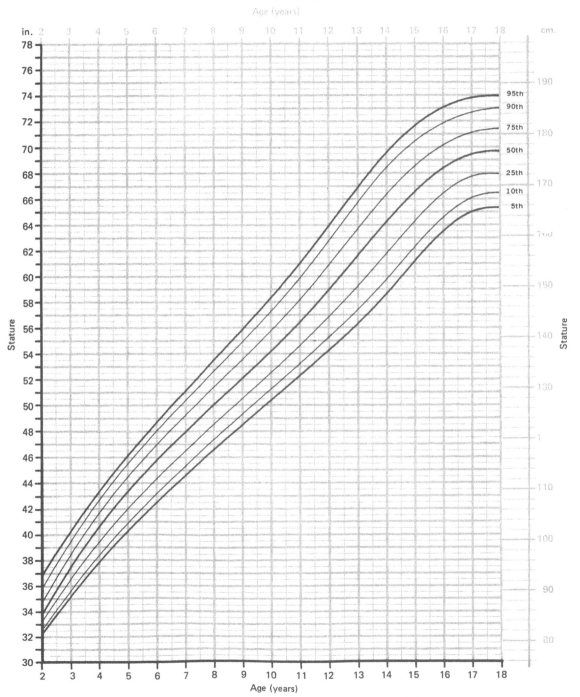

BOYS FROM 2 TO 18 YEARS

WEIGHT FOR AGE

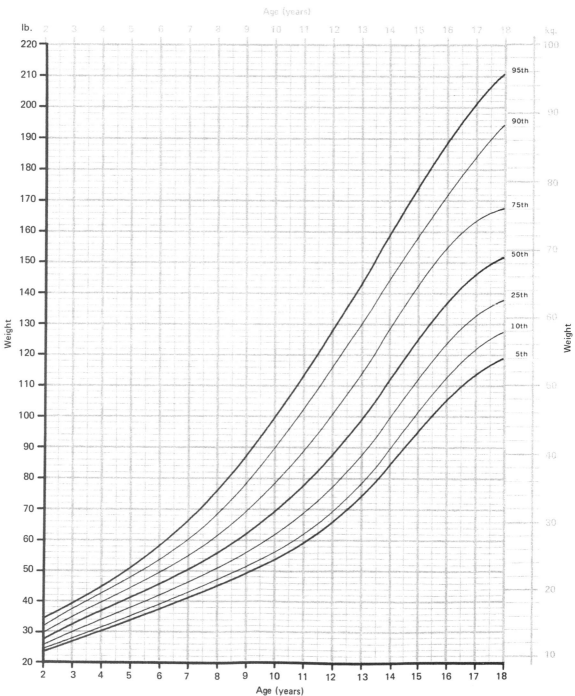

PRE-PUBERTAL BOYS FROM 2 TO 11½ YEARS

WEIGHT FOR STATURE

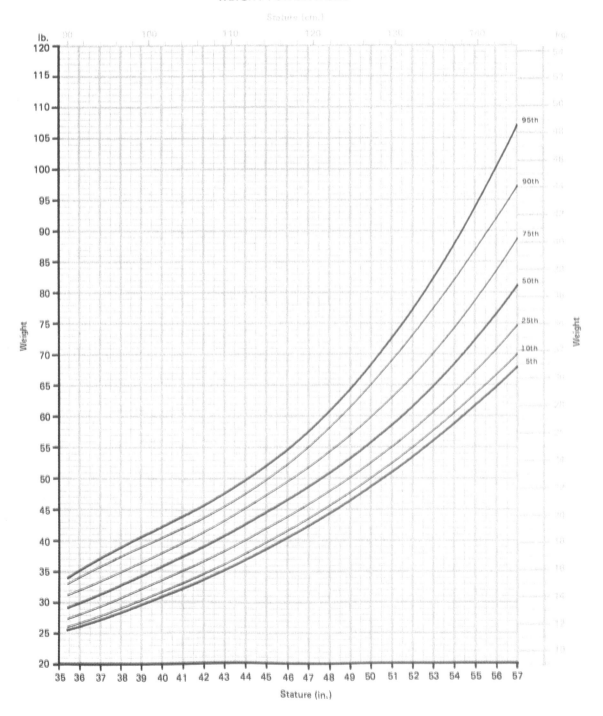

GIRLS FROM 2 TO 18 YEARS
STATURE FOR AGE

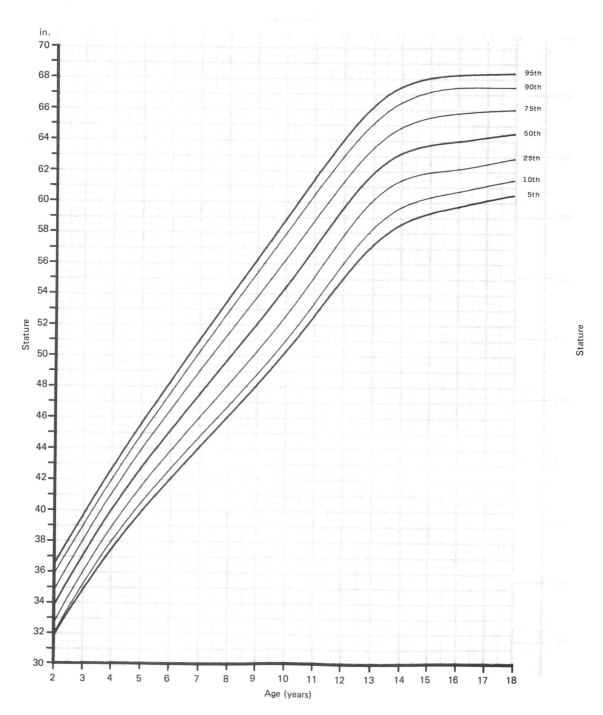

GIRLS FROM 2 TO 18 YEARS
WEIGHT FOR AGE

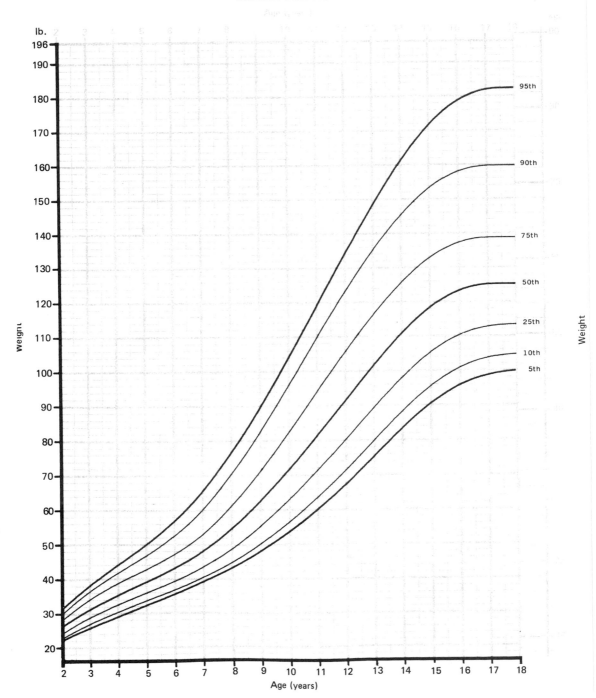

PRE-PUBERTAL GIRLS FROM 2 TO 10 YEARS

WEIGHT FOR STATURE

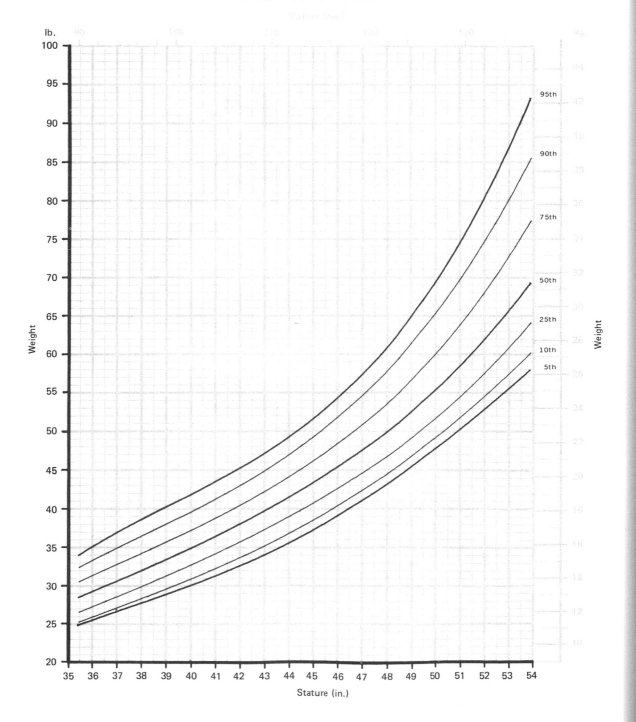

Appendix 11
Estimating Body Frame Size

1. Frame size may be determined by wrist circumference. Values are affected by variability of soft tissue. Wrist circumference is determined by measuring the smallest part of the wrist distal to the styloid process of the ulna and radius. The "r" value is then determined by this formula:

$$\frac{\text{height in centimeters}}{\text{wrist circumference in centimeters}}$$

Then refer to the following r value table to determine frame size:

Men r value	frame size	Women r value
10.4 or greater	small	11.0 or greater
9.6 to 10.4	medium	10.1 to 11.0
9.6 or less	large	10.1 or less

2. Elbow breadth is measured with the forearm upward at a 90-degree angle. The distance between the outer aspects of the two prominent bones on either side of the elbow is considered to be the elbow breadth. Elbow breadth less than that listed for medium frame indicates a small frame. Elbow breadth greater than that listed for medium frame indicates a large frame.

Frame Size for Women

Height in 1-inch heels	Elbow breadth for medium frames
4'10" to 4'11"	2¼" to 2½"
5'0" to 5'3"	2¼" to 2½"
5'4" to 5'7"	2⅜" to 2⅝"
5'8" to 5'11"	2⅜" to 2⅝"
6'0"	2½" to 2¾"

Frame Size for Men

Height in 1-in heels	Elbow breadth for medium frames
5'2" to 5'3"	2½" to 2⅞"
5'4" to 5'7"	2⅝" to 2⅞"
5'8" to 5'11"	2¾" to 3"
6'0 to 6'3"	2¾" to 3⅛"
6'4"	2⅞" to 3¼"

From Manual for Clinical Dietetics, The American Dietetic Association, 1996.

Appendix 12
Body Mass Index

Measure height to the nearest inch and weight to the nearest pound. Mark them on the body mass index (BMI) nomogram. Then use a straight edge (paper, ruler) to connect the two points and circle the spot where this straight line crosses the center line to obtain the BMI value. *Note:* When computing BMI with the equation weight ÷ height^2, kilograms and meters should be used.

NOMOGRAM FOR BODY MASS INDEX

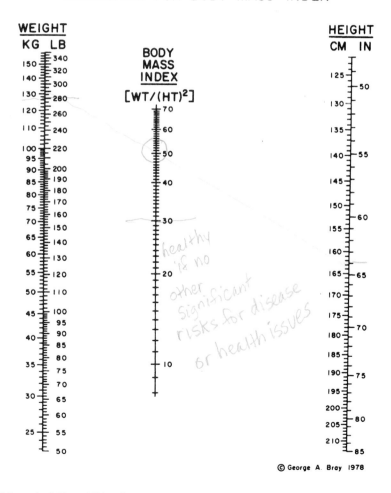

© George A. Bray 1978

From Manual of Clinical Dietetics, The American Dietetic Association, 5th edition, WB Saunders, Philadelphia, 1996.

Appendix 13

Nomogram to Estimate Stature from Knee Height in Persons Aged 60 to 90 Years

An elderly person's stature can be estimated from the following nomogram. To use this nomogram, locate the person's age on the left column and knee height on the middle column, and connect these two points. Mark where the connecting line crosses the stature column for the appropriate sex to find the estimated stature.

A knee-height caliper can be obtained from Ross Laboratory, 1-800-848-2607. In OH, PA, and WV, call 1-800-367-7677 or contact your local Ross representative.

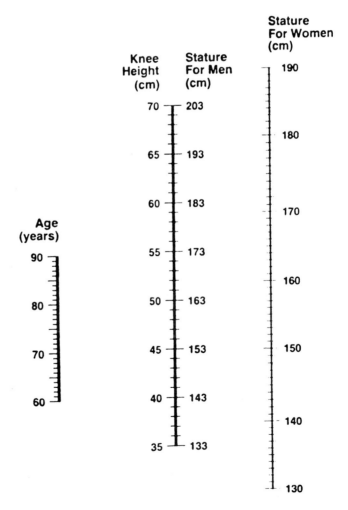

From Consultant Dietitians in Health Care Facilities, A Practice Group of the American Dietetic Association, Pocket Resource for Nutrition Assessment, 1990.

Appendix 14
Child Meal Patterns of the Child and Adult Care Food Program (CACFP)

Food Components	Food Items	REQUIRED MINIMUM QUANTITIES		
		Age: 1 up to 3	Age: 3 up to 6	Age: 6 up to 13
Breakfast				
Milk, fluid	Whole, low-fat, skim, or buttermilk	½ c	¾ c	1 c
Juice or fruit or vegetable		¼ c	½ c	½ c
Bread or bread alternate	Bread	½ sl	½ sl	1 sl
	Cold dry cereal	¼ c or ⅓ oz	⅓ c or ½ oz	¾ c or 1 oz
	Cooked cereal	¼ c	¼ c	½ c
	Biscuit or muffin	½ whole	½ whole	1 whole
	English muffin	¼ whole	¼ whole	½ whole
Snack (Serve 2 of 4 components)				
Milk, fluid		½ c	½ c	1 c
Juice[a] or fruit or vegetable		½ c	½ c	¾ c
Bread or bread alternate		½ sl	½ sl	1 sl
Meat or meat alternate		½ oz	½ oz	1 oz
	Yogurt, plain or flavored[b]	¼ c	¼ c	½ c
Lunch or Supper				
Milk, fluid		½ c	¾ c	1 c
Fruit or vegetable	2 or more servings of vegetables or fruits or both to total (must serve at least 2 different varieties)	¼ c total	½ c total	¾ c total
Bread or bread alternate	Bread	½ sl	½ sl	1 sl
	Graham crackers[c]	2 squares	2 squares	3½ squares
	Cooked pasta or noodle products	¼ c	¼ c	½ c
	Cooked cereal grains (i.e., rice)	¼ c	¼ c	½ c
	6-in Tortilla	½ whole	½ whole	1 whole
Meat or meat alternate (quantity of the edible portion as served)	Lean meat, poultry, or fish	1 oz	1½ oz	2 oz
	Cheese	1 oz	1½ oz	2 oz
	Cottage cheese	¼ c	⅜ c	½ c
	Large egg(s)	1	1	1
	Cooked dry beans, peas, or lentils	¼ c	⅜ c	½ c
	Peanut butter or other nut or seed butters	2 tbsp	3 tbsp	4 tbsp
	Peanuts, soy nuts, tree nuts, or seeds, as listed in program guidance.[d]	½ oz = 50%	¾ oz = 50%	1 oz = 50%

[a]Juice may not be served if milk is the only other component at snack.

[b]A serving of yogurt may be substituted for the meat or meat alternate.

[c]Refer to the "Crediting Food in CACFP" guide for serving sizes of other cracker types (available from CACFP).

[d]No more than 50 percent of the requirement and must be combined in the meal with at least 50 percent of other meat or meat alternatives. (1 oz of nuts/seeds = 1 oz of cooked lean meat, poultry, or fish.)

From the Child and Adult Care Food Program (CACFP), USDA, 1994.

Glossary

Absorption The passage of liquids and end products of digestion into the villi of the intestine.

Achalasia A condition in which the esophagus and gastrointestinal tract fail to relax, causing a feeling of fullness, vomiting, and possible aspiration of esophagael contents into the respiratory passages.

Acid-base balance A state of equilibrium between acidity and alkalinity of body fluids; problems with acidosis or alkalosis are determined by pH and blood gas analysis.

Activities of daily living (ADL) Activities that the average person performs routinely during a day.

Addison's disease A syndrome related to inadequate hormone secretion of the adrenal glands; may be associated with fluid and electrolyte imbalance and profound hypoglycemia unless treated with steroids.

Adipose tissue Body fat.

Adrenalin A hormone that works to raise blood sugar levels; also causes increased heart rate.

Aerobic exercise Any form of exercise that requires an increased intake of oxygen such as brisk walking or running.

AIDS Autoimmune deficiency syndrome; a disease caused by the human immunodeficiency virus (HIV) in which the immune system fails to function.

AIDS enteropathy A condition related to AIDS that causes malabsorption and resultant diarrhea.

Albumin A plasma protein responsible for regulating the osmotic force of blood.

Albuminuria Albumin in the urine.

Alimentary enzymes Enzymes in the digestive tract, such as sucrase, lactase, maltase, lipase, and others.

Alkali A chemical substance with a pH greater than 7.

Allergen A substance that induces hypersensitivity.

Amenorrhea The lack of menses.

Amino acids The substances that make protein. Essential amino acids must be supplied by the diet; nonessential amino acids can be synthesized by the body.

Amylase An enzyme that hastens the hydrolysis of starch into sugar.

Anabolism The constructive phase of metabolism, resulting in growth and repair; adj. anabolic.

Anaerobic exercise Any exercise that does not increase the intake of oxygen, such as weight lifting.

Anorexia   Loss of appetite.

Anorexia nervosa   A serious chronic condition with severe restriction of food intake unrelated to appetite and refusal to accept a normal weight as desirable; often associated with adolescent girls but also occurs with boys and athletes requiring a low body weight.

Anthropometry   The science that deals with body measurements, such as size, weight, and proportion.

Antibodies   Substances synthesized in the body that destroy bacteria or antigens.

Antidiuretic hormone   A hormone that suppresses the excretion of urine; stored and released by the pituitary gland.

Antigens   Substances that react with antibodies or help in the formation of antibodies.

Anuria   Lack of urinary excretion.

Arteriosclerosis   The hardening and thickening of the walls of the arteries.

Arthralgia   Joint pain.

Ascites   An accumulation of excess fluids in the abdomen.

Aspiration   Inhalation of food or liquid into the lungs; can cause pneumonia.

Atherosclerosis   A build-up of plaque inside the arteries and blood vessels that leads to heart disease.

Attention deficit hyperactivity disorder (ADHD)   The official term of the American Psychiatric Association that relates to a condition generally found in children who have an inability to pay attention and to sustain effort.

Autism   A syndrome beginning in infancy characterized by extreme withdrawal from the external environment and an obsessive desire to avoid change; the cause is unknown and affected children rarely recover.

Autonomic neuropathy   Nerve disease of the autonomic or involuntary system, such as the digestive or respiratory system.

Azotemia   Abnormally increased levels of nitrogen in the blood.

Basal metabolism   The lowest level of metabolism to support life; does not take into account physical activity.

Beriberi   A deficiency disease caused by lack of thiamine.

Beta carotene   The precursor to vitamin A which is found in plant products that are deep orange or dark-green leafy. An antioxidant that is believed to lower the risk of cancer and heart disease.

Beta cells   The cells of the pancreas, where insulin is produced.

Bile   A yellow fluid produced by the liver and stored in the gallbladder until needed in the small intestine for digestion of dietary fat.

Biological value of protein   Refers to the amount of essential amino acids in relation to the total quantity of protein. Animal protein sources (meat, eggs, milk) have a high biological value of protein.

Bipolar disorder   Formerly called manic depression, a condition marked by alternating periods of depression and mania (elation and agitation).

Biopsychosocial   The interplay between forces of biology, psychology, and social factors on one's health and health decisions.

Blood Urea Nitrogen (BUN)   The urea nitrogen concentration found in blood; an indicator of renal functioning.

Body Mass Index (BMI) Originally called the Quetelet Index, weight in kilograms divided by the square of the height in meters; felt to give a better indicator for appropriate height and weight measures than Metropolitan Life weight charts.

Botulism An often fatal form of food poisoning caused by a poisonous endotoxin.

Bulimarexia A condition vacillating between anorexic and bulimic eating patterns.

Bulimia A condition of overeating with purging or laxative abuse being common.

Cancer cachexia A condition of malnutrition associated with cancer.

Carbohydrate counting A meal planning strategy used in diabetes management.

Carbohydrate loading A strategy used by athletes to increase the amount of stored glycogen available to the muscles.

Cardiomyopathy A general term referring to heart disease.

Cariogenic Contributing to dental caries.

Carnitine A substance primarily synthesized in the kidneys with a role in fatty acid oxidation in tissue cells, especially those of cardiac and skeletal muscles.

Carotene Also referred to as beta carotene; the precursor to vitamin A found in dark-green leafy and deep orange vegetables and fruits.

Catabolism A destructive process that releases energy; adj. catabolic.

Celiac sprue An inflammatory condition of the villi of the jejunum related to gluten or gliadin found in wheat, oats, rye, barley, and triticale (a new hybrid grain); found more commonly among persons with British heritage.

Cellulose Structural fiber in fruits, vegetables, and grains.

Cerebral palsy A motor disorder caused by brain damage beginning in infancy that can involve muscle spasms, uncontrollable movements, or poor balance with a staggering gait.

Cerebrovascular accident (CVA) An embolus or blood clot; often called a "stroke."

Cheilosis A condition characterized by dry, scaly lips and cracks at the corners of the mouth; seen in riboflavin deficiency.

Chemotherapy A treatment for cancer; the provision of toxic chemicals to the system to destroy cancer cells.

Cholecystitis Inflammation of the gallbladder.

Cholelithiasis The presence of gallstones.

Cholesterol A fat-related compound that is produced in the livers of animals; found in animal fats but does not provide kilocalories.

Chyme The semiliquid form of digested food that passes from the stomach into the duodenum after undergoing the action of gastric juice.

Cirrhosis A disease of the liver often associated with alcoholism.

Cleft palate A condition in which there is an opening or hole in the roof of the mouth, sometimes extending to the lip, which needs to be surgically repaired.

Clostridium perfringens A type of bacteria that causes food poisoning.

Colostrum   The nutritious substance that precedes breast milk production in the first few days after delivery.

Complete protein   Protein containing all of the essential amino acids.

Coronary thrombosis   A condition of severe arteriosclerosis that cuts off blood supply to a part or parts of the heart; often fatal.

Cortisol   A hormone produced in the adrenal glands that works in the opposite manner to insulin to raise blood sugar levels.

Counter regulatory hormones   Hormones that work in the opposite manner to insulin; hormones that raise blood sugar levels principally through the release of stored glycogen in the liver or through the inhibition of insulin action.

Creatinine   A nitrogen compound used in a laboratory test to indicate renal function.

Cretinism   A condition of childhood caused by lack of thyroid gland secretion that leads to a dwarf size accompanied by mental retardation and sterility if not treated with thyroid extract for life.

Crohn's disease   A chronic condition of intermittant inflammation of the terminal portion of the ileum or other portion of the intestinal tract; usually treated with steroids, but attention to good nutrition is important. Also referred to as regional enteritis.

Cystic fibrosis   A hereditary disease with dysfunction of the exocrine glands resulting in thick mucus and abnormal secretion of sweat and saliva.

Daily Reference Values (DRV)   A system developed for use on food labels to indicate recommended nutrient intakes for 2000 and 2500 kilocalories.

Dawn phenomenon   Early morning phenomenon involving counter regulatory hormones that results in increased blood glucose levels.

Decubitus ulcer   Bed or pressure sore.

Dental enamel   The outside hard protective covering of teeth.

Dental plaque   A calcified coating on teeth that provides a perfect growing medium for bacteria; plaque needs to be removed regularly to prevent dental decay.

Depapillation   The smooth appearance of the papilla (elevations on the surface of the tongue containing taste buds) resulting from vitamin B deficiency.

Desirable weight   A body mass index (BMI) between 20 and 25; or a realistic weight that allows for good health for an individual.

DETERMINE check list   A tool to identify elderly persons who are at nutritional risk.

Diabetic coma   A condition of hyperglycemia with ketonuria; usually found in Type 1 diabetes. Also referred to as diabetic ketoacidosis.

Diabetic retinopathy   An eye disease found in persons with long-standing diabetes; prevented through good diabetes management.

Disaccharides   Double sugars such as sucrose and lactose.

Diuretic   A substance that promotes urine secretion.

Diverticulitis   Inflammation of the diverticula or outpouchings in the intestinal tract.

Diverticulosis   A permanent condition of the intestinal tract characterized by small pockets protruding from the intestinal wall; often associated with advancing age.

DNA   Deoxyribonucleic acid; part of the genetic material of body cells.

Down syndrome   A congenital condition characterized by physical malformations and some degree of mental retardation; caused by an extra chromosome. Also referred to as trisomy 21 syndrome because of the defect at chromosome 21; formerly referred to as mongolism because persons with this condition have facial characteristics resembling persons of the Mongolian race.

Dumping syndrome   A condition characterized by nausea, weakness, sweating, palpitation, fainting, often a warm feeling, and sometimes diarrhea. These symptoms occur after eating in people who have had a partial gastrectomy.

Duodenum   The first portion of the small intestine, about 10 inches long, connecting the pylorus to the jejunum.

Dysgeusia   Impaired sense of taste.

Dyslipidemia   Elevated triglycerides with low HDL-cholesterol levels.

Dyspepsia   Impaired digestion related to epigastric discomfort after meals.

Dysphagia   Difficulty in swallowing.

Edentulous   Without teeth.

Electrolyte   A mineral that disassociates into ions when fused or in solution so that electricity can be conducted.

Elemental feeding   A complete liquid nutrition supplement that does not require digestion.

Empty kilocalories   Foods that provide sugar or fat but few vitamins, minerals, or protein.

Encopresis   Incontinence of fecal material; often caused by a "plug" of solid fecal material that allows liquid fecal material to pass around the solid material.

End stage renal disease (ESRD)   A period in which BUN and creatinine levels are very high, with impairment to all body systems. Also known as uremia.

Endocrine system   The glands that secrete hormones directly into the circulation; a major control system of body functioning and metabolism.

Energy balance   The level of energy taken in (kilocalories) that equals that amount of energy expended (basal metabolism plus activity needs).

Enrichment   The replacement of nutrients lost in processing.

Enteral nutrition   A form of nutrition support usually with liquid nutrition supplements by way of the small intestine.

Enzyme   A protein that can hasten or produce a change in a substance.

Epilepsy   A group of symptoms related to abnormal electrical activity of the brain resulting in periodic seizure activity.

Epithelial   Pertaining to the cellular covering of the internal and external surfaces of the body.

Erythropoietin   A hormone produced in the kidneys that stimulates red blood cell production.

Esophageal reflux   A chronic disease with reflux of the stomach contents; may be associated with hiatal hernia.

Esophageal sphincter   The muscular connection between the esophagus and the stomach.

Esophageal varices   Enlargement of veins in the esophagus.

Essential amino acids   The substances that are turned into protein that must be supplied in the diet; found in animal protein sources but can be obtained from plant sources with careful food selection.

Essential fatty acids   Forms of fat needed for health that must be supplied by the diet; found in vegetable oils.

Estrogen   A female sex hormone produced primarily in ovaries but also in the adrenal glands and testes of males; allows for implantation of a fertilized egg.

Failure to thrive   A medical diagnosis that includes lack of physical growth (below the third percentile for weight and height for age); may be related to maternal deprivation.

Fetal alcohol syndrome   A group of symptoms characterized by mental and physical abnormalities of the infant linked to maternal alcohol intake during pregnancy.

Fifteen:fifteen rule (15:15 rule)   Treatment and re-evaluation of hypoglycemia; treatment with 15 grams of carbohydrate for someone who is still conscious, with a re-check of blood sugar levels in 15 minutes (procedure continues if blood sugar remains low).

Fifteen hundred rule (1500 rule)   The mathematical formula used to estimate point drop in blood glucose per one unit of regular insulin; the number 1500 divided by the total amount of insulin units regularly injected.

Fluoride   A mineral that promotes uptake of calcium by teeth and bones; currently used as a preventive measure against dental caries.

Food additives   Additives to food that are used for stabilization or to increase shelf-life and safety of food.

Food allergy   An abnormal hypersensitivity reaction to foods containing protein material called allergens.

Food exchange lists   A food guide that groups food based on equivalent amounts of carbohydrate, protein, and fat.

Food intolerance   A nonimmune intolerance to certain foods related to poor digestion or other factor.

Food jags   A term applied to childhood eating habits in which a few foods are eaten for days or weeks at a time.

Food quack   An untrained person who espouses potentially harmful nutrition practices.

Fore milk   Breast milk that is released from the front of the breasts; has a lower fat content than hind milk.

Fortification   The addition of nutrients to greater than the natural level found in a food; milk and margarine are often fortified.

Gastroparesis   A condition in which autonomic neuropathy of the stomach results in partial paralysis such that digestion and the propulsion of food through the digestive tract are impaired.

Gavage feeding   A form of feeding by tube.

Geriatrics   The branch of medicine concerned with the treatment and prevention of diseases affecting elderly individuals.

Gerontology   The study of the problems of aging.

Gestational   Related to pregnancy.

Gestational diabetes   A form of diabetes occurring during pregnancy, usually beginning between the 24th and 28th weeks of gestation.

Gingivitis   An inflammation of the gums.

Gliadin   A component of gluten that needs to be avoided in celiac disease.

Glomerular filtration rate (GFR)   Amount of glomerular filtrate in milliliters cleared through the kidneys in 1 minute. Rates less than 30 mL/min indicate that kidney disease may be present; lower rates call for aggressive management.

Glucagon   A counter regulatory hormone that is given by injection during severe bouts of hypoglycemia in an unconscious diabetic person.

Gluconeogenesis   The formation of glucose from protein.

Gluten   The protein portion of wheat, oats, rye, barley, and triticale (a hybrid grain); complete avoidance is often necessary in the control of celiac disease.

Glycated   The process in which glucose attaches to protein throughout body cells.

Glycemia   Blood glucose level.

Glycemic index   A means of rating food based on predictive impact on blood sugar levels; fats have the lowest and sugars have the highest glycemic index.

Glycerol   A component of fats.

Glycogen   The storage form of carbohydrate found in the liver and muscle tissues; released in the form of sugar as needed for energy or during times of physiological stress.

Glycogen loading   A process by which the glycogen stores in the liver are increased beyond normal levels to allow for the demands for endurance in athletic competition.

Glycogenolysis   The breakdown of stored carbohydrate in the liver from glycogen to glucose.

Glycosuria   Glucose in the urine; an outdated means of diabetes management; sometimes used for a simple means of diabetes screening.

Goiter   A swelling of the thyroid gland on the neck caused by iodine deficiency.

Gout   A hereditary form of arthritis in which uric acid is built up in the blood and may be deposited in joints and other tissues; usually treated with medication.

GRAS list   Generally recognized as safe; standards for acceptable levels of food additives.

Grazing   A term applied to a manner of continuous eating throughout the day rather than eating three meals.

Growth hormone   A substance that stimulates growth; works in the opposite manner to insulin to raise blood sugar levels.

Health   A relative state that includes physical, mental, social, and spirtual functioning such that an individual can meet ones's full potential.

Health Belief Model   A theory that stresses that an individual's perceived level of health risk and "cost" of behavior change contributes to health decisions.

Heat exhaustion   A disorder resulting from excessive loss of body fluids and electrolytes.

Hematocrit   The volume percentage of red blood cells in whole blood.

Hematuria   Blood in the urine.

Heme iron   The form of iron found in meat; iron that is readily absorbed.

Hemodialysis   A procedure used to remove toxic wastes from the blood of a patient with acute or chronic renal failure.

Hemoglobin   The oxygen-carrying pigment of the blood; the principal protein in the red blood cell.

Hemoglobin A$_{1C}$ (HbA$_{1C}$)   A test used to determine long-term diabetes management; indicates an average blood sugar reading over a two-month time period.

Hemorrhage   The loss of blood from a ruptured vessel.

Hepatic coma   Coma resulting from cerebral damage caused by liver disease.

Hepatitis   An inflammatory liver disease that has many forms and causes.

Hiatal hernia   Protrusion of part of the stomach through the opening of the esophageal hiatus of the diaphragm.

Hind milk   Milk released from the upper part of the breast in response to the hormone oxytocin; very rich in fat.

Histidinemia   A hereditary metabolic defect marked by excessive histidine in the blood and urine.

Holistic health   Having to do with the whole of one's health; considering all factors affecting one's state of health.

Homocystinuria   A lack of enzyme resulting in homocystine in the urine.

Homogenize   The process in which fat particles become so finely dispersed that they do not rise in a liquid.

Honeymoon period   Usually the first year after diagnosis of insulin-dependent diabetes mellitus; before the complete destruction of the beta cells.

Hormone   Chemicals produced by cells of the body to stimulate or retard certain life processes such as growth and reproduction.

Hospices   Organizations that support a natural process of death in one's home or in an institutional setting in which death and the grieving process are openly discussed.

Hydrogenated fat   A liquid vegetable oil that has the element hydrogen added to make a solid fat.

Hyperalimentation   Administration of all nutrients directly into the blood system. Also referred to as total parenteral nutrition (TPN).

Hypercalcemia   An excess of calcium in the blood.

Hypercalciuria   An excess of calcium in the urine.

Hyperchlorhydria   An excess of hydrochloric acid in gastic juice.

Hypercholesterolemia   An elevation of cholesterol in the blood.

Hyperemesis   Excessive vomiting.

Hyperglycemia   An elevation of glucose in the blood; diagnostic of diabetes with two fasting blood sugars over 126 mg/dL.

Hyperglycemic, Hyperosmolar Nonketotic Coma (HHNK)   A condition often associated with diabetes in an older person; blood sugars in the 500 mg/dL range or higher, with severe dehydration and confusion evident.

Hyperinsulinemia   High levels of insulin in the blood; often associated with obesity and insulin resistance.

Hyperkinesis   Abnormally increased motor activity or movement.

Hyperlipidemia   An elevation of specific lipoproteins, cholesterol, and triglycerides.

Hyperlipoproteinemia   An excess of lipoproteins in the blood.

Hyperosmotic diarrhea   A type of diarrhea caused by a high solute load that draws excess water into the intestinal tract.

Hyperplasty   A term related to the fat cell theory that describes a situation in which a person has an excess number of fat cells.

Hypertension   High blood pressure.

Hypertrophy   A term related to the fat cell theory that describes a situation in which a person has large-sized fat cells.

Hypertriglyceridemia   High levels of triglycerides in the blood; often associated with excess alcohol intake or the insulin resistance syndrome.

Hypoalbuminemia   Abnormally low levels of albumin in the blood.

Hypochlorhydria   A deficiency of hydrochloric acid in gastric juice.

Hypochromic   A lack of color in red blood cells as a result of decrease in hemoglobin.

Hypocupremia   Low copper levels in the blood.

Hypoglycemic unawareness   Low blood sugar without symptoms; generally occurs after years of uncontrolled diabetes.

IDDM (insulin dependent diabetes mellitus)   A form of diabetes that usually develops in children and young adults; once known as juvenile onset diabetes. Now referred to as Type 1 diabetes (in numerical versus arabic form).

IgE antibody   The immune factor related to food and other allergies.

Ileum   The lower part of the small intestine.

Immunoglobulin A (IgA)   Known to have antiviral properties; produced in nonvascular fluids such as saliva and intestinal secretions.

Inborn errors of metabolism   Conditions resulting in a lack of a hormone or other metabolic chemical that results in a build-up of toxic by-products in the system; often causes mental retardation unless the diet is altered beginning in infancy.

Ingestion   Eating; taking food into the digestive tract.

Insoluble fiber   A form of dietary fiber that does not dissolve in water; referred to as roughage. Whole wheat contains this type of fiber.

Insulin   A protein hormone formed in the pancreas and secreted into the blood for the purpose of regulating carbohydrate, lipid, and amino acid metabolism.

Insulin resistance   A condition in which the body cells resist the action of insulin; often found in obesity and with a high-fat diet; often a genetic predisposition exists.

Insulin resistance syndrome   A diagnosis is made by correlates, including central obesity, dyslipidemia, hypertension, Type 2 diabetes, gout, and polycystic ovary syndrome.

Insulin shock   Excess amounts of injected insulin result in profound hypoglycemia; glucose needed to treat either orally in a conscious state or via a venous route (IV dextrose).

Intermediate care facility (ICF)   A group home for persons with developmental disabilities; ICFs were developed in response to the deinstitutionalism of such persons.

Intrinsic factor   A substance produced in the stomach that helps absorption of vitamin B_{12}.

Iron overload   A rare disease of unknown origin characterized by widespread iron deposits in the body; can lead to pancreatic cirrhosis and other problems.

Irritable bowel syndrome (IBS)   A noninflammatory condition of the bowel, with altered bowel habits often alternating between diarrhea and constipation and with abdominal pain.

Islets of Langerhans   The portion of the beta cells found in the pancreas that produces insulin.

IU   Also known as international unit; a measure used for vitamin A amounts.

Jaundice   A condition related to hyperbilirubinemia, with the deposit of yellow bile pigments causing yellowness of skin.

Jejunostomy   A permanent opening performed by surgery between the jejunum and the surface of the abdominal wall.

Jejunum   The middle portion of the small intestine connecting the duodenum and the ileum.

Ketoacidosis   An accumulation of excess ketones (acid) that changes the pH of the blood; seen in uncontrolled diabetes mellitus.

Ketogenic diet   A diet containing large amounts of fat and minimal amounts of protein and carbohydrate; sometimes used in treating certain types of epilepsy in children.

Ketonuria   Ketones found in the urine; a test to help with diabetes management during illness, when blood sugars are over 240 mg/dL or during pregnancy.

Ketosis   The accumulation in the blood and tissues of large quantities of ketone bodies as a result of a complete oxidation of fats.

Kilocalorie (kcal)   A unit of measure used to describe food energy. One pound of body fat is equivalent to 3500 kcal of food.

Krebs cycle   The chemical process found at the cell level that converts food matter into energy.

Kwashiorkor   Protein deficiency disease.

Kyphosis   Also called hunchback; an abnormal curvature of the spine often related to osteoporosis.

Lactation   The breast-feeding period.

Lactobacillus culture   A culture containing a beneficial form of bacteria normally found in a healthy intestine; used in making yogurt.

Lactose intolerance   The inability to digest the milk sugar lactose due to inadequate amounts of the lactase enzyme; common symptoms are bloating of the abdomen with flatus and diarrhea.

Lean tissue   Muscle tissue.

Learned food aversion   An aversion to food that is learned through a negative association such as an illness.

Legumes   The fruit or seed of pod-bearing plants such as peas, beans, lentils, and peanuts.

Let-down reflex   A term used to describe the process whereby the hormone oxytocin allows the hind milk to flow during breast-feeding; characterized by a gentle "pins and needles" sensation.

Linoleic acid   An essential fatty acid.

Lipase   An enzyme that hastens the splitting of fats into glycerol and fatty acids.

Lipids   A term relating to all forms of fat.

Lipogenic   Related to substances that induce the promotion of body fat; insulin is a hormone that is lipogenic.

Lipolysis   The breakdown of body fat.

Lipoprotein   Lipid (fat) attached to protein; lipoproteins are the form of fats found in the blood.

Macrobiotic diet   A diet progressing in stages and consisting mainly of rice in the last stage. The diet is deficient in many nutrients, including some amino acids.

Macronutrient   The energy (kilocalorie) sources in food: carbohydrate, protein, and fat. Alcohol is also an energy source.

Malnutrition   A state of inadequate nutrient intake (such as marasmus) or an excess nutrient intake (such as obesity).

Marasmus   Protein-calorie malnutrition.

Medical Nutrition Therapy   A diet modified in nutrients and used as therapy for diabetes, renal and cardiovascular disease, and other diseases and conditions. Previously referred to as diet therapy or therapeutic diet.

Medium chain triglycerides (MCT)   A type of fat that does not require digestion; often used as a form of enteral nutrition support in conditions of fat malabsorption.

Megadose   Large doses; generally ascribed to supplements of vitamins and minerals that are greater than ten times the RDA.

Megaloblastic anemia   A form of anemia characterized by megaloblasts in the bone marrow or blood.

Ménière's disease   A disorder of the labyrinth of the inner ear that is treated with a low-sodium diet.

Micronutrient   A substance in food that is needed in small amounts; vitamins and minerals are examples.

Mid-arm circumference   A measurement used in anthropometry to help determine body fat percentage.

Milk anemia   A form of iron deficiency anemia attributable to an excess intake of milk, which replaces other iron sources such as meat.

Monosaccharides   The simplest form of carbohydrate; one unit of sugar molecules; glucose and fructose.

Morbid obesity   More than 30 percent overweight; Body Mass Index > 40.

Morbidity   Sickness rate.

Mortality   Death rate.

Myocardial infarct   Referred to as MI or heart attack.

Nasogastric   A term used in describing the placement of a feeding tube from the nose to the stomach.

Nasojejunal   A term used to describe the placement of a feeding tube from the nose to the jejunum.

Nephron   The functional part of the kidney that produces urine; about one million nephons make up each kidney.

Nephrosis   A general term for kidney disease.

Neurological impairment   Impairment related to a low level of consciousness or sensory or motor function.

Neuropathy   A condition characterized by functional disturbances and pathological changes outside the central region of the nervous system.

NIDDM (Non–insulin dependent diabetes mellitus)   A form of diabetes that is typically found in overweight adults. Insulin injection is sometimes necessary for good blood sugar control but is not required for survival. Now referred to as Type 2 diabetes (in numerical versus arabic form).

Nitrogen balance   A state in which nitrogen intake through protein ingestion equals the amount being excreted through the kidneys.

Nitrogenous wastes   Waste products of the body that contain nitrogen.

Nontropical sprue   Another term for celiac disease.

Nursing process   A goal-directed series of activities aimed at alleviating or preventing health problems; includes the five components of assessment, nursing diagnosis, planning, implementation, and evaluation.

Nutrient   A substance found in food that is essential for good health.

Nutrient density   The amount of nutrients per kilocalorie; high nutrient density means a large amount of nutrients per serving of food.

Nutrition   The sum of the processes by which the body uses food to support health.

Nutrition care process   Similar to the nursing process excluding the component of diagnosis.

Nutrition support   A term generally ascribed to the provision of enteral and parenteral nutrition; also includes the provision of liquid supplements for weight gain.

Nutritional status   The level at which a person meets their nutritional needs without deficiency or excess. People have good nutritional status when they have met all their nutritional needs.

Nutritionist   A term that has no legal definition. Registered dietitians are nutritionists in the sense that they are trained in the science of nutrition. Qualified nutritionists include persons with at least a four-year degree in the science of nutrition.

Obesity   The condition of weighing more than 20 percent of ideal body weight; a body mass index greater than 30.

Obstipation   Intractable constipation.

Oliguria   Decreased urinary output.

Omega-3 fatty acids   The type of fat found in fish oil and some plant products.

Oncology   The study of tumors.

Osmolality   The number of particles dissolved in a solution.

Osteodystrophy   A bone disease associated with renal disease, with elevated phosphorus and low or normal calcium levels found in the blood.

Osteomalacia   Softening of the bones often associated with vitamin D deficiency; in children the condition is known as rickets.

Osteoporosis   A condition characterized by a reduction in the quantity of bone.

Otitis media   An ear infection; often a chronic condition in infancy and childhood.

Overweight   An excess of 10 percent body weight over an ideal weight; Body Mass Index (BMI) > 27 is accepted as overweight; some authorities state that overweight is BMI > 24.

Oxidation A chemical process in which oxygen removes electrons from atoms; involved in energy metabolism.

Oxytocin A hormone that causes uterine contraction and promotes the let-down reflex of breast-feeding.

Palliative care Treatment to relieve or lessen pain or other uncomfortable symptoms but not to effect a cure.

Palmar grasp A hand grasp characterized by use of the palm.

Pancreas A gland behind the stomach that releases insulin, glucagon, and some enzymes of digestion for fats and proteins.

Pancreatitis Inflammation of the pancreas often associated with alcoholism and fat malabsorption.

Paraprofessional "Near" professional; a person who is not a professional but is trained to do a type of professional work.

Parenteral nutrition Provision of a liquid nutrition formula directly into the blood system via the subclavian vein or other site.

Pasteurization The heating of milk or other liquid to a temperature of 60° C (140° F) for 30 minutes, killing pathogenic bacteria and considerably delaying the development of other bacteria.

Pellagra A nutritional deficiency disease caused by long-term lack of niacin, resulting in a number of nervous, digestive, and skin symptoms.

Periodontal Around or near a tooth.

Peripheral Parts of the body away from the interior.

Peripheral nerves Nerves found in the arms, hands, legs, and feet.

Peripheral parenteral nutrition (PPN) Administration of nutrients through peripheral veins.

Peristalsis The wormlike movement by which the digestive tract propels its contents through waves of contraction.

Peritoneal dialysis A form of dialysis in which a dialysis solution is placed directly into the peritoneum surrounding the abdominal cavity and later removed.

Pernicious anemia A form of anemia caused by a lack of the intrinsic factor normally produced by the stomach mucosa leading to a deficiency in vitamin B_{12}.

Phenylketonuria (PKU) A congenital disease resulting from a deficit in the metabolism of the amino acid phenylalanine.

Physiological anemia One form of anemia often found in pregnancy as a result of an increase in plasma volume without an increase in red blood cells.

Pica An abnormal craving for nonfood substances.

Pincer grasp A hand grasp characterized by use of the thumb and index finger.

Placenta The organ developed prenatally in the uterus that transfers maternal nutrients to the fetus. Also known as afterbirth.

Polydipsia Excess thirst.

Polyphagia Excess appetite.

Polysaccharides The most complex form of carbohydrates; many units of sugar linked together.

Polyunsaturated fatty acids (PUFA) Liquid oils.

Polyuria Excessive excretion of urine.

Postpartum blues A period of depression, often brief, related to hormonal changes after pregnancy; often occurs two to three weeks after delivery.

Postprandial   After meals.

Pradar-Willi syndrome   A condition beginning in infancy characterized by hypotonicity and failure to thrive, with hyperphagia beginning in later childhood with a degree of mental retardation; the hyperphagia is often severe enough that food has to be locked away or highly controlled in order to prevent morbid obesity.

Preconceptual   Prior to conception.

Preeclampsia   An older term referring to a condition in late pregnancy related to increased blood pressure, edema, and proteinuria that can lead to eclampsia with convulsions and coma caused by cerebral edema; the current terminology is pregnancy-induced hypertension.

Pregnancy-induced hypertension   A condition of pregnancy characterized by elevated blood pressure, proteinuria, and abnormal fluid retention; the cause is unknown but the condition is associated with poor nutritional status (also known as toxemia).

Prenatal   Preceding birth; also referred to as perinatal.

Pre-term milk   Breast milk from a mother giving birth to a premature baby.

Products of conception   The sources of weight gain in pregnancy, including the weight of the baby, the placenta, increased uterine and breast size, increased blood volume weight, and an expected amount of increased maternal body fat that is equal to a minimum of 15 to 20 pounds.

Protein-calorie malnutrition   Also known as marasmus.

Proteinuria   Protein in the urine.

Prothrombin   A blood-clotting factor.

Prudent diet   A diet that is very low in fat.

P:S ratio   The amount of polyunsaturated to saturated fats found in the diet.

Public health   The field of health sciences concerned with the health of the community as a whole.

Purging   A term used in describing bulimic-type actions such as vomiting and laxative abuse.

Purines   A compound found in meat and meat extracts; sometimes avoided as a treatment for gout.

Radiation   Electromagnetic waves (as in ultraviolet waves, x-rays, gamma rays, and so on).

Radiation therapy   The treatment of cancer through the use of radiation to destroy cancer cells.

RAST test   Radioallergosorbent test; used to diagnose food allergies.

Reactive hypoglycemia   A form of low blood sugar that may be a precursor to diabetes; characterized by excess but delayed insulin production in response to simple carbohydrate intake.

Rebound scurvy   A type of vitamin C deficiency disease caused by rapid withdrawal from chronic ingestion of megadoses of vitamin C.

Receptor sites   The doors or entry ways into body cells.

Recommended Dietary Allowances (RDAs)   The recommended amount of nutrients to achieve health. The RDAs are felt to easily meet the nutritional needs of 95 percent of the population.

Refeeding syndrome Also called the nutrition recovery syndrome; occurs when nutritional support is undertaken too aggressively, resulting in decreased serum lab values as the cells increase their intake of minerals such as phosphorus.

Reference Dietary Intake (RDIs) A term developed for use with food labels; average amounts of the updated RDAs.

Renal insufficiency A stage of diminishing renal function when the glomerular filtration rate is reduced to about 30 mL/min and waste products begin to accumulate in the body.

Renal threshold The capacity for reabsorption by the kidneys.

Residue The undigested material found in food.

Retinol equivalents (RE) A means of measuring the vitamin A content of food.

Rickets A bone disease that begins in childhood, is caused by a lack of vitamin D, and results in bowing of legs.

Salmonella A form of gastroenteritis caused by a rod-shaped bacteria often associated with dairy products.

Saturated fat Solid fats; found in most animal fats in association with cholesterol and in hydrogenated fats.

Schizophrenia A large group of mental disorders characterized by mental deterioration, delusions, and withdrawal from the external world.

Sepsis The presence in the blood or other tissues of harmful microorganisms or their toxins.

Sickle cell disease A serious hereditary disease that causes red blood cells to have a sickle shape and to be rigid; found mainly in blacks but also occurs in persons with Mediterranean, Middle Eastern, and Asian Indian ancestry.

Sigmoid region A part of the intestinal tract.

Sodium The chief cation of extracellular body fluids.

Soluble fiber Forms of dietary fiber that dissolve in water and the digestive tract. Oat bran and legumes are high in soluble fiber.

Spastic Implying muscle spasms.

Specific dynamic action The increase in metabolism related to the process of digesting food.

Spina bifida Also known as neural tube defect; a developmental birth defect in which the spinal cord is not completely enclosed.

Sports anemia Anemia of athletes unrelated to iron intake.

Staphylococcus aureus A form of bacteria present on the skin and in the upper respiratory tract; often associated with a form of food poisoning when safe food handling procedures are not followed.

Steatorrhea Diarrhea characterized by excess fat in the stools.

Steroids An important group of body compounds that includes sex and adrenal hormones.

Sugar alcohols A form of sugar found in sugar substitutes that do not promote dental caries.

Tetany A condition with steady contraction of a muscle without distinct twitching caused by abnormal calcium metabolism.

Thrifty food plan A meal plan that can provide all necessary nutrients at the most minimal cost; the current basis for Food Stamp allotments.

Thrush   A bacterial infection often manifested with white blotches on the tongue and in the oral cavity.

Thyroxine   A hormone produced by the thyroid gland that increases the rate of metabolism.

Total parenteral nutrition (TPN)   Administration of nutrients through the superior vena cava.

Toxemia   General intoxication sometimes resulting from absorption of bacterial products formed at an infection site. Also a condition in late pregnancy characterized by elevated blood pressure, edema, and proteinuria; in reference to pregnancy the current terminology is pregnancy-induced hypertension.

Trans fatty acids   The form of fat found in hydrogenated fats.

Transferrin   A serum globulin or protein that binds and transports iron.

Tricep skinfold   An anthropometric measure in which calipers measure the fat on the back of the arm; such measuring requires training for accuracy.

Triglycerides   The form of food fat found in the blood and body tissues.

Tyramine   Related to tyrosine and found in ripe cheese; closely related structurally to epinephrine (a hormone), which has a similar but weaker effect.

Ulcerative colitis   A chronic condition manifested by abdominal pain and rectal bleeding; long-standing ulcerative colitis is a high-risk factor for the development of colon cancer.

Underweight   A body mass index less than 19.

Unsaturated fats   The form of fat with low levels of hydrogen; liquid or soft forms of fat.

Uremia   The final stage of renal disease associated with severe azotemia; includes symptoms of headache, muscular twitching, mental disturbances, nausea, and vomiting.

U.S. Dietary Guidelines   Guidelines aimed at reducing the mortality and morbidity of several diseases such as cardiovascular disease, hypertension, cancer, and diabetes mellitus. The guidelines recommend increased amounts of complex carbohydrates and dietary fiber, with reduced amounts of fat, sugar, salt, and alcohol. Maintaining or achieving desirable weight and including a variety of foods are also recommended.

Vegan   A person who does not eat animal products. Protein is derived from plant sources such as legumes, nuts, and seeds.

Vegetarian   A person who avoids eating meat for health or spiritual reasons. Some vegetarians avoid only red meat.

Videofluroscopy   A test done to determine a person's ability to swallow.

Villi   The hairlike projections inside the intestinal tract; involved in absorption of digested food matter.

Weaning   To discontinue breast-feeding and substitute other forms of feeding; may also relate to weaning off of nutrition support or other life support measures.

Xerophthalmia   Dryness and thickening of the membrane lining of the eyelid, eyeball, and cornea; results from vitamin A deficiency.

Xerostomia   Dryness of the mouth caused by dysfunctional salivary glands; often induced with radiation treatment for cancer near the oral cavity; can result in severe dental decay because of the absence of the neutralizing effect of saliva.

Index

Note: Page numbers in *italics* refer to figures; page numbers followed by t refer to tables.

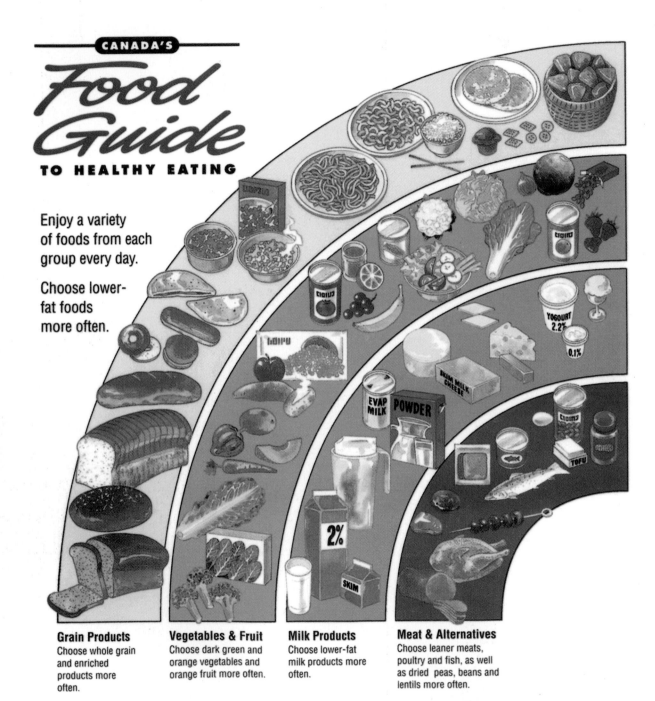

Health Canada **Santé Canada**

CANADA'S Food Guide TO HEALTHY EATING

Enjoy a variety of foods from each group every day.

Choose lower-fat foods more often.

Grain Products
Choose whole grain and enriched products more often.

Vegetables & Fruit
Choose dark green and orange vegetables and orange fruit more often.

Milk Products
Choose lower-fat milk products more often.

Meat & Alternatives
Choose leaner meats, poultry and fish, as well as dried peas, beans and lentils more often.

Canada

From Health Canada: Nutrition Recommendations: The Report of the Scientific Review Committee, 1990. Reproduced with the permission of the Minister of Public Works and Government Services Canada, 1998.